The Placebo

The Placebo

A READER

Edited by
FRANKLIN G. MILLER
Department of Bioethics,
Warren G. Magnuson Clinical Center,
National Institutes of Health,
Bethesda, Maryland

LUANA COLLOCA
National Center for Complementary
    and Alternative Medicine,
National Institute of Mental Health,
National Institutes of Health,
Bethesda, Maryland

ROBERT A. CROUCH
Bloomington, Indiana

TED J. KAPTCHUK
Program in Placebo Studies and
    the Therapeutic Encounter,
Beth Israel Deaconess Medical Center,
Harvard Medical School,
Boston, Massachusetts

THE JOHNS HOPKINS UNIVERSITY PRESS | Baltimore

© 2013 The Johns Hopkins University Press
All rights reserved. Published 2013
Printed in the United States of America on acid-free paper
1 2 3 4 5 6 7 8 9

The Johns Hopkins University Press
2715 North Charles Street
Baltimore, Maryland 21218-4363
www.press.jhu.edu

Library of Congress Cataloging-in-Publication Data

The placebo : a reader / edited by Franklin G. Miller . . . [et al.].
p. ; cm.
Includes bibliographical references and index.
ISBN 978-1-4214-0866-8 (pbk. : alk. paper) —
ISBN 1-4214-0866-x (pbk. : alk. paper)
I. Miller, Franklin G.
[DNLM: 1. Placebo Effect—Collected Works. 2. Placebos—
Collected Works. 3. Bioethical Issues—Collected Works. WB 330]
615.5—dc23   2012036698

A catalog record for this book is available from the British Library.

*Special discounts are available for bulk purchases of this book. For
more information, please contact Special Sales at 410-516-6936 or
specialsales@press.jhu.edu.*

The Johns Hopkins University Press uses environmentally friendly
book materials, including recycled text paper that is composed of at
least 30 percent post-consumer waste, whenever possible.

Contents

Preface

THE PLACEBO EFFECT has fascinated and perplexed scientists and scholars since at least the middle of the twentieth century. Although no standard definition of the "placebo effect" exists, it is generally understood as consisting of individuals' responses to the psychosocial context of medical treatments, "inert" interventions, or clinical encounters, as distinct from the inherent or characteristic physiological effects of medical interventions. Like many complex phenomena, the placebo effect has its dark side, known as the "nocebo effect"—the adverse effects of verbal and nonverbal communication by clinicians (and by investigators studying nocebo responses).

Research on what would come to be known as the placebo effect began with the pioneering studies of Stewart Wolf in the 1940s and has accelerated greatly since that time. Scientists have been interested in understanding the placebo phenomenon for three major reasons: (1) scientific curiosity concerning the impact of the mind or brain on bodily responses, (2) methodological concerns with the ability of randomized controlled trials to detect the efficacy of treatments and thus improve medical care, and (3) the hope to learn how clinicians can enhance the art of healing by promoting placebo responses (and by minimizing nocebo responses). As scientists have investigated the placebo effect, ethicists have engaged in a parallel investigation of the ethical issues raised by the use of placebo interventions in research and in clinical practice, for example, the ethics of deception, whether it is ethically justifiable to withhold proven effective treatment from those enrolled in placebo-controlled trials, and what ethical limits should be placed on the use of invasive sham-surgery interventions. Research on the placebo effect also intrigues journalists and the public, as reflected in the extensive attention in the news media devoted to the publication of new studies.

All inquiry is historically situated, whether or not researchers are aware of or appreciate the work of previous investigators and scholars. Prior research formulates the terminology and methods of inquiry that set the stage for contemporary inquiry. In compiling this anthology on the scientific, social, and ethical aspects of the placebo effect, we wanted to make available in one volume landmark articles, those which have framed the debates and which we believe are of enduring significance. We anticipate that this book will enlighten and stimulate scientists, scholars, and students who are engaged in research on the placebo and serve as a valuable reference for continuing inquiry.

We have divided the book into three sections: (1) the concept and significance of the placebo effect, (2) experimental studies of the placebo effect, and (3) ethical issues raised by the use of placebos in research and clinical practice. The articles in each section are preceded by introductions written by the editors, which aim to place these articles into context historically and with respect to current research. The reasons that have animated researchers to investigate the placebo effect in all its guises are those that have motivated us to prepare this anthology: pursuing scientific interest, enhancing the methodology of clinical trials, improving the art of healing, and promoting the ethical conduct of research and medicine.

Finally, a few quick words about the text. We have reproduced the articles below in their entirety, with the following exceptions: we have throughout removed abstracts, acknowledgments, conflict-of-interest statements, and other nonessential materials from the articles. Typos and other errors have been corrected silently. Where applicable, tables and figures have been renumbered to reflect the current chapter in which they are located. Unfortunately, because of the age of some articles, the reproduction quality of the images and figures could not be improved. When we intervened on the text in any substantive way (there are very few of these cases), it was designated by square brackets followed by "—eds." We hope that readers will find our editorial presence within the text to be minimal.

Acknowledgments

We have many people to thank for their assistance in creating this anthology. We would first like to thank the more than 170 authors of the articles reprinted here. Without their very fine work and their permission to reprint it, this book would not exist. We are also grateful to the publishers and copyright holders for granting permission to reprint these articles. Recognizing the purely pedagogic aims of this project, a few copyright holders kindly reduced their reprint fees for us; we thank them especially for this. At the Johns Hopkins University Press, we thank our editors, Wendy Harris, with whom we started this project, and Suzanne Flinchbaugh, with whom we finished it. Hearty thanks to both of them for their guidance and, especially, for their patience. We gratefully acknowledge the financial assistance provided by the Department of Bioethics at the National Institutes of Health, and we thank two of its outstanding program support specialists, Becky Chen and Tanya Vaughn, for their help with managing permissions issues. It is a pleasure to record these debts, but we alone are responsible for any errors that remain in the book.

We thank the following individuals for letting us reprint their work in this volume. Both articles listed below are open access, distributed under the terms of the Creative Commons public domain.

TED J. KAPTCHUK, ELIZABETH FRIEDLANDER, JOHN M. KELLEY, NORMA P. SANCHEZ, EFI KOKKOTOU, JOYCE P. SINGER, MAGDA KOWALCZYKOWSKI, FRANKLIN G. MILLER, IRVING KIRSCH, ANTHONY J. LEMBO, "Placebos without Deception: A Randomized Controlled Trial in Irritable Bowel Syndrome," *PLoS ONE* 2010;5(12):e15591.

FRANKLIN G. MILLER, DAVID WENDLER, AND LEORA C. SWARTZMAN, "Deception in Research on the Placebo Effect," *PLoS Medicine* 2005;2(9):e262.

We hereby thank and acknowledge the following publishers and copyright holders for permission to reprint the journal articles listed below.

1. The American Association for the Advancement of Science

RICHARD J. HERRNSTEIN, "Placebo Effect in the Rat," *Science* 1962;138:677–678. Copyright © 1962 AAAS. Reprinted with permission.

ROBERT ADER and NICHOLAS COHEN, "Behaviorally Conditioned Immunosuppression and Murine Systemic Lupus Erythematosus," *Science* 1982;215:1534–1536. Copyright © 1982 AAAS. Reprinted with permission.

RAÚL DE LA FUENTE-FERNÁNDEZ, THOMAS J. RUTH, VESNA SOSSI, MICHAEL SCHULZER, DONALD B. CALNE, and A. JON STOESSL, "Expectation and Dopamine Release: Mechanism of the Placebo Effect in Parkinson's Disease," *Science* 2001;293:1164–1166. Copyright © 2001 AAAS. Reprinted with permission.

PREDRAG PETROVIC, EIJA KALSO, KARL MAGNUS PETERSSON, and MARTIN INGVAR, "Placebo and Opioid Analgesia: Imaging a Shared Neuronal Network," *Science* 2002;295:1737–1740. Copyright © 2002 AAAS. Reprinted with permission.

TOR D. WAGER, JAMES K. RILLING, EDWARD E. SMITH, ALEX SOKOLIK, KENNETH L. CASEY, RICHARD J. DAVIDSON, STEPHEN M. KOSSLYN, ROBERT M. ROSE, and JONATHAN D. COHEN, "Placebo-Induced Changes in fMRI in the Anticipation and Experience of Pain," *Science* 2004;303:1162–1167. Copyright © 2004 AAAS. Reprinted with permission.

FALK EIPPERT, JÜRGEN FINSTERBUSCH, ULRIKE BINGEL, and CHRISTIAN BÜCHEL, "Direct Evidence for Spinal Cord Involvement in Placebo Analgesia," *Science* 2009;326:404. Copyright © 2009 AAAS. Reprinted with permission.

2. The American College of Neuropsychopharmacology

WALTER A. BROWN, "Placebo as a Treatment for Depression," *Neuropsychopharmacology* 1994;10:265–269. Copyright © 1994. Reprinted with permission from the American College of Neuropsychopharmacology (ACNP).

3. The American College of Physicians–American Society of Internal Medicine

HOWARD BRODY, "The Lie That Heals: The Ethics of Giving Placebos," *Annals of Internal Medicine* 1982;97:112–118. Copyright © 1982 American College of Physicians–American Society of Internal Medicine. Reprinted with permission.

ROBERT TEMPLE and SUSAN S. ELLENBERG, "Placebo-Controlled Trials and Active-Control Trials in the Evaluation of New Treatments: Part 1. Ethical and Scientific Issues," *Annals of Internal Medicine* 2000;133:455–463. Copyright © 2000 American College of Physicians–American Society of Internal Medicine. Reprinted with permission.

DANIEL E. MOERMAN and WAYNE B. JONAS, "Deconstructing the Placebo Effect and Finding the Meaning Response," *Annals of Internal Medicine* 2002;136:471–476. Copyright © 2002 American College of Physicians–American Society of Internal Medicine. Reprinted with permission.

TED J. KAPTCHUK, "The Placebo Effect in Alternative Medicine: Can the Performance of a Healing Ritual Have Clinical Significance?," *Annals of Internal Medicine* 2002;136:817–825. Copyright © 2002 American College of

Physicians–American Society of Internal Medicine. Reprinted with permission.

4. The American Medical Association

HENRY K. BEECHER, "The Powerful Placebo," *JAMA* 1955;159(17):1602–1606. Copyright © 1955 American Medical Association. Reprinted with permission.

5. The American Society for Clinical Investigation

STEWART WOLF, "Effects of Suggestion and Conditioning on the Action of Chemical Agents in Human Subjects: The Pharmacology of Placebos," *Journal of Clinical Investigation* 1950;29:100–109. Copyright © 1950 American Society for Clinical Investigation. Reprinted with permission.

6. The BMJ Publishing Group Ltd.

TED J. KAPTCHUK, JOHN M. KELLEY, LISA A. CONBOY, ROGER B. DAVIS, CATHERINE E. KERR, ERIC E. JACOBSON, IRVING KIRSCH, ROSA N. SCHNYER, BONG HYUN NAM, LONG T. NGUYEN, MIN PARK, ANDREA L. RIVERS, CLAIRE A. MCMANUS, EFI KOKKOTOU, DOUGLAS A. DROSSMAN, PETER GOLDMAN, and ANTHONY J. LEMBO, "Components of Placebo Effect: Randomised Controlled Trial in Patients with Irritable Bowel Syndrome," *BMJ* 2008;336:999–1003. Copyright © 2008. Reprinted with permission from BMJ Publishing Group Ltd.

JON C. TILBURT, EZEKIEL J. EMANUEL, TED J. KAPTCHUK, FARR A. CURLIN, and FRANKLIN G. MILLER, "Prescribing 'Placebo Treatments': Results of National Survey of U.S. Internists and Rheumatologists," *BMJ* 2008;337:a1938. Copyright © 2008. Reprinted with permission from BMJ Publishing Group Ltd.

7. Cambridge University Press

ADOLF GRÜNBAUM, "The Placebo Concept in Medicine and Psychiatry," *Psychological Medicine* 1986;16:19–38. Copyright © 1986 Cambridge Journals. Reproduced with permission.

8. Elsevier

LOUIS LASAGNA, FREDERICK MOSTELLER, JOHN M. VON FELSINGER, and HENRY K. BEECHER, "A Study of the Placebo Response," *American Journal of Medicine* 1954;16:770–779. Copyright © 1954. Reprinted with permission from Elsevier.

STEWART WOLF, CARL R. DOERING, MERVIN L. CLARK, and JAMES A. HAGANS, "Chance Distribution and the Placebo 'Reactor,'" *Journal of Laboratory and Clinical Medicine* 1957;49:837–841. Copyright © 1957. Reprinted with permission from Elsevier.

JON D. LEVINE, NEWTON C. GORDON, and HOWARD L. FIELDS, "The Mechanism of Placebo Analgesia," *Lancet* 1978;312(8091):654–657. Copyright © 1978. Reprinted with permission from Elsevier.

RICHARD H. GRACELY, RONALD DUBNER, WILLIAM R. DEETER, and PATRICIA J. WOLSKEE, "Clinicians' Expectations Influence Placebo Analgesia," *Lancet* 1985;325(8419):43. Copyright © 1985. Reprinted with permission from Elsevier.

GUNVER S. KIENLE and HELMUT KIENE, "The Powerful Placebo Effect: Fact or Fiction?" *Journal of Clinical Epidemiology* 1997;50:1311–1318. Copyright © 1997. Reprinted with permission from Elsevier.

LUANA COLLOCA, LEONARDO LOPIANO, MICHELE LANOTTE, and FABRIZIO BENEDETTI, "Overt versus Covert Treatment for Pain, Anxiety, and Parkinson's Disease," *Lancet Neurology* 2004;3:679–684. Copyright © 2004. Reprinted with permission from Elsevier.

9. The Hastings Center

PAUL S. APPELBAUM, LOREN H. ROTH, CHARLES W. LIDZ, PAUL R. BENSON, and WILLIAM J. WINSLADE, "False Hopes and Best Data: Consent to Research and the Therapeutic Misconception," *Hastings Center Report* 1987;17(2):20–24. Copyright © 1987 The Hastings Center. Reprinted with permission.

10. International Association for the Study of Pain® (IASP®)

NICHOLAS J. VOUDOURIS, CONNIE L. PECK, and GRAHAME COLEMAN, "The Role of Conditioning and Verbal Expectancy in the Placebo Response," *Pain* 1990;43:121–128. This article has been reproduced with permission of the International Association for the Study of Pain® (IASP®). The information may not be reproduced for any other purpose without permission.

GUY H. MONTGOMERY and IRVING KIRSCH, "Classical Conditioning and the Placebo Effect," *Pain* 1997;72:107–113. This article has been reproduced with permission of the International Association for the Study of Pain® (IASP®). The information may not be reproduced for any other purpose without permission.

DONALD D. PRICE, LEONARD S. MILLING, IRVING KIRSCH, ANN DUFF, GUY H. MONTGOMERY, and SARAH S. NICHOLLS, "An Analysis of Factors That Contribute to the Magnitude of Placebo Analgesia in an Experimental Paradigm," *Pain* 1999;83:147–156. This article has been reproduced with permission of the International Association for the Study of Pain® (IASP®). The information may not be reproduced for any other purpose without permission.

ANTONELLA POLLO, MARTINA AMANZIO, ANNA ARSLANIAN, CATERINA CASADIO, GIULIANO MAGGI, and FABRIZIO BENEDETTI, "Response Expectancies in Placebo Analgesia and Their Clinical Relevance," *Pain* 2001;93:77–84. This article has been reproduced with permission of the International Association for the Study of Pain® (IASP®). The information may not be reproduced for any other purpose without permission.

LUANA COLLOCA and FABRIZIO BENEDETTI, "Placebo Analgesia Induced by Social Observational Learning," *Pain* 2009;144:28–34. This article has been reproduced with permission of the International Association for the Study of Pain® (IASP®). The information may not be reproduced for any other purpose without permission.

ANDREA L. MARTIN and JOEL D. KATZ, "Inclusion of Authorized Deception in the Informed Consent Process Does Not Affect the Magnitude of the Placebo Effect for Experimentally Induced Pain," *Pain* 2010;149:208–215. This article has been reproduced with permission of the International Association for the Study of Pain® (IASP®). The information may not be reproduced for any other purpose without permission.

11. John Wiley and Sons Ltd.

CLEMENT J. MCDONALD, STEVEN A. MAZZUCA, and GEORGE P. MCCABE Jr., "How Much of the Placebo 'Effect' Is Really Statistical Regression?" *Statistics in Medicine* 1983;2:417–427. Copyright © 1983. Reprinted with permission.

BENJAMIN FREEDMAN, KATHLEEN CRANLEY GLASS, and CHARLES WEIJER, "Placebo Orthodoxy in Clinical Research II: Ethical, Legal, and Regulatory Myths," *Journal of Law, Medicine, and Ethics* 1996;24:252–259. Copyright © 1996. Reprinted with permission.

NICOLA MONDAINI, PAOLO GONTERO, GIANLUCA GIUBILEI, GIUSEPPE LOMBARDI, TOMMASO CAI, ANDREA GAVAZZI, and RICCARDO BARTOLETTI, "Finasteride 5 mg and Sexual Side Effects: How Many of These Are Related to a Nocebo Phenomenon?" *Journal of Sexual Medicine* 2007;4:1708–1712. Copyright © 2007. Reprinted with permission.

12. The Massachusetts Medical Society

LAWRENCE D. EGBERT, GEORGE E. BATTIT, CLAUDE E. WELCH, and MARSHALL K. BARTLETT, "Reduction of Postoperative Pain by Encouragement and Instruction of Patients: A Study of Doctor-Patient Rapport," *New England Journal of Medicine* 1964;270:825–827. Copyright © 1964 Massachusetts Medical Society. All rights reserved.

KENNETH J. ROTHMAN and KARIN B. MICHELS, "The Continuing Unethical Use of Placebo Controls," *New England Journal of Medicine* 1994;331:394–398. Copyright © 1994 Massachusetts Medical Society. All rights reserved.

ASBJØRN HRÓBJARTSSON and PETER C. GØTZSCHE, "Is the Placebo Powerless? An Analysis of Clinical Trials Comparing Placebo with No Treatment," *New England Journal of Medicine* 2001;344:1594–1602 [erratum in: *New England Journal of Medicine* 2001;345:304]. Copyright © 2001 Massachusetts Medical Society. All rights reserved.

EZEKIEL J. EMANUEL and FRANKLIN G. MILLER, "The Ethics of Placebo-Controlled Trials: A Middle Ground," *New England Journal of Medicine* 2001;345:915–919. Copyright © 2001 Massachusetts Medical Society. All rights reserved.

SAM HORNG and FRANKLIN G. MILLER, "Is Placebo Surgery Unethical?" *New England Journal of Medicine* 2002;347:137–139. Copyright © 2002 Massachusetts Medical Society. All rights reserved.

13. Medical Society of the State of New York

HAROLD G. WOLFF, EUGENE F. DUBOIS, MCKEEN CATTELL, OSKAR DIETHELM, MACK LIPKIN, HARRY GOLD, CHARLES H. WHEELER, and HENRY RICHARDSON, "Conferences on Therapy: The Use of Placebos in Therapy," *New York State Journal of Medicine* 1946;46:1718–1727. Reprinted with permission from the Medical Society of the State of New York.

14. Nature Publishing Group

FABRIZIO BENEDETTI, LUANA COLLOCA, ELENA TORRE, MICHELE LANOTTE, ANTONIO MELCARNE, MARINA PESARE, BRUNO BERGAMASCO, and LEONARDO LOPIANO, "Placebo-Responsive Parkinson Patients Show Decreased Activity in Single Neurons of Subthalamic Nucleus," *Nature Neuroscience* 2004;7:587–588. Copyright © 2004. Reprinted by permission from Nature Publishing Group.

15. SAGE Publications

ASBJØRN HRÓBJARTSSON and MICHAEL NORUP, "The Use of Placebo Interventions in Medical Practice: A National Questionnaire Survey of Danish Clinicians," *Evaluation and the Health Professions* 2003;26:153–165. Copyright © 2003. Reprinted by permission of SAGE Publications.

16. Scientific American

SISSELA BOK, "The Ethics of Giving Placebos," *Scientific American* 1974;231(5):17–23. Reproduced with permission. Copyright © 1974 Scientific American Inc. All rights reserved.

17. The Society for Neuroscience

MARTINA AMANZIO and FABRIZIO BENEDETTI, "Neuropharmacological Dissection of Analgesia: Expectation-Activated Opioid Systems versus Conditioning-Activated Specific Subsystems," *Journal of Neuroscience* 1999;19:484–494. Copyright © 1999. Reprinted with permission.

NORA D. VOLKOW, GENE-JACK WANG, YEMIN MA, JOANNA S. FOWLER, WEI ZHU, LAURENCE MAYNARD, FRANK TELANG, PAUL VASKA, YU-SHIN DING, CHRISTOPHER WONG, and JAMES M. SWANSON, "Expectation Enhances the Regional Brain Metabolic and the Reinforcing Effects of Stimulants in Cocaine Abusers," *Journal of Neuroscience* 2003;23:11461–11468. Copyright © 2003. Reprinted with permission.

JON-KAR ZUBIETA, JOSHUA A. BUELLER, LISA R. JACKSON, DAVID J. SCOTT, YANJUN XU, ROBERT A. KOEPPE, THOMAS E. NICHOLS, and CHRISTIAN S. STOHLER, "Placebo Effects Mediated by Endogenous Opioid Activity on μ-Opioid Receptors," *Journal of Neuroscience* 2005;25:7754–7762. Copyright © 2005. Reprinted with permission.

FABRIZIO BENEDETTI, MARTINA AMANZIO, SERGIO VIGHETTI, and GIOVANNI ASTEGGIANO, "The Biochemical and Neuroendocrine Bases of the Hyperalgesic Nocebo Effect," *Journal of Neuroscience* 2006;26:12014–12022. Copyright © 2006. Reprinted with permission.

18. Springer

IRVING KIRSCH and MICHAEL J. ROSADINO, "Do Double-Blind Studies with Informed Consent Yield Externally Valid

Results? An Empirical Test," *Psychopharmacology* 1993; 110:437–442. Copyright © 1993. Reprinted with permission.

19. Taylor & Francis Ltd.

FRANKLIN G. MILLER and LUANA COLLOCA, "The Legitimacy of Placebo Treatments in Clinical Practice: Evidence and Ethics," *American Journal of Bioethics* 2009;9(12):39–47. Reprinted by permission of Taylor & Francis Ltd., www.tandf.co.uk/journals.

20. Wolters Kluwer Health

THOMAS J. LUPARELLO, NANCY LEIST, CARY H. LOURIE, and PAULINE SWEET, "The Interaction of Psychologic Stimuli and Pharmacologic Agents on Airway Reactivity in Asthmatic Subjects," *Psychosomatic Medicine* 1970;32:509–513. Copyright © 1970. Reprinted with permission.

LOUIS W. BUCKALEW and KENNETH E. COFFIELD, "An Investigation of Drug Expectancy as a Function of Capsule Color and Size and Preparation Form," *Journal of Clinical Psychopharmacology* 1982;2:245–248. Copyright © 1982. Reprinted with permission.

ROBERT ADER, MARY GAIL MERCURIO, JAMES R. WALTON, DEBORRA JAMES, MICHAEL DAVIS, VALERIE E. OJHA, ALEXA BOER KIMBALL, and DAVID FIORENTINO, "Conditioned Pharmacotherapeutic Effects: A Preliminary Study," *Psychosomatic Medicine* 2010;72:192–197. Copyright © 2010. Reprinted with permission.

Contributors

† Robert Ader, Ph.D., M.D. (hc), Sc.D. (hc), Distinguished University Professor, Department of Psychiatry, University of Rochester School of Medicine and Dentistry, Rochester, New York, U.S.A.

Martina Amanzio, Ph.D., Assistant Professor of Psychobiology, Department of Psychology and Neuroscience Institute of Turin, University of Turin Medical School, Turin, Italy

Paul S. Appelbaum, M.D., Elizabeth K. Dollard Professor of Psychiatry, Medicine, and Law; Director, Division of Law, Ethics, and Psychiatry, Department of Psychiatry, Columbia University College of Physicians and Surgeons; and Research Scientist, New York State Psychiatric Institute, New York, New York, U.S.A.

Giovanni Asteggiano, M.D., Neurologist and Director, Department of Neurology, Alba Hospital, Alba, Italy

† Marshall K. Bartlett, M.D., Honorary Surgeon, Massachusetts General Hospital, Boston, Massachusetts, and Clinical Professor, Department of Surgery, Harvard Medical School, Boston, Massachusetts, U.S.A.

Riccardo Bartoletti, M.D., Associate Professor, Department of Urology, University of Florence, and Chief, Urology Unit, Santa Maria Annunziata Hospital, Florence, Italy

George E. Battit, M.D., Vice Chair Emeritus and Associate Professor, Department of Anesthesia, Critical Care and Pain Medicine, Massachusetts General Hospital and Harvard Medical School, Boston, Massachusetts, U.S.A.

† Henry K. Beecher, M.D., Henry Isaiah Dorr Professor of Anesthesia Research, Harvard Medical School, Boston, Massachusetts, U.S.A.

Fabrizio Benedetti, M.D., Professor of Physiology and Neuroscience, Department of Neuroscience and National Institute of Neuroscience, University of Turin Medical School, Turin, Italy

Paul R. Benson, Ph.D., Professor, Department of Sociology, and Senior Research Associate, Center for Social Development and Education, University of Massachusetts, Boston, Massachusetts, U.S.A.

Ulrike Bingel, Dr.med., Attending in Neurology, Department of Neurology, University Medical Center Hamburg-Eppendorf, Hamburg, Germany

Sissela Bok, Ph.D., Senior Visiting Fellow, Harvard Center for Population and Development Studies, Harvard University, Cambridge, Massachusetts, U.S.A.

Howard Brody, M.D., Ph.D., John P. McGovern Centennial Chair and Professor, Department of Family Medicine, and Director, Institute for the Medical Humanities, University of Texas Medical Branch, Galveston, Texas, U.S.A.

Walter A. Brown, M.D., Clinical Professor, Department of Psychiatry and Human Behavior, Alpert Medical School, Brown University, Providence, Rhode Island, and Clinical Professor, Department of Psychiatry, Tufts University School of Medicine, Boston, Massachusetts, U.S.A.

Christian Büchel, Dr.med., Head, Affective Neuroscience Working Group, University Medical Center Hamburg-Eppendorf, Hamburg, Germany

Joshua A. Bueller, M.B.A., Boulder, Colorado, U.S.A.

Tommaso Cai, M.D., Consultant Urologist, Department of Urology, Santa Chiara Hospital, Trento, Italy

Donald B. Calne, D.M., D.Sc., Professor Emeritus, Pacific Parkinson's Research Centre and National Parkinson Foundation Centre of Excellence, University of British Columbia and Vancouver Coastal Health, Vancouver, British Columbia, Canada

Caterina Casadio, M.D., Professor and Director, S.C.D.U. Thoracic Surgery, Faculty of Medicine, Surgery, and Health Science, University of Eastern Piedmont, Novara, Italy

Kenneth L. Casey, M.D., Professor Emeritus, Department of Neurology and Department of Molecular and Integrative Physiology, University of Michigan, Ann Arbor, Michigan, U.S.A.

† McKeen Cattell, M.D., Ph.D., Professor, Department of Pharmacology, Cornell University Medical College, New York, New York, U.S.A.

† Mervin L. Clark, M.D., Professor, Department of Medicine, University of Oklahoma School of Medicine, Oklahoma City, Oklahoma, U.S.A.

Jonathan D. Cohen, M.D., Ph.D., Eugene Higgins Professor of Psychology and Co-Director, Princeton Neuroscience Institute, Princeton University, Princeton, New Jersey, and Professor of Psychiatry, Western Psychiatric Institute and Clinic, University of Pittsburgh Medical Center, Pittsburgh, Pennsylvania, U.S.A.

Nicholas Cohen, Ph.D., Professor Emeritus, Department of Microbiology and Immunology, University of Rochester School of Medicine and Dentistry, Rochester, New York, U.S.A.

Grahame Coleman, Ph.D., Professor, School of Psychology and Psychiatry, Monash University, Victoria, Australia

Lisa A. Conboy, Sc.D., M.A., M.S., Instructor, Osher Research Center, Harvard Medical School, Boston, Massachusetts, and Co-Director of Research and Dean of Western Biomedicine, The New England School of Acupuncture, Newton, Massachusetts, U.S.A.

Farr A. Curlin, M.D., Associate Professor, Department of Medicine; Co-Director, Program on Medicine and Religion; and Faculty, MacLean Center for Clinical Medical Ethics, University of Chicago Medical Center, Chicago, Illinois, U.S.A.

Richard J. Davidson, Ph.D., Vilas Professor of Psychology and Psychiatry, University of Wisconsin–Madison, Madison, Wisconsin, U.S.A.

Roger B. Davis, Sc.D., Associate Professor of Medicine (Biostatistics), Division of General Medicine and Primary Care, Beth Israel Deaconess Medical Center, and Director of Statistics, Program in Placebo Studies and the Therapeutic Encounter, Beth Israel Deaconess Medical Center and Harvard Medical School, Boston, Massachusetts, U.S.A.

William R. Deeter, D.D.S., M.S., Oral Surgery Associates of Alaska, Anchorage, Alaska, U.S.A.

Raúl de la Fuente-Fernández, M.D., FRCPC, Section of Neurology, Hospital A. Marcide, Ferrol, Spain

† Oskar Diethelm, M.D., Chairman, Department of Psychiatry, Cornell University Medical College, and Chief, Payne Whitney Psychiatric Clinic, New York, New York, U.S.A.

Yu-Shin Ding, Ph.D., Professor, Department of Diagnostic Radiology; Director, PET Radiochemistry R&D; and Co-Director, PET Center, Yale University School of Medicine, New Haven, Connecticut, U.S.A.

† Carl R. Doering, M.D., D.Sc., Professor, Department of Preventive Medicine and Public Health, University of Oklahoma School of Medicine, Oklahoma City, Oklahoma, U.S.A.

Douglas A. Drossman, M.D., Professor of Medicine and Psychiatry, and Co-Director, UNC Center for Functional GI and Motility Disorders, Division of Gastroenterology and Hepatology, University of North Carolina at Chapel Hill, Chapel Hill, North Carolina, U.S.A.

Ronald Dubner, D.D.S., Ph.D., Professor, Department of Neural and Pain Sciences, University of Maryland Dental School, Baltimore, Maryland, U.S.A.

† Eugene F. Dubois, M.D., Professor, Department of Physiology, Cornell University Medical College, New York, New York, U.S.A.

Lawrence D. Egbert, M.D., M.P.H., Baltimore, Maryland, U.S.A.

Falk Eippert, Ph.D., Post-Doctoral Fellow, Institute for Systems Neuroscience, University Medical Center Hamburg-Eppendorf, Hamburg, Germany

Susan S. Ellenberg, Ph.D., Professor, Department of Biostatistics and Epidemiology; Senior Scholar, Center for Clinical Epidemiology and Biostatistics; and Associate Dean for Clinical Research, University of Pennsylvania School of Medicine, Philadelphia, Pennsylvania, U.S.A.

Ezekiel J. Emanuel, M.D., Ph.D., Diane v.S. Levy and Robert M. Levy University Professor and Vice Provost for Global Initiatives, University of Pennsylvania; Chair, Department of Medical Ethics and Health Policy; and Professor, Center for Bioethics, Perelman School of Medicine, University of Pennsylvania, Philadelphia, Pennsylvania, U.S.A.

Howard L. Fields, M.D., Ph.D., Professor of Neurology, University of California–San Francisco, San Francisco, California, U.S.A.

Jürgen Finsterbusch, Ph.D., Head, MR-Physics Working Group, University Medical Center Hamburg-Eppendorf, Hamburg, Germany

David Fiorentino, M.D., Ph.D., Associate Professor, Department of Dermatology, Stanford University School of Medicine, Palo Alto, California, U.S.A.

Joanna S. Fowler, Ph.D., Senior Scientist, Medical Department, Brookhaven National Laboratory, Upton, New York, U.S.A.

† Benjamin Freedman, Ph.D., Professor, Biomedical Ethics Unit, McGill University, and Clinical Ethicist, Sir Mortimer B. Davis–Jewish General Hospital, Montreal, Quebec, Canada

Elizabeth A. Friedlander, Ph.D., ANP-BC, FNP-C, Nurse Practitioner, Division of Gastroenterology, Beth Israel Deaconess Medical Center, Boston, Massachusetts, U.S.A.

Kathleen Cranley Glass, D.C.L., Professor, Biomedical Ethics Unit and Departments of Human Genetics and Pediatrics, McGill University, and Clinical Ethicist, Montreal Children's Hospital, McGill University Health Centre, Montreal, Quebec, Canada

† Harry Gold, M.D., Professor, Department of Pharmacology, Cornell University Medical College, New York, New York, U.S.A.

Peter Goldman, M.A., M.D., Maxwell Finland Professor of Biological Chemistry and Molecular Pharmacology, Emeritus, Harvard Medical School, Boston, Massachusetts, U.S.A.

Paolo Gontero, M.D., Associate Professor and Vice Chairman, Department of Urology, University of Turin and San Giovanni Battista Hospital, Turin, Italy

Newton C. Gordon, D.D.S., M.S., Professor Emeritus, Department of Oral and Maxillofacial Surgery, University of California–San Francisco School of Dentistry, San Francisco, California, U.S.A.

Peter C. Gøtzsche, M.D., Director, Nordic Cochrane Centre, and Professor, Institute of Medicine and Surgery, Faculty of Health Sciences, University of Copenhagen, Copenhagen, Denmark

Richard H. Gracely, Ph.D., Professor, Center for Neurosensory Disorders, University of North Carolina at Chapel Hill School of Dentistry, Chapel Hill, North Carolina, U.S.A.

Adolf Grünbaum, Ph.D., Andrew Mellon Professor of Philosophy of Science; Primary Research Professor, Department of History and Philosophy of Science;

Research Professor of Psychiatry; and Chair, Center for Philosophy of Science, University of Pittsburgh, Pittsburgh, Pennsylvania, U.S.A.

† James A. Hagans, M.D., M.S., Professor, Department of Preventive Medicine and Public Health, University of Oklahoma School of Medicine, Oklahoma City, Oklahoma, U.S.A.

† Richard J. Herrnstein, Ph.D., Edgar Pierce Professor of Psychology, Department of Psychology, Harvard University, Cambridge, Massachusetts, U.S.A.

Sam Horng, M.D., Ph.D., Medicine Intern, Yale–New Haven Hospital, New Haven, Connecticut, U.S.A.

Asbjørn Hróbjartsson, M.D., M.Phil., Ph.D., Senior Researcher, Nordic Cochrane Centre, Rigshospitalet, Copenhagen, Denmark

Martin Ingvar, M.D., Ph.D., Dean of Research, and Barbro and Bernard Osher Professor of Integrative Medicine, Osher Center for Integrative Medicine, Karolinska Institutet, Stockholm, Sweden

Lisa R. Jackson, Ph.D., Professor, Department of Psychology, Schoolcraft College, Livonia, Michigan, U.S.A.

Eric E. Jacobson, Ph.D., Lecturer, Department of Global Health and Social Medicine, Harvard Medical School, Boston, Massachusetts, U.S.A.

Deborra James, R.N., CCRC, DNC, Clinical Research Associate, Department of Dermatology, University of Rochester Medical Center, Rochester, New York, U.S.A.

Wayne B. Jonas, M.D., President and Chief Executive Officer, Samueli Institute, Alexandria, Virginia, and Professor, Department of Family Medicine, Georgetown University School of Medicine, Washington, D.C., U.S.A.

Eija Anneli Kalso, M.D., D.Med.Sci., Professor of Pain Medicine, Institute of Clinical Medicine, University of Helsinki, and Pain Clinic, Helsinki University Central Hospital, Helsinki, Finland

Joel D. Katz, Ph.D., C.Psych., Professor and Canada Research Chair in Health Psychology, Department of Psychology and School of Kinesiology and Health Science, York University, Toronto, Ontario, Canada

John M. Kelley, Ph.D., Associate Professor, Department of Psychology, Endicott College, Beverly, Massachusetts; Instructor, Department of Psychiatry, Harvard Medical School; Deputy Director, Program in Placebo Studies and the Therapeutic Encounter, Beth Israel Deaconess Medical Center and Harvard Medical School; and Staff Psychologist, Massachusetts General Hospital, Boston, Massachusetts, U.S.A.

Catherine E. Kerr, Ph.D., Assistant Professor, Department of Family Medicine; Director, Translational Neuroscience; and Core Faculty, Contemplative Studies Initiative, Alpert Medical School, Brown University, Providence, Rhode Island, U.S.A.

Helmut Kiene, M.D., Senior Research Scientist, Institute of Applied Epistemology and Medical Methodology, Freiburg, Germany

Gunver S. Kienle, Dr.med., Senior Research Scientist, Institute of Applied Epistemology and Medical Methodology, Freiburg, Germany

Alexandra Boer Kimball, M.D., M.P.H., Associate Professor, Department of Dermatology, Massachusetts General Hospital, Harvard Medical School, Boston, Massachusetts, U.S.A.

Irving Kirsch, Ph.D., Associate Director, Program in Placebo Studies and the Therapeutic Encounter, Beth Israel Deaconess Medical Center and Harvard Medical School, Boston, Massachusetts, U.S.A., and Professor Emeritus, University of Hull, Hull, UK, and University of Connecticut, Storrs, Connecticut, U.S.A.

Robert A. Koeppe, Ph.D., Professor, Department of Radiology, University of Michigan Medical School, Ann Arbor, Michigan, U.S.A.

Efi G. Kokkotou, M.D., Ph.D., D.Sc., Assistant Professor of Medicine, Harvard Medical School, and Director of Translational Research, Program in Placebo Studies and the Therapeutic Encounter, Beth Israel Deaconess Medical Center and Harvard Medical School, Boston, Massachusetts, U.S.A.

Stephen M. Kosslyn, Ph.D., Director, Center for Advanced Study in the Behavioral Sciences, Stanford University, Palo Alto, California, U.S.A.

Magda Kowalczykowski, B.A., Research Assistant, Division of Gastroenterology, Beth Israel Deaconess Medical Center, Boston, Massachusetts, U.S.A.

Michele Lanotte, M.D., Associate Professor of Neurosurgery, Department of Neuroscience, University of Turin Medical School, Turin, Italy

† Louis Lasagna, M.D., Dean Emeritus, Sackler School of Graduate Biomedical Sciences, Tufts University, Boston, Massachusetts, U.S.A.

Anthony J. Lembo, M.D., Associate Professor of Medicine, Harvard Medical School, and Director of Clinical Research, Program in Placebo Studies and the Therapeutic Encounter, Beth Israel Deaconess Medical Center and Harvard Medical School, Boston, Massachusetts, U.S.A.

Jon D. Levine, M.D., Ph.D., Professor of Medicine, University of California–San Francisco, San Francisco, California, U.S.A.

Charles W. Lidz, Ph.D., Research Professor, Department of Psychiatry, Center for Mental Health Services Research, University of Massachusetts Medical School, Worcester, Massachusetts, U.S.A.

† Mack Lipkin, M.D., Clinical Professor, University of North Carolina School of Medicine, Chapel Hill, North Carolina, U.S.A.

Leonardo Lopiano, M.D., Ph.D., Professor of Neurology, Department of Neuroscience, University of Turin Medical School, Turin, Italy

Thomas J. Luparello, M.D., Psychiatrist in Private Practice, Jamestown, New York, U.S.A.

Andrea L. Martin-Pichora, Ph.D., Psychologist (Supervised Practice), Ryerson University, Toronto, Ontario, Canada

Steven A. Mazzuca, Ph.D., Senior Research Professor, Division of Rheumatology, Department of Medicine, Indiana University School of Medicine, Indianapolis, Indiana, U.S.A.

George P. McCabe Jr., Ph.D., Professor, Department of Statistics, and Associate Dean for Academic Affairs, College of Science, Purdue University, West Lafayette, Indiana, U.S.A.

Clement J. McDonald, M.D., Director, Lister Hill National Center for Biomedical Communications, U.S. National Library of Medicine, Bethesda, Maryland, U.S.A.

Claire A. McManus, M.Ac., Licensed Acupuncturist, West Roxbury, Massachusetts; Spaulding Rehabilitation Hospital, Boston, Massachusetts; and Beth Israel Deaconess Medical Center, Boston, Massachusetts, U.S.A.

Mary Gail Mercurio, M.D., Associate Professor, Department of Dermatology, University of Rochester Medical Center, Rochester, New York, U.S.A.

Karin B. Michels, Sc.D., Ph.D., Associate Professor and Co-Director, Obstetrics and Gynecology Epidemiology Center, Department of Obstetrics, Gynecology and Reproductive Biology, Brigham and Women's Hospital, Harvard Medical School, and Associate Professor, Department of Epidemiology, Harvard School of Public Health, Boston, Massachusetts, U.S.A.

Leonard S. Milling, Ph.D., Associate Professor, Department of Psychology, University of Hartford, West Hartford, Connecticut, U.S.A.

Daniel E. Moerman, Ph.D., William E. Stirton Professor Emeritus, Department of Anthropology, University of Michigan–Dearborn, Dearborn, Michigan, U.S.A.

Nicola Mondaini, M.D., Consultant Urologist, Urology Unit, Santa Maria Annunziata Hospital, Florence, Italy

Guy H. Montgomery, Ph.D., Director, Integrative Behavioral Medicine Program, and Associate Professor, Department of Oncological Sciences, Division of Cancer Prevention and Control, Mount Sinai School of Medicine, New York, New York, U.S.A.

† Frederick Mosteller, Ph.D., Professor Emeritus, Department of Statistics, Harvard University, Cambridge, Massachusetts, U.S.A.

Sarah S. Nicholls, Ph.D., Associate Research Scientist, Yale Child Study Center, Yale University School of Medicine, and Psychologist in Private Practice, New Haven, Connecticut, U.S.A.

Thomas E. Nichols, Ph.D., Principal Research Fellow and Head of Neuroimaging Statistics, Department of Statistics and Warwick Manufacturing Group, University of Warwick, Coventry, U.K.

Michael Norup, M.D., Associate Professor, Department of Public Health, Faculty of Health Sciences, University of Copenhagen, Copenhagen, Denmark

Valerie E. Ojha, B.Sc.N., R.N., Clinical Research Nurse, Department of Anesthesia and Critical Care Medicine, Stanford University School of Medicine, Stanford, California, U.S.A.

Min Park, B.S.N., M.A.O.M., Seoul, South Korea

Connie L. Peck, Ph.D., A.O., Consultant, United Nations Institute for Training and Research, Geneva, Switzerland

Karl Magnus Petersson, M.D., Ph.D., Assistant Professor, Faculty of Human and Exact Sciences and Centre for Molecular and Structural Biomedicine, University of Algarve, Faro, Portugal, and Senior Scientist, Neurobiology of Language Department, Max Planck Institute for Psycholinguistics, Nijmegen, The Netherlands

Predrag Petrovic, M.D., Ph.D., Department of Clinical Neuroscience, Karolinska Institutet, Stockholm, Sweden

Antonella Pollo, M.D., Assistant Professor, Department of Neuroscience, University of Turin Medical School, Turin, Italy

Donald D. Price, Ph.D., Professor, Division of Neuroscience, Department of Oral and Maxillofacial Surgery, College of Dentistry, University of Florida, Gainesville, Florida, U.S.A.

† Henry Richardson, M.D., Professor, Department of Medicine, Cornell University Medical College, New York, New York, U.S.A.

James K. Rilling, Ph.D., Associate Professor, Department of Anthropology and Department of Psychiatry and Behavioral Sciences, Emory University, Atlanta, Georgia, U.S.A.

Andrea L. Rivers, M.D., M.P.H., Resident, St. Vincent's East Family Medicine Residency, Birmingham, Alabama, U.S.A.

Robert M. Rose, M.D., Clinical Professor, Department of Psychiatry and Behavioral Sciences, and Member, Institute for the Medical Humanities, University of Texas Medical Branch, Galveston, Texas, U.S.A.

Loren H. Roth, M.D., M.P.H., Professor, Department of Psychiatry, University of Pittsburgh School of Medicine, Pittsburgh, Pennsylvania, U.S.A.

Kenneth J. Rothman, Dr.P.H., Distinguished Fellow and Vice President for Epidemiologic Research, RTI Health Solutions, Research Triangle Park, North Carolina, and Professor, Departments of Epidemiology and Medicine, Boston University, Boston, Massachusetts, U.S.A.

Thomas J. Ruth, Ph.D., Senior Research Scientist, TRIUMF, Vancouver, British Columbia, Canada

Norma P. Sanchez, M.A., Boston, Massachusetts, U.S.A.

Rosa N. Schnyer, DAOM, L.Ac. Dipl. OM, Clinical Assistant Professor, College of Pharmacy, University of Texas at Austin, Austin, Texas, U.S.A.

Michael Schulzer, M.D., Ph.D., Professor Emeritus, Department of Statistics and Department of Medicine, and Biostatistician, Pacific Parkinson's Research Centre and National Parkinson Foundation Centre of Excellence,

University of British Columbia and Vancouver Coastal Health, Vancouver, British Columbia, Canada

David J. Scott, Ph.D., Research Scientist, Omneuron Inc., Menlo Park, California, U.S.A.

Edward E. Smith, Ph.D., William B. Ransford Professor of Psychology, Department of Psychology and Department of Psychiatry, Columbia University, and Chief, Division of Cognitive Neuroscience, New York State Psychiatric Institute, New York, New York, U.S.A.

Vesna Sossi, Ph.D., Professor and Michael Smith Foundation for Health Research Senior Scholar, Department of Physics and Astronomy, University of British Columbia, Vancouver, British Columbia, Canada

A. Jon Stoessl, C.M., M.D., FRCPC, FAAN, FCAHS, Professor and Head, Division of Neurology; Canada Research Chair in Parkinson's Disease; and Director, Pacific Parkinson's Research Centre and National Parkinson Foundation Centre of Excellence, University of British Columbia and Vancouver Coastal Health, Vancouver, British Columbia, Canada

Christian S. Stohler, D.M.D., Dr.Med.Dent., Dean, School of Dentistry, University of Maryland, Baltimore, Maryland, U.S.A.

James M. Swanson, Ph.D., Principal Investigator, Southern and Central California Study Center, National Children's Study, Department of Pediatrics, University of California, Irvine School of Medicine, Irvine, California, and Professor, Department of Psychiatry, Florida International University, Miami, Florida, U.S.A.

Leora C. Swartzman, Ph.D., Associate Professor, Department of Psychology, Western University, London, Ontario, Canada

Pauline Sweet, M.D., Psychiatrist in Private Practice, Brooklyn, New York, U.S.A.

Frank Telang, M.D., Staff Clinician, National Institute on Alcohol Abuse and Alcoholism, National Institutes of Health, Bethesda, Maryland, U.S.A.

Robert Temple, M.D., Deputy Director for Clinical Science, Center for Drug Evaluation and Research, Food and Drug Administration, Rockville, Maryland, U.S.A.

Jon C. Tilburt, M.D., M.P.H., Associate Professor of Medicine, Assistant Professor of Biomedical Ethics, Division of General Internal Medicine, Mayo Clinic, Rochester, Minnesota, U.S.A.

Elena Torre, M.D., Neurologist, Department of Neurology, Misericordia e Dolce Hospital, Prato, Italy

Paul Vaska, Ph.D., Medical Scientist, Medical Department, Brookhaven National Laboratory, Upton, New York, U.S.A.

Sergio Vighetti, Ph.D., Electrical Engineer, Department of Neuroscience, University of Turin Medical School, Turin, Italy

Nora D. Volkow, M.D., Director, National Institute on Drug Abuse (NIDA), National Institutes of Health, Bethesda, Maryland, U.S.A.

Nicholas J. Voudouris, Ph.D., MAPS, Senior Manager, Science & Education, The Australian Psychological Society Limited, Melbourne, Australia

Tor D. Wager, Ph.D., Associate Professor, Department of Psychology and Neuroscience, and Director, Cognitive and Affective Neuroscience Lab, University of Colorado at Boulder, Boulder, Colorado, U.S.A.

James R. Walton, M.S., Information Analyst II, Nursing Practice Administration, University of Rochester Medical Center–Strong Memorial Hospital, Rochester, New York, U.S.A.

Gene-Jack Wang, M.D., Senior Scientist and Chair, Medical Department, Brookhaven National Laboratory, Upton, New York, U.S.A.

Charles Weijer, M.D., Ph.D., Professor and Canada Research Chair in Bioethics, Rotman Institute of Philosophy, Department of Philosophy, Western University, London, Ontario, Canada

† Claude E. Welch, M.D., Senior Surgeon, Massachusetts General Hospital, and Clinical Professor of Surgery, Emeritus, Harvard Medical School, Boston, Massachusetts, U.S.A.

David Wendler, Ph.D., Head, Unit on Vulnerable Populations, Department of Bioethics, National Institutes of Health, Bethesda, Maryland, U.S.A.

† Charles H. Wheeler, M.D., Professor, Department of Medicine, Cornell University Medical College, New York, New York, U.S.A.

William J. Winslade, Ph.D., J.D., Ph.D., James Wade Rockwell Professor of Philosophy of Medicine, Institute for the Medical Humanities, University of Texas Medical Branch, Galveston, Texas, and Director, Health Law and Policy Institute, University of Houston Law Center, Houston, Texas, U.S.A.

† Stewart Wolf, M.D., Professor and Head, Department of Medicine, University of Oklahoma, Oklahoma City, Oklahoma, U.S.A.

† Harold G. Wolff, M.D., Anne Parrish Titzel Professor of Medicine (Neurology), Cornell University Medical College, and Director, Neurological Service, New York Hospital, New York, New York, U.S.A.

Patricia J. Wolskee, Ph.D., General Faculty, College of Mind-Body Medicine, Saybrook University, San Francisco, California, U.S.A.

Christopher T. Wong, M.S., Research Associate, Medical Department, Brookhaven National Laboratory, Upton, New York, U.S.A.

Yanjun Xu, Ph.D., Computer Scientist, Information and Computing Sciences Division, SRI International, Princeton, New Jersey, U.S.A.

Wei Zhu, Ph.D., Professor and Deputy Chair, Department of Applied Mathematics and Statistics, Stony Brook University, Stony Brook, New York, U.S.A.

Jon-Kar Zubieta, M.D., Ph.D., Phil F. Jenkins Endowed Professor and Associate Chair for Research, Department of Psychiatry; Professor, Department of Radiology; and Research Professor, Molecular and Behavioral Neuroscience Institute, University of Michigan, Ann Arbor, Michigan, U.S.A.

Note

Despite our best efforts, we were unable to collect sufficient information about the following authors to include them in the list of contributors. We apologize for this omission.
Anna Arslanian, †Bruno Bergamasco, Louis W. Buckalew, Kenneth E. Coffield, Michael Davis, Ann Duff, Andrea Gavazzi, Gianluca Giubilei, Nancy Leist, Giuseppe Lombardi, Cary H. Lourie, Yemin Ma, Giuliano Maggi, Laurence Maynard, Antonio Melcarne, Bong Hyun Nam, Long T. Nguyen, Marina Pesare, Michael J. Rosadino, Joyce P. Singer, Alex Sokolik, and †John M. von Felsinger.

† — deceased

PART I

The Concept and Significance of the Placebo Effect

Setting the Agenda for Placebo Studies: A Historical Analysis

Before 1946, placebos served what were considered to be two marginal roles in medicine. First, they were used to placate "malingerers" and "ignorant" patients (Kaptchuk 1998a). While commonly used, physicians seemed embarrassed by their "pious fraud" (Jefferson 1898), and the few published discussions about placebos gave little indication regarding their widespread use. They were considered harmless and devoid of any clinical effectiveness. Second, placebos were used in experiments as controls for debunking mostly unorthodox and controversial therapies such as mesmerism and homeopathy (Kaptchuk 1998b). Here, the role of the placebo was to define a boundary between legitimate and illegitimate medicine. In both cases, placebos were not themselves of any scientific or intellectual interest.

In 1946, at a conference devoted to the use of placebos in therapy held at Cornell University Medical School, ideas about placebos underwent a paradigm shift. Famous medical researchers openly declared that "the placebo is a potent agent and in its actions can resemble almost any drug" and further that the study of placebos is "the most important step to be taken in scientific therapy" (Wolff et al. 1946, 1718). Those who participated in the Cornell conference thus declared that what would come to be known as the "placebo effect" was a central agenda of medicine. The issues discussed in the conference foreshadowed the questions, debates, and discussions that are still central concerns in the study of placebos: What is the magnitude of the placebo response? What kinds of medical conditions respond to placebos? What are the characteristics of people who respond to placebos? What emotional states predict placebo responses? What is the role of the patient–physician relationship, and of the physician's personality, in the placebo response? What is the importance of no-treatment controls when examining the effects of suggestion? What is the link between the placebo effect and the perceived efficacy of unconventional therapies? What psychological mechanisms are involved in the placebo effect: suggestion, symbols, the psychotherapeutic action of giving a "medicine" to a patient, and/or conditioning? Why is the "blind-test," as Harry Gold, a participant in the Cornell conference, put it (quotes in the original), so critical for evaluating new therapies? What are the best placebos to use clinically? Is there an ethical difference between using a "pure" placebo (i.e., a totally inert substance) versus using

an "impure" placebo (i.e., a substance that has no effect but has traces of something that in larger dosages conceivably has physiological effects)? Is it ethical to use placebos in therapy? Would such use undermine a patient's trust in his or her physician? What do placebo effects say about an integrated vision of the "psychobiological" unity of human beings?

If one adds to the previous list research into the neurobiology of placebo effects, the issues discussed at the 1946 conference would arouse excitement at any contemporary scientific meeting on placebos. Given the then-unprecedented focus on placebos, we thus begin our anthology of landmark studies with the groundbreaking publication that emerged from the 1946 meeting at Cornell, "Conferences on Therapy: The Use of Placebos in Therapy." This introduction tells the story leading up to the Cornell conference and, in fact, the history leading up to all the articles in this anthology. We also discuss Henry Beecher's 1955 landmark article "The Powerful Placebo," along with recent critical appraisals of Beecher's data and methods. We close with a discussion and review of several major conceptual articles that help to frame the issues that arise in the rest of the anthology.

The Medical World before "Bogus" Treatments

Before the early modern era (late seventeenth and early eighteenth centuries), literate European physicians did not prescribe "bogus" or "simulated" treatments. Specific diseases—ontologically isolated entities—were rarely the focus of a physician's attention nor was there much interest in specific treatments for particular conditions. Rather, illness was primarily a metaphoric description of a person's appearance, personality, behaviors, and bodily and mental symptoms, and was described in terms of elemental (air, fire, water, and earth) or temperamental (sanguine, phlegmatic, choleric, and melancholy) imbalances (dyscrasia) (Ackerknecht 1982). In the scholarly Galenic medical tradition (and, in fact, in all the literate humoral traditions such as Chinese or Ayurveda medicine), an extreme dichotomy of soma (body) and psyche (mind), much less their separate existence, was not conceivable (Kaptchuk 2000; Temkin 1973). A treatment targeted the "person" who manifested as a singular "gestalt." An appropriate treatment—including regimes, behaviors, herbs, and/or words—always existed for a humoral disorder; there was never a need for a simulated or fake treatment. When incurable and mortal diseases were recognized (such as leprosy or plague), therapeutics directed at the humors (or temperaments) were still available (Conrad et al. 1995; Siraisi 1990). Physicians were rarely without therapeutic options, though they might refuse to "override nature" in a hopeless situation (Amundsen 1978; Edelstein 1967). For magico-religious healers, bogus treatment was even more unthinkable. The supernatural realm provided an endless source of potential healing possibilities, and one could always engage in "performative speech acts, and ritual action" until death (Tambiah 1990, 108). Religious healing was always a source of relief in this world or the next. Self-defined dummy treatments were simply unnecessary.

Modernity and Placebo Treatment

The scientific revolution of Galileo, Descartes, and Newton discredited scholastic Aristotelian philosophy. In a parallel phenomenon, new findings in anatomy and new mechanistic theories of disease causation led to a gradual displacement of Galenic medicine. The anatomical basis of certain pathologies discovered by such pioneers as Malpighi, Morgagni, Auenbrugger, Willis, and van Haller initiated a major shift in medical thinking from a concentration on the "gestalt" of a person's humors to the isolation of localized changes in organs and tissue. The Galenic pharmacy was often equally condemned because it lacked specific or mechanistically defined remedies. Physicians attuned to the new developments of modernity felt an acute absence of effective armaments corresponding to these newly understood afflictions. Patients needed responses. During this long transition, undoubtedly with some desperation, physicians self-consciously adopted placebo treatment.

The earliest known description of placebo treatment appears in William Cullen's medical lecture notes (Kerr et al. 2008). Writing in 1772, Cullen (1710–1790), the most famous physician of the Scottish Enlightenment and a teacher to countless students from throughout Europe, describes two cases of placebo treatment. In one case, the patient, described "as absolutely incurable, and as hastening very fast to his fate," was in need of comfort; in the second case, the patient was a paralytic to whom, as Cullen puts it, "I gave it because it is necessary to give a medicine, and as what I call a placebo" (Cullen 1772, 218–219 300). Both treatments involved "impure" placebos, that is, tiny and useless amounts of ingredients that would have, at much higher doses, some purported pharmacological activity. Cullen regarded a placebo treatment not only as one given to please the patient but also as one without any curative intent or possibility. Given that Cullen nowhere hints that this is an innovative procedure, it seems likely that physicians previously and elsewhere also administered placebos as treatments. In fact, one already finds "placebo" defined "as a commonplace method or medicine" in prominent medical dictionaries by 1785 (Shapiro 1968; White 1985).

Placebo treatment was common throughout the nineteenth century, and patients routinely quaffed a "polychromatic assortment of sugar pills" (Anon. 1885, 577). Thomas Jefferson, for example, penned one of the earliest observations of what he called the "pious fraud." In his letter of June 21, 1807, to Dr. Caspar Wistar, Jefferson writes:

> One of the most successful physicians I have ever known, has assured me, that he used more bread pills, drops of colored water, & powders of hickory ashes, than of all other medicines put together. It was certainly a pious fraud. (Jefferson 1898, 82)

Richard Cabot (1890–1920), an eminent professor at Harvard Medical School, described how in the late nineteenth century he used placebos "by the bushel" (Cabot 1903, 349). This practice continued into the middle of the twentieth century. For example, a 1954 *Lancet* article, entitled "The Humble Humbug," depicted the final effort for this soon-to-be-antiquated understanding of the placebo:

> a means of reinforcing a patient's confidence in his recovery, when the diagnosis is undoubted and no more effective treatment is possible; that for some unintelligent or inadequate patients life is made easier by a bottle of medicine to comfort their ego; that to refuse a placebo to a dying incurable patient may be simply cruel; and that to decline to humour an elderly "chronic" brought up on the bottle is hardly within the bounds of possibility. (Anon. 1954, 321)

In almost all known descriptions of placebo treatment (until the 1950s in the English medical literature and until the 1890s in the French and German literatures) placebo meant an innocuous treatment without any consequences for the patient's medical condition. Placebos were useful in managing patients, but they had no discernible effects on pathophysiology. Placebos belonged to the "moral" dimension of medicine (Flint 1863), a comfort to the patient and his family (Rosenberg 1967), and a small but indispensable concession to the "superstition of the patient . . . to strengthen his confidence" (Wunderlick 1852, 75). When patients improved with placebo treatment it was thought to be because of spontaneous remission and the "tendency to a natural cure" that came as a result of "rest in bed, a well-regulated diet, and good nursing" (Sutton 1865, 428, 393). Physicians believed that placebos would helpfully "appeal to the imagination" of the patient, but would have no effect on pathophysiology or physical symptoms (Hall 1887, 145). The early modern emphasis on "monistic mechanistic materialism" (Ledermann 1970) could concede little to an imitation treatment that had no basis in the science of the day.

Despite the increasing purchase of more modern ideas, a small group of physicians still adhered to premodern notions of mind–body interactions or to alternative vitalist theories of medicine (Kaptchuk 2005). As the Scottish surgeon James Braid wrote in the 1850s:

> with implicit faith, hope, and confidence on the part of the patient, many disorders may be recovered from, even whilst the patients are merely taking a drop of plain water occasionally, or a particle of bread, or *any other harmless substances*, . . . (Braid 1852, 38; cf., e.g., Lisle 1861; Naval Surgeon 1847; Tuke 1873)

But these voices were a decided minority and not part of elite academic medicine.

Placebo Controls in Medical Research

The transition of the placebo from innocuous humble humbug to potent agent was gradual and connected to its increasing use as a control in medical experiments.

The 1784 Royal Commission appointed by the King of France, Louis XVI, to investigate "animal magnetism" or "mesmerism" performed the first known scientific placebo-controlled experiments. The panel of experts included the American scientist Benjamin Franklin, Antoine Lavoisier, the French discoverer of oxygen, and the renowned French physician Joseph-Ignace Guillotin. The commissioners were concerned with establishing whether the mesmeric treatment changed the "natural history of disease" (Franklin et al. 1785 [1784]). They considered that

> nature alone and without our interferences, cures a great
> number of persons. . . . by attributing to it [magnetism] all
> the cures performed by nature, would tend to prove that it had
> an action useful and curative, when in reality it might have
> no action at all. (Franklin et al. 1785 [1784], 16)

The commission seems to have adopted a well-known sixteenth-century methodology that was originally used to test the veracity of religious exorcisms with "trick trials" using fake exorcist procedures (Kaptchuk et al. 2009). Between March and June 1784, the commission performed a series of both genuine and sham exposures to animal magnetism. Some of the experiments included genuine and bogus "mesmerized" water or a "mesmerized" tree. Whether they actually received genuine or fake treatment, if subjects believed it was real, they experienced the effects of magnetism. The short version of the commission's conclusion was twofold: first, that "[t]his agent, this fluid, has no existence," and second, that any observed effects were due to the research subject's "imagination" and to nature's "power of operating without medicine" (Franklin et al. 1785 [1784], 40, 15).

The placebo-controlled experiment became a common component in the nineteenth-century tug-of-war between orthodox and unorthodox medicine (such as homeopathy and hypnosis, which was merely a relabeled form of mesmerism). Practitioners of orthodox medicine used placebo controls to debunk the outsiders, while practitioners of unconventional medicine used such controls to demonstrate the authenticity of their techniques (Kaptchuk 1998b). In the overwhelming number of reports, researchers and physicians credited the observed effects of both the placebo controls and the unorthodox therapies to:

> the spontaneous course of most natural diseases . . . and it
> is easy to attribute to our therapeutic experience what the
> spontaneous disease course can produce by itself and to look
> for a cause in an agent whose power is totally non-existent.
> (Trousseau and Gouraud 1834, 239)

Suggestion in Fin de Siècle French and Germanic Medical Research

Orthodox acceptance of the idea that the mind could exert an effect on bodily symptoms gained its first general mainstream support in fin de siècle France and very quickly thereafter in German-speaking Europe. The opportunity for such a shift came about almost single-handedly because of the involvement of one of Europe's most famous physicians, Jean-Martin Charcot (1825–1893), the founder of modern clinical neurology. His supreme self-confidence in his "anatomo-clinical epistemology" (Goetz et al. 1995, 206) led him to believe that hypnotism was not a mental phenomenon but an abnormal physiological phenomenon allied to hysteria and describable in neurological terms with objective and mechanical indices. In the widely followed uproar of the ensuing debate, interpretations of mental phenomenon underwent a major transformation (Hillman 1965). Hippolyte Bernheim (1840–1919), a teacher of Freud, argued that the paralyses, mutisms, and coxalgia that Charcot had demonstrated to audiences of physicians, the European elite, and in the popular press were not due to physical pathways but rather to "suggestion." For Bernheim, suggestion meant "influence exerted by an idea . . . received by the mind," which could translate into action, sensation, or movement (Bernheim 1889 [1886], 125). Many placebo-controlled experiments were undertaken during this debate and eventually Charcot, in his last publication, conceded at least partial defeat when he wrote that faith healing relied on the "powerful force of auto-suggestion" enhanced with "a confidence, a credulity, a receptivity of suggestion," and seemed to especially affect "nervous disease[s]" (Charcot 1893, 22, 19, 25). (For a full discussion of the many experiments and debates during this controversy, see Ellenberger 1970; Gauld 1992; Goetz et al. 1995; Kaptchuk 1998b.)

Bernheim went on to develop his ideas of suggestion and hypnotism, and his influence on psychiatry was enormous especially through his impact on Freud. While not a central theme in his work, Bernheim, on occasion, mentioned that he used bread pills to treat patients with somatic complaints (Bernheim 1891). Besides Freud, Bernheim influenced such psychiatrists as Pierre Janet (1859–1947) who did not hesitate "to think that bread pills are medically indicated in certain [medical] cases . . . [especially] if I deck them out with impressive names" (Janet 1925, 338). At least in French psychiatry, orthodox French physicians could argue that placebos had some medical consequences beyond the disease's natural history. But the placebo was discussed primarily as a psychological issue of suggestion that needed to be addressed by a relatively small audience of psychiatrists.

The next major debate about the power of suggestion quickly moved to German-speaking Europe after a second French episode that began with Édouard Brown-Séquard (1817–1894), one of the most prominent scientists of his time and the successor to Claude Bernard's chair in physiology at the Collège de France. In 1889, Brown-Séquard declared that subcutaneous injections of animal testicles could rejuvenate physical and mental health. The therapy quickly became an international sensation (Borell 1976). But just as quickly, mostly German-speaking scientists—influenced by the Charcot-Bernheim debates—began to call for blind trials to assess the effects of suggestion on Brown-Séquard's results. For example, Auguste Forel (1848–1931), a famous professor of psychiatry in Zurich, denounced the "senile-erotic ideas started by Brown-Séquard's spermatotherapy" and insisted that the reported outcomes must have resulted from suggestion (Forel 1894, 388). (Rare discussions of these ideas can be found in the English-language literature; see, e.g., Graves 1920; Kaptchuk 1998b.)

Most important, pharmacologists, especially German-speaking ones, began to perform n-of-1 placebo-controlled experiments in individual patients and noticed the profound effects of bogus treatment on outcomes (Kaptchuk 1998b). At the same time, the German government and pharmaceutical industry became intensely interested in stimulants— such as cola, caffeine, cocaine, mate, and tea—which might be used to create "super-soldiers." Pharmacologists worried that the observed effects of such substances might be due to suggestion. Paul Martini (1889–1964), Germany's leading interwar pharmacologist, was one of the key figures who helped establish that the concern about the effects of suggestion on disease outcomes were quite general and should be rigorously assessed for all drugs. His 1932 manual *Methodenlehre der therapeutischen Untersuchung* (never translated into English, but renderable as *Methodology of Therapeutic Investigation*), although ignored (or at least never cited) in the English-language literature, explicitly and meticulously described the methodological safeguards, including blinding and concurrent controls, needed to exclude the causal effects of suggestion from investigations of a drug's efficacy. Martini's methodological arguments led to the widespread adoption of placebo controls in Germany in the interwar period (Shelley and Baur 1999). For the first time, the need to separate the effects of suggestion from the effects of so-called active interventions was applicable to all drugs. At least in orthodox pharmacologist circles, the control of suggestion became the rationale for blind experiments.

The Background to the 1946 Cornell Conference on Therapy: Harry Gold, Harold G. Wolff, and Stewart Wolf

The turn-of-the-century English-language literature had scattered references to the concrete German methodology of treatment evaluation but never seems to have mentioned the word "suggestion" (Kaptchuk 1998b). In the United States, the most influential person early on who championed this emerging methodology was Torald Sollmann (1874–1965), who emigrated from Germany at the age of thirteen but later returned to his homeland to obtain his medical and pharmacy degrees. After returning to the United States, he still frequently traveled to Europe and did several stints of postgraduate work in Germany and in France. In his position as head of the American Medical Association's Council on Pharmacy and Chemistry, he made early English-language pleas for "blind-test" assessment in the pages of JAMA, yet he only wrote of the dangers of failing to control for natural history and studiously avoided any mention of the German-language discussion of suggestion with which he was undoubtedly familiar (Sollmann 1917, 1930). It would seem that researchers within the United States were still uncomfortable with the idea of mind–body interactions.

During the 1930s, at least two dozen placebo-controlled pharmaceutical studies were undertaken in the United States (Kaptchuk 1998b). Patients improved in the placebo arms of the trials, and researchers almost invariably attributed this improvement to "natural history" or "spontaneous remission." The innovative 1937 placebo-controlled study of the effect of xanthines on cardiac pain by Harry Gold and his colleagues deserves special note. The study had a high placebo response rate and, at the end of the article, Gold et al. (1937) list ten factors that could possibly have contributed to the placebo response. They included spontaneous remission, changes in the weather, work, diet, domestic affairs, bowels, medical adviser, and emotional stress. The final two reasons, which seem ad hoc, were "confidence" and "encouragement" aroused by a new procedure (Gold et al. 1937). Gold (1899–1973) was a key figure in the 1946 Cornell conference and a leading member of the Department of Pharmacology at Cornell University Medical School. Given that he was Russian born and fluent in German and Russian (besides his native Yiddish), it is almost inconceivable that he was unfamiliar with Martini's work (S. Wolf, personal communication to T. J. Kaptchuk, November 9, 1999). Why did Gold not mention suggestion as a cause of the placebo response in this study? A further question is whether the other leaders of the 1946 Cornell conference were aware of the empirical research into the power of suggestion within the European literature.

Harold G. Wolff (1898–1962) was one of America's most prominent neurologists and a faculty member at Cornell University Medical School. In the prewar period, his interests were drawn to the emerging field of psychosomatic medicine. Wolff sought to "develop a unitary concept of man" that integrated the "psychobiology" of Pavlov and classical conditioning with the "concept of unconscious mental activities . . . [formulated by] Janet, Morton Prince, Freud, and Jung (notably Freud)" (Wolff 1947, 944–945). Also born in New York to immigrant parents from Russia, he was fluent in German, Russian, and probably Yiddish, and deeply committed to a new synthesis of neurology, conditioning, and psychodynamic, psychosomatic, and psychosocial theories of illness and health. In fact, he spent a year doing postgraduate work in Pavlov's laboratory in Petrograd in 1931–1932 and was one of the founders of the American Psychosomatic Society in 1942. During World War II, Wolff and his colleagues performed analgesia n-of-1 experiments on "suggestible" and "non-suggestible" subjects and found that "suggestible" subjects responded similarly to both placebo and aspirin (Wolff and Goodell 1943). The results of some of these experiments were presented at the 1946 Cornell conference.

Besides Wolff and Gold, the 1946 conference brought together other leaders from Cornell University's Medical School. Eugene DuBois (1882–1959), a well-known professor of clinical physiology, was given the honor of delivering the opening remarks. It is hard to imagine that he was not familiar with German theories of suggestion since he had held several fellowships in Germany. Also present at the Cornell conference was Oskar Diethelm (1898–1993), who directly observed Wolff's World War II experiments with placebos. Diethelm was a graduate of the University of Zurich Medical School and a student of Auguste Forel. He revealed his commitment to Germanic theories of suggestion before World War II when he wrote in his psychiatry textbook that "suggestions play a role in every treatment" (Diethelm 1936, 45). It would seem that the speakers at the 1946 conference were already deeply informed of European theories of suggestion and conditioning. Evidence of this shift can also be found in the different way that Gold presented the findings from his 1937 study at the 1946 meeting. Instead of a laundry list of ten possible factors, Gold succinctly says that responses to placebo are "the psychotherapeutic action of just giving a 'medicine'" (Wolff et al. 1946, 1723). A fully psychological explanation of the placebo response is for the first time an acceptable analysis at an American medical meeting.

But the 1946 discussion of placebos at Cornell involved much more than the addition of one further example of a psychological phenomenon—the placebo effect—that can accompany medication. Rather, an understanding of the role and action of placebos in an emerging theory of the "psychobiological unity" of health and illness emerges from this conference. Henceforward, the study of placebos becomes a critical issue for validating and investigating this new theory of medicine. Going beyond the French psychiatric notions of suggestion or the Germanic pharmacologists' concern to disentangle the effects of suggestion from those of medications, the Cornell conference participants, clearly showing the influence of Continental European medicine, in effect declare that understanding the placebo response is a central agenda of medicine. A milestone has been reached.

To read the publication that emerged from the 1946 Cornell conference is to witness the first public declaration of a new research agenda on placebos. While other topics such as blind testing with placebo controls, the influence of suggestion on treatment outcomes, and the ethics of placebo treatment had already been extensively discussed in Continental Europe (but not in Great Britain), this 1946 forum represents the first declaration of a research agenda investigating "the placebo [as] a potent agent . . . [which] in its actions can resemble almost any drug" (Wolff et al. 1946, 1718). An American placebo phenomenon has thus been born and a new research agenda defined.

Placebos became the critical link in a meta-agenda "to abandon dualisms and dichotomies such as are exhibited when body and mind are used as opposing terms, and to develop a unitary concept of man" (Wolff 1947, 944). Stewart Wolf (1914–2005), who was later recruited by Harold Wolff to join the Cornell faculty, was a key participant in the development of this meta-agenda and produced early results in his study of the effects of suggestion and conditioning on the action of chemical agents, effects Wolf called "placebo effects" (Wolf 1950). (Interestingly, Wolf was fluent in French and German and, in fact, was an accomplished historian of fin de siècle France and early-twentieth-century German medicine and was thus familiar with all the details of the German and French debates on suggestion [Wolf 1993].) Moreover, Wolf was in the audience at the 1946 conference (S. Wolf, personal communication to T. J. Kaptchuk, 1999) and would go on to do foundational studies on the placebo effect, two of which are included in Part II, Section A of this anthology.

Henry K. Beecher, the Powerful Placebo, and His Critics

If pioneers such as Wolff, Gold, and Wolf created an American placebo effect, Henry Beecher's watershed 1955 JAMA publication, "The Powerful Placebo," popularized the idea and made it a central feature of general medical knowledge. Beecher (1904–1976) was a distinguished anesthesiologist researcher and medical reformer at Harvard Medical School. (Later he would make significant contributions in such diverse areas as measuring subjective health outcomes, ethical standards for research, and defining brain death [Lowenstein and McPeek 2007].) Unlike the Cornell University group, his agenda had little to do with psychosomatics and instead focused primarily on the new methodology of the randomized controlled trial (RCT) being developed by the English Statistical School of R. A. Fisher and Austin Bradford Hill (Kaptchuk 1998b). The British agenda was primarily concerned with concurrent controls, random assignment to treatment arms, and statistical inference. For the British researchers, when placebos were discussed it was because their use could be a recruitment and retention device and help with blinding (Kaptchuk 1998b; Kaptchuk and Kerr 2004).

Beecher's awareness of the impact of the psychological factors on pain perception began with his observations of wounded soldiers at Anzio beachhead during World War II (Beecher 1946, 1956). At some point, he became aware of the work coming out of Cornell University but did not actively communicate with this group (S. Wolf, personal communication to T. J. Kaptchuk, 1999). Some years after the war, Beecher estimated that, at least for subjective symptoms, "a third to a half of [patients] will be relieved of their symptoms by a placebo" (Beecher 1952, 161). Later, Beecher performed what could be called the first proto-meta-analysis of placebo effects to provide concrete data. This was his landmark study from 1955, and it is the second article included in Part I. Beecher aggregated 1,082 patients in fifteen randomized trials and found that the "average significant effectiveness of [the placebo was] $35.2 \pm 2.2\%$" (Beecher 1955, 1603). He extensively references Wolf's 1950 study (the first chapter in

Part II, Section A of this anthology) and quotes Wolf's claim that placebo effects "include objective changes at the end organ which may exceed those attributable to potent pharmacological action" (Wolf 1950, 108). The article emphasizes that uncontrolled placebo effects are an overwhelming threat to the proper evaluation of medication efficacy. Beecher inserted the new American understanding of "placebo effects" into the British imperative to adopt RCTs and helped create the normative rationale for the design and conduct of RCTs (Kaptchuk 1998b). To date, Beecher's paper remains the most cited article on the placebo effect.

Until recently, there was no serious debate about Beecher's 1955 article (although some of his main collaborators declined to co-author the publication because they felt uncomfortable with the methods [L. Lasagna, personal communication to T. J. Kaptchuk, 2000; F. Mosteller, personal communication to T. J. Kaptchuk, 2002]). Many of the criticisms had to do with Beecher's failure to mention the role of natural history in the observed results, especially given that some of the eighteen trials actually had no-treatment natural history controls. Beecher also did not consider that people worsened while taking placebos. Interestingly, Louis Lasagna (1923–2003), a close collaborator of Beecher's, simultaneously published an article on clinical trials that, unlike Beecher's article, emphasized the importance of natural history as a confounder in understanding genuine pharmaceutical effects (Lasagna 1955).

In 1983, a team of statisticians, Clement McDonald, Stephen Mazzuca, and George McGabe Jr., published the first systematic criticism of Beecher's paper and concluded that most of the improvement attributable to the placebo effect was actually regression to the mean (McDonald et al. 1983). (This is the third chapter in Part I.) This important article seems to have been largely ignored by the medical community (McDonald 2001). In 1997, Gunver Kienle and Helmut Kiene reanalyzed the fifteen trials in Beecher's historic paper and concluded that there were no demonstrable placebo effects but only the effects of such phenomenon as spontaneous improvement, fluctuation of symptoms, scaling bias, and experimental subordination; some of Beecher's errors, Kienle and Kiene maintain, were even due to simple misquotation of his sources. Kienle and Kiene's paper, included as the fourth chapter in Part I, seems to have had little impact on placebo orthodoxy.

It was only in 2001 when Asbjørn Hróbjartsson and Peter Gøtzsche published a highly publicized article in the *New England Journal of Medicine* that genuine doubts about Beecher's claims received a widespread audience. (This is the fifth chapter in Part I.) In a sophisticated meta-analysis of 114 RCTs that included both a placebo treatment and a no-treatment control, Hróbjartsson and Gøtzsche found that placebo treatment in RCTs had no significant effect on objective and binary measures. For continuous subjective measures, and especially for pain, a "possible small benefit" may exist but they found "little evidence that placebos in general

have powerful clinical effects" (Hróbjartsson and Gøtzsche 2001, 1594, 1599). In 2010, Hróbjartsson and Gøtzsche published a larger follow-up study with the same methodology that both confirmed and modified the earlier study. They confirmed that placebo treatment does not have "large effects" but found that there is a placebo effect with patient-reported outcomes, especially pain, and that higher placebo effects were associated with device placebos (such as acupuncture), trials with the explicit purpose of studying placebos, small (and likely statistically underpowered) trials, and trials that falsely informed patients that the trial did not have a placebo treatment (Hróbjartsson and Gøtzsche 2010). Not unexpectedly, there was an avalanche of criticism directed at their methodology and at their interpretation of the results following their 2001 article (Spiegel et al. 2001; Vase et al. 2002; Wampold et al. 2005). Nonetheless, their analysis has transformed the field of placebo studies and made no-treatment controls (or some equivalent) an indispensable requirement for legitimate research in the field.

Philosophic Confusion

Understanding and appreciating the placebo effect has been hampered by conceptual confusion and by value judgments imported into supposedly value-neutral terminology. The etymological meaning of "placebo"—I shall please—suggests that placebo treatments merely please the patient who is seeking a treatment without the possibility of having any biologically or clinically significant effect. In the context of placebo-controlled trials, the placebo is seen as a fake, a dummy, or a sham intervention, in contrast with the *verum*, the *real* treatment. This creates the impression, especially in biomedical circles, that responses associated with placebo interventions must be unreal artifacts, or, if real, at best unimportant. Moreover, typical placebo controls, such as sugar pills and saline injections, are often described as "inert." Strictly speaking, this is mistaken, as both sugar and saline have biochemical properties. They are instead inert in the sense that there is no reason to think that these agents have a targeted therapeutic effect on the conditions under investigation in placebo-controlled trials. But if the placebo is inert, how can a placebo effect be a real phenomenon? A further confusion is the contrast drawn between real treatments with "specific efficacy" and placebo treatments that produce "nonspecific" effects. Since effects must be produced by some specific mechanism, how can any real effect be nonspecific? Indeed, many of the landmark articles in Part II of this anthology describe a variety of specific neurobiological mechanisms underlying placebo effects. And because specificity in diagnosis and treatment is highly valued in scientific medicine, so-called nonspecific phenomena, such as placebo responses, are treated as unimportant, both in therapeutic and research contexts. Much conceptual and normative work thus remains to be done on placebos.

In his classical article on the placebo response, included as the sixth chapter in Part I, philosopher of science Adolf

Grünbaum notes that "the medical and psychiatric literature on placebos and their effects is conceptually bewildering, to the point of being a veritable Tower of Babel" (Grünbaum 1986, 19). Grünbaum attempts to bring clarity to the understanding of the placebo phenomenon by explicating placebo effects in a conceptual model that contrasts them with the "characteristic" factors of medical therapies. These characteristic factors are defined (often only implicitly) by a "therapeutic theory," which hypothesizes that a given treatment intervention for a target disorder will produce beneficial clinical outcomes by virtue of its characteristic factors. By contrast, placebo effects are beneficial outcomes that derive from the "incidental" treatment factors—those factors that are not specified by the therapeutic theory as potentially productive of beneficial clinical outcomes. For example, arthroscopic surgery to treat osteoarthritis of the knee was hypothesized, in accordance with an implicit therapeutic theory, to relieve arthritic pain by virtue of lavage (rinsing out the knee joint) or debridement (removal of unhealthy joint tissue) applied by means of the surgical intervention. The implicit therapeutic theory assumed that the characteristic treatment factors—lavage and debridement—were the mechanisms by which reduced arthritic knee pain was achieved. However, when a sham-controlled trial of this treatment showed that the surgical procedures were no better than a sham intervention (consisting merely of a skin incision and no other manipulation of the knee), the authors concluded that the observed benefits from arthroscopic knee surgery were placebo effects (Moseley et al. 2002). Incidental factors, such as positive expectations of patients undergoing an invasive procedure for a painful and disabling condition not responsive to medical therapy, may have been responsible, at least in part, for the observed clinical outcomes in patients in both the surgical and sham procedure groups.

Grünbaum's analysis remains the best analytical account of the placebo effect from a mainstream biomedical perspective. It avoids the misleading conceptual baggage that continues to predominate in the medical literature and helps to clearly differentiate potential placebo effects from therapeutic effects that derive from the characteristic factors of a treatment intervention. But it tells us almost nothing about what placebo effects distinctively are. Instead, Grünbaum's aim is to clearly distinguish placebo effects from the "characteristic" pharmacological or physiological effects of medical therapies. Various fruitful perspectives have been developed by others, such as explaining placebo effects as the product of classical conditioning (Ader 1997), as reflecting the meaning that patients attribute to clinical interventions (Moerman and Jonas 2002), and as the outcome of medical rituals (Kaptchuk 2011). (The discussion of the "meaning response" by Daniel Moerman and Wayne Jonas is included here as the seventh and penultimate chapter in Part I.) To date, however, robust and comprehensive theoretical accounts that aim to integrate and explain the diversity of placebo effects have yet to be developed (Miller et al. 2009).

The New Placebo–Alternative Medicine Link

"Placebo treatment" has always been the accusation directed at unconventional therapies (e.g., Hooker 1849). In the early history of placebo use, this meant that alternative therapies were thought to have no effect on clinical outcomes and that they did little but mask the natural course of the patient's condition (Kaptchuk 1998a). From the time of the 1946 Cornell conference, however, critics of alternative therapies adopted a different rhetorical strategy. One of the claims made by the Cornell conference participants was that the "success and therapeutic results" of unconventional medicines, such as homeopathy, "are probably better than those in the case of some of the regular drugs"; this demonstrates, they concluded, "very clearly what can be done by placebos" (Wolff et al. 1946, 1718). To the extent that placebo effects were legitimized, critics were provided with another way to attack alternative medicine: the acceptance of placebo effects became yet another insult to be hurled against alternative medicine. Now, if they acknowledged that alternative medicine treatments produce positive results at all, critics of alternative medicine claimed that they did so only because they are placebos dressed up as therapies (Kaptchuk and Eisenberg 1998). The article by Ted Kaptchuk, our eighth and final chapter in Part I, takes up this issue with a new twist (Kaptchuk 2002). Is it possible that alternative medicine, because of its elaborate rituals, provides "enhanced" placebo effects? Is it possible that the placebo effects of some alternative therapies may have clinical significance and be superior to mainstream treatments? This question has become especially prominent in recent years, as some alternative therapies have been shown to be superior to conventional care but no different from placebo controls (Li and Kaptchuk 2011).

Summary

The first part of this book includes articles that helped bring about the new placebo agenda of mid-twentieth-century American medicine. The 1946 Cornell conference brought together the American (but often European-born) pioneers in placebo research and established the placebo agenda for the second half of the twentieth century, one that has expanded in the twenty-first century. The conference participants argued for the importance of placebo controls in experiments and debated the question of treating patients with placebos. Importantly, they also argued that a better understanding of placebo phenomena was of crucial scientific importance and deserving of research attention. Researchers took up this challenge and produced important results in the decades following the Cornell conference. A collection of these important articles are collected in Part II of this volume.

REFERENCES

Ackerknecht EH. *A Short History of Medicine*, rev. edition. Baltimore: Johns Hopkins University Press, 1982.

Ader R. The role of conditioning in pharmacotherapy. In: Harrington A (ed.). *The Placebo Effect: An Interdisciplinary Exploration*. Cambridge, Mass.: Harvard University Press, 1997, pp. 138–165.

Amundsen DW. The physician's obligation to prolong life: A medical duty without classical roots. *Hastings Center Report* 1978;8(4):23–31.

Anonymous. Placebos. *Medical Record* 1885;27:576–577.

Anonymous. The humble humbug. *Lancet* 1954;264:321.

Beecher HK. Pain in men wounded in battle. *Bulletin of the U.S. Army Medical Department* 1946;5:445–454.

Beecher HK. Experimental pharmacology and measurement of the subjective response. *Science* 1952;116:157–162.

Beecher HK. The powerful placebo. *JAMA* 1955;159:1602–1606.

Beecher HK. Relationship of significance of wound to pain experienced. *JAMA* 1956;161:1609–1613.

Bernheim H. *Suggestive Therapeutics: A Treatise on the Nature and Uses of Hypnotism*. Herter CA (trans.). New York: G. P. Putnam's Sons, 1889 [1886].

Bernheim H. *Hypnotisme, suggestion, psychothérapie: Études nouvelles*. Paris: Octave Doin, 1891.

Borell M. Brown-Séquard's organotherapy and its appearance in America at the end of the nineteenth century. *Bulletin of the History of Medicine* 1976;50:309–320.

Braid J. *Magic, Witchcraft, Animal Magnetism, Hypnotism, and Electro-Biology; being a digest of the latest views of the author on these subjects*. London: John Churchill, 1852.

Cabot RC. The use of truth and falsehood in medicine: An experimental study. *American Medicine* 1903;5:344–349.

Charcot JM. The faith-cure. *The New Review* 1893;8:18–31.

Conrad LI, Neve M, Nutton V, Porter R, Wear A. *The Western Medical Tradition: 800 BC to AD 1800*. New York: Cambridge University Press, 1995.

Cullen W. *Cullen Clinical Lectures 1772–1773*. Edinburgh: Royal College of Physicians of Edinburgh Manuscript, 1772.

Diethelm O. *Treatment in Psychiatry*. New York: Macmillan, 1936.

Edelstein L. The Hippocratic physician. In: Temkin O, Temkin C (eds.). *Ancient Medicine: Selected Papers of Ludwig Edelstein*. Baltimore: Johns Hopkins Press, 1967.

Ellenberger HF. *The Discovery of the Unconscious: The History and Evolution of Dynamic Psychiatry*. New York: Basic Books, 1970.

Flint A. A Contribution toward the Natural History of Articular Rheumatism; consisting of a report of thirteen cases treated solely with palliative measures. *American Journal of the Medical Sciences* 1863;46:17–36.

Forel A. Das Verhältnis gewisser therapeutischer Methoden zur Suggestion. *Zeitschrift für Hypnotismus, Suggestionstherapie, Suggestionslehre und verwandte psychologische Forschungen*. 1894;2:385–390.

Franklin B, Majault, Le Roy, Sallin, Bailly, D'Arcet, De Bory, Guillotin, and Lavoisier. *Report of Dr. Benjamin Franklin and Other Commissioners, Charged by the King of France with the Examination of Animal Magnetism, as Now Practiced at Paris; translated from the French, with an historical introduction*. London: J. Johnston, 1785 [1784].

Gauld A. *A History of Hypnotism*. New York: Cambridge University Press, 1992.

Goetz CG, Bonduelle M, Gelfand T. *Charcot: Constructing Neurology*. New York: Oxford University Press, 1995.

Gold H, Kwit NT, Otto H. The xanthines (theobromine and aminophylline) in the treatment of cardiac pain. *JAMA* 1937;108:2173–2179.

Graves TC. Commentary on a case of hystero-epilepsy with delayed puberty. *Lancet* 1920;196:1134–1135.

Grünbaum A. The placebo concept in medicine and psychiatry. *Psychological Medicine* 1986;16:19–38.

Hall GS. Psychological literature. *American Journal of Psychology* 1887;1:128–146.

Hillman RG. A scientific study of mystery: The role of the medical and popular press in the Nancy-Salpêtrière controversy on hypnotism. *Bulletin of the History of Medicine* 1965;39:163–182.

Hooker W. *Physician and Patient; or, a Practical View of the Medical Duties, Relations and Interests of the Medical Profession and the Community*. New York: Baker and Scribner, 1849.

Hróbjartsson A, Gøtzsche PC. Is the placebo powerless? An analysis of clinical trials comparing placebo with no treatment. *New England Journal of Medicine* 2001;344:1594–1602.

Hróbjartsson A, Gøtzsche PC. Placebo interventions for all clinical conditions. *Cochrane Database of Systematic Reviews* 2010; Issue 1, Art. No.: CD003974. doi: 10.1002/14651858.CD003974.pub3.

Janet PM. *Psychological Healing: A Historical and Clinical Study*. Paul E, Paul C (trans.). New York: Macmillan, 1925.

Jefferson T. *The Writings of Thomas Jefferson*. Vol. 9 (1807–1815). Ford PL (ed.). New York: G. P. Putnam's Sons, 1898.

Kaptchuk TJ. Powerful placebo: The dark side of the randomised controlled trial. *Lancet* 1998a;351:1722–1725.

Kaptchuk TJ. Intentional ignorance: A history of blind assessment and placebo controls in medicine. *Bulletin of the History of Medicine* 1998b;72:389–433.

Kaptchuk TJ. *The Web That Has No Weaver: Understanding Chinese Medicine*. Chicago: Contemporary Books (McGraw-Hill), 2000.

Kaptchuk TJ. The placebo effect in alternative medicine: Can the performance of a healing ritual have clinical significance? *Annals of Internal Medicine* 2002;136:817–825.

Kaptchuk TJ. Vitalism. In: Micozzi MS (ed.). *Fundamentals of Complementary and Integrative Medicine*, 3rd edition. St. Louis, Mo.: Saunders, 2005.

Kaptchuk TJ. Placebo studies and ritual theory: A comparative analysis of Navajo, acupuncture and biomedical healing. *Philosophical Transactions of the Royal Society B, Biological Sciences* 2011;366:1849–1858.

Kaptchuk TJ, Eisenberg, DM. The persuasive appeal of alternative medicine. *Annals of Internal Medicine* 1998;129:1061–1065.

Kaptchuk TJ, Kerr CE. Unbiased divination, unbiased evidence, and the patulin clinical trial. *International Journal of Epidemiology* 2004;33: 247–251.

Kaptchuk TJ, Kerr CE, Zanger A. Placebo controls, exorcisms, and the devil. *Lancet* 2009;374:1234–1235.

Kerr CE, Milne I, Kaptchuk TJ. William Cullen and a missing mind-body link in the early history of placebos. *Journal of the Royal Society of Medicine* 2008;101:89–92.

Kienle, GS, Kiene H. The powerful placebo effect: Fact or fiction? *Journal of Clinical Epidemiology* 1997;50:1311–1318.

Lasagna L. The controlled clinical trial: Theory and practice. *Journal of Chronic Diseases* 1955;1:353–367.

Ledermann EK. *Philosophy and Medicine*. Aldershot, UK: Gower Publishing, 1970.

Li A, Kaptchuk TJ. The case of acupuncture for chronic low back pain: When efficacy and comparative effectiveness conflict. *Spine* 2011;36: 181–182.

Lisle E. Feuilleton de l'homoeopathie orthodoxe. *L'Union médicale* 1861;128:11–72.

Lowenstein E, McPeek B (eds.). *Enduring Contributions of Henry K. Beecher to Medicine, Science, and Society*. Philadelphia: Lippincott, Williams and Wilkins, 2007.

Martini P. *Methodenlehre der therapeutischen Untersuchung*. Berlin: Verlag von Julius Springer, 1932.

McDonald CJ. Is the placebo powerless? [correspondence] *New England Journal of Medicine* 2001;345:1276–1277.

McDonald CJ, Mazzuca SA, McCabe GP Jr. How much of the placebo "effect" is really statistical regression? *Statistics in Medicine* 1983; 2:417–427.

Miller FG, Colloca L, Kaptchuk TJ. The placebo effect: Illness and interpersonal healing. *Perspectives in Biology and Medicine* 2009;52: 518–539.

Moerman DE, Jonas WB. Deconstructing the placebo effect and finding the meaning response. *Annals of Internal Medicine* 2002;136:471–476.

Moseley JB, O'Malley K, Petersen NJ, et al. A controlled trial of arthroscopic surgery for osteoarthritis of the knee. *New England Journal of Medicine* 2002;347:81–88.

Naval Surgeon. Notes of some Experiments, illustrating the influence of the Vis Medicatrix, and of the Imagination, in the Cure of Diseases. *British and Foreign Medical Review* 1847;23:265–269.

Rosenberg C. The practice of medicine in New York a century ago. *Bulletin of the History of Medicine* 1967;41:223–253.

Shapiro AK. Semantics of the placebo. *Psychiatric Quarterly* 1968;42:653–695.

Shelley JH, Baur MP. Paul Martini: The first clinical pharmacologist? *Lancet* 1999;353:1870–1873.

Siraisi NG. *Medieval and Early Renaissance Medicine: An Introduction to Knowledge and Practice.* Chicago: University of Chicago Press, 1990.

Sollmann T. The crucial test of therapeutic evidence. *JAMA* 1917;69:198–199.

Sollmann T. The evaluation of therapeutic remedies in the hospital. *JAMA* 1930;94:1279–1281.

Spiegel D, Kraemer H, Carlson RW. Is the placebo powerless? [correspondence] *New England Journal of Medicine* 2001;345:1276.

Sutton HG. Cases of Rheumatic Fever, Treated for the most part by Mint Water. Collected from the Clinical Books of Dr. Gull, with some Remarks on the Natural History of that Disease. *Guy's Hospital Reports* 1865;11:392–428.

Tambiah SJ. *Magic, Science, Religion, and the Scope of Rationality.* New York: Cambridge University Press, 1990.

Temkin O. *Galenism: Rise and Decline of a Medical Philosophy.* Ithaca, N.Y.: Cornell University Press, 1973.

Trousseau A, Gouraud H. Répertoire clinique: Expériences homoeopathiques tentées à l'Hôtel-Dieu de Paris. *Journal des connaissances médico-chirurgicales* 1834;8:238–241.

Tuke DH. *Illustrations of the Influence of the Mind Upon the Body in Health and Disease: Designed to Elucidate the Action of the Imagination.* Philadelphia: Henry C. Lea, 1873.

Vase L, Riley JL, III, Price DD. A comparison of placebo effects in clinical analgesic trials versus studies of placebo analgesia. *Pain* 2002;99:443–452.

Wampold BE, Minami T, Tierney SC, Baskin TW, Bhati KS. The placebo is powerful: Estimating placebo effects in medicine and psychotherapy from randomized clinical trials. *Journal of Clinical Psychology* 2005;61:835–854.

White S. Medicine's humble humbug: Four periods in the understanding of the placebo. *Pharmacy in History* 1985;27:51–60.

Wolf S. Effects of suggestion and conditioning on the action of chemical agents in human subjects—the pharmacology of placebos. *Journal of Clinical Investigation* 1950;29:100–109.

Wolf S. *Brain, Mind, and Medicine: Charles Richet and the Origins of Physiological Psychology.* New Brunswick, N.J.: Transaction, 1993.

Wolff HG, DuBois EF, Cattell M, et al. Conferences on therapy: The use of placebos in therapy. *New York State Journal of Medicine* 1946;46:1718–1727.

Wolff HG, Goodell H. The relation of attitude and suggestion to the perception of and reaction to pain. *Research Publications, Association for Research in Nervous and Mental Disease* 1943;23:434–448.

Wolff HG. Protective reaction patterns and disease. *Annals of Internal Medicine* 1947;27:944–969.

Wunderlick CA. *Handbuch der Pathologie und Therapie.* Stuttgart: Verlag von Ebner & Seubert, 1852.

I

Conferences on Therapy

The Use of Placebos in Therapy

Harold G. Wolff, Eugene F. DuBois, McKeen Cattell, Oskar Diethelm, Mack Lipkin, Harry Gold, Charles H. Wheeler, and Henry Richardson

Harold G. Wolff, Eugene F. DuBois, McKeen Cattell, Oskar Diethelm, Mack Lipkin, Harry Gold, Charles H. Wheeler, and Henry Richardson, "Conferences on Therapy: The Use of Placebos in Therapy," *New York State Journal of Medicine* 1946;46:1718–1727.

These are stenographic reports, slightly edited, of conferences by the members of the Departments of Pharmacology and of Medicine of Cornell University Medical College and the New York Hospital, with collaboration of other departments and institutions. The questions and discussions involve participation by members of the staff of the college and hospital, students, and visitors. [. . .].

DR. HAROLD G. WOLFF: This afternoon we are going to discuss a very important therapeutic device, the use of the placebo. Dr. DuBois will make the opening remarks.

DR. EUGENE F. DUBOIS: I think it is high time that we devoted a therapeutic conference to placebos. They have been considered the humblest, the most unscientific, and, perhaps, the most dishonest group of drugs that are used by doctors.

As a matter of fact, I think we can show that the study of the placebos is the most important step to be taken in scientific therapy. I am going to make several statements which will probably be challenged because they are drastic.

The first one is that, although placebos are scarcely mentioned in the literature, they are administered more than any other group of drugs. The second statement is that, although few doctors admit that they give placebos, there is a placebo ingredient in practically every prescription. The third statement is that the placebo is a potent agent and in its actions can resemble almost any drug.

As for the literature, we first ought to have a definition of placebo. It comes from the Latin word meaning "I will please," and its definition is "a medicine adapted rather to pacify than to benefit the patient." That is the definition given in the dictionary, adapted to pacify rather than benefit the patient. Well, does anyone believe that it is not benefiting the patient if we can pacify him?

I found extraordinarily little in the old literature about placebos. The *Index Medicus* for the last ten years does not mention it. Practically none of the books on therapy mentioned it in their indices, but, I note that Clark in his 1940 edition of *Applied Pharmacology* states that drugs can be divided into two classes: placebos, which are given to tranquilize the patient, and substances which are intended to produce a definite pharmacologic action. He goes on to state that the use

of placebos is psychotherapy and not pharmacology. I think that statement can be challenged.

Jackson states that the physician may prescribe such preparations sometimes to patients who are malingering, and thus play one deception against the other until a correct diagnosis can be made. That is a statement that can be challenged. He implies that the placebo has no pharmacologic action, has no effect on the patient.

The best discussion, in fact, the only good one I found, is in Fantus' text, the 1939 edition. He states that the modern tendency is no doubt away from placebos. It is not only more economical but more efficient to employ skilled, pure psychotherapy. He states that the lower the degree of the patient's intelligence, the more he may be benefited by a placebo. He goes on to state that millions are wasted by prescribing vitamins and fancy tonics. This brings out the point that there is a placebo element in most of the prescriptions of vitamins and fancy tonics. He adds that if one wishes to prescribe placebos, one should remember that iron and calcium are not very abundant in food. They might be deficient. They are cheap and inoffensive. He believes it is not right to cause anyone to pay for articles that have no value, and that it is best to write the prescription for something that has a recognized though slight remedial value. I am going to bring up that point later. Then he states that in the case of patients whose disordered imaginations torture them with affliction from which they suffer quite as truly as they would from any real ill, it is clearly as much the physician's duty to employ such remedies as are likely to relieve the deluded imaginations as it is to give certain medicines for a better-defined disease.

Of course, the history of placebos goes back, way, way back, beyond Hippocrates. They are the most ancient of drugs, and we are safe in saying that in older times and in backward communities at the present time, about 90 per cent of the drugs which are given are placebos. They are inert drugs which please the patient and benefit the patient, and satisfy the doctor. The enormous success of homeopathy, where drugs are given in great dilution, in sugar pills, drugs so dilute that they could not possibly have any pharmacologic action, is a good example. Its success and therapeutic results are probably better than those in the case of some of the regular drugs that are given in huge doses by the rival practitioners. At least, it has demonstrated very clearly what can be done by placebos.

I thought I would look at our *New York Hospital Pharmacopoeia* of the year 1816. That was the first pharmacopoeia issued, and it was not a bad one, by the way. There are lots of good drugs in it, and, apparently, these drugs were considered carefully by the doctors in this hospital over a hundred years ago. There is a list of about 160 drugs. If one examines these in the light of our present knowledge, I think about one third of them would be considered inert. How about that Dr. Cattell? Did you have a chance to go over that?

DR. MCKEEN CATTELL: Dr. Gold and I looked it over. That seems to be approximately correct.

DR. DUBOIS: I had hoped to examine the *New York Hospital Formulary* of twenty years ago. I remember we gave it a pretty careful searching in the committee, and I think that one third to one sixth of those drugs were inert. What is going to happen to our present hospital formulary when someone goes over it a hundred years from now? Well, I think most of the drugs have actions, but better drugs will be found by that time.

We can divide placebos into three classes and I suggest this division. The first is the pure placebo, that is, the bread pill or the lactose tablet. Those lactose tablets have been found to be more effective if they are colored either pink or blue, or, better still, mottled. Then there is the impure placebo, that is, it is adulterated with a drug which might have some pharmacologic action, such as tincture of gentian, or a very small dose of nux vomica. That is the adulterated placebo, the false placebo, the bastard placebo, you might call it. I don't know the best term. Then, for the third group, there is the universal pleasing element which accompanies every prescription. You cannot write a prescription without the element of the placebo. A prayer to Jupiter starts the prescription. It carries weight, the weight of two or three thousand years of medicine. The fact that it is signed by a doctor, that it has required a doctor to write out the prescription, that the prescription has to be taken to a drug store to be made up, that the patient has to pay for it, that it has, perhaps, a bad taste, all of those things are placebo elements in a prescription.

The pure placebo relieves only the patient. The impure placebo relieves the doctor's symptoms as well as those of the patient. The doctor wants to give something that he thinks will help the patient so he prescribes a drug of doubtful value, vitamins or, as Dr. Fantus suggests, iron or calcium with the hope that they might help the patient. This is somewhat more effective, because in time it deceives the doctor. He begins to think that he is giving a potent drug and he can sell this better to the patient because he believes in it. He tells the patient with more conviction that the patient is going to be helped by this particular drug, but it deceives the doctor, and all of us have been so deceived. This is the basis of unscientific unorthodoxy, the worship of strange gods, the giving of these placebos and thinking that they are potent drugs. It is like the heathen in his blindness. He takes a block of stone and he hews out of it an image of a god and then he worships that god. The doctor takes a drug which he thinks is probably inactive or may be inactive, or it may be potent, and he gives it and gets good results, and, finally, he comes to believe that it is a good drug. I think that is responsible for a very large proportion of our therapeutic literature. It may be said that the effects of placebos resemble, to a certain extent, the effects of potent agents. The extent of the placebo action has only recently been appreciated. We thought we were making a big advance in scientific therapy when we began to study a drug by comparing, we will say, 100 cases given the drug with 100 cases that were given no drug or no treatment. That was considered satisfactory a few years ago, but now we realize that one has to compare a group receiving these drugs with a group receiving placebos. If you take three groups, one given no treatment, a second given placebos, and a third given the test drug, you will very often find that the group given the placebos get along very much better, have a much higher percentage of cures than those without treatment, and, perhaps, almost as many as those with the test drug, in some cases more. For example, we found recently that placebos have a marked effect in preventing seasickness, not quite as good an effect as some of the drugs which are used, but, nevertheless, they brought about a very distinct improvement. In a recent study, Seidel and Abrams found that hypodermics of saline were just as effective as vaccines against chronic rheumatoid arthritis.

I think you are familiar with the work of Wolff and Goodell, who have studied the pharmacologic effects of placebos. I trust, Dr. Wolff, you are going to show us some of those.

DR. WOLFF: The giving of a pill by the physician to the patient is the symbol for the statement, "I will take care of you," and the very force of the statement gives support and reassurance and often relief from pain. It has been possible in the laboratory to demonstrate the effect of placebos on the pain threshold in suggestible and nonsuggestible subjects. Such experiments illuminate the effectiveness of placebos often observed in patients.

The pain threshold can be measured by exposing an area of skin, blackened with India ink, to heat from a 1,000-watt lamp. It is expressed as that amount of heat in gram calories per second per square centimeter which just elicits a sensation of pain at the end of a three-second exposure. This threshold is approximately uniform from individual to individual. With this method, it was found that 0.3 Gm. of acetylsalicylic acid predictably raised the pain threshold approximately 35 to 40 per cent above its control level before the administration of the analgesic agent. It was also observed, however, that it was sometimes possible to raise the pain threshold by administering a sucrose tablet to an individual who believed that he was receiving a tablet of acetylsalicylic acid. A series of experiments using capsules of acetylsalicylic acid and placebo capsules of sucrose were therefore performed, with laboratory workers as the subjects.

Series 1.—The effects of placebos and analgesics on a relatively "nonsuggestible" man. The subject was a 27-year-old professional psychologist with a lively interest in the procedure and a good deal of experience with experiments on sensation. He was given 0.3 Gm. of acetylsalicylic acid in a capsule, and measurements of the pain threshold were made at intervals of ten minutes. The threshold was elevated 30 per cent above its control level within ninety minutes. Four days later this same subject was given a capsule containing 0.3 Gm. sodium bicarbonate and was told that he was receiving an analgesic agent similar to that of the previous experiment. The operator was aware of the contents of the capsule and tried throughout the experiment to persuade the subject to choose a higher threshold. These efforts to change the attitude and judgment of the subject were unsuccessful, and the pain threshold was not elevated. On the next day, another placebo capsule, whose contents were unknown to both the subject and the operator, was similarly ineffective in raising the pain threshold. A week later, the subject was given a third placebo capsule and was told that the contents were a potent analgesic, and the hope was expressed that he would suffer no ill effects. He was thanked for his cooperation in what might prove to be a troublesome experience. All of these suggestions had no effect in raising the pain threshold in this relatively nonsuggestible man.

Series 2.—The effects of placebos and analgesics on the pain threshold of a "suggestible" woman. The subject was a 21-year-old chemist, well trained in analytic methods, but without experience in sensory testing methods. She was extremely cooperative, suggestible, and anxious to perform in a manner which she believed was "expected" of her. On the first day of the experiment, she was given 0.9 Gm. acetylsalicylic acid which raised the pain threshold 31 per cent within two hours. The results of the experiment and the usual pain-threshold-raising effects of analgesics were explained to her. Two weeks later, she was given a capsule containing lactose, but which she suspected was again acetylsalicylic acid. Within ninety minutes, her pain threshold was elevated 20 per cent. She was informed that she had received a placebo, that she had nevertheless reported her pain threshold as elevated, and that she must be more careful in her observations. She was disturbed by her poor performance so that the next week, in her third experiment, she was extremely cautious and somewhat suspicious of the contents of the capsule. Although the capsule contained 0.6 Gm. acetylsalicylic acid, during the next three hours there was no elevation of her pain threshold. The subject was given a two weeks' holiday, and on her return she was reassured of her ability to make careful observations. Thereafter, there was the expected elevation of her pain threshold following administration of acetylsalicylic acid, and no elevation of the threshold following placebos.

Series 3.—The interplay between attitudes of the subject and the suggestion of the physician. The subject was a 40-year-old physicist, well trained in reporting pain threshold and other sensory data. On one day, she was given a placebo which the operator made every effort to convince her was an effective analgesic agent, but the subject stated that she herself was convinced that the capsule was a placebo. Her threshold was not elevated. On a subsequent day, the experiment repeated with administration of another placebo, and this time the subject thought she had received an analgesic. This conviction the operator upheld with enthusiasm, and the pain threshold was elevated 30 per cent within ninety minutes.

It has been clearly demonstrated in these experiments and elsewhere that the pain-threshold-elevating effect of an agent such as acetylsalicylic acid is appreciable and reproducible. However, these experiments show that a similar threshold-raising effect can be obtained with a placebo, if the subject can be convinced by suggestion that he has received an agent which will raise the pain threshold. Whether this measurable effect is truly a raising of the pain threshold or merely an alteration in attention is hard to say. For example, the pain threshold has been shown also to be elevated in the subject of Series 3 by concentration on a difficult arithmetic problem, by hypnosis in which it was suggested that the subject no longer felt pain, and by distracting, loud noises. On the other hand, an individual can be made to believe that a light will be painful, and then experience photophobia, which does not mean that the threshold for light is lowered. It merely means that the individual's reaction to a situation has been changed by suggestion, and he may even report a sensation before he feels it. Another well-known example of this phenomenon is that of the man who "jumps the gun" at a race. It is obvious that he cannot have a lowered threshold for sound, but because of his previous experience, reacts before the stimulus is given. Dogs who are given morphine in rather large doses will vomit following the injection, and if this is done regularly, for two or three weeks, and then sterile saline is substituted for the morphine, the dogs will also vomit following the injection of the sterile saline. The needle and the injection without any morphine are sufficiently potent symbols to set off the physiologic response to the morphine.

It would be a great loss to patients not to make use of the facts described above. Obviously, there is a great force in our hands which ought to be turned to account in giving patients relief from sickness and pain. Every physician should learn to understand that every pill he gives his patient is a powerful agent, whether the pill be sugar, digitalis, phenobarbital, or a vitamin.

There are several psychologic factors inherent in the placebo which are the forces used when someone is given a pill, a tablet, or a bottle of medicine by his physician. They may be briefly summarized. First of all, any pill, whether it be sugar or medication, is in part placebo because it is a symbol of the doctor. In his absence the patient needs his support. When he has a little pill box with tablets to take, that is an interpolation of the doctor. He can carry that much of the doctor with him, and it is effective. It is a symbol of being cared for, an emotional support or endorsement, because the doctor in writing out his prescription for pills, and in giving his directions for their use has signified his interest in the patient and his problems. The pill is the symbol of the doctor's unspoken or spoken words, "I will take care of you." A whole body of knowledge, experience, and wisdom is epitomized in that little pill for the patient. When he takes it, he can feel that his doctor has used his trained judgment in choosing a particular tablet out of a great number of other possible tablets. It represents to the patient a focal point of his physician's education and experience. He can put his faith in such a pill, which helps to fill his need to have a belief that he will be made stronger and get well. The pill also helps to fulfill a patient's need to feel dependent. He wants to feel supported, or he will get very shaky. To be sure, it not the best kind of support, but it is often a help. A bitter or even nauseating placebo medicament fills a need for punishment. Everyone feels the need for punishment at some time. Guilt is a universal feeling at some time or other, and it is a satisfaction to have justice doled out. Last of all, the pill supports the desire to get well. The patient is very anxious to be pushed in that direction and to feel that his progress is being made speedier and more comfortable.

DR. OSKAR DIETHELM: To put it into my own words, Dr. DuBois and Dr. Wolff have stressed that we have to consider the patient, the drug, and the physician in evaluating the effect of a drug. In evaluating the patient we have made very little progress. We know little about the meaning of suggestibility. It refers to the ability of a person to react in a positive way to suggestions. This concept is no doubt very valuable, but little progress has been made in understanding what factors permit the person to be more suggestible from the truly psychobiologic point of view; the emotions as well as the physiologic functions are involved.

No doubt, the factor of belief is very important in the reaction to a drug, but again, when we try to understand from a medical point of view what belief means, we are considerably handicapped. The older formulation is that the person reacts to suggestion because what is suggested to him becomes a reality within that person; he believes in it, and, therefore, the expected result will take place. This is obviously possible only within a very limited range, but within this range it is definitely a fact. Just what factors play a role in it is hard to say.

Dr. Wolff brought in the factor of attention. From experimental work there is much to support Dr. Wolff's suggestion that attention is one of the main factors. On the other hand, it is also true that the role of emotions is very important and the various emotions seem to play a far greater role than is generally suspected.

We know that certain emotions, such as fear, can have a more far-reaching effect than the other emotions, as for instance, depression or sadness. Why this is so we do not know, nor do we know why emotions should be so important in circumstances in which belief plays so dominant a role.

Dr. Wolff has stressed one symbolic value of the drug. There is no doubt that there is a great deal in what he said, and I cannot add anything to his very clear analysis from that point of view. However, a drug may have many other meanings to the patient, of which we may not be aware.

The personality of the physician is of the utmost importance, and, as Dr. Wolff has demonstrated very beautifully in his experiments, when a person believes in the drug he is given, the results are much more far-reaching. That, however, also means that the physician, who has the best results with any drug in which he highly believes, is the one who is least in a position to evaluate the results critically. This is so because he is naturally involved with his own personality, not merely in the administration of the drug but also in any scientific investigation. We are often surprised that an investigator fails to notice certain mistakes, while somebody of far less training or far less imagination can point them out.

I think that our present trend to use placebos in investigations of drugs has much to be said for it, but I do not think it answers the problem completely from a scientific angle, because we usually do not have time to study all the individual reactions involved. We have a certain safety factor in statistical methodology. On the other hand, it is questionable whether we have the right to depend so much on statistical results.

DR. WOLFF: Dr. Lipkin, would you say a word or two about the use of the apparatus as a placebo?

DR. MACK LIPKIN: What we did was to take a group of patients with Raynaud's syndrome and used an apparatus similar to that employed for mecholyl iontophoresis. Instead of mecholyl, we applied saline or dry bandages, and did not turn on the current, but simply clicked the dials. We used two milliamperes of current with saline, which is very little. Some improvement was reported in every case, and the results were excellent in six cases. Suggestion was undoubtedly responsible for the results in these. In one case the patient was so treated three times a week without our knowledge by a clinic nurse for a period of a year. The result was excellent. Previously, she had been unable to go out in the cold weather without suffering spasm, unless she used fur-lined gloves and carried a muff.

DR. WOLFF: What was the treatment?

DR. LIPKIN: That particular patient received saline iontophoresis, two milliamperes once a week, and an intramuscular injection of sterile saline twice a week. Before treatment, she was unable to work for the first hour after she reached the office. Just touching the typewriter keys would throw her fingers into spasm. After treatment, she could dispense with the muff and could work as soon as she reached the office during a record cold winter.

DR. WOLFF: Dr. Gold, would you tell us of your experience with placebos?

DR. HARRY GOLD: The statement that the lower the degree of the patient's intelligence, the more he may be benefited by a placebo, interested me very much. I should like to challenge it. I don't believe there is much relationship between the state of the intelligence and the responsiveness to a placebo. There is no closer relationship here than there is between the state of the intelligence and the state of the emotions, for the placebo exerts its actions through the mechanism of suggestion. Anyone who has ever had to treat physicians as patients has undoubtedly learned the difficulties encountered in the use of those agents which give us almost no trouble in the case of nonmedical patients. One is forever being vexed by the account of therapeutic or disagreeable results, obtained from very intelligent people, teachers, professors, businessmen in high places and the like, in relation to medicaments which could by no possibility exert such actions through their pharmacologic properties. I have made it a rule to distrust so-called intelligent people, who are eager to be informed about the details of a treatment on the grounds that they are "intelligent" and can be depended upon to cooperate better with a complete understanding. I need only to be perfectly frank with one of these patients and tell him, for example, that we need to guard against digitalis toxicity, that toxicity makes its appearance with a loss of appetite, spots before the eyes, nausea, vomiting, or premature contractions, when I am promptly confronted by all of these symptoms long before enough of the drug has been taken to exert any effect. I am likely to tell these "intelligent" people much less than the so-called unintelligent ones. The case of a distinguished New York physician who was involved in a problem which brought him frequently to our laboratory some years ago always sticks in my mind. I noticed him breathing very heavily when he walked up the stairs, and when I asked him what was the matter with him, he said that for many years he had had heart failure with auricular fibrillation and proceeded to show me that his legs were almost twice their normal size. He carried a bottle of tincture of digitalis in his back pocket and took a few drops now and then. When I asked him why he didn't take more of it, and take it more regularly, he said that he was very sensitive to digitalis; it irritated his stomach and made him uncomfortable. He had become somewhat addicted to heroin by its continued use to control his attacks of nocturnal dyspnea and cough. Here was a very "intelligent" scientist in advanced heart failure, virtually without treatment, with the only drug that could possibly put him in order. On the condition that he was not to ask me what I was giving him, I undertook to manage him. I made up a bottle of medicine containing a teaspoonful of the tincture of digitalis in a tablespoonful of the tincture of valerian. The taste as well as the large quantity per dose threw him off the track completely. He took a daily dose containing a teaspoonful of the tincture of digitalis. During the first few days, he carried on almost without a moment of sleep because he was too busy passing urine. He lost some 40 pounds. All symptoms of failure subsided. He remained actively engaged in his scientific work for the next three years and was free of failure when he died suddenly of a coronary thrombosis. When he knew that he was receiving a few drops of tincture of digitalis it made him so sick to his stomach that he couldn't continue with it, but when he was kept in the dark about the nature of the medication, he took a teaspoonful daily without the slightest trouble. I am sure that every one of us could multiply the numbers of such experiences which show that the efficacy of the placebo bears little relationship to the "intelligence" of the patient.

As Dr. DuBois indicated, every medicinal agent which is prescribed or administered to a patient carries with it the element of suggestion. The element of suggestion reinforces the specific action of the agent. The improvement which results is, in part, the consequence of a specific action and, in part, that of the element of suggestion. In the usual way in which a medicinal agent is administered, there are, in point of fact, three elements, the specific action of the drug, the element of suggestion inherent in the very fact that an agent is administered, and, also, the element of optimism of the physician which is conveyed to the patient. These three reinforce each other. Physicians seem to have no objection to prescribing medication with these three elements, but there seems to be a good deal of resistance to the prescribing of an agent associated only with the latter two elements, that is, an agent devoid of specific action on the cells of the body, an agent without pharmacologic properties in the ordinary sense. We appear to have a sense of guilt about prescribing such an agent. It seems to suggest a kind of frivolous therapy to many people.

In the special classes on ambulant therapy with groups of the fourth-year clinical clerks, we often begin with the placebos. I remember discussing this matter with one group of students. A visitor was present. He said that he also uses placebos, but that he prescribes yeast tables for that purpose since it also supplies them with vitamins. I have no objection to yeast tablets as placebos, but I do object to the principle involved. I believe that a placebo does not have to be legitimized by the inclusion of a useless amount of potent material. The placebo is not only a symbol of the patient being cared for in the sense in which Dr. Wolff has referred to it, being cared for by a special technic, namely, by the use of a medicine. The placebo is a specific psychotherapeutic device with values of its own. It possesses therapeutic virtues independent of any reinforcements by optimistic expressions on the part of the physician.

A paper appeared in the April 1941 issue of the *Journal of the American Pharmaceutical Association* in which the author deplored the fact that only one of eighteen candidates taking the state board examinations knew of Basham's mixture, a defunct preparation of iron which undergoes decomposition on standing and which provides about 25 mg. of iron in a tablespoonful, so that about 20 tablespoonfuls a day have to be given in order to attain a satisfactory iron intake for the treatment of anemia. He also deplored the fact that not one man could write a prescription correctly containing fluidextract of senega, fluidextract of squill, camphorated tincture of opium, and syrup of tolu for a case of chronic bronchitis with cough, and that none could write, correctly, a prescription for grippe containing acetphenetidin, quinine sulfate, camphor monobromate, caffeine citrate, and codeine sulfate. The author of this paper was Leighton, the secretary of the State of Maine Board of Registration of Medicine. Here are good examples of an outworn and decadent materia medica. Physicians have a large share of the responsibility for its survival. I believe that its survival is linked up with the physician's lack of reverence for the placebo. In one of our previous conferences, someone made the statement that unless the physician believes in the efficacy of the medicament, it is not likely to prove efficacious, and "honest" doctors are not likely to find it easy to give evidence of enthusiasm for coated sugar pills. They, therefore, prescribe such mixtures as elixir of iron, quinine, and strychnine, or a few tablets of yeast, preparations containing either useless agents or quantities of agents without a vestige of evidence of pharmacologic value. Such prescribing has the effect of promoting self-delusion on the part of the physician, for, since patients improve during their use, the physician soon begins to suspect that there may be some kind of pharmacologic potency in them. What is more, they miss the opportunity of learning the full power of the chemical agent as a psychotherapeutic device.

The importance of the placebo in the investigation of drug action in man can hardly be overestimated. In one of our previous conferences, I called attention to a study which we had made in the clinic on the effect of aminophylline and theobromine on cardiac pain in ambulant patients with coronary artery disease. There, the results showed that sugar of milk brought about improvement in 25 per cent of the cases and theobromine in 22 per cent of the cases. The "blind-test" was an important aspect of that study, namely, the fact that neither the patient nor the doctor knew when it was a placebo or a potent agent that the patient was taking. These are the only conditions under which it is possible to ascertain how much of the improvement is due to the specific action of the drug and how much to the psychotherapeutic action of just giving a "medicine."

The conviction which some patients acquire regarding the value of the placebo is sometimes disturbing. We have at times gone back to check on whether a potent agent might not have been put into the prescription by mistake, because of the patient's unshakable devotion to the medicine.

Dr. DuBois referred to the similarity in the effects of potent agents and placebos. I went back to a series of charts of ambulant clinic patients for some of the effects which patients attributed to the placebo. Here they are: I sleep better; my appetite is improved; my breathing is better; it makes me stronger; the bowels are better; I can walk further without pain in the chest; my nerves are more steady; it causes me more pain in the chest; it makes my heart flutter. This is a fairly representative list of the kinds of effects placebos produce.

I should like to mention four placebos which I find very useful. One is the lactose tablet. The druggist sometimes gets you into trouble with that, since he occasionally tells the patient what it is. The compound tincture of gentian is a useful placebo in cases in which a bitter medicine is appropriate. Aromatic elixir has a place in those cases in which a well-flavored, pleasant placebo is desirable. Ammoniated tincture of valerian as a placebo has a great many uses. The riot of tastes and smells in this preparation is very effective in creating illusions of an efficacious medicine. It may be given in teaspoonful doses in water or without water, or in drops in such numbers and at such intervals as seem desirable. It has the further advantage that its utility is not likely to be disturbed by information which the patient obtains from the pharmacist. If the pharmacist looks up its actions in his favorite source of information, the dispensatory, he is apt to find a very long list of conditions for which it has been recommended, uses for which not a vestige of scientific evidence exists.

DR. WOLFF: Does that demonstrate the patient's need for punishment?

DR. GOLD: It might very well fall into that group. The fact is that the tincture of valerian requires no embellishments. It requires no suggestion on the part of the physician, other than that associated with the very act of counting drops or measuring out teaspoonful and swallowing an agent with tastes and smells traditionally associated with potent medicaments.

These few placebos which I have mentioned serve most purposes, although it is obvious that a list could be made almost without limit. It is the principle which I should like to urge that we keep in mind, namely, that placebo therapy, without potent pharmacologic agents in the sense of agents directly acting on the cells of the body, is a very useful type of medication. It is much more legitimate in my way of thinking than the practice of loading patients with barbiturates and other sedatives as is the common practice in situations in which the physician is hard pressed for something to prescribe.

It goes without saying that the selection of patients for placebo therapy is as important as the proper selection of patients for any other type of therapy. Certainly, not every patient presenting a psychotherapeutic problem should be managed with a placebo medicine. The placebo should rarely, if ever, take the place of long-range psychotherapeutic management. It is particularly applicable to those situations in which it is the physician's judgment that the patient will not tolerate a course of treatment which does not include the taking of a medicine. There are, for example, many patients with complex problems who have already been under medications of various kinds for long periods of time and in whom there is need for reorientation with the patient free of the effects of potent agents. It is often much easier to carry on in this period of temporizing and study with the patient under the influence of a placebo medication.

DR. WOLFF: Dr. Gold, suppose in this ideal community that we are going to have in the future, the doctor had enough time and energy, do you think it would still be a good idea to use this particular therapeutic device? There is no quarrel with its effectiveness. It is a question whether it is the best device if you had an optimum relation with the patient.

DR. GOLD: Yes, I think the placebo as a chemical device for psychotherapy has a definite place which cannot be filled by anything else in many cases.

DR. WOLFF: Are there other questions or comments?

DR. DIETHELM: Dr. Gold, in your studies did you also pay attention to the negative suggestive attitude of the patient to a placebo or any drug, or the negative attitude of the physician who is a therapeutic nihilist?

DR. GOLD: What you mean is not quite clear to me.

DR. WOLFF: May I illustrate? For example, we give a man aspirin. He thinks it is a placebo. It fails to raise the pain threshold. The reason for the failure is presumably the negative suggestive attitude. Another example, Dr. A gives a patient a potent medicament, but it does not work as well as when Dr. B gives it.

DR. DIETHELM: To come back to what I said, there are in all people both aspects of suggestibility, the positive and the negative. The positive is the ability to react in such a way as to believe what is suggested. The negative is the tendency to reject the suggestion. It is a well-known fact that the stronger the negative suggestibility, if one can break through it, the stronger will be the positive suggestibility in that person. There is, then, apparent suggestibility which is positive in the sense of rejection as well as positive in the sense of believing.

DR. GOLD: Would the negative type of reaction be revealed, for example, in the fact that the placebo made the person worse?

DR. WOLFF: Yes.

DR. DIETHELM: It might be well to consider that point.

DR. GOLD: We have some information on negative suggestibility in that sense. In the study of the effect of xanthines for the relief of cardiac pain to which I referred, 15 per cent of the patients maintained that the theobromine increased their pain and 6 per cent maintained that the lactose tablets increased their pain. In another study in which we investigated the question of whether digitalis constricts the coronary arteries and increases pain in patients with angina pectoris, the results showed that sugar of milk tablets increased the pain in 15 per cent of the cases, the same for digitalis. You will recall that these studies were made with the "blind-test" in which neither the doctor nor the patient knew at the time which medicine was being given, so that the only element of suggestion came from that inherent in the taking of a tablet or capsule. The fact that the patients were quite convinced that the medicines made them worse is, I presume, the negative suggestibility reaction. Is that your point?

DR. DIETHELM: Yes.

DR. CATTELL: This problem of negative attitude toward therapy worries me in relation to establishing potency in investigative work because you cannot use placebo or any control against that. I have particularly in mind an experience in studying analgesic action in a group of subjects who may have had the conviction that aspirin was without effect. In these experiments, we could not demonstrate a rise in threshold from aspirin. We used the placebo, and this also gave negative results. I am wondering whether suggestion may not have vitiated the conclusions.

DR. WOLFF: I think there is a real possibility of obscuring effects from an analgesic agent under such circumstances.

DR. C. H. WHEELER: I think we all agree that placebos are useful and should be used. But I would like to call attention to the fact that many of the placebos which are used are dangerous to the patient, and that many doctors, when they want to give a patient something, instead of giving him something harmless, like to inject something into the veins or muscles, as calcium, or vitamins, or sodium cacodylate. I think that is a practice which cannot be sufficiently condemned. It is horrifying to find how commonly that is done. I know one physician who gives his patients arsphenamine injections as a placebo. He finds that when a person needs a tonic, arsphenamine injections work better than anything else.

DR. HENRY RICHARDSON: Could I comment? I have been trying to formulate this subject during the discussion, a thing which is very familiar to me in practice. I don't like the association of psychotherapy with adultery, or of placebos with purity. I have not been able to work out in my mind any pure action of a placebo. If there were such an action, you should be able to set up an apparatus like a slot machine, with labels for headache, stomach, or bowels. You could then push the right lever and get a placebo which would have the required effect on the diseased organ.

Everyone here has commented on the action of the placebo through suggestion. In other words, it always involves some personal relationship, or else the prestige of the medical profession as exerted directly or through the effect of medical discoveries as purveyed by the drug stores.

I am not one of those who have given placebos as such, except perhaps as a control in experimental work. With the ordinary medication, there is always the chance of hitting on some effective remedy, even when the physician has little confidence in the preparation which he gives. Moreover, there are a great many medications which are on the borderline between pharmacology and placebos. I don't like the element of deception in a placebo, apart from the fact that it is disastrous to get found out. I think that if there is to be a deception it should be the one which the patient demands and which, also, I think he needs.

Patients come in, for instance, to an endocrine clinic with a preconceived notion of what they need, which may be very concrete and definite. Some of them are suspicious individuals who want to know all about the preparation, the theory of its action, the application to their case, and whether it is freshly manufactured or not. Such individuals often have some basic insecurity which they do not wish to reveal, and occasionally one of them is found to have paranoid ideas. There is another type. I am thinking of a young woman, who was probably neurotic, who had a strong drive to become an actress. The obstacle to this ambition, according to her, was her premature gray hair. She said that she would commit suicide if it were not cured, and I took this threat seriously. At that time, vitamins were being given for this purpose. It was a very delicate point to decide just how much improvement I might see in the hair at any one time, because the change was infinitesimal, and I did not want to use up the improvement all at once. So I had to see just enough red hair at the roots of the gray to keep up the psychotherapy of suggestion.

We kept on that way for several months and we got by the crisis.

Similar things happen a great number of times. I regard the use of medicine, whether an active preparation or placebo, as inseparable from its psychotherapeutic effect. It is a means of giving the patient moral support through medical care, and it is chiefly important because it gives opportunity to move on to something better. It is like the experience of the social workers, who find that the problem which the patient first presents is not the fundamental one. After two or three interviews, it turns out to be subordinate to something more vital. In this way, people who keep on coming back to a doctor for more medicine will often reveal bit by bit what it is that is bothering them. In this way the physician who will listen to his patients can move from the psychotherapy of medication or placebo to something which is much more effective.

DR. GOLD: Dr. Richardson's comments indicate the need for the proper selection of a placebo. In the case he cited, it is clear that the successful outcome was not due to the so-called antigray hair vitamins which were given, but to the placebo aspect of such a preparation. That was, perhaps, a fortunate choice of a placebo in this particular case. In the absence of satisfactory evidence that such a preparation had much of a chance of changing the color of her hair, the administration of that material became little more than a chemical device for psychotherapy, and that is what a placebo is.

I would like to take exception to applying the term "deception" to the use of the placebo. If deception is involved in the case of the pure placebo, it applies to only one person, namely, the patient, for the physician knows that the agent is devoid of all but psychotherapeutic properties. But when we use an agent of questionable pharmacologic activity, or in amounts that can, by no possibility, exert pharmacologic action, there is the danger of deceiving two people, both the patient and the physician. The doctor may come to think that the agent has potency when, in fact, it has none. That danger is real. Isn't that the trouble with a large share of our drug therapy? Physicians prescribe useless agents and ascribe false values to them because they have had no experience with unequivocal placebos in their place. Whether we regard the use of the placebo as deception or not depends on where we start. If we start with the proposition that there are certain patients who profit by the very act of taking a medicine, if we grant that premise, then certainly no deception is involved in their taking something in a teaspoon which makes them better. Nothing is gained by having the physician deceived in the bargain.

DR. RICHARDSON: The point is very obscure. Usually the situation is such that some drug may do good but one cannot be certain. I don't see how one can rationalize the giving of sugar of milk. It is difficult to lie out of that situation.

DR. GOLD: I have no more difficulty coming to terms with the use of sugar of milk which I know has only psychotherapeutic values, than with the use of elixir of iron, qui-

nine, and strychnine as a "tonic." The latter has all the support of traditional misinformation, but not of a vestige of scientific evidence. Both are placebos. I object to the latter type of placebo because it contains potent agents which have played a large part in deceiving physicians into believing that its merits are more than psychotherapeutic. As long as we encourage the use of preparations falling into that class, the development of rational therapeutics will continue to lag. Of course, there is always the danger of the patient charging you with the use of innocuous medication in the case of a pure placebo, but one is not entirely free of that danger when, for example, one employs some kind of advertised medication for which unjustified claims have been made. It probably won't be very long before one of your colleagues will call the matter to the patient's attention, or the patient may come upon the information in his reading, that the preparation which you used hadn't a ghost of a chance of producing the effects you ascribed to it. As I mentioned, the choice of a placebo is important. There are many situations in which the use of sugar of milk would be very unwise, for example, when the patient is likely to read the prescription, or is one who is likely to have the curiosity to try to learn what you are prescribing. You are quite free of that danger in situations in which you dispense rather than prescribe. That is how it comes about that the sugar of milk tablet has proved so useful in our clinics. I am less interested, however, in the question as to what placebo one should use, than I am in the viewpoint that the use of a placebo is highgrade therapeutics, and that to try to validate a placebo by a useless amount of some potent material, is a substandard practice.

Dr. DuBois called my attention to a paper by O. H. Perry Pepper in the *American Journal of Pharmacy*, volume 117, page 409, 1945. It is entitled "A Note on the Placebo." It pays tribute to the placebo as a therapeutic agent in the art of medicine. Those three pages reveal some of the clearest thinking on the subject of the placebo that I have ever heard or read. You should all read it.

Summary

DR. GOLD: The use of placebos in therapeutics was explored in the conference this afternoon. We may briefly summarize some of the major statements although this falls short of conveying the full force of the views which were set forth. Suggestion is a vital part of treatment. The suggestive reaction may be positive in which case it reinforces the action of a drug, or negative in which case it detracts from its specific activity. The negative reaction is a source of error in the analysis of drug action in man. The power of suggestion in influencing the action of a drug was shown in the pain threshold experiments of Dr. Wolff. It had the effect of conferring analgesic properties on sugar of milk and removing those properties from aspirin.

Therapeutic agents exert their effects in three ways, namely, by specific pharmacologic activity, suggestion inherent in the use of a medicine, and the element of optimism or personality of the physician. They reinforce each other.

The placebo as a chemical device for psychotherapeutic treatment has been largely neglected in the literature. The existence of an extensive materia medica of agents largely devoid of pharmacologic properties is due to the failure to appreciate fully the power of suggestion inherent in the giving of a medicine. The placebo produces many of the therapeutic effects of potent pharmacologic agents. Several examples were cited of the efficacy of the placebo. An experience in the successful control of Raynaud's syndrome by means of an iontophoresis apparatus with only saline and without sufficient current to exert any specific action was an interesting illustration of what such measures can achieve. The use of the placebo is an important contribution to the method of scientific study of drug action.

There was general agreement on the utility of a placebo, but opinion divided sharply on the question of what kind of an agent should serve that purpose. It was pointed out that the "pure" placebo is an inert material and exerts its effects only by the mechanism of suggestion, while the "impure or adulterated" placebo possesses, also, pharmacologic properties in the more usual sense. There were those who maintained that the prescribing of an inert agent such as sugar of milk was unjustified, and that some kind of pharmacologic properties, however slight or doubtful, should be represented in the prescription for a placebo. The opposing view took the position that the use of a chemical agent as a psychotherapeutic device is proper therapy and maintained that it gained no validity by the inclusion of materials of doubtful indication, of equivocal actions, or in ineffectual amounts. It was urged that the inclusion of such materials be discouraged for they frequently deceive the physician into believing that the particular agent possesses other than psychotherapeutic properties.

It was indicated that successful management with a placebo depends on the proper selection of cases and choice of placebo materials.

2

The Powerful Placebo

HENRY K. BEECHER

Henry K. Beecher, "The Powerful Placebo," JAMA 1955;159:1602–1606.

Placebos have doubtless been used for centuries by wise physicians as well as by quacks, but it is only recently that recognition of an enquiring kind has been given the clinical circumstance where the use of this tool is essential ". . . to distinguish pharmacological effects from the effects of suggestion, and . . . to obtain an unbiased assessment of the result of experiment." It is interesting that Pepper could say as recently as 10 years ago "apparently there has never been a

paper published discussing [primarily] the important subject of the placebo." In 1953 Gaddum[1] said:

Such tablets are sometimes called placebos, but it is better to call them dummies. According to the Shorter Oxford Dictionary the word placebo has been used since 1811 to mean a medicine given more to please than to benefit the patient. Dummy tablets are not particularly noted for the pleasure which they give to their recipients. One meaning of the word dummy is a "counterfeit object." This seems to me the right word to describe a form of treatment which is intended to have no effect and I follow those who use it. A placebo is something which is intended to act through a psychological mechanism. It is an aid to therapeutic suggestion, but the effect which it produces may be either psychological or physical. It may make the patient feel better without any obvious justification, or it may produce actual changes in such things as the gastric secretion . . . Dummy tablets may, of course, act as placebos, but, if they do, they lose some of their value as dummy tablets. They have two real functions, one of which is to distinguish pharmacological effects from the effects of suggestion, and the other is to obtain an unbiased assessment of the result of experiment.

One may comment on Gaddum's remarks: Both "dummies" and placebos are the same pharmacologically inert substances; i.e., lactose, saline solution, starch. Since they appear to be differentiable chiefly in the reasons for which they are given and only at times distinguishable in terms of their effects, it seems simpler to use the one term, placebo, whose two principal functions are well stated in Professor Gaddum's last sentence quoted above. Finally, I do not understand how a dummy tablet could be prevented from having a psychological effect that, if pleasing, would make it a placebo. One term seems to fill the bill. If it falls a bit short of precision, perhaps the language will have to grow a little to include the new use.

To the increasingly well-recognized uses of the placebo I would add its use as a tool to get at certain fundamental mechanisms of the action of drugs, especially those designed to modify subjective responses. This use will be illustrated here. Strong evidence will be presented to support the view that several classes of drugs have an important part of their action on the reaction or processing component of suffering, as opposed to their effect on the original sensation.

The opportunities opened up by the placebo are unique, for it cannot possibly enter into any process by virtue of its chemical composition. It has, so to speak, neither the reactivity nor the physical dimensions required of an "effective" drug. It does not matter in the least what the placebo is made of or how much is used so long as it is not detected as a placebo by the subject or the observer. Thus the placebo provides an indispensable tool for study of the reaction or processing component of suffering. This will be referred to later on in this paper. I have discussed it extensively elsewhere.[2]

Reasons for Use

Reasons for the use of the placebo can be indicated by summarizing, then, its common purposes: as a psychological instrument in the therapy of certain ailments arising out of mental illness, as a resource of the harassed doctor in dealing with the neurotic patient, to determine the true effect of drugs apart from suggestion in experimental work, as a device for eliminating bias not only on the part of the patient but also, when used as an unknown, of the observer, and, finally, as a tool of importance in the study of the mechanisms of drug action. Moreover, as a consequence of the use of placebos, those who react to them in a positive way can be screened out to advantage under some circumstances and the focus sharpened on drug effects. For example, Jellinek (1946) in studying 199 patients with headache found, that 79 never got relief from a placebo, whereas 120 did.[1] His data for these numbers can be tabulated as follows: While differences between A, B, and C do not emerge in the "mean success rate," it appears in the placebo-nonreactor group that A is definitely more effective than the other agents (Table 2.1). He thus demonstrated (validated with statistical methods) that when the placebo reactors are screened out more useful differentiations can be made than otherwise is the case. Jellinek is not on such sure ground when he seems to dismiss the placebo reactors as those having "imagined pain, psychological headaches." From work on postoperative wound pain done by me and my associates it appears that placebos can relieve pain arising from physiological cause. (Certainly the reverse is true: psychological cause in promoting a flow of gastric juice can produce ulcer pain, etc.) This matter of the place of reaction to unpleasant sensory phenomena has been discussed elsewhere.[2]

We can take an example from our own work where placebos have relieved pain arising from physiological cause (surgical incision) and show how useful the screening out of placebo reactors can be. I, with Keats, Mosteller, and Lasagna,[3] in 1953, administered analgesics by mouth to patients having steady, severe postoperative wound pain, and we found that when we took all patients and all data we could not differentiate between certain combined acetylsalicylic acid data and narcotic (morphine and codeine) data; however, when we screened out the placebo reactors, a sharp differential

Table 2.1.
Percentage of relief from placebo in 199 patients with headaches

Agent	Effective Mean Success Rate, % (n=199)	Effectiveness in Placebo-Nonreactor Group, % (n=79)	Effectiveness in Placebo-Reactor Group, % (n=120)
A	81	88	82
B	80	67	87
C	80	77	82
Placebo	52	0	—

[Note: Data from Jellinek (1946)[1]—eds.]

emerged in favor of the acetylsalicylic acid administered orally as opposed to the narcotics administered orally. Observations of this kind were enough to give us an interest in the placebo reactor as such. We made a study of him and of the placebo response[4] in 1954 in a group of 162 patients having steady, severe postoperative wound pain. We found that there were no differences in sex ratios or in intelligence between reactors and nonreactors. There are however significant differences in attitudes, habits, educational background, and personality structure between consistent reactors and nonreactors. These have been described in the report of this study.[4] (There was a significantly higher incidence of relief from morphine in the placebo reactors than in the nonreactors.)

Lasagna, Mosteller, von Felsinger, and I[4] found in a study of severe postoperative wound pain that the number of placebo doses was correlated highly with the total number of doses of all kinds. Fifteen patients with one placebo dose showed 53% relief from the placebo; 21 patients with two placebo doses got 40% relief from the placebo; in 15 patients with three placebo doses 40% gave relief; and of 15 patients with four or more placebo doses 15% gave relief. There was a significant correlation between number of doses and percentage relief. This same study gave an opportunity to examine the consistency of the placebo response. Sixty-nine patients received two or more doses of a placebo. Fifty-five per cent (38 patients) of these behaved inconsistently, that is to say, sometimes the placebo produced relief and sometimes not. Fourteen per cent (10 patients) were consistent reactors, that is, all placebo doses were effective. Thirty-one per cent (21 patients) were consistent nonreactors; the placebo doses were never effective. It is impossible to predict the efficacy of subsequent placebos from the response to the initial dose of saline. It must not be supposed that the action of placebos is limited to "psychological" responses. Many examples could be given of "physiological" change, objective change, produced by placebos. Data on this will be presented below.

Magnitude of the Therapeutic Effect of Placebos

Notwithstanding the keen interest of a number of individuals in placebo reactors and the placebo response, there is too little scientific as well as clinical appreciation of how important unawareness of these placebo effects can be and how devastating to experimental studies as well as to sound clinical judgment lack of attention to them can be. This problem exists in many laboratories and in many fields of therapy. Its size and pervasiveness can best be illustrated by quantitative data from the studies of others as well as our own. Fifteen illustrative studies have been chosen at random (doubtless many more could have been included) and are shown in Table 2.2. These are not a selected group: all studies examined that presented adequate data have been included. Thus in 15 studies (7 of our own, 8 of others) involving 1,082 patients, placebos are found to have an average significant effectiveness of

Table 2.2.
Therapeutic effectiveness of placebos in several conditions

Condition	Study	Placebo			Patients, No.		% Satisfactorily Relieved by a Placebo	
		Agent	Route*					
Severe post-operative wound pain	Keats and Beecher (1950)[J]	Saline	I.V.		118		21	
	Beecher et al. (1951)[A]	Saline	S.C.		29		31	
	Keats et al. (1951)[K]	Saline	I.V.		34		26	
	Beecher et al. (1953)[3]	Lactose	P.O.		52		40 ⎫	
					36		26 ⎬ 33 (mean)	
					44		34 ⎭	
					40		32	
	Lasagna and others (1954)[4]	Saline	S.C.		14		50 ⎫	
					20		37	
					15		53 ⎬ 39 (mean)	
					21		40	
					15		40	
					15		15 ⎭	
Cough	Gravenstein et al. (1954)[F]	Lactose	P.O.		22		36 ⎫ 40 (mean)	
					22		43 ⎭	
Drug-induced mood changes	Lasagna et al. (1955)[L]	Isotonic sodium chloride	S.C.	Normal "Post-addicts"	20		30	
					30		30	
Pain from angina pectoris	Evans and Hoyle (1933)[D] Travell et al. (1949)[M]	Sodium bicarbonate	P.O.		66		38	
		"Placebo"	P.O.		19		26	
	Greiner et al. (1950)[G]	Lactose	P.O.		27		38	
Headache	Jellinek (1946)[I]	Lactose	P.O.		199		52	
Seasickness	Gay and Carliner (1949)[E]	Lactose	P.O.		33		58	
Anxiety and tension	Wolf and Pinsky (1954)[5]	Lactose	P.O.		31		30	
Experimental cough	Hillis (1952)[H]	Isotonic sodium chloride	S.C.	Many experiments	1		37	
Common cold	Diehl (1933)[C]	Lactose	P.O.	Cold acute	110		35	
				Subacute chronic	48		35	
				Total patients	1,082	Average relieved	35.2±2.2%	

Note: * I.V., Intravenous; S.C., subcutaneous; P.O., oral.

$35.2 \pm 2.2\%$, a degree not widely recognized. The great power of placebos provides one of the strongest supports for the view that drugs that are capable of altering subjective responses and symptoms do so to an important degree through their effect on the reaction component of suffering.[2]

Toxic and Other Subjective Side-Effects of Placebos

Not only do placebos produce beneficial results, but like other therapeutic agents they have associated toxic effects. In a consideration of 35 different toxic effects of placebos that we had observed in one or more of our studies, there is a sizable incidence of effect attributable to the placebo as follows: dry mouth, 7 subjects out of 77, or 9%; nausea, 9 subjects out of 92, or 10%; sensation of heaviness, 14 subjects out of 77, or 18%; headache, 23 subjects out of 92, or 25%; difficulty concentrating, 14 subjects out of 92, or 15%; drowsiness, 36 subjects out of 72, or 50%; warm glow, 6 subjects out of 77, or 8%; relaxation, 5 subjects out of 57, or 9%; fatigue, 10 subjects out of 57, or 18%; sleep, 7 subjects out of 72, or 10%. The effects mentioned were recorded as definite but without the subject's or observer's knowledge that only a placebo had been administered.

Wolf and Pinsky[5] reported in 1954 on an interesting study of placebos and their associated toxic reactions. They found, in studying a supposedly effective drug and a placebo (lactose) in patients with anxiety and tension as prominent complaints, that these symptoms were made better in about 30% of 31 patients. It is interesting to observe that the improvement rate was greater on the subjective side as just given than it was when objective signs of anxiety such as tremulousness, sweating, and tachycardia were considered. In this case (objective signs) about 17% were made better.

In these patients of Wolf and Pinsky there were various minor complaints, but 3 of the 31 patients had major reactions to the placebo: one promptly had overwhelming weakness, palpitation, and nausea both after taking the placebo and also after the tested (therapeutically ineffective) drug. A diffuse rash—itchy, erythematous, and maculopapular—developed in a second patient after the placebo. It was diagnosed by a skin consultant as dermatitis medicamentosa. The rash quickly cleared after the placebo administration was stopped. Since the placebo was a small quantity of lactose taken orally, it is hardly possible that it could have produced a real dermatitis. In a third patient, within 10 minutes after taking her pills, epigastric pain followed by watery diarrhea, urticaria, and angioneurotic edema of the lips developed. These signs and symptoms occurred twice more after she received the pills and again when the batch of pills was shifted; thus she had the reaction after both the (therapeutically ineffective) drug as well as after the placebo. These powerful placebo effects are objective evidence that the reaction phase[2] of suffering can produce gross physical change.

Objective Effects of Placebos

Abbot, Mack, and Wolf[6] found in 13 experiments with placebos on a subject with a gastric fistula that the gastric acid level decreased in 8 experiments, increased in 2, and was unchanged in 3. Whereas, in a second group of 13 experiments with no agent used, the gastric acid level increased in 1 case, decreased in 4, and remained the same in 8. The gastric acid level fell apparently about twice as often when a placebo was used as when no agent was administered. In the section above on toxic effects, reference was made to the patients of Wolf and Pinsky[5] who developed objective toxic signs following placebo administration: palpitation, erythematous rash, watery diarrhea, urticaria, angioneurotic edema. Wolf[7] has pointed out ". . . 'placebo effects' include objective changes at the end organ which may exceed those attributable to potent pharmacologic action."

During work with narcotics, Keats and I observed that 7 subjects out of 15, or 47%, were recorded as having constricted pupils, believed at the time (using "unknowns" technique) to be a drug effect, although later it was found that a placebo had been used. Even though this observed effect possibly might not have been related to the placebo adminis-

tration in this case, it illustrates the kind of error that can get into uncontrolled drug experiments.

Cleghorn, Graham, Campbell, Rublee, Elliott, and Saffran studied the adrenal cortex in psychoneurotic patients where anxiety requiring hospitalization was the most prominent feature.[B] They found that a placebo (isotonic sodium chloride) injection produced a response in patients with severe anxiety similar to that given by corticotropin (ACTH) in normal patients. (As criteria of adrenal cortical activity, they used the following indexes: increase in circulating neutrophils, decrease in lymphocytes, decrease in eosinophils, and an increase in the ratio of uric acid to creatinine. And more recently they have added: potassium, sodium, 17-ketosteroids, and neutral reducing lipids determinations.) The amount of change was recorded in several types of experiments on normals (labeled O) as well as on patients. The patients have been divided arbitrarily into three categories, mild effect (labeled $\frac{1}{2}$), moderate (labeled 1), marked (labeled 2) and the numerical range limits for these groups set down. The label numbers in a given case were added together to give a composite index of adrenal cortical activity. Normal subjects who received a small dose of corticotropin always reacted more than the $\frac{1}{2}$ class; class 1 was the range of change never observed in normal controls but was common in stress and with corticotropin; class 2 presented a degree of change that was unusual for doses of corticotropin not exceeding 25 units. The response increased with the dose of corticotropin. Twenty-five of the subjects received a saline placebo injection. From the data it is evident that the patients with the severest anxiety states have a greater disturbance of their adrenal cortical activity by the placebo than is true of patients with less anxiety.

These objective changes show that placebos can set off the adrenals and mimic drug action. They also show that the severer the disease state the greater is their effect. (This is in line with our long-standing thesis that, for sound information concerning the effectiveness of certain drugs designed to alter subjective responses ordinarily arising in disease, it is sounder than otherwise to go to the pathological situation for answers as to drug effectiveness.)

In work in progress I have found strong evidence that placebos are far more effective in relieving a stressful situation (early postoperative wound pain) when the stress is severe than when it is less so. Thus subjective and objective (Cleghorn and others) data both support the view of a differential effectiveness of placebos.

Comment

An interesting discussion of the use of the placebo in therapy was presented by Gold and others in one of the Cornell Conferences on Therapy in 1946.[8] Gold was one of the very earliest investigators to understand the use and significance and importance of the placebo. Not enough attention has been given to his sensible comments over the years. At this particular conference, DuBois commented that, although scarcely mentioned in the literature, placebos are more used than any other class of drugs. He objected to the definition of a placebo as an agent designed to pacify rather than to benefit and held, reasonably enough, that to pacify is to benefit. DuBois recalled that Fantus claimed that the lower the intelligence of the patient the more he is benefited by a placebo. Gold strongly disagreed and provided support for his disagreement. We agree with Gold on the basis of our own evidence.[4] Wolff pointed out that the placebo as a symbol of the doctor says in effect "I will take care of you." Diethelm suggested that the person reacts to suggestion because what is suggested becomes to him reality. He believes it and consequently the expected result occurs. (In believing, the expected reaction takes place.) Gold made a strong plea for "pure" placebos; i.e., placebos that do not contain any element that could conceivably have a direct effect on the body's cells, otherwise the physician is likely to deceive himself. He comes to believe that these unlikely agents are nevertheless, by virtue of the specific drug included, effective, when really all the power they have is as a placebo.

In studies of severe, steady postoperative wound pain extending over a considerable number of years, we have found that rather constantly 30% or more of these individuals get satisfactory pain relief from a placebo. The effectiveness of a placebo does vary in this work as shown in Table 2.2, from one group to another, but is always at an impressively high level, generally above the 30% mentioned. Certainly, in these and the other studies shown in Table 2.2, the validity of the thesis presented here (namely, that the placebo can have powerful therapeutic effect) hinges largely on the definition of "satisfactory relief." In each study referred to, this has been carefully defined. For example, in our pain work, satisfactory relief is defined as "50 per cent or more relief of pain" at two checked intervals, 45 and 90 minutes after administration of the agent. (This is a reproducible judgment patients find easy to make.) Each author has been explicit, and some have required even greater success than indicated above. For example, Gay and Carliner (1949) required, for a positive effect, complete relief of seasickness within 30 minutes of administration of the placebo.[E] The important point here is that in each of these representative studies, patients and observers alike, working with unknowns (usually "double blind" technique) have concluded that a real therapeutic effect has occurred. The implication of this for an uncontrolled study is clear.

The constancy of the placebo effect ($35.2 \pm 2.2\%$), as indicated by the small standard error of the mean in a fairly wide variety of conditions, including pain, nausea, and mood changes, suggests that a fundamental mechanism in common is operating in these several cases, one that surely deserves further study.

With placebos having an average high effectiveness of 35% (Table 2.2) in the variety of conditions dealt with here, it should be apparent that "clinical impression" is hardly a dependable source of information without the essential safeguards of the double unknowns technique, the use of placebos also as unknowns, randomization of administration, the use of correlated data (all agents are studied in the same patients), and mathematical validation of any supposed differences. These safeguards are essential when matters of judgment enter into decision. Many "effective" drugs have power only a little greater than that of a placebo. To separate out even fairly great true effects above those of a placebo is manifestly difficult to impossible on the basis of clinical impression. Many a drug has been extolled on the basis of clinical impression when the only power it had was that of a placebo.

Not only does the use (and study) of placebos offer much of practical value, but it is important to recognize that use of this tool promises to give access to an understanding of certain basic problems of mechanism of action of narcotics and other agents that modify subjective responses. A detailed discussion has been given elsewhere[2] of the two phases of suffering: the original pain sensation, for example, and then the reaction to it or the processing of it by the central nervous system. The evidence for the importance of the reaction phase as the site of drug action has been assembled,[2] and in that account the effectiveness of placebos stands as one of the principal supports of the concept. We can learn still more from placebos along this line. Consider the following statement: If, against all of the evidence to the contrary, one were to hold the view that the placebo is a feeble or useless therapeutic agent, then the placebo should appear most effective when the test condition is mild and less effective when pitted against severe conditions. There are two kinds of evidence, subjective and objective, referred to above, that just the opposite is the case: placebos are most effective when the stress (anxiety or pain, for example) is greatest.

Two other views fit well with these findings. For some years we have held to the working hypothesis that subjective responses must be studied in man where they arise in pathology, that they cannot be usefully contrived experimentally in man. There is considerable factual evidence to support this view.[2] We believe the reason for this is that in pathology the significance, the reaction, is greatest and of a kind and degree that cannot adequately be produced experimentally. Where the significance is greatest, one can expect the greatest reaction, the greatest (more extensive) processing of the original sensations, and, in a parallel way, the greatest response to therapy both of "active" drugs (like morphine) and of placebos insofar as they act on the reaction phase. This may explain why morphine fails to block the experimental pain of the Hardy-Wolff procedures.[2] The greater effectiveness of the placebo where the stress and reaction are greatest, taking into account that the placebo can only act on the reaction facet, supports the view that placebos being chiefly effective as indicated when there is great significance, great reaction, do indeed act by altering the reaction.

Placebos provide an opportunity for attacking problems not possible to study with specifically effective drugs (like morphine on pain), since with these drugs one can never be sure that the original sensation was not altered by drug action. The placebo effect of active drugs is masked by their active effects. The power attributed to morphine is then presumably a placebo effect plus its drug effect. The total "drug" effect is equal to its "active" effect plus its placebo effect: 75% of a group in severe postoperative pain are satisfactorily relieved by a large dose of morphine (15 mg of the salt per 70 kg of body weight), but 35% are relieved by the placebo.

Summary and Conclusions

It is evident that placebos have a high degree of therapeutic effectiveness in treating subjective responses, decided improvement, interpreted under the unknowns technique as a real therapeutic effect, being produced in $35.2 \pm 2.2\%$ of cases. This is shown in over 1,000 patients in 15 studies covering a wide variety of areas: wound pain, the pain of angina pectoris, headache, nausea, phenomena related to cough and to drug-induced mood changes, anxiety and tension, and finally the common cold, a wide spread of human ailments where subjective factors enter. The relative constancy of the placebo effect over a fairly wide assortment of subjective responses suggests that a fundamental mechanism in common is operating, one that deserves more study. The evidence is that placebos are most effective when the stress is greatest. This supports the concept of the reaction phase as an important site of drug action.

Placebos have not only remarkable therapeutic power but also toxic effects. These are both subjective and objective. The reaction (psychological) component of suffering has the power to produce gross physical change. It is plain not only that therapeutic power of a drug under study must in most cases be hedged about by the controls described below but also that studies of side-effects must be subjected to the same controls.

When subjective responses, symptoms, are under study, it is apparent that the high order of effectiveness of placebos must be recognized. Clearly, arbitrary criteria of effectiveness of a drug must be set up. Preservation of sound judgment both in the laboratory and in the clinic requires the use of the "double blind" technique, where neither the subject nor the observer is aware of what agent was used or indeed when it was used. This latter requirement is made possible by the insertion of a placebo, also as an unknown, into the plan of study. A standard of reference should be employed for comparison with new agents or techniques. Randomization of administration of the agents tested is important. The use of correlated data (the agents compared are tested in the same patients) is essential if modest numbers are to be worked with. Mathematical validation of observed difference is often necessary. Whenever judgment is a component of appraisal of a drug or a technique, and this is often the case, conscious or unconscious bias must be eliminated by the procedures just mentioned. These requirements have been discussed in detail elsewhere.[9]

REFERENCES

1. Gaddum, J.H.: Walter Ernest Dixon Memorial Lecture: Clinical Pharmacology, Proc. Roy. Soc. Med. **47**: 195–204, 1954.

2. Beecher, H.K.: The Subjective Response and Reaction to Sensation: The Reaction Phase as the Effective Site for Drug Action, Am. J. Med. **20**: 107–113, 1956.

3. Beecher, H.K.; Keats, A.S.; Mosteller, F., and Lasagna, L.: The Effectiveness of Oral Analgesics (Morphine, Codeine, Acetylsalicylic Acid) and the Problem of Placebo "Reactors" and "Non-Reactors," J. Pharmacol. & Exper. Therap. **109**: 393–400, 1953.

4. Lasagna, L.; Mosteller, F.; von Felsinger, J.M.; and Beecher, H.K.: A Study of the Placebo Response, Am. J. Med. **16**: 770–779, 1954.

5. Wolf, S. and Pinsky, R.H.: Effects of Placebo Administration and Occurrence of Toxic Reactions, J.A.M.A. **155**: 339–341, 1954.

6. Abbot, F.K.; Mack, M.; and Wolf, S.: The Action of Banthine on the Stomach and Duodenum of Man with Observations on the Effects of Placebos, Gastroenterology **20**: 249–261, 1952.

7. Wolf, S.: Effects of Suggestion and Conditioning on the Action of Chemical Agents in Human Subjects—The Pharmacology of Placebos, J. Clin. Invest. **29**: 100–109, 1950.

8. Wolff, H.G.; DuBois, E.F.; and Gold, R., in Cornell Conferences on Therapy: Use of Placebos in Therapy, New York J. Med. **46**: 1718–1727, 1946.

9. Beecher, H.K.: Appraisal of Drugs Intended to Alter Subjective Responses, Symptoms (Report to Council on Pharmacy and Chemistry), J.A.M.A. **158**: 399–401, 1955.

[Note: We have provided full citation information for articles that Beecher either incompletely cited or for which he provided no citation information. We list them below in alphabetical order and they appear in the text and/or tables as superscripted letters in square brackets.—eds.]

[A]. Beecher HK, Deffer PA, Fink FE, Sullivan DB. Field use of methadone and levo-iso-methadone in a combat zone (Hamhung-Hungnam, North Korea). *United States Armed Forces Medical Journal* 1951;2: 1269–1276.

[B]. Cleghorn RA, Graham BF, Campbell RB, Rublee NK, Elliott FH, Saffran M. Anxiety states: their response to ACTH and to isotonic saline. In: Mote JR (ed.). *Proceedings of the First Clinical ACTH Conference.* Philadelphia, Penn.: J.R. Blakiston Co., 1950, pp. 561–565.

[C]. Diehl HS. Medicinal treatment of the common cold. JAMA 1933;101: 2042–2049.

[D]. Evans W, Hoyle C. The comparative value of drugs used in the continuous treatment of angina pectoris. *Quarterly Journal of Medicine* 1933;2:311–338.

[E]. Gay LN, Carliner PE. The prevention and treatment of motion sickness. I. Seasickness. *Bulletin of the Johns Hopkins Hospital* 1949;84:470–487.

[F]. Gravenstein JS, Devloo RA, Beecher HK. Effect of antitussive agents on experimental and pathological cough in man. *Journal of Applied Physiology* 1954;7:119–139.

[G]. Greiner T, Gold H. Cattell M, et al. A method for the evaluation of the effects of drugs on cardiac pain in patients with angina of effort; a study of khellin (visammin). *American Journal of Medicine* 1950;9:143–155.

[H]. Hillis BR. The assessment of cough-suppressing drugs. *Lancet* 1952;259:1230–1235.

[I]. Jellinek EM. Clinical tests on comparative effectiveness of analgesic drugs. *Biometrics Bulletin* 1946;2:87–91.

[J]. Keats AS, Beecher HK. Pain relief with hypnotic doses of barbiturates and a hypothesis. *Journal of Pharmacology and Experimental Therapeutics* 1950;100:1–13.

[K]. Keats AS, D'Alessandro GL, Beecher HK. Controlled study of pain relief by intravenous procaine. JAMA 1951;147:1761–1763.

[L]. Lasagna L, von Felsinger JM, Beecher HK. Drug-induced mood changes in man. I. Observations on healthy subjects, chronically ill patients, and postaddicts. JAMA 1955;157:1006–1020.

[M]. Travell J, Rinzler SH, Bakst H, et al. Comparison of effects of alpha-tocopherol and matching placebo on chest pain in patients with heart disease. *Annals of the New York Academy of Sciences* 1949;52: 345–353.

3

How Much of the Placebo "Effect" Is Really Statistical Regression?

CLEMENT J. McDONALD, STEVEN A. MAZZUCA, AND
GEORGE P. McCABE JR.

Clement J. McDonald, Steven A. Mazzuca, and George P. McCabe Jr., "How Much of the Placebo 'Effect' Is Really Statistical Regression?," *Statistics in Medicine* 1983;2:417–427.

Investigators have variously claimed that the placebo is powerful,[1] that it meters its curative effects in proportion to the severity of the illness[1] and that it influences both objective and subjective outcomes.[2–4] Some authors have advocated a legitimate place for placebo therapy in patient care.[2] Patients do tend to improve in association with placebo treatment. This association, however, does not by itself prove that the placebo treatment causes the improvement. This paper considers the degree to which statistical regression toward the mean could account for the improvements associated with placebo therapy.

We exclude from the scope of our discussion placebo therapy associated with intense conditioning[5,6] or body invasion, i.e., needle sticks or surgical incisions. In the first case, the improvements can be attributed to Pavlovian mechanisms and in the second, to neuroendocrine mechanisms.[7] Most medical prescribing is not associated with either of these circumstances. At the outset, we emphasize that our question regarding the strength of the placebo effect does not diminish the requirements for placebo-treated controls in clinical trials. Such controls are imperative to prevent bias and ensure proper assignment of cause.

Statistical Regression

Statistical regression describes a tendency of extreme measures to move closer to the mean when they are repeated. It is a well-known phenomenon first described by Galton in 1885[8] and since reviewed and described in medical settings by many authors.[9–12] It explains such diverse phenomena as the observations that individuals who score high in tests tend to do less well in repeat tests and the observation that sons of tall fathers tend, on the average, to be shorter than their progenitors.[8] The amount of improvement due to regression can be large and statistically significant.[13] Given observations about paired random variables, X_1 and X_2, regression toward the mean occurs whenever the two variables are positively correlated and have identical distributions.[14]

For bivariate normal random variables with common mean μ, common variance, and correlation ρ (often referred to as the test/retest or reliability coefficient), regression toward the mean is usually expressed as follows:[15]

$$E(X_2 \mid X_1 = x_1) = \mu + \rho(x_1 - \mu) \tag{1}$$

The expected change between baseline and repeat observations is thus,

$$\Delta = E(X_2 - X_1 \mid X_1 = x_1) = (\mu - x_1)(1 - \rho) \tag{2}[15A]$$

To convince oneself that Δ always represents a change toward the mean, consider the following. Under the assumption that X_1 and X_2 are positively correlated, the sign of Δ is determined by $(\mu - x_1)$. If the initial measure, x_1, is below the mean, $(\mu - x_1)$ is positive. Therefore, Δ represents an increase toward the mean. If the initial measure is above the mean, $(\mu - x_1)$ is negative. Consequently, Δ represents a decrease toward the mean. Only when $\rho = 1$, implying perfect reliability of the measure, does no change occur.

Two other aspects of equation (2) deserve attention. First, the amount of 'improvement' is proportional to $(1 - \rho)$. Thus, the less reliable the measure, the greater the expected improvement. Secondly, statistical regression is proportional to $(\mu - x_1)$, the distance between the mean and the baseline measure, i.e., the more abnormal the initial measure, the larger is the expected improvement.

What we have described for a single variable has multivariate extensions. Here, multiple observations about a patient can be described as a point in multidimensional space. For a population of patients there is a mean point. The distance between any point and the mean point can be measured in terms of a distance function such as the Euclidean norm. In many cases, individuals whose distance from the mean is extreme on first observation will move closer to the mean upon repeat observation. For example, this will occur when each of many measurements are mutually independent and have the properties required for univariate regression. In this case equation (2) will apply to each measure individually and therefore the repeat measure will be closer to the mean point than the initial measure. Discussion of the general multivariate case is complex and beyond the scope of this paper.

The variables used to judge the success of therapy are especially susceptible to statistical regression. By definition, the pretreatment values of these measures will be extreme (abnormal). Because the pre- and post-measures are taken in the same individual, they will tend to be positively, but imperfectly, correlated. Finally, under many circumstances (for example, when the treatment has no effect and the disease process is not rapidly progressive), the statistical distribution of the before and after observations will be the same. (Note that the requirements for regression refer to the distribution of the larger population from which we draw patients for treatment, not the smaller population we treat.) Thus, the conditions for statistical regression to occur are often satisfied. We emphasize that this does not mean that all treated populations improve, nor that all improvement is due to regression. What it means is that regression may provide the illusion of efficacy when a drug has no effect.

The question posed in the introduction now becomes a question of size. Is the regression 'effect' large enough to account for the improvements observed in placebo-treated patients? To answer this question, we obtain respective estimates of the size of the improvement expected from regression and that observed with placebo treatment.

The Estimated Amount of Improvement Observed with Placebo Treatment

Most information about the size of the placebo 'effect' comes from observations with placebo-treated patients in clinical trials. In a widely quoted article, Beecher[1] reviewed the effect of placebo therapy in 15 different studies and reported that 35.2 per cent of the pooled population of patients from all these studies improved after placebo therapy. This is neither the average improvement per patient nor the average direction of change. The percentage reported is the number of patients who improved divided by the number treated, and contains no information about patients who worsened under placebo treatment. (Using the same technique, a clinic weighing patients with a scale accurate to the gram could demonstrate a 50 per cent weight loss each visit when there was no change in the average weight.) Thus, this measure is not a useful one for our purpose. The magnitude of improvement and the number of patients who worsened under placebo therapy were not reported in many of the papers of that era.

Since we were unable to find published estimates of the *average* amount of improvement in placebo-treated patients, we obtained our own estimate from a random sample of 30 placebo-controlled clinical trials reported in the 1979 *Abridged Index Medicus*. We obtained the mean percentage change in placebo-treated patients by comparing the last reported baseline measure with the last measure obtained during treatment. The signs of these changes were adjusted to ensure that improvements were always represented by a positive, and deteriorations by a negative, value. When more than one variable was reported in the study, we used the variable with the median percentage change as our index variable. We included papers reporting both subjective and objective variables because the literature about placebos emphasizes the positive effect of placebo treatment in both classes of observations.

The index variable in 17 of our articles was a biological, physiological, or anatomical measurement, i.e., an objective measure. In the remaining 13 articles, it was a measure of behaviour, perception or pain, i.e., a subjective measurement. Many of these studies employed techniques that would tend to reduce the effect of statistical regression on the placebo-treated patients. Half of the studies took two or more pretreatment measures and used either the average or the last of these measures as their baseline for measuring improvement. Most of the subjective measurements were averages of multipoint measurements (e.g., psychological scales). Such averages are more reliable than comparable single point measures.

Over the period of placebo treatment, the index variable improved in 16, remained the same in 1 and worsened in 13 of the selected reports (see Table 3.1). The mean improvement was 9.9 per cent and the median—a more reliable measure of central tendency in skewed samples such as this—was 0.3 per cent. A number of factors could account for the difference between the size of the improvement in our, and in Beecher's sample of papers. First, our estimate took into account patients who worsened as well as those who improved, providing a valid estimate of the magnitude of the improvement.

Secondly, our sample of papers included only three reports about pain. Beecher's included nine. Placebos may have a greater effect on pain than on other conditions. Finally, the differences in the study design of the modern papers compared to the older papers would tend to mute the effect of statistical regression in the newer papers and thus reduce the total improvement observed compared with the older papers.

The inclusion of objective measurements in our report did not account for the lesser overall effect, since the average improvement observed in subjective parameters was actually less than that in the objective parameters.

The Size of the Regression Effect

The ideal way to judge the relative contribution of statistical regression to the improvement observed in placebo treatment would be to compute the expected amount of regression (using equation (2)) for the patient data reported in the cited studies and compare it with the observed improvement. Such an approach, however, would require information about the mean, μ, for the population from which the treated patients were selected and the test/retest reliability coefficient, ρ, of the measures reported. This information was not available in any of the cited papers. In fact, except for biochemical tests and blood pressure measures, we could find little information about the test/retest reliability of clinical measures in general.

The alternative was to obtain an order of magnitude estimate of the size of the regression effect by using data available in the medical literature. Harris[46] and Cotlove[47] reported detailed information about the mean (μ), S.D. (σ), and test/retest reliability (ρ) of 15 biochemical measures. Specimens for their study were obtained in a standardized fashion from normal volunteers on a weekly basis for 10 weeks. Because these were biochemical measurements obtained in a highly standardized fashion in a reference laboratory, these data will yield conservative estimates of the size of the regression 'effect' expected in ordinary practice.

Using Harris and Cotlove's data for each of the 15 variables and equation (3) [derived from equation (2) by dividing by X_1, multiplying by 100 per cent and substituting ($\mu + 3\sigma$) for X_1], we determined the percentage change expected when we selected for repeat observation results that exceeded the usual upper normal limits (i.e., greater than $\mu + 3\sigma$).

$$percentage\ improvement = \frac{3\sigma(1-\sigma) \times 100}{\mu + 3\sigma} \qquad (3)$$

Table 3.1.
Percentage change observed during placebo treatment in 30 randomly selected placebo-controlled drug trials

Median variable	Source*	Length of study	Number of subjects	Baseline average†	Adjusted percentage change
Menstrual pain rating[16]	F2	6 mo	5	2.7	−11.1
Serum alkaline phosphatase[17]	F2	48 mo	10	4.4	−6.8‡
Work done (treadmill)[18]	T2	24 hr	11	10.2	−3.9‡
Plasma tocopherol[19]	Tx, F2	7 day	14	0.250	216.0‡
Schizophrenia severity rating[20]	F3	3–7 day	6	2.3	−17.4
Papule grading[21]	F1	11 wk	20	3.1	35.5‡
Plasma growth hormone[22]	T1	5 hr	12	28.3	−3.2‡
Arterial pH[23]	T5	5 hr	7	7.35	0.3‡
Raskin depression scale[24]	T5	6 mo	17	8.8	25.0
Hamilton depression scale[25]	T2	3 mo	17	30.6	0.3
Drug craving scale[26]	T4	8 wk	51	−18.4	−32.6
Pain rating[27]	T3	4 mo	16	4.0	5.0
Systolic blood pressure (standing)[28]	F2	3 wk	22	150.0	−2.7‡
Diastolic blood pressure (standing)[29]	F4	10 day	27	120.0	−1.3‡
Bunney-Hamburg psychosis scale[30]	F2, F3	5 wk	13	7.5	10.7
Agitation rating[31]	F2	2 day	12	43.0	11.2
Acne cyst grading[32]	T2	12 wk	24	0.3	33.3‡
Systemic vascular resistance[33]	T1	1 hr	10	2.33	1.2‡
Hyperactivity rating by mother[34]	F1	6 wk	5	15.3	12.4
Number of spells of nocturnal enuresis/2wks[35]	T2	2 wk	22	10.6	−3.8
Healing peptic ulcer rating (endoscopy)[36]	T2	4 wk	24	4.0	24.0‡
Cardiothoracic ratio[37]	T1	6 wk	12	0.58	0.0‡
LDL cholesterol[38]	T4	2 wk	15	325.5	1.2‡
Arterial PO_2[39]	F1	6 hr	5	58.2	5.5‡
Pulmonary wedge pressure[40]	T1	6 hr	8	29.1	−9.6‡
Maximum expiratory flow[41]	T2	7 wk	21	0.43	37.2‡
Pain rating (post tooth extraction)[42]	F1	2 hr	17	3.4	−58.8
Opiate withdrawal rating[43]	F1	2 hr	5	12.6	−4.8
Foot infections[44]	Tx	6 wk	20	1.0	50.0‡
Rhinitis severity rating[45]	F2	8 wk	31	2.0	−15.0

* F indicates figure in article; T=table; Tx=taken from text.
† Percentage change from placebo group baseline mean; positive values indicate change toward normal range; negative, away from normal range.
‡ Indicates objective measurement.

We looked at the high rather than the low end of the normal range to ensure a conservative percentage estimate. We set our threshold at one standard deviation above the usual upper normal limit of 2σ to reflect usual treatment practices: we usually do not treat patients until they are well into the abnormal range. The first column of Table 3.2 shows the results of these computations. The sizes of the improvements range from 2.5 per cent for serum sodium to 26 per cent for serum lactate hydrogenase. The median of the 15 tests improved by 10 per cent.

Do changes of this size really occur in practice? To answer this question, we reviewed the computer-stored records for 12,000 patients who visited the Wishard Memorial Hospital General Medicine Clinic between August 1978 and August 1980. For each biochemical variable, we selected patients who had two or more observations and examined only the first (T_1) and the last (T_2) measurements. For each biochemical variable, the T_1 and T_2 measures were positively correlated

and their distributions were approximately the same. Thus, the conditions for occurrence of statistical regression are satisfied. Statistical regression is independent of time's arrow and can be observed whether we look forward or backward in time. Because we were concerned that changes from T_1 to T_2 might be too readily attributed to physician's interventions, we selected patients whose values were three standard deviations above the mean at T_1 and computed the percentage change backward in time to T_2. The results are listed in Table 3.3. Every one of the 15 tests improved (became less abnormal from T_2 to T_1). The median percentage change of the 15 measurements was 9.5, a rate comparable to our theoretic estimates.

For completeness, we performed the same analysis selecting patients who were abnormal at T_1, and computed the amount of change forward to T_2. Again, we saw improvement in all 15 parameters. In the case of each of the biochemical measurements, the change obtained in the forward direc-

Table 3.2.
Percentage improvement expected from regression for 15 biochemical variables with the given mean (μ), standard deviation (σ), and test/retest correlation (ρ) when initial measures are 3 standard deviations above the mean (see text)

Test	Percentage improvement	μ*	σ*	ρ†
1. Sodium	2.5	139.4	1.9	0.34
2. Potassium	10.6	4.1	0.29	0.38
3. Chloride	4.2	104.6	2.2	0.29
4. Carbon dioxide	10.4	27.3	1.9	0.40
5. Calcium	7.8	2.55	0.12	0.37
6. Magnesium	8.4	0.81	0.07	0.59
7. Inorganic phosphorus	13.0	3.49	0.51	0.56
8. Total protein	6.7	6.97	0.50	0.62
9. Albumin	8.8	4.2	0.35	0.56
10. Uric acid	15.0	4.62	1.16	0.63
11. Urea nitrogen	16.6	13.5	3.1	0.60
12. Glucose	10.0	94.5	9.7	0.57
13. Cholesterol	6.9	205	36	0.8
14. SGOT	19.0	14.5	4.7	0.47
15. LDH	26.0	328	72.0	0.51

Note: * From Table 1 of Reference 47.
† Computed from the equation

$$\rho = \frac{1}{1 + (S_p/S_g)}$$

where S_p/S_g is obtained from Table 5 of Reference 46.

tion was comparable to that in the backward direction. Although it is possible to conceive of a causal mechanism that could explain the observed changes in some of these variables, the most reasonable explanation for the improvement seen in all 15 variables, when examined both forward and backward in time, is statistical regression.

Discussion

The numerical size of the improvement we observed in placebo-treated patients and that of the estimate that would occur in biochemical variables due to statistical regression were remarkably similar. Because these estimates are based upon different clinical variables and different patient populations, we cannot determine the true proportion of the improvement due to statistical regression. Observations used to judge the success of therapy, however, are ripe for statistical regression toward the mean. Moreover, improvements of as much as 26 per cent could be expected, even from biochemical variables measured under highly standardized conditions. Together, these two facts suggest that regression accounts for an important share of the improvement observed with placebo treatment.

Many of the unusual characteristics of the placebo 'effect' could be explained by assuming that statistical regression is responsible for the observed improvements. By definition, statistical regression is a random phenomenon and therefore could explain the observation that the placebo effect is "not uniform, constant or predictable" in individual patients.[48] Regression is proportional to the degree of the baseline abnormalcy and therefore could explain the observation that the placebo effect is "most effective when stress (anxiety or pain, for example) is greatest."[1] Statistical regression is proportional to measurement unreliability [(1 − ρ) of equation (2)] and single point human observations tend to be less reliable than comparable objective measurements. This could explain the traditional wisdom that subjective measurements are more susceptible to placebo influence than objective measurements.

Finally, conclusive proof of a causal role of placebo treatment requires a controlled trial comparing placebo treated with non-treated patients. One of the early proponents of the importance of the placebo effect noted the lack of studies making direct comparisons between these two groups.[49] We found one modern trial that did compare placebo-treated and untreated control groups.[50] In this study of blood pressure control, both control groups improved by the same amount. One could argue that the improvements were the same because the investigator contact required in obtaining follow-up had a placebo effect equal to that of the placebo treatment itself. However, the results are more easily explained by statistical regression operating equally in the two control groups.

Some have argued that placebo treatment causes negative as well as positive effects. Clearly, side effects such as nausea, vomiting and drowsiness occur in association with placebo treatment. A few studies have reported that placebo-treated patients had unusual rates of adverse effects, of a kind unique to the experimental treatment. These observations may be examples of the causal effects of placebo therapy but they can also be explained by ascertainment bias in such studies.

Regardless of the relative importance of statistical regression to the placebo effect, regression is important in its own right. It can produce improvements in biochemical variables that are large enough to be important. Similar or larger regression induced improvements are likely to occur in clinical observations that tend to be less reliable than analytical biochemical measurements. In fact, we can even expect regression to yield improvement in imagining findings, since such findings also vary spontaneously. For example, in a study of serial barium swallows, oesophageal varices disappeared on one or more occasions in 25 per cent of patients who had biopsy-proven cirrhosis and manometry-proven hypertension.[51]

It is also important because it extracts a price of increased sample size requirements from the clinical researcher and an increased risk of judging a clinical therapy effective when it is not from the clinician. This price can be minimized by taking steps to reduce intrapatient measurement variability. There are three approaches. The first, and most obvious, is to select the most reliable measures from among those that are practical. The second is to use the average of a number of different measures of similar reliability rather than a single

Table 3.3.
Observed change in patients selected for 3–standard deviation abnormalcy

Test name	Number in total population	Average of total population at T_1	Average of total population at T_2	Average in selected population at T_2*	Percentage change from T_1 to T_2
Sodium	8373	139.3	139.0	153.7	6.2
Potassium	8946	4.13	4.05	6.6	27.1
Chloride	8365	102.3	101.9	110.0	3.8
Bicarbonate	8352	25.7	26.1	30.7	9.5
Calcium	7197	9.83	9.75	11.6	7.0
Magnesium	905	2.07	2.0	3.0	20.8
Phosphorus	1017	3.57	3.72	7.0	37.3
Total protein	7128	7.81	7.80	9.0	6.9
Albumin	7096	4.29	4.27	5.2	11.3
Uric acid	7417	6.21	6.23	9.7	13.7
Blood-urea-nitrogen	9340	15.6	15.8	36.0	21.2
Glucose	5968	154.7	155.4	224.5	8.7
Cholesterol	7243	223.0	219.6	367.3	13.0
SGOT	7267	43.5	38.5	117.5	25.6
Lactate dehydrogenase	6097	222.7	220.8	279.8	8.9

* Selected population consists of patients selected for values >3 standard deviations above mean at T_2.

measure, since such an average is more reliable than any of its components. The last is to observe the chosen measures more than once, preferably at different points in time before beginning therapy. By using the average of enough pretreatment measures, one can reduce the size of regression to any predetermined level.[9,10] When the baseline variation in the observation is due only to random noise, and not to drifts in the baseline, circadian rhythms or other cycles, the regression effect can be eliminated entirely by two pretreatment observations of the outcome variables. In this case, the first observation is used to select patients for treatment, and the second to measure the change due to treatment.[12]

Proper use of these techniques will reward the clinical researcher with smaller sample size requirements and the clinician with better judgements.

[. . .]

REFERENCES

1. Beecher, H. "The powerful placebo," *Journal of the American Medical Association*, **159**, 1602–1606 (1955).
2. Vogel, A.V., Goodwin, J.S., and Goodwin, J.M. "The therapeutics of placebo," *American Family Physician*, **22**, 105–109 (1980).
3. Gallimore, R.G. and Turner, J.L. "Contemporary studies of placebo phenomenon," *Psychopharmacology in the Practice of Medicine*, Edited by M.E. Jarvick. Appleton-Century-Crofts, New York, 47–57, (1977).
4. Benson, H. and McCallie, D.P., Jr. "Angina pectoris and the placebo effect," *New England Journal of Medicine*, **300**, 1424–1429 (1979).
5. Lown, B. "Verbal conditioning of angina pectoris during exercise testing," *American Journal of Cardiology*, **40**, 630–634 (1977).
6. Wolf, S. "Effects of suggestion and conditioning on the action of chemical agents in human subjects—the pharmacology of placebos," *Journal of Clinical Investigation*, **29**, 100–109 (1950).
7. Wintrobe, M., Lee, G., Boggs, D., *et al. Clinical Hematology*, 7th Edition, Lea & Febiger, Philadelphia, 1974, p. 252.
8. Galton, F. "Regression towards mediocrity in hereditary stature," *Journal of the Anthropological Institute of Great Britain and Ireland*, **15**, 246–263 (1886).
9. David, C.E. "The effect of regression to the mean in epidemiologic and clinical studies," *American Journal of Epidemiology*, **104**, 493–498 (1976).
10. Gardner, M.J. and Heady, J.A. "Some effects of within-person variability in epidemiologic studies," *Journal of Chronic Diseases*, **26**, 781–795 (1973).
11. Shepard, D.S. "Reliability of blood pressure measurements: implications for designing and evaluating programs to control hypertension," *Journal of Chronic Diseases*, **34**, 191–209 (1981).
12. Ederer, F. "Serum cholesterol changes: effects of diet and regression toward the mean," *Journal of Chronic Diseases*, **25**, 277–289 (1972).
13. Silverman, G. "Placebo effect and changes in response set with retesting: a further source of bias," *Neuropharmacology*, **18**, 1019–1021 (1979).
14. Tversky, A. and Kahneman, D. "Judgement under uncertainty: heuristics and biases," *Science*, **185**, 1124–1131 (1974).
15. Anderson, T.W. *Introduction to Multivariate Statistical Analysis*, Wiley, New York, 1958, p. 29.
[15a. Note: Please see the correspondence between Stephen Senn and McDonald, Mazzuca, and McCabe regarding equations (1) and (2). Senn discovered a typographical error in equation (2), which was acknowledged and further discussed by McDonald et al. Equation (2) as it appears here is now correct. For further details, see Senn SJ. Letter to the Editor. *Statistics in Medicine* 1988;7:1203; and McDonald CJ, Mazzuca SA, and McCabe GP. Letters to the Editor. *Statistics in Medicine* 1989;8:1301–1302—eds.]
16. Chan, W., Dawood, M., and Fuchs, F. "Relief of dysmenorrhea with the prostaglandin synthetase inhibitor ibuprofen: effect on prostaglandin levels in menstrual fluid," *American Journal of Obstetric Gynecology*, **135**, 102–108 (1979).
17. Kershenobich, D., Uribe, M., Suarez, G., *et al.* "Treatment of cirrhosis with colchicine: a double-blind randomized trial," *Gastroenterology*, **77**, 532–536 (1979).
18. Thadani, U. and Parker, J. "Propranolol in angina pectoris: duration of improved exercise tolerance and circulatory effects after acute oral administration," *American Journal of Cardiology*, **44**, 118–125 (1979).
19. Bell, E., Brown, E., Milner, R., Sinclair, J., and Zipursky, A. "Vitamin E absorption in small premature infants," *Pediatrics*, **63**, 830–832 (1979).

20. Shopsin, B., Klein, H., Aaronsom, M., and Collora, M. "Clozapine, chlorpromazine, and placebo in newly hospitalized, acutely schizophrenic patients," *Archives of General Psychiatry*, **36**, 657–664 (1979).

21. Cook, C., Center, R., and Michaels, S. "An acne grading method using photographic standards," *Archives of Dermatology*, **115**, 571–575 (1979).

22. Liuzzi, A., Chiodini, P., Oppizzi, G. *et al.* "Lisuride hydrogen maleate: evidence for a long lasting dopaminergic activity in humans," *Journal of Clinical Endocrinology and Metabolism*, **46**, 196–202 (1978).

23. Danahy, D., Tobis, J., Aronow, W., Chetty, K., and Glauser, F. "Effects of isosorbide dinitrate on pulmonary hypertension in chronic obstructive pulmonary disease," *Clinical Pharmacology and Therapeutics*, **25**, 541–548 (1979).

24. Prusoff, A., Williams, D., Weissman, M., and Astrachan, B. "Treatment of secondary depression in schizophrenia: a double-blind, placebo-controlled trial of amitriptyline added to perphenazine," *Archives of General Psychiatry*, **36**, 569–575 (1979).

25. Klaiber, E., Broverman, D., Vogel, W., and Kobayashi, Y. "Estrogen therapy for severe persistent depressions in women," *Archives of General Psychiatry*, **36**, 550–554 (1979).

26. Report of the National Research Council Committee on Clinical Evaluation of Narcotic Antagonists. "Clinical evaluation of naltrexone treatment of opiate-dependent individuals," *Archives of General Psychiatry*, **35**, 335–340 (1978).

27. Morrison, J. and Jennings, J. "Primary dysmenorrhea treated with indomethacin," *Southern Medical Journal*, **72**, 425–428 (1979).

28. Miller, S. and Vertes, V. "Ticrynafen and hydrochlorothiazide: a double-blind study of antihypertensive properties with an open crossover," *Journal of the American Medical Association*, **241**, 2174–2176 (1979).

29. Olivari, M., Bartorelli, C., Polese, A., *et al.* "Treatment of hypertension with nifedipine, a calcium antagonistic agent," *Circulation*, **59**, 1056–1062 (1979).

30. Alexander, P., Van Kammen, D., and Bunney, W. "Antipsychotic effects of lithium in schizophrenia," *American Journal of Psychiatry*, **136**, 283–287 (1979).

31. Carman, J. and Wyatt, R. "Use of calcitonin in psychotic agitation or mania," *Archives of General Psychiatry*, **36**, 72–75 (1979).

32. Weimar, V., Puhl, S., Smith, W., and tenBroeke, J. "Zinc sulfate in acne vulgaris," *Archives of Dermatology*, **114**, 1776–1778 (1978).

33. Strumza, P., Rigaud, M., Mechmeche, R., *et al.* "Prolonged hemodynamic effects (12 hours) or orally administered sustained-release nitroglycerin," *American Journal of Cardiology*, **43**, 272–277 (1979).

34. Harley, J., Matthews, C., and Eichman, P. "Synthetic food colors and hyperactivity in children: a double-blind challenge experiment," *Pediatrics*, **62**, 975–983 (1978).

35. Birkasova, M., Birkas, O., Flynn, M., and Cort, J. "Desmopressin in the management of nocturnal enuresis in children: a double-blind study," *Pediatrics*, **62**, 970–974 (1978).

36. Lam, S., Lam, K., Lai, C., *et al.* "Treatment of duodenal ulcer with antacid and sulpiride: a double-blind controlled study," *Gastroenterology*, **76**, 315–322 (1979).

37. Aronow, W., Lurie, M., Turbow, M., *et al.* "Effect of prazosin vs placebo on chronic left ventricular heart failure," *Circulation*, **59**, 344–350 (1979).

38. Kuo, P.T., Hayase, K., Kostis, J.B., and Moreyra, A.E. "Use of combined diet and colestipol in long-term (7–7½ years) treatment of patients with type II hyperlipoproteinemia," *Circulation*, **59**, 199–211 (1979).

39. Marks, K.H., Berman, W., Friedman, Z., *et al.* "Furosemide in hyaline membrane disease," *Pediatrics*, **62**, 785–788 (1978).

40. Orlando, J.R., Danahy, D.T., Lurie, M., and Aronow, W.S. "Effect of trimazosin on hemodynamics in chronic heart failure," *Clinical Pharmacology and Therapeutics*, **24**, 531–536 (1978).

41. Little, J.W., Hall, W.J., Douglas, R.G., *et al.* "Airway hyperreactivity and peripheral airway dysfunction in influenza A infection," *American Review of Respiratory Diseases*, **118**, 295–303 (1978).

42. Levine, J.D., Gordon, N.C., and Fields, H.L. "The mechanism of placebo analgesia," *Lancet*, **1**, 654–657 (1978).

43. Gold, M.S., Redmond, D.E., and Kleber, H.D. "Clonidine blocks acute opiate-withdrawal symptoms," *Lancet*, **2**, 599–601 (1978).

44. Ongley, R.C. "Efficacy of topical miconazole treatment of tinea pedis," *Canadian Medical Association Journal*, **119**, 353–354 (1978).

45. Horan, J.D. and Johnson, J.D. "Flunisolide nasal spray in the treatment of perennial rhinitis," *Canadian Medical Association Journal*, **119**, 334–338 (1978).

46. Harris, E., Kanofsky, P., Shakarji, G., and Cotlove, E. "Biological and analytic components of variation in long-term studies of serum constituents in normal subjects. II. Estimating biological components of variation," *Clinical Chemistry*, **16**, 1022–1027 (1970).

47. Cotlove, E., Harris, E., and Williams, G. "Biological and analytic components of variation in long-term studies of serum constituents in normal subjects. III. Physiological and medical implications," *Clinical Chemistry*, **16**, 1028–1032 (1970).

48. Shapiro, A.K. "Factors contributing to the placebo effect and their implications for psychotherapy," *American Journal of Psychotherapy*, **18**, Suppl. 1, 73–88 (1964).

49. Liberman, R. "An analysis of the placebo phenomenon," *Journal of Chronic Diseases*, **15**, 761–783 (1962).

50. Medical Research Council Working Party, "Randomized controlled trial of treatment for mild hypertension. Design of a pilot trial," *British Medical Journal*, **1**, 1437–1440 (1977).

51. Palmer, E. "On the natural history of esophageal varices which are secondary to portal cirrhosis," *Annals of Internal Medicine*, **47**, 18–26 (1957).

4

The Powerful Placebo Effect

Fact or Fiction?

GUNVER S. KIENLE AND HELMUT KIENE

Gunver S. Kienle and Helmut Kiene, "The Powerful Placebo Effect: Fact or Fiction?," *Journal of Clinical Epidemiology* 1997;50:1311–1318.

Placebo effects have gained great popularity. Within the last three years hardly any major medical journal failed to have publications about placebo effects and their scientific basis. The tradition of placebo research goes back to the fifties. It was in 1955 that Henry K. Beecher, with his famous and seminal article "The Powerful Placebo" [1], was the first author to quantify the effects of placebos in a variety of diseases. He claimed that the symptoms of 35% of 1082 patients in 15 studies [2–16] were satisfactorily relieved by placebos alone [1]. Today placebos are supposed to be effective in almost every disease, and estimates of the extent of the placebo effect even go far beyond Beecher's 35% [17–20].

This paper fundamentally questions the claimed extent of the placebo effect. A reanalysis of placebo literature was carried out, with surprising results: A wide range of errors was found in the placebo literature, which produced false impressions of placebo effects.

To illustrate these errors it is most appropriate to refer to the classic "The Powerful Placebo" [1] itself, because it is still the most frequently cited paper on placebo and because its mistakes are still prevalent in placebo literature today (as far as we can judge from 800 articles on the placebo effect we have analyzed [21,22]). In the following article, the results of the analysis of the 15 trials reported in Beecher's article are described. The analysis is based on two questions: 1. Is the existence of the placebo effect demonstrated in those 15 trials that Beecher had surveyed in "The Powerful Placebo"? 2. If not, what are the factors that can create the false impression of a placebo effect?

Definition and Methods

It seems easy to define placebos: They are imitations of specific treatments, with the absence of the specific therapeutic constituents. However, defining placebos is a very controversial topic [22–24]. Gøtzsche even concluded, "The placebo concept as presently used cannot be defined in a logically consistent way and leads to contradictions" [25]. From reading Beecher's own article, he refers to "pharmacologically inert substances" [1], the administration of which he considers can have "real therapeutic effects" [1]. Based on this, the criteria for acknowledging a placebo *effect* taken for this present paper are as follows: (1) A *placebo* had to be given. (2) The event had to be an *effect* of the placebo treatment, i.e., the event would not have happened without placebo administration. (3) The event had to be relevant for the disease or symptom, i.e., it had to be a *therapeutic* event.

Besides these three criteria there were no other predefined criteria for the analysis. Basic medical knowledge and common sense were the only scientific tools.

Result

For 14 out of the 15 trial publications [2–16] detailed analysis was possible. (One publication [4] did not give account of the study design.) The overall result was that for none of these trials was there any reason to assume the existence of the slightest placebo effect. These studies were placebo-controlled drug trials. Although they were not carried out in order to investigate placebo effects, Beecher retrospectively attributed the improvements in the placebo groups to *effects* of the placebo administration. However, on the basis of the published data, in all of these trials the reported outcome in the placebo groups can be fully, plausibly, and easily explained *without* presuming any therapeutic placebo effect. The published data of these trials make it quite obvious that there were a variety of reasons for the reported results, such as spontaneous improvements, additional treatments, methodological artifacts, etc. In some of the original trial publications even the authors themselves had explicitly written that there were *no* placebo effects.

Beecher completely neglected all obvious reasons for the outcome in the placebo groups, simply calling the reported results "real therapeutic effects" of placebo administration. Thus, he totally misinterpreted the trials.

Factors that have caused false impressions of placebo effects—not only in Beecher's but in other publications as

Table 4.1.
Factors that can cause the false impression of a placebo effect

- Natural course of a disease
  - Spontaneous improvement
  - Fluctuation of symptoms
  - Regression to the mean
  - Habituation
- Additional treatment
- Observer bias
  - Conditional switching of treatment
  - Scaling bias
  - Poor definition of drug efficacy
- Irrelevant response variables
- Subsiding toxic effect of previous medication
- Patient bias
  - Answer of politeness and experimental subordination
  - Conditioned answers
  - Neurotic or psychotic misjudgment
- No placebo given at all
  - Psychotherapy
  - Psychosomatic phenomena
  - Voodoo medicine
- Uncritical reporting of anecdotes
- Misquotation
- False assumption of toxic placebo effects created by
  - Everyday symptoms
  - Misquotation
  - Persistence of symptoms

well—are listed in Table 4.1. Most of these factors are relevant in the 15 studies surveyed by Beecher; their distribution is shown in Table 4.2 [1–16,21].

Beecher's "The Powerful Placebo"—presenting a quantitative "proof" of the existence of real therapeutic placebo effects—created a cognitive framework for further placebo research in which all kinds of phenomena were registered as therapeutic placebo effects in a rather uncritical fashion (for further details, see [21,22]). Therefore, in order to avoid such obvious misinterpretations, it is important to know those factors that can create illusions of placebo effects. They will be described in the following. Examples will be taken from Beecher's "The Powerful Placebo"; for further illustration a few examples will be taken from a similarly classic German placebo survey [17].

Factors That Can Create False Impressions of Placebo Effects
Spontaneous Improvement

Spontaneous improvement of a disease does not occur as a result of a placebo administration; it is *not* an *effect* of a placebo. This often seems to be disregarded in the placebo literature.

In a placebo-controlled drug trial on acute common cold, described as mild and of short duration, 35% of the patients receiving placebos felt better within 6 days (2 days after the onset of placebo administration) [2]. Beecher interpreted

Table 4.2.
Factors that created the illusion of a placebo effect in H. K. Beecher's study list (quoted from [21])

	Study [see references]														
	[2]	[3]	[4]	[5]	[6]	[7]	[8]	[9]	[10]	[11]	[12]	[13]	[14]	[15]	[16]
Percent of patients who were "satisfactorily relieved by a placebo," according to Beecher [1]	35	38	52	58	26	38	21	26	31	37	26–40	30	15–53	36–43	30
Factors creating illusions of placebo effect:															
• Spontaneous improvement	x	x		x	x		x	x	x		x	x	x		
• Spontaneous fluctuation of symptoms		x			x	x			x				x		
• Conditional switching of treatment	x	x				x			x	x	x				
• Scaling bias	x	x				x									
• Additional treatment	x				x										
• Irrelevant response variables					x	x									x
• Answer of politeness										x	x		x		
• Conditional answers											x		x		
• Neurotic or psychotic misjudgment												x			
• Misquotation		x	x		x		x	x	x	x	x	x	x	x	
• Everyday symptoms misinterpreted as placebo side effects												x			x
• Habituation			x							x					
• Poor definition of drug efficacy					x	x									x
• Subsiding toxic effect of previous medication								x							x
Demonstration of placebo effect?	No	No	a	No	No	No	No	No	No	No	No	No	No	No	No

Note: a — The publication [4] gives no account of the study design.

these improvements as an effect of the placebo administration [1]. However, he did not consider that many patients with a mild common cold improve spontaneously within 6 days (as already pointed out in the original publication [2]).

Other examples: Four [8,9,12,14] of the trials in Beecher's list evaluated treatment of post-operative pain. Reanalyzing these trials, it was possible in two [8,9] of these studies to determine the spontaneous diminishing of postoperative pain on the basis of published data on the decrease of patients' demand for analgesics. This diminishing rate was equal to that of Beecher's claimed "placebo effect" [21]. Therefore, there is no reason to assume a placebo effect.

Spontaneous improvement was a major factor in Beecher's misinterpretation of 10 of the 15 trials. This error is widespread in the placebo literature.

Fluctuation of Symptoms

In chronic diseases (or with chronic pain [26,27]) *fluctuation of symptoms* should be taken into account. Patients feel better one day and worse the next. Therefore, looking at a number of chronically ill patients, one will simply *always* see some patients improving. Because of this, it is a mistake to forget to mention the rate of deterioration, and only report the rate of improvement and call the latter a placebo "effect."

For example, Beecher referred to patients with diseases such as ulcer, migraine, muscle tension, or headache who suffered from anxiety and tension and were treated for eight 2-week periods alternately with mephenesin and placebo [13]. Beecher claimed a placebo effect of 30% since "roughly" 20–30% of the patients improved. However, 10–20% of the

patients deteriorated. As can be seen in a published figure, there was only a net improvement of 5–10% [21]. This seems a rather low rate, considering the observation period (16 weeks), the kind of diseases (ulcer, muscle tension, headache, etc.) and possible improvement through the intermediate mephenesin treatment. Therefore, there was no reason to assume any placebo effect. (Besides, no information about patient compliance was supplied in the publication, and it was not ruled out that patients had other medical support.)

Neglecting spontaneous fluctuations of symptoms was the main reason why Beecher also misinterpreted three other trials [3,6,7]. This is a very common mistake also in other literature about placebos: A 20% placebo effect is claimed [17] for a placebo-controlled drug trial on patients with angina pectoris. However, in the same trial, 72% [28] of the placebo-treated patients deteriorated.

A 21% placebo effect is claimed [17] for a trial on cerebral infarction, because 21% of the patients improved in the placebo group. However, in that trial [29], 53% of the patients on placebo died, even though every patient received the best supportive medical care. (Of course, neither the improvement of 21%, nor the death of 53% of the patients can be reasonably attributed to placebo administration.)

Spontaneous improvement of diseases and the spontaneous fluctuation of symptoms are special forms of *regression to the mean*, i.e., the tendency of extreme values to move closer to the average on repeated measurement. In their interesting article, "How much of the placebo 'effect' is really statistical regression?" McDonald *et al.* [30] have argued that "most improvements attributed to the placebo effect are actually instances of statistical regression."

Additional Treatment

So-called placebo effects often occur under *additional* treatment. Of course there is no justification to call such improvements a "placebo effect."

In one of the angina pectoris trials in Beecher's list [6], the placebo group additionally received nitrates. In another trial concerning the common cold [2], the patients were allowed to take rest, hot baths, gargles, diets, etc.

Many other examples can be found in the literature about placebo effects. For instance, a study [31] supposedly shows placebo effects in irritable colon treatment [17], but all patients had been put on a special diet. In another study [32], taken as a showcase for placebo effects in alcoholism [17], patients in the placebo group received specialized medical and psychosocial support.

Conditional Switching of Treatment

In some of the trials in Beecher's list, the "placebo effect" was further amplified by selecting patients in the following manner: When the patients felt well, they received a placebo; when they felt worse, they were switched to active treatment, or they were excluded from evaluation until they felt better again.

In a study on angina pectoris [3], patients got placebos as long as they only had a few episodes of angina; when the episodes increased, they received one of the test drugs. Thus good periods were selected for placebo treatment, and bad periods were selected for drug treatment. Consequently, the extent of the placebo effect was grossly overestimated. Similarly, in one of the trials concerning treatment of postoperative pain [12], patients were only included when they had already improved to the degree that they could take oral medication. When patients got worse again (pain increase, regurgitation, etc.), they were excluded from evaluation until they improved again.

Scaling Bias

In three of Beecher's trials [2,3,7] there were false augmentations of placebo effects due to asymmetrical measurement scales [21]. The scales included two or more categories for improvement, and only one or even none for deterioration. Thus the scales tempted patients to falsely give too many positive reports.

Irrelevant or Questionable Response Variables

Immense placebo effects can be claimed when they are based on response variables which are irrelevant for the condition in question [21]:

There is the claim of a 73% placebo effect in multiple sclerosis [17]. The facts in the original publication [33] were that no objective change in the neurological condition was found in any patient on placebo, yet 73% of the patients had the subjective feeling of increased euphoria, strength, and agility. However, euphoria is itself a symptom of multiple sclerosis; therefore an increase of euphoria is not necessarily a sign of improvement. Spontaneous variation of euphoria and optimistic answers are typical for this disease and therefore are inappropriate response variables for demonstrating placebo effects.

Supposedly there is a 61% placebo effect in hypertension [17]. The facts in the original trial [34] were that there was no significant change in blood pressure under placebo, but 61% of the patients subjectively felt better. However, all patients had first received veratrum, which caused severe toxic symptoms in 64% of the patients. It was then substituted by placebos. Therefore the relief of symptoms in 61% of placebo-treated patients can be explained by the cessation of veratrum toxicity [21]. There is no reason to assume any placebo effect.

Answers of Politeness and Experimental Subordination

In one of the trials on postoperative pain [8] the authors discuss the "exceedingly difficult" criteria of pain relief. They had observed that patients often claimed pain relief in contrast to the physician's impression. This observation is only peripherally related to the trials surveyed by Beecher, but it is of great importance in many other placebo reports [22]. The issue was recently described by Roberts [35]: "The word 'placebo' means 'to please' but this applies to both the patient and the doctor. For example, patients may report positive outcomes to their physicians out of a need to 'be polite' to them." The same issue was addressed by Sackett [36]: "Finally, when the patient is grateful for clinician's time and effort in trying to help them, this gratitude (plus simple good manners) often is reflected in an exaggeration of the benefits of the latest prescription when they are asked 'Did that medicine help you?'"

The same phenomenon was called a *verbal* (in contrast to a *real* therapeutic) placebo effect by Kiene [37]. He also mentioned the phenomenon of *experimental subordination*, i.e., in an experiment the subject says what he thinks he is expected to say, rather than what he really observes or experiences [37]. Similar phenomena have been described by several other authors [38–41].

To differentiate polite answers or experimental subordination from *true therapeutic* placebo effects and to develop appropriate methods for this differentiation [22] is a key issue in placebo research.

Conditioned Answers

It seems difficult to differentiate therapeutic placebo effects and conditioned effects. Numerous authors closely associate them or even presume that conditioning is the basic constituent of placebo effects [42–46]. However, a differentiation is necessary. Conditioned effects need *specific* presuppositions: First, a specific unconditioned stimulus and, second, a specific setting, which is a very close temporal pairing of the unconditioned and the conditioned stimulus. In many instances, conditioning even seems to work only when it superimposes biological rhythms. These specific presuppositions are usually not present in clinical placebo situations.

Since Pavlov, many experiments on drug-conditioned responses in animals were carried out. But from these experiments one cannot conclude that *healing* or a real *therapeutic* drug effect also can be provoked as a conditioned reflex. Surely, in cancer patients nausea and vomiting can be conditioned by repeated chemotherapy. But this does not mean that tumor remissions can be conditioned as well. Unfortunately, it is just the other way round: While conditioned vomiting often increases during chemotherapy cycles, there is generally a decrease in the therapeutic sensitivity of the tumor.

In fact, clinical experience contradicts the assumption that healing can be conditioned. Episodes of chronic disease are usually more difficult to treat than the acute or first manifestation of an illness, even if this first manifestation has been treated successfully. (Classical conditioning paradigm would predict just the opposite.) Moreover, there are many severe symptoms that are treated effectively by regular and repeated drug administration. These therapeutic settings are similar to conditional settings, and therefore should be adequate for the conditioning of therapeutic effects. Yet when interrupting such regular therapies, a rapid deterioration of patients is observed in practice.

Nevertheless, conditioning may be important when giving placebos, in that it can produce answers of politeness, verbal placebo effects, and experimental subordination rather than effecting a true placebo effect. This realm of communication seems far more susceptible to influences such as conditioning than the realm of effective healing. It is easier to provoke such communicative and behavioral reactions than true therapeutic placebo effects. This seems to have happened in one of the pain trials [14] in Beecher's list. It had a typical conditioning setting: Morphine and placebo were either alternated, or series of morphine administrations were interrupted by placebos. In this setting the "placebo effect" decreased after repeated placebo administration. One can find an easy explanation for this decrease, because it was just like in Pavlov's classic experiments. When, in Pavlov's experiments, the ringing of the bell repeatedly was not combined with real food, the salivation decreased. Similarly, when in those patients the drug application ("ringing of the bell") was not combined repeatedly with real pain relief ("food"), the patients' positive answers ("salivation") decreased. This means that the patients gradually recognized that they were receiving inactive treatments, and that only *verbal* placebo effects had been conditioned, *not* real ones [21]. A key issue when judging placebo effects is to decide whether a patient's report is true or not.

In an example of a crossover placebo-controlled study on hypertension, a conditioned reduction of blood pressure was shown; however, it was short term (a few days). Notably, when placebos were given as first treatment within this crossover design, no antihypertensive effect occurred, although 83% of the patients had previously been treated with antihypertensive remedies [47]. Thus, in this trial only a short-term conditioned effect occurred, due to the specific conditioning setting, while there was no placebo effect. These findings concur with several trials on placebo in hypertension [48–51]; they did not show any placebo effect either.

Neurotic or Psychotic Misjudgment

The reliability of a patient's report is often particularly difficult to assess in neurotic or psychotic disturbances [21]. Here the placebo literature offers fascinating stories [52]. However, one should not forget that a common feature in psychosis or neurosis is disturbed interpretation of reality. Therefore one clearly has to differentiate between a psychotic or neurotic misjudgment, on the one hand, and a correct observation of a therapeutic effect, on the other hand. (This differentiation is difficult, but not impossible; in fact, it is the psychiatrist's daily work.) Neurotic or psychotic misjudgments can hardly give any valid evidence for the existence of placebo effects.

No Placebo Given at All

There is a class of anecdotal reports in the placebo literature, which have nothing to do with placebos, because no placebos were given at all [21].

The purpose of these anecdotes is to demonstrate the possible power of "nonspecific" causes. Beecher himself reported adventurous episodes from the voodoo culture, when supposedly dying people recovered immediately, or when magic rituals brought about the death of apparently healthy people [53].

Another classic example is an anecdote in Stewart Wolf's well-known "The Pharmacology of Placebos" [54]: A woman with a gastric ulcer could not respond with gastric acid production during provocative tests with even the most powerful secretory drugs. Yet, immediate acid secretion occurred when she was asked about her husband who, as she had just recently discovered, had been sexually abusing her 12-year-old daughter. Wolf used this story to demonstrate the possible range of placebo effectiveness. However, this is misleading. This was an example of a psychosomatic effect, not the effect of placebo application. The example does not show that the mere ritual of giving a pill can be equated with the effect of discovering the sexual abuse of one's daughter by one's husband.

Uncritical Reporting of Anecdotes

One needs to be cautious about claims of placebo effects not only in clinical trials, but also in case reports. While most scientists are reasonably skeptical regarding therapeutic benefits from drugs, they welcome reports about placebo effects with uncritical enthusiasm [55]. For example, Beecher demonstrates the power of nonspecific effects by the following story [53]: A middle-aged woman underwent surgical exploration because of cancer, which was then found to be inoperable. When she had recovered from anesthesia, one of her relatives told her the truth about her illness. Within the next hour the woman went into cardiovascular shock and died after a few hours.

This story, however, does not testify for nonspecific effects. Before diagnosing such a mysterious "placebo" death, every rational doctor must first rule out the most likely causes: postoperative complications, such as bleeding or pulmonary embolism. These are frequent hazards after operations and in cancer patients.

Many such uncritical placebo anecdotes, although impressive, come to nothing when they are looked at a little closer [21].

Misquotation

A particular problem of placebo literature seems to be that of misquotations. An example is Beecher's claim that in a study of antitussive agents [15] there was a placebo effect in 36% of 22 patients and in 43% of another 22 patients. However, the actual result was that under *none* of the placebo administrations could any significant change be demonstrated. Besides, there were not 22 placebo-treated patients (the groups were much smaller), and there were no reports about any 36% or 43% of patients. Thus, Beecher's quotation was wrong (which is amazing, as Beecher himself had been one of the authors of the original publication).

Beecher misquoted 10 of the 15 trials listed in "The Powerful Placebo." He sometimes inflated the percentage or the number of patients, or he cited as a percentage of patients what in the original publications is referred to as something completely different, such as the number of pills given, the percentage of days treated, the amount of gas applied in an experimental setting, or the frequency of coughs after irritating a patient [21]. The main effects of these errors were false inflations of the alleged placebo effect. A multitude of misquotations can also be found in other placebo literature [21].

False Assumptions of Toxic Placebo Effects

Beecher did not only write about "real therapeutic effects" of placebo administration; he also wrote about "toxic and other side-effects of placebos." He states that in various trials there had been 35 different toxic effects of placebos such as dry mouth, nausea, headache, drowsiness, warm glow, fatigue, and sleep. The frequency ranged from 8% to 50%. For this, Beecher did not quote any references.

When judging toxic placebo effects one needs to take into account the studies by Green [57] and by Reidenberg et al. [58]. They demonstrated that many people experience *everyday symptoms* such as dry mouth, headache, drowsiness, fatigue, etc. The frequency of these symptoms is similar to the frequency of Beecher's so-called placebo side-effects. Therefore, it is very likely that these everyday symptoms are documented in a trial situation and are then misinterpreted as "side-effects" of the placebos.

With respect to "toxic placebo effects," one always has to consider the possibility of misquotations. In one of the publications in Beecher's trial list, the authors [13] reported an impressive finding that 61% of the placebo patients in a streptomycin trial showed the specific toxic effects of streptomycin, including high-tone and low-tone hearing loss, eosinophilia, and impairment of urea clearance. This remarkable placebo toxicity has been passed on in the medical literature. However, going back to the original publication [56] one will find that *none* of the patients in the streptomycin trial ever received a placebo.

Finally, symptoms are called "side effects" of placebo treatment, only because they do not disappear or because they get worse [21]. For example, in a trial on chronic pain, 13% of the patients in the placebo group improved, and 20% deteriorated. While the improvement was interpreted as a therapeutic placebo effect, the deterioration was interpreted as a *toxic* placebo effect [19,59].

Discussion

Beecher's "The Powerful Placebo," published in 1955, has been a seminal and most influential paper. It is still the most frequently cited placebo reference. This is amazing, as none of the original trials cited by Beecher gave grounds to assume the existence of placebo effects. The reanalysis of a similar classic German placebo survey [17] gave the same results. No placebo effects could be found [21].

The conceptual and methodological mistakes of Beecher's classic paper are still prevalent today. Although some modern experimental placebo research is of better methodological quality, a valid demonstration of therapeutic placebo effects still appears lacking. Having analyzed a total of 800 articles on placebo, we have not found any reliable demonstration of the existence of placebo effects. (In bronchial asthma, effects of suggestion are documented under experimental conditions. This, however, does not imply the existence of an efficacious placebo therapy of bronchial asthma [22].)

Comparing placebo-treated and untreated patients might be a valid method for investigating placebo effects. (In one of the trials [5] in Beecher's list, there was an untreated control group; it showed the same result as the placebo group.) As these trials, however, do not control for factors such as answers of politeness, experimental subordination, and additional treatment they can create false positive results. For instance, Ernst and Resch [60] systematically collected trials that included both a placebo-treated and an untreated group. They found four trials that showed superior outcomes in the placebo groups. The best trials were two 5-arm randomized trials on ultrasound treatment of postoperative swelling. As there were better results in the placebo group (i.e., turned off ultrasound apparatus) than in the untreated groups [61,62], the results were categorized as "true" and "substantial" placebo effects [60]. However, in the placebo groups, a coupling cream was also applied, the humidity and cooling effect of which possibly reduced the postoperative swelling. Consequently, the existence of a placebo effect is questionable in these trials, too. A possibility to do placebo research lies within balanced study designs [63,64] (2 × 2 factorial designs: verum vs. placebo, strong vs. weak suggestion of efficacy). However, variations of outcome do not indicate true therapeutic placebo effects as long as experimental subordination has not been ruled out [37].

There can be no doubt that the extent and frequency of placebo effects as published in most of the literature are gross exaggerations. Some placebo experts have had some awareness of these issues. For example, Shapiro and Shapiro [65] wrote: "In our opinion, the belief that placebos and psychological factors have a specific and clinically meaningful effect on physical illness is not supported by a critical, data-oriented review of the literature." Even more drastically, Roberts [35] said: "The so-called placebo effect is a myth born of misperception, misunderstanding, mystery and hope." However, these comments remained isolated even in the Shapiros' and Roberts' own publications.

Undoubtedly, psychosomatic effects exist. Hence, clear differentiation between placebo and non-placebo components in therapeutical settings [22] is essential for valid placebo research and for research in complementary medicine. Many factors and phenomena have been summed up under the terms "placebo" and "placebo effect," without being *placebos* or *effects* of placebo administrations. Those factors and phenomena were taken as evidence of "true therapeutic placebo effects," although they are not. Thus, the Powerful Placebo turns out to be a fiction.

One might consider substituting the term "placebo effect" by the term "non-specific effects." Changing of words, however, does not change the situation that the existence of therapeutic effects of placebo administration seems questionable. Besides, as Peek [66] and Grünbaum [67] have already pointed out, there is no such thing as "non-specific effects." The term is a *contradictio in adjecto*: a contradiction in itself.

Finally, these factors that can create false impressions of placebo effects might seem to be compelling reasons for randomization and blinding. However, analyses indicate that these factors are not necessarily distributed equally in drug and control groups, thus challenging the validity of randomized double-blind trials [37,68–70]. This issue needs further investigation.

REFERENCES

1. Beecher HK. The powerful placebo. **J Am Med Assoc** 1955;159: 1602–1606.
2. Diehl HS. Medicinal treatment of the common cold. **J Am Med Assoc** 1933;101:2042–2049.
3. Evans W, Hoyle C. The comparative value of drugs used in the continuous treatment of angina pectoris. **Quart J Med** 1933;2:311–338.
4. Jellinek EM. Clinical tests on comparative effectiveness of analgesic drugs. **Biometrics Bull** 1946;2:87–91.
5. Gay LN, Carliner PE. The prevention and treatment of motion sickness. I. Seasickness. **Bull Johns Hopkins Hosp** 1949;84:470–487.
6. Travell J, Rinzler SH, Bakst H, Benjamin ZH, Bobb A. Comparison of effects of alpha-tocopherol and a matching placebo on chest pain in patients with heart disease. **Ann New York Acad Sci** 1949;52:345–353.
7. Greiner T, Gold H, Cattell M, *et al.* A method for the evaluation of the effects of drugs on cardiac pain in patients with angina of effort; a study of khellin (visammin). **Am J Med** 1950;9:143–155.
8. Keats AS, Beecher HK. Pain relief with hypnotic doses of barbiturates and a hypothesis. **J Pharmacol Exp Ther** 1950;100:1–13.
9. Keats AS, D'Alessandro GL, Beecher HK. A controlled study of pain relief by intravenous procaine. **J Am Med Assoc** 1951;147:1761–1763.
10. Beecher HK, Deffer PA, Fink FE, Sullivan DB. Field use of methadone and levo-iso-methadone in a combat zone (Hamhung-Hungnam, North Korea). **U S Armed Forces Med J** 1951;2:1269–1276.
11. Hillis BR. The assessment of cough-suppressing drugs. **Lancet** 1952;259(6721):1230–1235.
12. Beecher HK, Keats AS, Mosteller F, Lasagna L. The effectiveness of oral analgesics (morphine, codeine, acetylsalicylic acid) and the problem of placebo "reactors" and "non-reactors." **J Pharmacol Exp Ther** 1953;109:393–400.
13. Wolf S, Pinsky RH. Effects of placebo administration and the occurrence of toxic reactions. **J Am Med Assoc** 1954;155:339–341.
14. Lasagna L, Mosteller F, von Felsinger JM, Beecher HK. A study of the placebo response. **Am J Med** 1954;16:770–779.
15. Gravenstein JS, Devloo RA, Beecher HK. Effect of antitussive agents on experimental and pathological cough in man. **J Appl Physiol** 1954;7: 119–139.
16. Lasagna L, von Felsinger JM, Beecher HK. Drug-induced mood changes in man. 1. Observations on healthy subjects, chronically ill patients, and "postaddicts." **J Am Med Assoc** 1955;157:1006–1020.
17. Netter P, Classen W, Feingold E. Das Placeboproblem. In: Dölle W, Müller-Oerlinghausen B, Schwabe U, Eds. **Grundlagen der Arzneimitteltherapie–Entwicklung, Beurteilung und Anwendung von Arzneimitteln.** Mannheim, Wien, Zürich: Wissenschaftsverlag; 1986: 355–366.
18. Roberts AH, Kewman DG, Mercier L, Hovell M. The power of nonspecific effects in healing: Implications for psychosocial and biological treatments. **Clin Psychol Rev** 1993;13:375–391.
19. Turner JA, Deyo RA, Loeser JD, Von Korff M, Fordyce WE. The importance of placebo effects in pain treatment and research. **J Am Med Assoc** 1994;271:1609–1614.
20. Bodem SH. Bedeutung der Placebowirkung in der praktischen Arzneitherapie. **Pharm Ztg** 1994;139(51/52):9–19.
21. Kienle GS. **Der *sogenannte* Placeboeffekt; Illusion, Fakten, Realität.** Stuttgart: Schattauer Verlag GmbH; 1995.
22. Kienle GS, Kiene H. Placebo effect and placebo concept: A critical methodological and conceptual analysis of reports on the magnitude of the placebo effect. **Altern Ther Health Med** 1996;2(6):39–54. [Reprint from: Kienle GS, Kiene H. Placeboeffekt und Placebokonzept—eine kritische methodologische und konzeptionelle Analyse von Angaben zum Ausmaß des Placeboeffekts. **Forsch Komplementärmed** 1996;3:121–138.]
23. White L, Tursky B, Schwartz GE, Eds. **Placebo—Theory, Research, and Mechanisms.** New York, London: Guilford Press; 1985.
24. Hornung J. Was ist ein Placebo? Die Bedeutung einer korrekten Definition für die klinische Forschung. **Forsch Komplementärmed** 1994;1:160–165.
25. Gøtzsche PC. Is there logic in the placebo? **Lancet** 1994;344:925–926.
26. Whitney CW, Von Korff M. Regression to the mean in treated versus untreated chronic pain. **Pain** 1992;50:281–285.
27. Deyo RA. Practice variations, treatment fads, rising disability. **Spine** 1993;18:2153–2162.
28. LeRoy GV. The effectiveness of the xanthine drugs in the treatment of angina pectoris. **J Am Med Assoc** 1941;116:921–925.
29. Dyken M, White PT. Evaluation of cortisone in the treatment of cerebral infarction. **J Am Med Assoc** 1956;162:1531–1534.

30. McDonald C, Mazzuca S, McCabe G Jr. How much of the placebo 'effect' is really statistical regression? **Stat Med** 1983;2:417–427.

31. Lichstein J, DeCosta Mayer J, Hauch EW. Efficacy of methantheline (banthine) bromide in therapy of the unstable colon. **J Am Med Assoc** 1955;158:634–637.

32. Wells RE. Use of reserpine (Serpasil) in the management of chronic alcoholism. **J Am Med Assoc** 1957;163:426–429.

33. Blomberg LH. Treatment of disseminated sclerosis with active and inactive drugs. **Lancet** 1957;1:431–432.

34. Coe WS, Best MM, Kinsman JM. Veratrum viride in the treatment of hypertensive vascular disease. **J Am Med Assoc** 1950;143:5–7.

35. Roberts AH. The powerful placebo revisited: The magnitude of nonspecific effects. **Mind/Body Medicine** 1995;(March):1–10.

36. Sackett DL. Randomized trials in individual patients. In: Antes G, Edler L, Holle R, Köpcke W, Lorenz R, Windeler J, Eds. **Biometrie und unkonventionelle Medizin.** Münster–Hiltrup: Landwirtschaftsverlag GmbH; 1995: pp. 19–33.

37. Kiene H. A critique of the double-blind clinical trial. Parts 1 & 2. **Altern Ther Health Med** 1996;2(1):74–80 and 1996;2(2):59–64. [Reprint from: Kiene H. **Kritik der klinischen Doppelblindstudie. MMW-Taschenbuch.** München: MMW Medizin;1993: 35.]

38. Barber TX. The effects of "hypnosis" on pain. **Psychosom Med** 1963;25: 303–333.

39. Clark WC. Sensory-decision theory analysis of the effect on the criterion for pain and thermal sensitivity. **J Abnorm Psychol** 1969; 74:363–371.

40. Fordyce WE, Lansky D, Calsyn DA, et al. Pain measurement and pain behavior. **Pain** 1984;18:53–69.

41. Tedeschi JT, Schlenker BR, Bonoma TV. Cognitive dissonance: Private ratiocination or public spectacle? **Amer Psychol** 1971;26:685–695.

42. Ader R. Conditioned immunopharmacological effects in animals: Implications for a conditioning model of pharmacotherapy. In: White L, Tursky B, Schwartz GE, Eds. **Placebo—Theory, Research, and Mechanisms.** New York: Guilford Press; 1985.

43. Peck C, Coleman G. Implications of placebo theory for clinical research and practice in pain management. **Theor Med** 1991;12: 247–270.

44. Voudouris NJ, Peck CL, Coleman G. The role of conditioning and verbal expectancy in the placebo response. **Pain** 1990;43:121–128.

45. Wall PD. Pain and the placebo response. **Ciba Found Symp** 1993;174:187–211.

46. Wickramasekera I. A conditioned response model of the placebo effect: Predictions from the model. In: White L, Tursky B, Schwartz GE, Eds. **Placebo—Theory, Research, and Mechanisms.** New York: Guilford Press; 1985.

47. Suchman AL, Ader R. Classic conditioning and placebo effects in crossover studies. **Clin Pharmacol Ther** 1992;52:372–377.

48. Iacono P, Drici MD, De Lunardo C, Salimbeni B, Lapalus P. Placebo effect in cardiovascular clinical pharmacology. **Int J Clin Pharmacol Res** 1992;12(2):53–56.

49. Mancia G, Omboni S, Parati G, et al. Lack of placebo effect on ambulatory blood pressure. **Am J Health** 1995;8:311–315.

50. Weber MA, Neutel JM, Smith DHG. Controlling blood pressure throughout the day: Issues in testing a new anti-hypertensive agent. **J Hum Hypertens** 1995;9(Suppl.5):S29–S35.

51. Report of Medical Research Council Working Party on Mild to Moderate Hypertension. Randomised controlled trial of treatment for mild hypertension: Design and pilot trial. **Br Med J** 1977;1:1437–1440.

52. Schindel L. Placebo und Placebo-Effekte in Klinik und Forschung. **Arzneimittelforschung** 1967;17:892–918.

53. Beecher HK. Die Placebowirkung als unspezifischer Wirkungsfaktor im Bereich der Krankheit und der Krankenbehandlung. In: Gross F, Beecher HK, Eds. **Placebo—das universelle Medikament? Paul-Martini-Stiftung der Medizinisch Pharmazeutischen Studiengesellschaft e.V.** Mainz: Eggebrecht-Presse; 1984.

54. Wolf S. The pharmacology of placebos. **Pharmacol Rev** 1959;11: 689–704.

55. Hollister L. Placebology: Sense and nonsense. **Curr Ther Res** 1960;2: 477–483.

56. Veterans Administration. Minutes of the Fifth Streptomycin Conference; Knickerbocker Hotel, Chicago, Illinois; April 15–18, 1948.

57. Green DM. Pre-existing conditions, placebo reactions, and "side effects." **Ann Intern Med** 1964;60:255–265.

58. Reidenberg MM, Lowenthal DT. Adverse nondrug reactions. **N Engl J Med** 1968;279:678–679.

59. Long DM, Uematsu S, Kouba RB. Placebo responses to medical device therapy for pain. **Stereotact Funct Neurosurg** 1989;53:149–156.

60. Ernst E, Resch KI. Concept of true and perceived placebo effects. **Br Med J** 1995;311:551–553.

61. Ho KH, Hashish I, Salmon P, Freeman R, Harvey W. Reduction of post-operative swelling by a placebo effect. **J Psychosom Res** 1988;32: 197–205.

62. Hashish I, Harvey W, Harris M. Anti-inflammatory effects of ultrasound therapy: Evidence for a major placebo effect. **Br J Rheumatol** 1986;25: 77–81.

63. Ross S, Krugman A, Lyerly S, Clyde D. Drugs and placebos: A model design. **Psychol Rep** 1962;10:382–392.

64. Marlatt A, Rohsenow D. Cognitive processes in alcohol use: Expectancy and the balanced placebo design. **Adv Subst Abuse** 1980;1: 159–199.

65. Shapiro AK, Shapiro E. Patient-provider relationships and the placebo effect. In: Matarazzo JD, Weiss SM, Herd JA, Miller NE, Eds. **Behavioral Health: A Handbook of Health Enhancement and Disease Prevention.** New York: Wiley-Interscience; 1984: 371–383.

66. Peek CJ. A critical look at the theory of placebo. **Biofeedback Self-Regul** 1977;2:327–335.

67. Grünbaum A. Explications and implications of the placebo concept. In: White L, Tursky B, Schwartz GE, Eds. **Placebo—Theory, Research, and Mechanisms.** New York: Guilford Press; 1985.

68. Kirsch I, Weixel LJ. Double blind versus deceptive administration of a placebo. **Behav Neurosci** 1988;102:319–323.

69. Hornung J. Zur Problematik der Doppelblindstudien. **Therapeutikon** 1989;3:696–701.

70. Kirsch I, Rosadino MJ. Do double-blind studies with informed consent yield externally valid results? **Psychopharmacology** 1993;110:437–442.

5

Is the Placebo Powerless?

An Analysis of Clinical Trials Comparing Placebo with No Treatment

Asbjørn Hróbjartsson and Peter C. Gøtzsche

Asbjørn Hróbjartsson and Peter C. Gøtzsche, "Is the Placebo Powerless? An Analysis of Clinical Trials Comparing Placebo with No Treatment," *New England Journal of Medicine* 2001;344:1594–1602.

Placebos have been reported to improve subjective and objective outcomes in up to 30 to 40 percent of patients with a wide range of clinical conditions, such as pain, asthma, high blood pressure, and even myocardial infarction.[1,2,3] In his 1955 article "The Powerful Placebo," Beecher concluded, "It is evident that placebos have a high degree of therapeutic effectiveness in treating subjective responses, decided improvement, interpreted under the unknowns technique as a real therapeutic effect, being produced in 35.2±2.2% of cases."[1]

Beecher's article and the 35 percent figure are often cited as evidence that a placebo can be an important medical treatment. The vast majority of reports on placebos, including Beecher's article, have estimated the effect of placebo as the difference from base line in the condition of patients in the placebo group of a randomized trial after treatment. With this approach, the effect of placebo cannot be distinguished from the natural course of the disease, regression to the mean, and the effects of other factors.[4-6] The reported large effects of placebo could therefore, at least in part, be artifacts of inadequate research methods.

Despite the reservations of many physicians,[7] the clinical use of placebo has been advocated in editorials and articles in leading journals.[3,8,9] To understand better the effects of placebo as a treatment, we conducted a systematic review of clinical trials in which patients with various clinical conditions were randomly assigned to placebo or to no treatment. We were primarily interested in the clinical effect of placebo as a treatment for disease, rather than the role of placebo as a comparison treatment in clinical trials. A secondary aim was to study whether the effect of placebo differed for subjective and objective outcomes.

Methods

Definition of Placebo

Placebo is difficult to define satisfactorily.[5] In clinical trials, placebos are generally control treatments with a similar appearance to the study treatments but without their specific activity. We therefore defined placebo practically as an intervention labeled as such in the report of a clinical trial.

Literature Search

We searched Medline, EMBASE, PsycLIT, Biological Abstracts, and the Cochrane Controlled Trials Register for trials published before the end of 1998. The search was developed iteratively for synonyms of "placebo," "no treatment," and "randomized clinical trial" (the exact search strategy is available as Supplementary Appendix 1 with the full text of this article at http://www.nejm.org and was based on a published protocol[10]). We systematically read the reference lists of included trials and selected books and review articles. We also asked researchers in the field to provide lists of relevant trials.

Selection of Studies

We included studies if patients were assigned randomly to a placebo group or an untreated group (often there was also a third group that received active treatment). We excluded studies if randomization was clearly not concealed—that is, if group assignment were predictable[11] (e.g., patients were assigned to treatment groups according to the day of the month). We also excluded studies if participants were paid or were healthy volunteers, if the person who assessed objective outcomes was aware of group assignments, if the dropout rate exceeded 50 percent, or if it was very likely that the alleged placebo had a clinical effect not associated with the treatment ritual alone (e.g., movement techniques for postoperative pain). All potentially eligible trial reports were read in full by both authors. Disagreements concerning eligibility were resolved by discussion.

Extraction of Data

Data were extracted from the report of each trial with the use of forms tested in pilot studies. We contacted the authors of the included studies when reported outcome data were inadequate for meta-analysis. We noted how the randomization was conducted and whether the therapist responsible for the administration of placebo (as distinct from the observer) was unaware of group assignments. Furthermore, we noted the purpose of the trial, the dropout rate, whether the placebo was given in addition to the standard treatment, and whether the main outcome was clearly indicated.

We noted whether the placebo was pharmacologic (e.g., a tablet), physical (e.g., a manipulation), or psychological (e.g., a conversation); whether clinical problems reported by the patients could have been observed by others (i.e., whether the symptoms were observable outcomes such as cough); and whether objective outcomes were laboratory data, were derived from examinations that required the cooperation of the patients (i.e., objective outcomes such as forced expiratory volume), or did not require such cooperation (e.g., edema).

Both reviewers independently selected outcomes by referring only to the methods sections of articles; any disagreements were resolved by discussion. As the primary outcome, we selected the main objective or subjective outcome of each trial (preferably a characteristic symptom). If a main outcome was not indicated, we used the outcome that we felt was most relevant to patients. Binary outcomes (e.g., the proportions of smokers and nonsmokers) were preferred to continuous ones (e.g., the mean number of cigarettes smoked). Data recorded immediately after the end of treatment were preferred to follow-up data, although end-of-treatment data were not always available. For crossover trials, we extracted data from the first treatment period only; if that was not possible, we used the summary data as if they had been derived from a parallel-group trial (i.e., using the between-group standard deviations and total number of participants for both groups).

Synthesis of Data

For each trial with binary outcomes, we calculated the relative risk of an unwanted outcome, defined as the ratio of the number of patients with an unwanted outcome to the total number of patients in the placebo group, divided by the same ratio in the untreated group. Thus, a relative risk below 1.0 indicates a beneficial effect of placebo.

For trials with continuous outcomes, we calculated the standardized mean difference, which was defined as the difference between the mean value for an unwanted outcome in the placebo group and the corresponding mean value in the untreated group divided by the pooled standard deviation.[12] A value of −1 signifies that the mean in the placebo group was 1 SD below the mean in the untreated group, indicating a beneficial effect of placebo.

We calculated the pooled relative risk of an unwanted outcome for trials with binary outcomes and the pooled standardized mean difference for those with continuous outcomes.[13] Because of the different clinical conditions and settings, we expected that the data sets would be heterogeneous—that is, that the effects of individual trials would vary more than expected by chance alone. The variance and statistical significance of the differences were therefore assessed with the use of random-effect calculations.[13] We calculated the pooled effects for subjective and objective outcomes and for specific clinical problems that had been investigated in at least three trials by different research groups.[14]

We performed preplanned analyses of subgroups to see whether our findings were sensitive to the type of placebo or the type of outcome involved. Furthermore, for each trial, we plotted the effect against the inverse of its standard error (which increases with the number of trial participants). Since the variation in the estimated effect decreases with increasing sample size, the plot is expected to resemble a symmetrical funnel. If there is significant asymmetry in such funnel plots, it is usually caused by small trials' reporting greater effects, on average, than large trials, which can reflect publication bias[15] or other biases. We also performed several preplanned sensitivity analyses to determine whether our findings were sensitive to variations in the quality of the trials.

In trials with continuous outcomes, we used F tests to check whether the standard deviations of the placebo group and the untreated group were significantly different.[16] We regarded the distributions of either group as non-Gaussian if 1.64 SD exceeded the mean for positive outcomes.[17] Chi-square tests were used to test for heterogeneity on the basis of the DerSimonian and Laird Q statistic.[13,18] Results are reported with 95 percent confidence intervals. All P values are two-tailed.

Results

Selection and Characteristics of Studies

We identified 727 potentially eligible trials. We subsequently excluded 597 trials for the following reasons: 404 were nonclinical or nonrandomized, 129 were missing a placebo group or an untreated group, 29 were reported in more than one publication, 11 had clearly unblinded assessment of objective outcomes, and 24 met other criteria for exclusion, such as dropout rates over 50 percent. No relevant outcome data were available for 16 of the remaining 130 trials. The analysis therefore included 114 trials.[19–132]

There were 10 crossover trials, of which 7 (which included a total of 182 patients) were handled as parallel trials. In 112 trials, there was a third group assigned to active treatment in addition to the placebo and the untreated groups. In 88 of these, determining the effect of placebo was not mentioned as an objective of the study. The trial reports were published in five languages between 1946 and 1998. The outcomes were binary in 32 trials[19–50] and continuous in 82.[51–132] In 76 trials, the outcome in the data we extracted was identified as a main outcome by the authors of the trials. If only patients in the placebo and untreated groups were counted, the trials with binary outcomes included 3795 patients with a median of 51 patients per trial (interquartile range, 26 to 72), and the trials with continuous outcomes included 4730 patients with a median of 27 patients per trial (interquartile range, 20 to 52).

The typical pharmacologic placebo was a lactose tablet. The typical physical placebo was a procedure performed with a machine that was turned off (e.g., sham transcutaneous electrical nerve stimulation). The typical psychological placebo was a nondirectional, neutral discussion between the patient and the treatment provider, referred to as an "attention placebo." No treatment typically entailed observation only or standard therapy; in the latter case, all patients in the trial received standard therapy, and the placebo was additional.

The results for the individual trials are available as Supplementary Appendix 2 and Supplementary Appendix 3 with the full text of this article at http://www.nejm.org. The trials investigated 40 clinical conditions: hypertension, asthma, anemia, hyperglycemia, hypercholesterolemia, seasickness, Raynaud's disease, alcohol abuse, smoking, obesity, poor oral hygiene, herpes simplex infection, bacterial infection, common cold, pain, nausea, ileus, infertility, cervical dilatation, labor, menopause, prostatism, depression, schizophrenia, insomnia, anxiety, phobia, compulsive nail biting, mental handicap, marital discord, stress related to dental treatment, orgasmic difficulties, fecal soiling, enuresis, epilepsy, Parkinson's disease, Alzheimer's disease, attention-deficit–hyperactivity disorder, carpal tunnel syndrome, and undiagnosed ailments.

Binary Outcomes

As compared with no treatment, placebo did not have a significant effect on binary outcomes (overall pooled relative risk of an unwanted outcome with placebo, 0.95; 95 percent confidence interval, 0.88 to 1.02). The pooled relative risk was 0.95 for trials with subjective outcomes (95 percent confidence interval, 0.86 to 1.05) and 0.91 for trials with objective outcomes (95 percent confidence interval, 0.80 to 1.04) (Table 5.1).

There was significant heterogeneity among the trials with binary outcomes (P = 0.003), indicating that the variation in the effect of placebo among trials was larger than would be

Table 5.1.

Effect of placebo in trials with binary or continuous outcomes*

Outcome	No. of Participants	No. of Trials	Pooled Relative Risk (95% CI)[†]
Binary			
Overall	3795	32	0.95 (0.88 to 1.02)
Subjective	1928	23	0.95 (0.86 to 1.05)
Objective	1867	9	0.91 (0.80 to 1.04)
			Pooled Standardized Mean Difference (95% CI)[‡]
Continuous			
Overall	4730	82	−0.28 (−0.38 to −0.19)
Subjective	3081	53	−0.36 (−0.47 to −0.25)
Objective	1649	29	−0.12 (−0.27 to 0.03)

* CI denotes confidence interval.

[†] The relative risk was defined as the ratio of the number of patients with an unwanted outcome to the total number of patients in the placebo group, divided by the same ratio in the untreated group. A value below 1.0 indicates a beneficial effect of placebo.

[‡] The standardized mean difference was defined as the difference between the mean values for unwanted outcomes in the placebo and untreated groups divided by the pooled standard deviation. A negative value indicates a beneficial effect of placebo.

Table 5.2.

Effect of placebo on specific clinical problems*

Outcome	No. of Participants	No. of Trials	Pooled Relative Risk (95% CI)[†]
Binary			
Nausea	182	3	0.94 (0.77 to 1.16)
Smoking	887	6	0.88 (0.71 to 1.09)
Depression	152	3	1.03 (0.78 to 1.34)
			Pooled Standardized Mean Difference (95% CI)[‡]
Continuous			
Pain	1602	27	−0.27 (−0.40 to −0.15)
Obesity	128	5	−0.40 (−0.92 to 0.12)
Asthma	81	3	−0.34 (−0.83 to 0.14)
Hypertension	129	7	−0.32 (−0.78 to 0.13)
Insomnia	100	5	−0.26 (−0.66 to 0.13)
Anxiety	257	6	−0.06 (−0.31 to 0.18)

* Only problems addressed by at least three trials are included. CI denotes confidence interval.

[†] The relative risk was defined as the ratio of the number of patients with an unwanted outcome to the total number of patients in the placebo group, divided by the same ratio in the untreated group. A value below 1.0 indicates a beneficial effect of placebo.

[‡] The standardized mean difference was defined as the difference between the mean values for unwanted outcomes in the placebo and untreated groups divided by the pooled standard deviation. A negative value indicates a beneficial effect of placebo.

expected to result from chance alone. The heterogeneity was not due to small trials' showing more pronounced effects of placebo than large trials (P = 0.56).[15]

Three clinical problems had been investigated in at least three independent trials with binary outcomes: nausea, relapse after the cessation of smoking, and depression. Placebo had no significant effect on these outcomes, but the confidence intervals were wide (Table 5.2).

Continuous Outcomes

The overall pooled standardized mean difference was −0.28 (95 percent confidence interval, −0.38 to −0.19). Thus, there was a beneficial effect of placebo, because the pooled mean of the placebo groups was 0.28 SD lower than the pooled mean of the untreated groups (P < 0.001). The pooled standardized mean difference was significant for trials with subjective outcomes (−0.36; 95 percent confidence interval, −0.47 to −0.25) but not for trials with objective outcomes (−0.12; 95 percent confidence interval, −0.27 to 0.03) (Table 5.1).

There was significant heterogeneity among the trials with continuous outcomes (P<0.001). The magnitude of the effect of placebo decreased with increasing sample size (P = 0.05), indicating a possible bias related to the effects of small trials.

Pain, obesity, asthma, hypertension, insomnia, and anxiety were each investigated in at least three independent trials. Only the 27 trials involving the treatment of pain (including a total of 1602 patients) showed a significant effect of placebo as compared with no treatment (pooled standardized mean difference, −0.27; 95 percent confidence interval, −0.40 to −0.15). There was no significant effect of placebo on

the other conditions, although the confidence intervals were wide (Table 5.2).

Expressing the standardized mean differences in terms of clinical outcomes indicates that the effect of placebo on pain corresponds to a reduction in the mean intensity of pain of 6.5 mm (95 percent confidence interval, 3.6 to 9.6) on a 100-mm visual-analogue scale. The nonsignificant effect of placebo on obesity corresponds to a reduction in mean weight of 3.2 percent (95 percent confidence interval, 7.4 to −1.2 percent); on hypertension, a reduction in mean diastolic blood pressure of 3.2 mm Hg (95 percent confidence interval, 7.8 to −1.3); and on insomnia, a decrease in the mean time required to fall asleep of 10 minutes (95 percent confidence interval, 25 to −5). For asthma and anxiety, the measurement scales were too variable to allow clinical interpretation of the results.

Small trials involving the treatment of pain did not have significantly greater effects than large trials (P = 0.20), but the power of the test was low.[15] There was no significant heterogeneity among the nine sets of data on specific clinical problems (P > 0.10), but the power of these analyses was also low.

Sensitivity Analyses

The number of trials compared in the sensitivity analyses was in most cases nine or more, and they included more than 1000 patients. There was no difference in the effect of placebo between subcategories of objective and subjective binary outcomes (Table 5.3). The effect of placebo among

Table 5.3.
Effect of placebo in trials with specific types of outcomes*

Outcome	No. of Participants	No. of Trials	Pooled Relative Risk (95% CI)[†]
Binary			
Laboratory data	1423	4	0.92 (0.73 to 1.17)
Objective, not involving patient's cooperation	320	2	0.89 (0.66 to 1.20)
Objective, involving patient's cooperation	124	3	0.84 (0.52 to 1.36)
Subjective and observable	586	15	0.93 (0.77 to 1.11)
Subjective and nonobservable	1342	8	0.97 (0.89 to 1.07)
			Pooled Standardized Mean Difference (95% CI)[‡]
Continuous			
Laboratory data	649	4	0.18 (0.02 to 0.33)
Objective, not involving patient's cooperation	641	15	−0.25 (−0.50 to −0.01)
Objective, involving patient's cooperation	359	10	−0.21 (−0.44 to 0.02)
Subjective and observable	958	13	−0.41 (−0.61 to −0.20)
Subjective and nonobservable	2123	40	−0.35 (−0.48 to −0.22)
Subjective and nonobservable with pain excluded[§]	521	13	−0.55 (−0.87 to −0.23)

* Observable outcomes were clinical problems reported by the patients that could have been observed by others (e.g., cough). CI denotes confidence interval.
[†] The relative risk was defined as the ratio of the number of patients with an unwanted outcome to the total number of patients in the placebo group, divided by the same ratio in the untreated group. A value below 1.0 indicates a beneficial effect of placebo.
[‡] The standardized mean difference was defined as the difference between the mean values for unwanted outcomes in the placebo and untreated groups divided by the pooled standard deviation. A negative value indicates a beneficial effect of placebo.
[§] The 27 trials involving the treatment of pain comprised 72 percent of the information in the analysis of subjective and nonobservable continuous outcomes; therefore, an unplanned calculation excluding these trials was performed.

subcategories of continuous outcomes did not differ significantly, except for a negative effect of placebo in four trials with laboratory data[66,67,75,76] (Table 5.3). For both continuous and binary outcomes, there were no significant differences among the various types of placebos (Table 5.4).

The effect of placebo on continuous or binary outcomes was not influenced by the dropout rate (≤ 15 percent vs. > 15

Table 5.4.
Effect of three types of placebo*

Outcome	No. of Participants	No. of Trials	Pooled Relative Risk (95% CI)[†]
Binary			
Pharmacologic	3099	21	0.97 (0.88 to 1.07)
Physical	479	4	0.94 (0.83 to 1.08)
Psychological	217	7	0.88 (0.72 to 1.08)
			Pooled Standardized Mean Difference (95% CI)[‡]
Continuous			
Pharmacologic	2363	24	−0.20 (−0.37 to −0.04)
Physical	1378	22	−0.31 (−0.50 to −0.13)
Psychological	989	36	−0.34 (−0.49 to −0.19)

* CI denotes confidence interval.
[†] The relative risk was defined as the ratio of the number of patients with an unwanted outcome to the total number of patients in the placebo group, divided by the same ratio in the untreated group. A value below 1.0 indicates a beneficial effect of placebo.
[‡] The standardized mean difference was defined as the difference between the mean values for unwanted outcomes in the placebo and untreated groups, divided by the pooled standard deviation. A negative value indicates a beneficial effect of placebo.

percent) or by whether the observers were aware of group assignments, but only two trials with binary objective outcomes (involving 316 patients) included observers who were clearly unaware of the group assignments[39,40] (data not shown). The effects of placebo were also unrelated to whether the care providers were unaware of the treatment type (placebo or experimental), whether placebos were given in addition to standard treatments, whether the effect of placebo was an explicit research objective, or whether we had identified the main outcome on the basis of clinical relevance (data not shown). The size of the effect in trials with clearly concealed randomization did not differ from that in other trials, but only four trials with continuous outcomes[84,95,97,107] (involving 523 patients) and one with binary outcomes[40] (involving 54 patients) reported clearly concealed randomization (data not shown). For continuous outcomes, the effect was not influenced by non-Gaussian distributions in the placebo or the untreated groups (data not shown).

Discussion

We did not detect a significant effect of placebo as compared with no treatment in pooled data from trials with subjective or objective binary or continuous objective outcomes. We did, however, find a significant difference between placebo and no treatment in trials with continuous subjective outcomes and in trials involving the treatment of pain.

Several types of bias may have affected our findings. Blinded evaluation of subjective outcomes was not possible in the trials we reviewed. Patients in an untreated group would know they were not being treated, and patients in a placebo group would think they had received treatment. It is difficult to distinguish between reporting bias and a true effect of placebo on subjective outcomes, since a patient may tend to try to please the investigator and report improvement when none has occurred. The fact that placebos had no significant effect on objective continuous outcomes suggests that reporting bias may have been a factor in the trials with subjective outcomes.

If patients in the untreated groups sought treatment outside the trials more often than patients in the placebo groups, the effects of placebo might be less apparent. Very few trials provided information on concomitant treatment. The risk of bias is expected to be larger in trials in which placebo is the only treatment and is not given in addition to standard therapy. We did not, however, find a difference in effect between the two types of trials.

There was some evidence that placebos had greater effects in small trials with continuous outcomes than in large trials. This could indicate that some small trials with negative outcomes have not been published or that we did not identify them.[15] It is difficult to identify relevant trials in this field; another systematic search for trials involving placebo groups versus untreated groups found only 12 studies.[133] We identified 114 trials from which the outcomes could be extracted, but 88 of these trials investigated the effect of active treatment in a third group of patients and did not explicitly study the effect of placebo. Because the publication of such trials is not directly associated with the effect of placebo, it is unlikely that the existence of unpublished trials could explain the higher effects reported in small studies.

Poor methodology in small trials could also explain the large effects of placebo. It surprised us that we found no association between measures of the quality of a trial and placebo effects. However, the statistical power of our sensitivity analyses may have been too low. Furthermore, it is possible that small trials tended to investigate clinical conditions in which placebos truly had greater effects. Thus, although we found an effect of placebos on subjective continuous outcomes, the inverse relation between trial size and effect size implies that the estimates of pooled effect should be interpreted cautiously.

It can also be difficult to interpret whether a pooled standardized mean difference is large enough to be clinically meaningful. Some individual trials reported clinically relevant effects with standardized mean differences of less than −0.6,[91] but such "outlier" values may be spurious. If the possible biases we have discussed are disregarded, the pooled effect of placebo on pain corresponds to one third of the effect of nonsteroidal anti-inflammatory drugs, as compared with placebo, in double-blind trials.[134] It is uncertain whether such an effect is important for patients.

Our study has other limitations. We did extensive analyses of predefined subgroups according to the type of placebo, disease, and outcome without identifying a subgroup of trials in which the effect of placebo was large. However, we cannot exclude the possibility that, in the pooling of heterogeneous trials, the existence of such a subgroup was obscured. Our conclusions are also limited to the clinical conditions and outcomes that were investigated. It should be noted that few trials reported on the quality of life or patients' well-being.

We reviewed the effect of placebos but not the effect of the patient-provider relationship. We could not rule out a psychological therapeutic effect of this relationship, which may be largely independent of any placebo intervention.[20]

Moreover, the use of placebos in blinded, randomized trials is a precaution directed against many forms of bias and not only a way of controlling for the effects of placebo. Patients who are aware of their treatment assignment may differ from unaware patients in their way of reporting beneficial and harmful effects of treatment, in their tendency to seek additional treatment outside the study, and in their risk of dropping out of the study. Furthermore, staff members who are aware of treatment assignments may differ in their use of alternative forms of care and in their assessment of outcomes. Thus, even if there was no true effect of placebo, one would expect to find differences between placebo and untreated groups because of bias associated with a lack of double-blinding.

We were unable to detect any such significant difference in trials with subjective or objective binary or continuous objective outcomes. This surprising finding can possibly be explained by our selection of trials. Since our goal was to study the clinical effect of placebos, we reduced the influence of observer bias and bias due to dropouts by excluding trials with clearly unblinded objective outcomes and by attempting to analyze post-treatment data instead of follow-up data. In addition, since most trials we included did not primarily address the effect of a placebo but, rather, evaluated that of an active treatment, our study may have underestimated bias associated with the interests of the investigators. Since the design of our review precludes estimation of the overall influence of bias due to a lack of double-blinding, our results do not imply that control groups that receive no treatment can be substituted for control groups that receive placebo without creating a risk of bias. This result is in accordance with an empirical study of 33 meta-analyses, which found that randomized trials that were not double-blinded yielded larger estimates than blinded trials, with odds ratios that were exaggerated by 17 percent.[11]

In conclusion, we found little evidence that placebos in general have powerful clinical effects. Placebos had no significant pooled effect on subjective or objective binary or continuous objective outcomes. We found significant effects of placebo on continuous subjective outcomes and for the treatment of pain but also bias related to larger effects in small trials. The use of placebo outside the aegis of a controlled, properly designed clinical trial cannot be recommended.

REFERENCES

1. Beecher HK. The powerful placebo. JAMA 1955;159:1602–1606.
2. Lasagna L. The placebo effect. J Allergy Clin Immunol 1986;78: 161–165.

3. Brown WA. The placebo effect. Sci Am 1998;278:90–95.

4. Kienle GS, Kiene H. The powerful placebo effect: fact or fiction? J Clin Epidemiol 1997;50:1311–1318.

5. Gøtzsche PC. Is there logic in the placebo? Lancet 1994;344:925–926.

6. Hróbjartsson A. The uncontrollable placebo effect. Eur J Clin Pharmacol 1996;50:345–348.

7. Rawlinson MC. Truth-telling and paternalism in the clinic: philosophical reflections on the use of placebos in medical practice. In: White L, Tursky B, Schwartz GE, eds. Placebo: theory, research, and mechanisms. New York: Guilford Press, 1985:403–418.

8. Oh VMS. The placebo effect: can we use it better? BMJ 1994;309:69–70.

9. Chaput de Saintonge DM, Herxheimer A. Harnessing placebo effects in health care. Lancet 1994;344:995–998.

10. Hróbjartsson A, Gøtzsche PC. Placebo intervention compared with no treatment (protocol for a Cochrane review). In: The Cochrane library. No. 1. Oxford, England: Update Software, 1999 (software).

11. Schulz KF, Chalmers I, Hayes R, Altman DG. Empirical evidence of bias: dimensions of methodological quality associated with estimates of treatment effects in controlled trials. JAMA 1995;273:408–412.

12. Estimation of a single effect size: parametric and nonparametric methods. In: Hedges LV, Olkin I. Statistical methods for meta-analysis. Orlando, Fla.: Academic Press, 1985:75–106.

13. DerSimonian R, Laird N. Meta-analysis in clinical trials. Control Clin Trials 1986;7:177–188.

14. Linde K, Clausius N, Ramirez G, et al. Are the clinical effects of homeopathy placebo effects? A meta-analysis of placebo-controlled trials. Lancet 1997;350:834–843. [Erratum: Lancet 1998;351:220.]

15. Egger M, Davey Smith G, Schneider M, Minder C. Bias in meta-analysis detected by a simple, graphical test. BMJ 1997;315:629–634.

16. Comparing groups—continuous data. In: Altman DG. Practical statistics for medical research. London: Chapman and Hall, 1991:179–228.

17. Cochrane Consumers & Communication Group. Statistical policy. In: The Cochrane library. No. 1. Oxford, England: Update Software, 1999 (software).

18. Comparing groups—categorical data. In: Altman DG. Practical statistics for medical research. London: Chapman and Hall, 1991:229–276.

19. Tyler DB. The influence of a placebo, body position and medication on motion sickness. Am J Physiol 1946;146:458–466.

20. Thomas KB. General practice consultations: is there any point in being positive? BMJ 1987;294:1200–1202.

21. Hutton N, Wilson MH, Mellits D, et al. Effectiveness of an antihistamine-decongestant combination for young children with the common cold: a randomized, controlled clinical trial. J Pediatr 1991;118:125–130.

22. Guglielmi RS, Roberts AH, Patterson R. Skin temperature biofeedback for Raynaud's disease: a double-blind study. Biofeedback Self-Regul 1982;7:99–120.

23. Watzl H, Olbrich R, Rist F, Cohen R. Placebo-Injektionen und Alkoholkontrollen in der stationären Behandlung alkoholkranker Frauen—eine experimentelle Untersuchung Zweier Behandlungsmerkmale. Z Klin Psychol 1986;15:333–345.

24. Wilson A, Davidson WJ, Blanchard R. Disulfiram implantation: a trial using placebo implants and two types of controls. J Stud Alcohol 1980;41:429–436.

25. Killen JD, Fortmann SP, Newman B, Varady A. Evaluation of a treatment approach combining nicotine gum with self-guided behavioral treatments for smoking relapse prevention. J Consult Clin Psychol 1990;58:85–92.

26. Malcolm RE, Sillett RW, Turner JAM, Ball KP. The use of nicotine chewing gum as an aid to stopping smoking. Psychopharmacology (Berl) 1980;70:295–296.

27. Jacobs MA, Spilken AZ, Norman MM, Wohlberg GW, Knapp PH. Interaction of personality and treatment conditions associated with success in a smoking control program. Psychosom Med 1971;33:545–556.

28. Williams JM, Hall DW. Use of single session hypnosis for smoking cessation. Addict Behav 1988;13:205–208.

29. Hyman GJ, Stanley RO, Burrows GD, Horne DJ. Treatment effectiveness of hypnosis and behaviour therapy in smoking cessation: a methodological refinement. Addict Behav 1986;11:355–365.

30. Elliott CH, Denney DR. A multiple-component treatment approach to smoking reduction. J Consult Clin Psychol 1978;46:1330–1339.

31. Faas A, Chavannes AW, van Eijk JTM, Gubbels JW. A randomized, placebo-controlled trial of exercise therapy in patients with acute low back pain. Spine 1993;18:1388–1395.

32. Walton RE, Chiappinelli J. Prophylactic penicillin: effect on posttreatment symptoms following root canal treatment of asymptomatic periapical pathosis. J Endod 1993;19:466–470.

33. McMillan CM. Transcutaneous electrical stimulation of Neiguan anti-emetic acupuncture point in controlling sickness following opioid analgesia in major orthopaedic surgery. Physiotherapy 1994;80:5–9.

34. Najningier B, Patowski W, Zieniewicz K, et al. Zofran w zapobieganiu nudnosciom i wymiotom po cholecystektomii laparoskopowej. Acta Endosc Pol 1997;7:125–128.

35. Dundee JW, Chestnutt WN, Ghaly RG, Lynas AGA. Traditional Chinese acupuncture: a potentially useful antiemetic? BMJ 1986;293:583–584.

36. Adriaanse AH, Kollée LAA, Muytjens HL, et al. Randomized study of vaginal chlorhexidine disinfection during labor to prevent vertical transmission of group B streptococci. Eur J Obstet Gynecol Reprod Biol 1995;61:135–141.

37. Harrison RF, de Louvois J, Blades M, Hurley R. Doxycycline treatment and human infertility. Lancet 1975;1:605–607.

38. Aune A, Alræk T, Huo L, Barheim A. Kan akupunktur forebygge blærekatarr hos kvinner? Tidsskr Nor Laegeforen 1998;118:1370–1372.

39. Heinzl S, Andor J. Preoperative administration of prostaglandin to avoid dilatation-induced damage in first-trimester pregnancy terminations. Gynecol Obstet Invest 1981;12:29–36.

40. Tarrier N, Yusupoff L, Kinney C, et al. Randomised controlled trial of intensive cognitive behaviour therapy for patients with chronic schizophrenia. BMJ 1998;317:303–307.

41. Whittaker CB, Hoy RM. Withdrawal of perphenazine in chronic schizophrenia. Br J Psychiatry 1963;109:422–427.

42. Frank E, Kupfer DJ, Perel JM, et al. Three-year outcomes for maintenance therapies in recurrent depression. Arch Gen Psychiatry 1990;47:1093–1099.

43. Klerman GL, Dimascio A, Weisman M, Prusoff B, Paykel ES. Treatment of depression by drugs and psychotherapy. Am J Psychiatry 1974;131:186–191.

44. Rabkin JG, McGrath PJ, Quitkin FM, et al. Effects of pill-giving on maintenance of placebo response in patients with chronic mild depression. Am J Psychiatry 1990;147:1622–1626.

45. Roughan PA, Kunst L. Do pelvic floor exercises really improve orgasmic potential? J Sex Marital Ther 1981;7:223–229.

46. Berg I, Forsythe I, Holt P, Watts J. A controlled trial of 'Senokot' in faecal soiling treated by behavioral methods. J Child Psychol Psychiatry 1983;24:543–549.

47. Blackman S, Benton AJ, Cove LM. The effect of imipramine on enuresis. Am J Psychiatry 1964;120:1194–1195.

48. Double DB, Warren GC, Evans M, Rowlands RP. Efficacy of maintenance use of anticholinergic agents. Acta Psychiatr Scand 1993;88:381–384.

49. Stransky M, Rubin A, Lava NS, Lazaro RP. Treatment of carpal tunnel syndrome with vitamin B6: a double-blind study. South Med J 1989;82:841–842.

50. Tan S, Bruni J. Cognitive-behavior therapy with adult patients with epilepsy: a controlled outcome study. Epilepsia 1986;27:225–233.

51. Antivalle M, Lattuada S, Salvaggio M, et al. Placebo effect and adaptation to noninvasive monitoring of BP. J Hum Hypertens 1990;4:633–637.

52. Bosley F, Allen TW. Stress management training for hypertensives: cognitive and physiological effects. J Behav Med 1989;12:77–89.

53. Canino E, Cardona R, Monsalve P, et al. A behavioral treatment program as a therapy in the control of primary hypertension. Acta Cient Venez 1994;45:23–30.

54. Frankel BL, Patel DJ, Horwitz D, Friedewald WT, Gaarder KR. Treatment of hypertension with biofeedback and relaxation techniques. Psychosom Med 1978;40:276–293.

55. Rossi A, Ziacchi V, Lomanto B. The hypotensive effect of a single daily dose of labetalol: a preliminary study. Int J Clin Pharmacol Ther Toxicol 1982;20:438–445.

56. Seer P, Raeburn JM. Meditation training and essential hypertension: a methodological study. J Behav Med 1980;3:59–71.

57. Yates RG, Lamping DL, Abram NL, Wright C. Effects of chiropractic treatment on blood pressure and anxiety: a randomized, controlled trial. J Manipulative Physiol Ther 1988;11:484–488.

58. Block J. Effects of rational emotive therapy on overweight adults. Psychother Theory Res Pract 1980;17:277–280.

59. Hall RG, Hanson RW, Borden BL. Permanence of two self-managed treatments of overweight in university and community populations. J Consult Clin Psychol 1974;42:781–786.

60. Hanson RW, Borden BL, Hall SM, Hall RG. Use of programmed instruction in teaching self-management skills to overweight adults. Behav Ther 1976;7:366–373.

61. Murphy JK, Williamson DA, Buxton AE, et al. The long-term effects of spouse involvement upon weight loss and maintenance. Behav Ther 1982;13:681–693.

62. Senediak C, Spence SH. Rapid versus gradual scheduling of therapeutic contact in a family based behavioral weight control programme for children. Behav Psychother 1985;13:265–87.

63. Godfrey S, Silverman M. Demonstration of a placebo response in asthma by means of exercise testing. J Psychosom Res 1973;17:293–297.

64. May O, Hansen NCG. Comparison of terbutaline, isotonic saline, ambient air and non-treatment in patients with reversible chronic airway obstruction. Eur Respir J 1988;1:527–530.

65. Morton AR, Fazio SM, Miller D. Efficacy of laser-acupuncture in the prevention of exercise-induced asthma. Ann Allergy 1993;70:295–298.

66. Lindholm LH, Ekbom T, Dash C, Isacsson Å, Scherstén B. Changes in cardiovascular risk factors by combined pharmacological and nonpharmacological strategies: the main results of the CELL Study. J Intern Med 1996;240:13–22.

67. Tuomilehto J, Voutilainen E, Huttunen J, Vinni S, Homan K. Effect of guar gum on body weight and serum lipids in hypercholesterolemic females. Acta Med Scand 1980;208:45–48.

68. Diamond L, Dockhorn RJ, Grossman J, et al. A dose-response study of the efficacy and safety of ipratropium bromide nasal spray in the treatment of the common cold. J Allergy Clin Immunol 1995;95:1139–1146.

69. Hayden FG, Diamond L, Wood PB, Korts DC, Wecker MT. Effectiveness and safety of intranasal ipratropium bromide in common colds: a randomized, double-blind, placebo-controlled trial. Ann Intern Med 1996;125:89–97.

70. Stabholz A, Shapira J, Shur D, et al. Local application of sustained-release delivery system of chlorhexidine in Down's syndrome population. Clin Prev Dent 1991;13:9–14.

71. Stewart JE, Jacobs-Schoen M, Padilla MR, et al. The effect of a cognitive behavioral intervention on oral hygiene. J Clin Periodontol 1991;18:219–222.

72. Sipich JF, Russell RK, Tobias LL. A comparison of covert sensitization and "nonspecific" treatment in the modification of smoking behavior. J Behav Ther Exp Psychiatry 1974;5:201–203.

73. Spanos NP, Mondoux TJ, Burges CA. Comparison of multi-component hypnotic and non-hypnotic treatments for smoking. Contemp Hypn 1995;12:12–9.

74. Longo DJ, Clum GA, Yaeger NJ. Psychosocial treatment for recurrent genital herpes. J Consult Clin Psychol 1988;56:61–66.

75. Crosby L, Palarski VA, Cottington E, Cmolik B. Iron supplementation for acute blood loss anemia after coronary artery bypass surgery: a randomized, placebo-controlled study. Heart Lung 1994;23:493–499.

76. Karunakaran S, Hammersley MS, Morris RC, Turner RC, Holman RR. The Fasting Hyperglycaemia Study. III. Randomized controlled trial of sulfonylurea therapy in subjects with increased but not diabetic fasting plasma glucose. Metabolism 1997;46:Suppl. 1:56–60.

77. Nawrocki JD, Bell TJ, Lawrence WT, Ward JP. A randomized controlled trial of transurethral microwave thermotherapy. Br J Urol 1997;79:389–393.

78. GRECHO, U292 INSERM, ARC, GREPA. Evaluation de deux produits homéopathiques sur la reprise du transit après chirurgie digestive: un essai contrôlé multicentrique. Presse Med 1989;18:59–62.

79. Nyboe Andersen A, Damm P, Tabor A, Pedersen IM, Harring M. Prevention of breast pain and milk secretion with bromocriptine after second-trimester abortion. Acta Obstet Gynecol Scand 1990;69:235–238.

80. Benedetti F, Amanzio M, Maggi G. Potentiation of placebo analgesia by proglumide. Lancet 1995;346:1231–1231.

81. Benedetti F, Amanio M, Casadio C, et al. Control of postoperative pain by transcutaneous electrical nerve stimulation after thoracic operations. Ann Thorac Surg 1997;63:773–776.

82. Chenard JR, Marchand S, Charest J, Jinxue L, Lavignolle B. Évaluation d'un traitement comportemental de la lombalgie chronique: l'école interactionelle du dos. Sci Comportement 1991;21:225–239.

83. Classen W, Feingold E, Netter P. Influence of sensory suggestibility on treatment outcome in headache patients. Neuropsychobiology 1983;10:44–47.

84. Conn IG, Marshall AH, Yadav SN, Daly JC, Jaffer M. Transcutaneous electrical nerve stimulation following appendicectomy: the placebo effect. Ann R Coll Surg Engl 1986;68:191–192.

85. Coyne P, MacMurren M, Izzo T, Kramer T. Transcutaneous electrical nerve stimulator for procedural pain associated with intravenous needlesticks. J Intraven Nurs 1995;18:263–267.

86. Forster EL, Kramer JF, Lucy SD, Scudds RA, Novick RJ. Effects of TENS on pain, medications, and pulmonary function following coronary artery bypass graft surgery. Chest 1994;106:1343–1348.

87. Frega A, Stentella P, Di Renzi F, et al. Pain evaluation during carbon dioxide laser vaporization for cervical intraepithelial neoplasia: a randomized trial. Clin Exp Obstet Gynecol 1994;21:188–191.

88. Goodenough B, Kampel L, Champion GD, et al. An investigation of the placebo effect and age-related factors in the report of needle pain from venipuncture in children. Pain 1997;72:383–391.

89. Gracely RH, Dubner R, Wolskee PJ, Deeter WR. Placebo and naloxone can alter post-surgical pain by separate mechanisms. Nature 1983;306:264–265.

90. Hargreaves A, Lander J. Use of transcutaneous electrical nerve stimulation for postoperative pain. Nurs Res 1989;38:159–161.

91. Hashish I, Harvey W, Harris M. Anti-inflammatory effects of ultrasound therapy: evidence for a major placebo effect. Br J Rheumatol 1986;25:77–81.

92. Hashish I, Hai HK, Harvey W, Feinmann C, Harris M. Reduction of postoperative pain and swelling by ultrasound treatment: a placebo effect. Pain 1988;33:303–311.

93. Helms JM. Acupuncture for the management of primary dysmenorrhea. Obstet Gynecol 1987;69:51–56.

94. Hong CZ, Chen YC, Pon CH, Yu J. Immediate effects of various physical medicine modalities on pain threshold of an active myofascial trigger point. Musculoskeletal Pain 1993;1(2):37–53.

95. Lander J, Fowler-Kerry S. TENS for children's procedural pain. Pain 1993;52:209–216.

96. Levine JD, Gordon NC. Influence of the method of drug administration on analgesic response. Nature 1984;312:755–756.

97. Moffett JAK, Richardson PH, Frost H, Osborn A. A placebo controlled double blind trial to evaluate the effectiveness of pulsed short wave therapy for osteoarthritic hip and knee pain. Pain 1996;67:121–127.

98. Parker JC, Smarr KL, Buckelew SP, et al. Effects of stress management on clinical outcomes in rheumatoid arthritis. Arthritis Rheum 1995;38:1807–1818.

99. Reading AE. The effects of psychological preparation on pain and recovery after minor gynaecological surgery: a preliminary report. J Clin Psychol 1982;38:504–512.

100. Rowbotham MC, Davies PS, Verkempinck C, Galer BS. Lidocaine patch: double-blind controlled study of a new treatment method for post-herpetic neuralgia. Pain 1996;65:39–44.

101. Sanders GE, Reinert O, Tepe R, Maloney P. Chiropractic adjustive manipulation on subjects with acute low back pain: visual analog pain scores and plasma beta-endorphin levels. J Manipulative Physiol Ther 1990;13:391–395.

102. Sprott H, Mennet P, Stratz T, Müller W. Wirksamkeit der Akupunktur bei Patienten mit generalisierter Tendomyopathie (Fibromyalgie). Aktuel Rheumatol 1993;18:132–135.

103. Tan S, Poser EG. Acute pain in a clinical setting: effects of cognitive-behavioural skills training. Behav Res Ther 1982;20:535–545.

104. Vlaeyen JWS, Teeken-Gruben NJG, Goossens MEJB, et al. Cognitive-educational treatment of fibromyalgia: a randomized clinical trial. I. Clinical effects. J Rheumatol 1996;23:1237–1245.

105. Wojciechowski FL. Behavioral treatment of tension headache: a contribution to controlled outcome research methodology. Gedrag Tijdschrift Voor Psychol 1984;12(5):16–30.

106. Hawkins PJ, Liossi C, Ewart BW, et al. Hypnotherapy for control of anticipatory nausea and vomiting in children with cancer: preliminary findings. Psycho-Oncology 1995;4:101–106.

107. O'Brien B, Relyea MJ, Taerum T. Efficacy of P6 acupressure in the treatment of nausea and vomiting during pregnancy. Am J Obstet Gynecol 1996;174:708–715.

108. Tremeau ML, Fontanie-Ravier P, Teurnier F, Demouzon J. Protocole de maturation cervicale par acupuncture. J Gynecol Obstet Biol Reprod (Paris) 1992;21:375–380.

109. Irvin JH, Domar AD, Clark C, Zuttermeister PC, Friedman R. The effects of relaxation response training on menopausal symptoms. J Psychosom Obstet Gynaecol 1996;17:202–207.

110. Ascher LM, Turner RM. Paradoxical intention and insomnia: an experimental investigation. Behav Res Ther 1979;17:408–411.

111. Espie CA, Lindsay WR, Brooks DN, Hood EM, Turvey T. A controlled comparative investigation of psychological treatments for chronic sleep-onset insomnia. Behav Res Ther 1989;27:79–88.

112. Lick JR, Heffler D. Relaxation training and attention placebo in the treatment of severe insomnia. J Consult Clin Psychol 1977;45:153–161.

113. Nicassio P, Bootzin R. A comparison of progressive relaxation and autogenic training as treatments for insomnia. J Abnorm Psychol 1974;83:253–260.

114. Turner RM, Ascher LM. Controlled comparison of progressive relaxation, stimulus control, and paradoxical intention therapies for insomnia. J Consult Clin Psychol 1979;47:500–508.

115. Kendall PC, Williams L, Pechacek TF, et al. Cognitive-behavioral and patient education interventions in cardiac catheterization: the Palo Alto Medical Psychology Project. J Consult Clin Psychol 1979;47:49–58.

116. Lorr M, McNair DM, Weinstein GJ, Michaux WW, Raskin A. Meprobamate and chlorpromazine in psychotherapy: same effects on anxiety and hostility of outpatients. Arch Gen Psychiatry 1961;4:381–389.

117. Macaluso AD, Connelly AM, Hayes WB, et al. Oral transmucosal fentanyl citrate for premedication in adults. Anesth Analg 1996;82:158–161.

118. Markland D, Hardy L. Anxiety, relaxation and anaesthesia for day-case surgery. Br J Clin Psychol 1993;32:493–504.

119. Rybarczyk BD, Auerbach SM. Reminiscence interviews as stress management interventions for older patients undergoing surgery. Gerontologist 1990;30:522–528.

120. Theroux MC, West DW, Corddry DH, et al. Efficacy of intranasal midazolam in facilitating suturing of lacerations in preschool children in the emergency department. Pediatrics 1993;9:624–627.

121. Lick J. Expectancy, false galvanic skin response feedback, and systematic desensitization in the modification of phobic behavior. J Consult Clin Psychol 1975;43:557–567.

122. Rosen GM, Glasgow RE, Barrera M. A controlled study to assess the clinical efficacy of totally self-administered systematic desensitization. J Consult Clin Psychol 1976;44:208–217.

123. Fuchs CZ, Rehm LP. A self-control behavior therapy program for depression. J Consult Clin Psychol 1977;45:206–215.

124. Nandi DN, Ajmany S, Ganguli H, et al. A clinical evaluation of depressives found in a rural survey in India. Br J Psychiatry 1976;128:523–527.

125. Davidson AM, Denney DR, Elliott CH. Suppression and substitution in the treatment of nailbiting. Behav Res Ther 1980;18:1–9.

126. Bramston P, Spence SH. Behavioural versus cognitive social-skills training with intellectually-handicapped adults. Behav Res Ther 1985;23:239–246.

127. Jacobson NS. Specific and nonspecific factors in the effectiveness of a behavioral approach to the treatment of marital discord. J Consult Clin Psychol 1978;46:442–452.

128. Nocella J, Kaplan RM. Training children to cope with dental treatment. J Pediatr Psychol 1982;7:175–178.

129. Weingaertner AH. Self-administered aversive stimulation with hallucinating hospitalized schizophrenics. J Consult Clin Psychol 1971;36:422–429.

130. Crapper McLachlan DR, Dalton AJ, Kruck TPA, et al. Intramuscular desferrioxamine in patients with Alzheimer's disease. Lancet 1991;337:1304–1308. [Erratum: Lancet 1991;337:1618.]

131. Quayhagen MP, Quayhagen M, Corbeil RR, Roth P, Rodgers JA. A dyadic remediation program for care recipients with dementia. Nurs Res 1995;44:153–159.

132. Pelham WE, Murphy DA, Vannatta K, et al. Methylphenidate and attributions in boys with attention-deficit hyperactivity disorder. J Consult Clin Psychol 1992;60:282–292.

133. Ernst E, Resch KL. Concept of true and perceived placebo effects. BMJ 1995;311:551–553.

134. Gøtzsche PC. Sensitivity of effect variables in rheumatoid arthritis: a meta-analysis of 130 placebo controlled NSAID trials. J Clin Epidemiol 1990;43:1313–1318. [Erratum: J Clin Epidemiol 1991;44:613.]

Correction

"Is the Placebo Powerless? An Analysis of Clinical Trials Comparing Placebo with No Treatment"

In the Web-only Supplementary Appendix 3, the point estimates for Hall et al. (1974) and Davidson et al. (1980) should have read, "−0.17" and "−0.94," respectively, not "−1.17" and "0.94" as published. The confidence interval for Rybarczyk and Auerbach (1990) should have read, "−0.73 to 0.40," not "−0.40 to 0.13," as published.

6

The Placebo Concept in Medicine and Psychiatry

Adolf Grünbaum

Adolf Grünbaum, "The Placebo Concept in Medicine and Psychiatry," *Psychological Medicine* 1986;16:19–38.

Introduction

Just what is the problem of identifying an intervention or treatment t of one sort or another as a placebo for a target disorder D? One set of circumstances, among others, in which the need for such an identification may arise is the following. After the administration of t to some victims of D, some of them recover from their affliction to a significant extent. Now suppose that there is cogent evidence that this improvement can indeed be causally attributed at all to some factors or other among the spectrum of constituents comprising the dispensation of t to a patient. Then it can become important to know whether the therapeutic gain that ensued from t in the alleviation of D was due to *those particular factors* in its dispensation that the advocates of t have theoretically designated as deserving the credit for the positive treatment outcome. And one aim of this paper is to articulate in detail the bearing of the answer to this question on whether t qualifies generically as a placebo or not. For, as will emerge, the medical and psychiatric literature on placebos and their effects is conceptually bewildering, to the point of being a veritable Tower of Babel.

The proverbial sugar pill is hardly the sole placebo capable of producing therapeutic benefits for ailments other than hypoglycemia and other glucose deficits. Indeed, the long-term history of medical treatment has been characterized as largely the history of the placebo effect (Shapiro and Morris, 1978). After all, it is not only the patients who can be unaware that the treatments they are receiving are just placebos for their disorders; the physicians as well may mistakenly believe that they are administering nonplacebos for their patients' ailments, when they are actually dispensing placebos, while further enhancing the patients' credulity by communicating their own therapeutic faith. For example, as we shall see, surgery for angina pectoris performed in the United States during the 1950s turned out to be a mere placebo. Unbeknown to the physicians who practiced before the present century, most of the medications they dispensed were at best pharmacologically ineffective, if not outright physiologically harmful or even dangerous. Thus, during all that time, doctors were largely engaged in the unwitting dispensation of placebos on a massive scale. Even after the development of contemporary scientific medicine some 80 years ago, "the placebo effect flourished as the norm of medical treatment" (Shapiro and Morris, 1978, p. 371).

The psychiatrist Jerome Frank (1973) has issued the sobering conjecture that those of the roughly 200 psychotherapies whose gains exceed those from spontaneous remission do *not* owe such remedial efficacy to the *distinctive* treatment factors credited by their respective therapeutic advocates, but succeed for other reasons. Nonetheless, Frank admonishes us not to disparage such placebogenic gains in therapy, at least as long as we have nothing more effective. And even in internal medicine and surgery, a spate of recent articles has inveighed against downgrading placebogenic benefits, the grounds being that we should be grateful even for small mercies. Yet the plea not to forsake the benefits wrought by placebos has been challenged on ethical grounds: the injunction to secure the patient's informed consent is a demand whose fulfilment may well render the placebo ineffective, though perhaps not always (Park and Covi, 1965).

The physician Arthur K. Shapiro is deservedly one of the most influential writers in this field of inquiry. He has been concerned with the history of the placebo effect (1960) and with the semantics of the word "placebo" (1968), no less than with current empirical research on placebogenic phenomena in medical and psychological treatments (Shapiro and Morris, 1978). Thus, in his portion of the last-cited paper, he has refined (1978, p. 371) his earlier 1971 definition of "placebo" in an endeavour to codify the current uses of the term throughout medicine and psychiatry. The technical vocabulary employed in A. K. Shapiro's earlier and most recent definitions is standard terminology in the discussion of placebo therapies and of experimental placebo controls, be it in pharmacology, surgery, or psychiatry. Yet just this standard technical vocabulary, I submit, generates confusion by being misleading or obfuscating, and indeed cries out for conceptual clarification. Hence it is my overall objective to revamp Shapiro's definitions substantially so as to provide a clear and rigorous account of the placebo notion appropriate to current medicine and psychiatry.

Critique, Explication, and Reformulation of A. K. Shapiro's Definition

Critique

While some placebos are known to be such by the dispensing physician—though presumably not by the patient—other placebo therapies are mistakenly believed to be nonplacebos by the physician as well. Mindful of this dual state of affairs, A. K. Shapiro's definition of a placebo therapy makes it clear that, at any given stage of scientific knowledge, a treatment modality actually belonging to the genus placebo can be of the latter kind rather than of the traditionally recognized first sort. To capture both of these two species of placebo therapy, he casts his definition into the following general form, in which the expression "$=_{def.}$" stands for the phrase "is definitionally equivalent to":

> Therapy t is a placebo therapy $=_{def.}$ t is of a kind A OR t is of kind B.

Any definition of this "either-or" form is called a "disjunctive" definition, and *each* of the two independent clauses connected by the word "or" is called a "disjunct." For example, suppose we define a "parent" by saying:

Person X is a parent = $_{def.}$ X is a father OR X is a mother.

This is clearly a *disjunctive* definition. And it is convenient to refer to each of the separate clauses "X is a father" and "X is a mother" as a "disjunct." Thus, the sentence "X is a father" can obviously be regarded as the first of the two disjuncts, while the sentence "X is a mother" is the second disjunct. Hence, for brevity, I thus refer respectively to the corresponding two parts of Shapiro's actual disjunctive definition (Shapiro and Morris, 1978):

> A *placebo* is defined as any therapy or component of therapy that is deliberately used for its nonspecific, psychological, or psychophysiological effect, or that is used for its presumed specific effect, but is without specific activity for the condition being treated. (p. 371)

Shapiro goes on to point out at once that the term "placebo" is used not only to characterize a treatment modality or therapy, but also a certain kind of experimental control:

> A *placebo*, when used as a control in experimental studies, is defined as a substance or procedure that is without specific activity for the condition being evaluated [*sic*]. (p. 371)

And then he tells us furthermore that

> A *placebo effect* is defined as the psychological or psychophysiological effect produced by placebos. (p. 371)

All of the conceptual puzzlement warranted by these three statements arises in the initial disjunctive definition of a "placebo therapy." For it should be noted that this definition employs the tantalizing words "nonspecific effect," "specific effect," and "specific activity" in unstated *technical* senses. Once these terms are elucidated, the further definitions of a "placebo control" and of a "placebo effect" become conceptually unproblematic. Hence let us now concentrate on the disjunctive definition of a "placebo therapy," and see what help, if any, Shapiro gives us with the technical terms in which he has expressed it. Contrary to the belief of some others, I contend that his explicit comments on their intended construal still leaves them in an unsatisfactory logical state for the purposes at hand.

In the joint 1978 paper, A. K. Shapiro and Morris elaborate quite vaguely on the key concept of "specific activity" as follows:

> Specific activity is the therapeutic influence attributable solely to the contents or processes of the therapies rendered. The criterion for specific activity (and therefore the placebo effect) should be based on scientifically controlled studies. (p. 372)

They provide this characterization as part of a longer but very rough delineation of the complementary notions denoted by the terms "specific" and "nonspecific," locutions that are as pervasive as they are misleading or confusing in the literature on placebos. Thus, they make the following comment on the definition of "placebo" given above, which I amplify within brackets:

> Implicit in this definition is the assumption that active treatments [i.e., nonplacebos] may contain placebo components. Even with specific therapies [i.e., nonplacebos] results are apt to be due to the combination of both placebo and nonplacebo effects. Treatments that are devoid of active, specific components are known as pure placebos, whereas therapies that contain nonplacebo components are called impure placebos . . . Treatments that have specific components but exert their effects primarily through nonspecific mechanisms are considered placebo therapies . . .
>
> The key concept in defining placebo is that of "specific activity." In nonpsychological therapies, specific activity is often equated with nonpsychological mechanisms of action. When the specific activity of a treatment is psychological [i.e., in psychotherapies that derive therapeutic efficacy from those particular factors in the treatment that the pertinent theory singles out specifically as being remedial] this method of separating specific from nonspecific activity is no longer applicable. Therefore, a more general definition of specific activity is necessary. Specific activity is the therapeutic influence attributable solely to the contents or processes of the therapies rendered [i.e., the therapeutic influence, if any, that derives solely from those component factors of the therapy that are specifically singled out by its advocates as deserving credit for its presumed efficacy]. The criterion for specific activity (and therefore the placebo effect) should be based on scientifically controlled studies . . . In behavior therapy, some investigators have utilized "active placebo" control groups whereby some aspects of the therapy affect behavior but those aspects differ from the theoretically relevant ingredients of concern to the investigator. (pp. 371–372)

This passage urgently calls for clarification beyond what I have supplied within brackets. In particular, the terms "specific activity" and "nonspecific effect," though standard, are anything but clear. Yet, as the authors emphasize further on, it is by virtue of a treatment's *lack* of so-called specific activity for a given target disorder that this treatment *objectively* qualifies as a placebo, regardless of whether the dispensing physician believes the treatment to have actual placebo status or not. They import this emphasis on the irrelevance of belief to generic placebo *status* into their definition. There, in its first paragraph, a disjunction makes explicit provision for the presence of such belief on the part of the dispenser, as well as for its absence. In the first disjunct, it is a placebo that the physician *believes* himself or herself to be giving the patient, and the doctor is right in so believing. In the second disjunct, the physician believes himself or herself to be administering a *non*placebo, but he or she is definitely mistaken in so believing.

In either case, a placebo is actually being dispensed, be it wittingly or unwittingly. For brevity, I distinguish between the two situations to which these disjuncts pertain by saying that the treatment is an "intentional placebo" in the former case, while being an "inadvertent placebo" in the latter. Note that if a treatment *t* is actually not a placebo generically while its dispenser or even the whole professional community of practitioners believes *t* to be one, then *t* is precluded from qualifying as a "placebo" by the definition. To earn the label "intentional placebo," a treatment not only must be *believed* to be a placebo by its dispenser, but must also actually *be* one generically. Thus, therapists have administered a nonplacebo in the erroneous belief that it is a placebo. For example, at one time, some psychoanalysts used phenothiazines to treat schizophrenics in the belief that these drugs were mere (anger-reducing, tranquillizing) placebos; they presumed them to be ineffective for the psychic dissociation and the pathognomonic symptoms of schizophrenia. But controlled studies showed that these medications possessed a kind of therapeutic efficacy for the disorder that was not placebogenic (Davis and Cole, 1975*a*, *b*).

Incidentally, besides not being placebos for schizophrenia, the phenothiazines turned out to be capable of inducing the negative side effects of parkinsonism, at least transiently (Blakiston's *Gould Medical Dictionary*, 1972, p. 1130). But the motor impairment manifested in parkinsonism is attributed to a deficiency of brain dopamine. Thus the unfavourable parkinsonian side effect of the phenothiazine drugs turned out to have *heuristic* value because it suggested that these drugs block the dopamine receptors in the brain. And since the drugs were also effective nonplacebos for schizophrenia, the parkinsonian side effect raised the possibility that an excess of dopamine might be implicated in the aetiology of schizophrenia. In this way, a *biochemical* malfunction of the brain was envisioned quite specifically as causally relevant to this psychosis (Kolata, 1979).

Let me now specify the terminology and notation that I employ in my rectifying explication of "placebo," using the diagram shown in Figure 6.1. Overall, there is some stated or tacit therapeutic theory, which I call "ψ." Now ψ designs or recommends a particular treatment or therapy *t* for a particular illness or target disorder D. In the left-hand box of Figure 6.1, I generically depict a treatment modality or therapy *t*. Note

that it contains a spectrum of ingredients or treatment factors. For example, the theory ψ may insist that if it is to recommend surgery for the treatment of gallstones, then the surgical process must obviously include the removal of the gallstones, rather than a mere sham abdominal incision. I want a name for those treatment factors that a given theory ψ thus picks out as the defining characteristics of a given type of therapy *t*. And I call these factors the "characteristic factors F" of *t*. But ψ recognizes that besides the characteristic factors F, the given therapy normally also contains other factors which it regards as just incidental. For example, a theory that deems the removal of gallstones to be therapeutic for certain kinds of pains and indigestion will assume that this abdominal surgery includes the administration of anesthesia to the patient. To take a quite different example, when Freud recommended psychoanalytical treatment, he insisted on the payment of a hefty fee, believing it to be perhaps a catalyst for the patient's receptivity to the therapeutic task. Furthermore, a therapeutic theory may well allow that a given therapy includes not only known incidental factors, but also others that it has failed to recognize. And the letter C in the diagram, which labels "incidental treatment factors," is intended to apply to both known and unknown factors of this type.

Turning to the right-hand box in Figure 6.1, we note that the patient's life functions and activities are generically subdivided into two parts: the target disorder D at which the therapy *t* is aimed, and then the rest of his or her functions. But there may well be some vagueness in the circumscription of D. Both its pathognomonic symptoms and the presumed aetiological process responsible for them will surely be included in the syndrome D. Yet some nosologists might include, while others exclude, certain accessory manifestations of D that are quite secondary, because they are also present in a number of other, nosologically distinct syndromes. Somewhat cognate conceptual problems of taxonomic circumscription arose in chemistry upon the discovery of isomerism, and even in the case of chemical isotopy.

Finally, in the middle of Figure 6.1, arrows represent some of the interesting possible causal influences or effects that may result from each of the two sets of treatment factors.

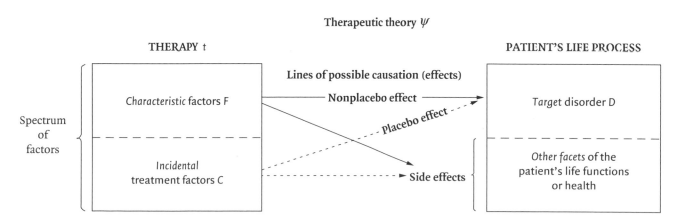

Figure 6.1. Illustration of therapeutic theory, ψ, used in clarifying the definition of "placebo."

Thus, one or more of the characteristic factors F may be remedial for the target disorder D, or the F factors may have no effect on D, or the F factors conceivably could make D even worse. By the same token, these factors F may have these three kinds of influence on other facets of the patient's health. And any of these latter effects—whether good or bad—will be called "side effects." Now *if (and only if) one or more of the characteristic factors do have a positive therapeutic effect on the target disease D, then the therapy as a whole qualifies generically as a nonplacebo for D.* This is the situation that is depicted in the diagram by the words "nonplacebo effect" in the horizontal solid arrow from F to D.

It is vital to realize that, in Figure 6.1, the causal arrows are intended to depict *possible* (imaginable) effects, such that the given treatment factors may have various sorts of positive or adverse effects on the target disorder, or on other facets of the patient's health. Thus, the diagram can be used to depict a nonplacebo therapy as well as a placebo therapy. In the former case, there is an actual beneficial causal influence by the characteristic factors on D, whereas in the latter case such an influence does not—as a matter of actual fact—exist, though it is imaginable (logically possible).

Similarly, the incidental treatment factors C may or may not have positive or negative effects on D. Furthermore, these factors C may have desirable or undesirable effects *outside of* D, which we again call side effects. If the incidental factors do have an effect on D, we can refer to that effect as a "placebo effect," even if the therapy qualifies overall as a generic nonplacebo by containing therapeutically effective characteristic factors. For example, suppose that the characteristic factors in a certain chemotherapy are effective against a given kind of cancer, at least for a while, so that this chemotherapy is a nonplacebo for this affliction. Then this therapeutic effectiveness may well be *enhanced*, if the dispensing physician communicates his or her confidence in this therapy to the patient. And if there is such enhancement, the treatment factors C do indeed produce a positive placebo effect on D, a situation depicted in the diagram by the broken diagonal arrow. Thus we can say that *whether a given positive effect on D is or is not a placebo effect depends on whether it is produced by the incidental treatment factors or the characteristic ones.*

Let me now use the preceding informal preliminary account to give a more systematic and precise characterization of the genus placebo as well as of two of its species, thereby also revamping A. K. Shapiro's definitions.

A treatment process normally has a spectrum of constituent factors as well as a spectrum of effects when administered for the alleviation of a given target disorder D. Effects on the patient's health not pertaining to D are denominated "side effects." Though the term "side effects" often refers to *undesirable* effects outside D, there is neither good reason nor general agreement to restrict it in this way. As I soon illustrate, the therapeutic theory ψ that advocates the use of a particular treatment modality t to remedy D demands the inclusion of certain characteristic constituents F in any treatment process that ψ authenticates as an application of t. Any such process, besides qualifying as an instance of t according to ψ, will typically have constituents C other than the characteristic ones F singled out by ψ. And when asserting that the factors F are remedial for D, ψ *may* also take cognizance of one or more of the noncharacteristic constituents C, which I denominate as "incidental." Thus, ψ may perhaps attribute certain side effects to either F or C. Indeed, it may even maintain that one or another of the incidental factors affects D—say, by enhancing the remedial effects that it claims for F. In short, if a doctor is an adherent of ψ, it may well furnish him or her with a therapeutic rationale for administering t to a patient afflicted by D, or for refraining from doing so.

For instance, consider pharmacological treatment, such as the dispensation of digitoxin for congestive heart dysfunction or of nitroglycerin for angina pectoris. Then it is perfectly clear that the water with which such tablets are swallowed, and the patient's awareness of the reputation of the prescribing cardiologist, for example, are incidental treatment factors, while the designated chemical ingredients are characteristic ones. But Freud also specified these two different sorts of treatment factors in the nonpharmacological case of psychoanalytical treatment, while recognizing that some of the incidental factors may serve initially as catalysts or icebreakers for the operation of the characteristic ones. Thus, he identified the characteristic constituents as the educative and affect-discharging lifting of the patient's presumed repressions, effected by means of overcoming ("working through") the analysand's resistance to their conscious recognition in the context of "resolving" his or her "transference" behaviour towards the doctor. And Freud depicted the patient's faith in the analyst, and the derivation of emotional support from that authority figure, as mere catalysts or icebreakers in the initial stage of treatment—factors that are incidental, because they are avowedly quite incapable of extirpating the pathogenic causes, as distinct from producing merely cosmetic and temporary relief.

Hence Freud stressed tirelessly that the patient's correct, affect-discharging insight into the aetiology of his or her affliction is the one quintessential ingredient that distinguishes the remedial dynamics of his treatment modality from any kind of treatment by suggestion. Treatments by suggestion, he charged, leave the pathogenic repressions intact, and yield only an ephemeral cosmetic prohibition of the symptoms (see Grünbaum, 1984). In the same vein, Freud came to maintain early in his career that the characteristic factors of Erb's electro-therapy for nervous disorders were therapeutically unavailing, and that any gains from treatment with that electric apparatus were achieved by its incidental factors.

Explications and Reformulations

The schematic diagram in Figure 6.1 can serve as a kind of glossary for the notations ψ, t, F, and C that I have introduced. Using this notation, I shall offer several explications, which supersede those I have offered earlier (Grünbaum, 1981). In the first of these explications, which pertains to the "intentional" species of placebo, the fourth condition (d) is somewhat tentative:

(1) A treatment process t characterized by a given therapeutic theory ψ as having constituents F, but also possessing other, perhaps unspecified incidental constituents C, will be said to be an "intentional placebo" with respect to a target disorder D, suffered by a victim V and treated by a dispensing practitioner P, just when the following conditions are jointly satisfied: (a) none of the characteristic treatment factors F are remedial for D; (b) P believes that the factors F indeed all fail to be remedial for D; (c) but P also believes that—at least for a certain type of victim V of D—t is nonetheless therapeutic for D by virtue of containing some perhaps even unknown incidental factors C different from F; and (d) yet—more often than not—P abets or at least acquiesces in V's belief that t has remedial efficacy for D by virtue of some constituents that belong to the set of characteristic factors F in t, provided that V is aware of these factors.

Note that the first of these four conditions explicates what it is for a treatment type t to have the objective generic property of being a placebo with respect to a given target disorder D. The objective property in question is just that the characteristic constituents F of t are actually not remedial for D. On the other hand, the remaining three of the four conditions describe the property of belonging to the species of intentional placebo, over and above being a placebo generically. And, clearly, these three further conditions pertain to the beliefs and intentions of the practitioners who dispense t and of the patients who receive it. In particular, they render whether the therapist is *intentionally* administering a generic placebo to the patient, rather than unaware of the placebo status of the treatment. But notice that the fourth condition would require modification, if there were enough cases, as has been suggested, in which a patient may benefit therapeutically even after being told that he or she is receiving a generic placebo. On the other hand, the fourth condition apparently still suffices to cover those cases in which surgeons perform appendectomies or tonsillectomies solely at the behest of their patients, who, in turn, may be encouraged by their families. The need to accommodate such interventions has been stressed by Piechowiak (1982, 1983).

The caveat regarding the fourth condition (d) is occasioned by a report (Park and Covi, 1965) on an exploratory and "paradoxical" study of 15 adult neurotic out-patients, who presented with anxiety symptoms. The treating therapists did provide support and reassurance, yet "the responsibility for improvement was thrown back to the patient by means of the paradoxical statement that he needed treatment but that he could improve with a [placebo] capsule containing no drug" (p. 344). Of the 14 patients who remained willing to receive the capsules for a week, 6 *disbelieved* the purported pharmacological inertness of the capsules, and 3 of them even experienced "side-reactions," which they attributed to the pills (p. 342). But the three patients who did

firmly believe in the doctor's candid disclosure of inertness improved after 1 week, no less than the "sceptics," who thought they were receiving an effective nonplacebo after all. Hence Park and Covi concluded that "unawareness of the inert nature of the placebo is not an indispensable condition for improvement on placebo" (p. 342). Yet, as these authors acknowledged at once, in so small a sample of patients, improvement may have occurred "in spite of" the disclosure as a matter of course, under *any* sort of treatment or even as a matter of spontaneous remission. And since it is quite unclear whether the moral drawn by Park and Covi is at all generalizable beyond their sample, I have let the fourth condition stand.

Piechowiak (1983) also calls attention to uses of diagnostic procedures (e.g., endoscopy, stomach X-rays) when deemed unnecessary by the physician, but demanded by the anxious patient suffering from, say, cancerphobia, who may even believe them to be therapeutic. In the latter sort of instance, the gastroenterologist may justify an invasive procedure to himself or herself and the patient, because when the expected negative finding materializes, it may alleviate the patient's anxiety as well as the vexatious somatic effects of that anxiety. In some cases (e.g., Wassermann test for syphilis), the patient may be under no illusions as to the dynamics by which this relief was wrought, any more than the doctor. But Piechowiak is concerned to point out that in other cases (e.g., angiography), the patient may well conceptualize the diagnostic intervention as *itself* therapeutic. And hence this author suggests the assimilation of these latter cases to intentional placebos. In this way, he suggests, account can be taken of the cognizance taken by doctors of the therapeutic beliefs of their patients—beliefs that are psychological realities, even if they are scientifically untutored.

As we have seen, a particular treatment modality t derives its identity from the full set of its characteristic treatment factors, as singled out by the therapeutic theory that advocates the use of t in stated circumstances. Hence therapies will be distinct, provided that they differ in at least one characteristic factor. By the same token, therapies whose distinct identities are specified in each case by two or more characteristic factors can have at least one such factor in common without detriment to their distinctness, just as they can thus share one or more incidental factors. Indeed, as I illustrate later, a shared factor that counts as characteristic of one therapy may qualify as merely incidental to another. And clearly these statements concerning factors common to distinct therapies hold for somatic medicine and psychotherapy alike.

Thus, in *either* of these two classes of healing interventions, a therapy that qualifies as a nonplacebo for a certain target D derives precisely this therapeutic status from the remedial efficacy of some or all of its characteristic factors. Yet it may share these efficacious ingredients with other, distinct therapies that differ from it in at least one characteristic factor. In fact, one or all of the common factors may count as only incidental to some of the other therapies. And it is to be borne in mind that a therapy having at least one remedial characteristic ingredient is generically a nonplacebo, even if the remaining characteristic factors are otiose. Hence a therapy t can be a nonplacebo with respect to a particular D, even if all of its efficacious characteristic treatment ingredients are common to both t and distinct other therapies!

Unfortunately, Critelli and Neumann (1984) run afoul of this important state of affairs by concluding incorrectly that "the common-factors criterion . . . appears to be the most viable current definition of the placebo for the study of psychotherapy" (p. 35). They see themselves as improving on A. K. Shapiro's explication of the placebo concept, at least for psychotherapy. Yet they actually impoverish it by advocating the so-called common-factors definition (for psychotherapy), which they do not even *state*, and by altogether failing to render the two species of placebo adumbrated in the 1978 definition given by Shapiro and Morris. Besides, Critelli and Neumann contend that Shapiro's explication of the notion of a generic placebo suffers from his abortive attempt to encompass somatic medicine and psychotherapy simultaneously. But once I have completed my thorough recasting of Shapiro's pioneering definition below, it will be clear that—contrary to Critelli and Neumann—his endeavour to cover medicine and psychotherapy with one definitional stroke is *not* one of the defects of his explication.

Turning now to placebo *controls*, we must bear in mind that to assess the remedial merits of a given therapy t* for some D, it is imperative to disentangle from each other two sorts of possible positive effects as follows: (1) those desired effects on D, if any, actually wrought by the characteristic factors of t*; and (2) improvements produced by the expectations aroused in both the doctor and the patient by their belief in the therapeutic efficacy of t*. To achieve just such a disentanglement, the baseline measure (2) of expectancy effect can be furnished by using a generic placebo t in a control group of persons suffering from D. For ethical reasons, informed consent has presumably been secured from a group of such patients to be "blindly" allocated to either the control group or the experimental group.

Ideally, this investigation should be a triply blind one. To say that the study is triply blind is to say the following: (a) the patients do not know to which group they have been assigned; (b) the dispensers do not know whether they are administering t* or t; and (c) the outcome assessors do not know which patients were the controls. But there are treatment modalities—such as surgery and psychotherapy—in which the *second* of these three sorts of blindness obviously cannot be achieved.

By subtracting the therapeutic gains with respect to D in the control group from those in the experimental group, investigators can obtain the sought-after measure (1) of the incremental remedial potency of the characteristic factors in t*. And, for brevity, one can then say that with respect to D, the generic placebo t functions as a "placebo control" in the

experimental evaluation of the therapeutic value of t* as such. More briefly, the placebo served in a controlled clinical trial of t*.

As will be recalled, the relevant definition of that term given by A. K. Shapiro and Morris (1978, p. 371) reads as follows: "A placebo, when used as a control in experimental studies, is defined as a substance or procedure that is without specific activity for the condition being evaluated." But just this characterization of a "placebo control," as used in experimental studies in medicine or psychotherapy, is in dire need of emendation. As they would have it, "the condition" D is "being evaluated" in an experimental study employing a placebo control. But surely what is being evaluated instead is the conjectured therapeuticity of a designated treatment t* (substance, procedure) for D. And I suggest that their definition of a placebo control be recast as follows. A treatment type t functions as a "placebo control" in a given context of experimental inquiry, which is designed to evaluate the characteristic therapeutic efficacy of another modality t* for a target disorder D, just when the following requirements are jointly satisfied: (1) t is a *generic placebo* for D, as defined under the first condition (a) in the definition above of "intentional placebo"; (2) the experimental investigator conducting the stated controlled trial of t* believes that t is not only a generic placebo for D, but also is generally quite harmless to those victims of D who have been chosen for the control group. And, as I have noted, the investigator's reason for using t as a placebo control when evaluating the characteristic therapeutic value of t* for D is as follows: especially if t* is expensive or fraught with negative side effects, clinicians wish to know to what extent, if any, the beneficial effects on D due to its characteristic treatment factors *exceed* those produced by its incidental ones.

When schematized in this way, some of the complexities inherent in the notion of a placebo control are not apparent. To their credit, Critelli and Neumann (1984) have perceptively called attention to some of the essential refinements in psychotherapy research:

> [I]t is imperative that test procedures be compared to realistic placebo controls. Too often in the past, false claims of incremental effectiveness have resulted from the experimental use of placebos that even the most naïve would not mistake for genuine therapy. There appears to be a tendency for experimental placebos to be in some sense weaker, less credible, or applied in a less enthusiastic manner than treatments that have been offered as actual therapies. At a minimum, placebo controls should be equivalent to test procedures on all major recognized common factors. These might include induced expectancy of improvement; credibility of rationale; credibility of procedures; demand for improvement; and therapist attention, enthusiasm, effort, perceived belief in treatment procedures, and commitment to client improvement. (p. 38)

Having issued this salutary caveat, these authors claim that "current [psycho]therapies have yet to meet the challenge of demonstrating incremental effects" (p. 38). Yet one of the reasons they go on to give for posing this challenge relies on their belief that treatment factors common to two or more therapies *must* be—in my parlance—incidental rather than characteristic ingredients. As I have pointed out, however, formulations invoking this belief tend to darken counsel. Here too, placebo controls cannot be *doubly* blind.

Suedfeld (1984) likewise addresses methodological (and also ethical) problems arising in the employment of placebo controls to evaluate psychotherapy. As he sees it, "the necessity for equating the expectancy of the active [nonplacebo] and placebo treatment groups implies the acceptance of the null hypothesis, a position that is better avoided" (p. 161). To implement this avoidance, he advocates the use of a "subtractive expectancy placebo," which he describes as follows:

> It consists of administering an active, specific therapeutic procedure but introducing it with the orientation that it is inert with respect to the problem being treated. In other words, the client is led to expect less of an effect than the treatment is known to produce. The Subtractive Expectancy Procedure avoids the need to invent or find an inert technique, attempts to create initial differences in expectancy which can be substantiated by the rejection of the null hypothesis, and also makes it feasible to assess the specific effect of an active treatment in a design with one treated and one untreated (control) group. (p. 161)

Here I am not concerned with the pros and cons of the subtractive expectancy placebo procedure advocated by Suedfeld, *qua* alternative to the null hypothesis on which my definition above of a "placebo control" is implicitly predicated. Whatever that balance of investigative cogency, there can be little doubt that some of the ideas in Suedfeld's paper are illuminating or at least suggestive. Besides, I appreciate his several citations of my initial paper, "The Placebo Concept" (Grünbaum, 1981). There I made concrete proposals for the replacement of the standard technical vocabulary used in the placebo literature, precisely because of the Tower of Babel confusion that is engendered by it.

Alas, in criticism of Suedfeld, I must point out that his exposition is genuinely marred by just the penalties of ambiguity, obscurity, and confusion exacted by the received placebo vocabulary, because he unfortunately chooses to retain that infelicitous terminology for the formulation of his ideas. As we shall see in due course, the terms "active," "specific," and "nonspecific" are especially insidious locutions in this context. Yet these ill-fated terms, and their cognates or derivatives, abound in Suedfeld's presentation. In any case, so much for the notion of a placebo control.

Recently there have been interesting conjectures as to the identity of the incidental constituents C that confer somatic remedial potency on medications qualifying as intentional placebos for some Ds with respect to certain therapeutic theories. It has been postulated (J. Brody, 1979) that, when present, such therapeutic efficacy derives from the placebo's psy-chogenic activation of the secretion of substances as follows: (1) pain-killing endorphins, which are endogenous opiate-like substances; (2) interferon, which counters viral infections; and (3) steroids, which reduce inflammations. Indeed, the physiological mechanisms involved are believed to be operative as well in the so-called miracle cures by faith healers, holy waters, and so-called quacks. As an example, there is evidence from a study of dental postoperative pain (Levine *et al.*, 1978) that endorphin release does mediate placebo-induced analgesia. And this suggests analgesic research focusing on variables that affect endorphin activity (Levine *et al.*, 1979).

So far I have explicated only one of the two species of placebo *therapy* adumbrated in the disjunctive definition given by A. K. Shapiro and Morris (1978). Hence let me now explicate their second disjunct, which pertains to the second species of placebo.

(2) A treatment process t characterized by a given therapeutic theory ψ as having constituents F will be said to be an "inadvertent placebo" with respect to a target disorder D, suffered by a victim V and treated by a dispensing practitioner P, just when each of the following three conditions is satisfied: (a) none of the characteristic treatment factors F are remedial for D; (b) but—at least for a certain type of victim V of D—P credits these very factors F with being therapeutic for D, and indeed he or she deems at least some of them to be causally *essential* to the remedial efficacy of t; also (c) more often than not, V believes that t derives remedial efficacy for D from constituents belonging to t's characteristic factors, provided that V is aware of these factors.

It is to be clearly understood that, as before, the first condition (a) codifies the *generic* property of being a placebo. The second condition (b) of this second explication renders the following: P denies that t's efficacy, if any, might derive mainly from its incidental constituents. Here the third condition (c) is subject to the same caveat (Park and Covi, 1965) that I have issued for the fourth condition (d) in my first explication above.

Clarifying Comments

Let me now add four sets of clarifying comments on my explications, because of questions put to me by Edward Erwin (personal communication, 1981), a philosopher of psychology.

(1) Clearly, it was the intentional species of placebo that was denoted by the term "placebo" in its original pharmacological use. And its use in A. K. Shapiro's definition to denote as well what I have called the inadvertent species constitutes a *generalization* of the genus placebo, prompted by the sobering lesson of the history of medicine that most treatments were inadvertent rather than intentional placebos, and often harmful to boot! But the tacit intuitions of many people as to what a placebo is are strongly geared to its original status in pharmacology. No wonder that these intuitions call for identifying the intentional species of placebo with the entire genus. Consequently, some people will be ruffled by the fact that, in my explication of the *generalized* use of the term, the

generic property of being a placebo is, of course, considerably less restrictive than the property of being an intentional placebo. For, as is clear from the codification of the generic placebo property in the first condition (a) of both of my explications, any treatment t qualifies generically as a placebo for a given target disorder D merely on the strength of the failure of all of its characteristic factors F to be remedial for D.

But once the source of the counterintuitiveness is recognized, it should be dispelled and should occasion no objection to my explication of the generic property. Furthermore, in the generalized generic sense of "placebo," a treatment t does belong to the genus placebo even if its characteristic factors exacerbate D, since exacerbation is a particularly strong way of failing to be remedial for D. Surely it is the failure of the *characteristic* treatment factors to be *remedial* for D that is at the heart of the notion of a placebo therapy, *not* their failure to have an *effect* on D, either bad or good. And the failure of a practitioner who dispenses a harmful inadvertent placebo t to be cognizant of its ill effect hardly detracts from t's objective status as a generic placebo. Nor does the malaise of those who would invoke the favourable etymological significance of the term "placebo" in order to forbid a generalized generic concept that fails to exclude the envisaged untoward case. Either species of placebos can *undesignedly* exacerbate D! History teaches that many well-intended treatments were *worse than useless*.

Finally, note that if one were to define a generic placebo therapy t *alternatively* as one whose characteristic factors are *without effect* on D, it would have the consequence that a nonplacebo t would either exacerbate D or be remedial for it, or would have a merely neutral effect on it. But in my definitional scheme, the characteristic factors of a nonplacebo must be positively therapeutic.

(2) There are treatments only *some* of whose characteristic factors F are therapeutic for a given D, while the therapeutic theory ψ that advocates their dispensation claims that *all* of the factors F are thus remedial. For example, it has recently been claimed (Kazdin and Wilson, 1978) that in the systematic desensitization brand of behaviour therapy, which is an effective treatment for certain phobias, only one of its three F factors is thus therapeutic, while the other two appear unavailing. What, it might be asked, is the classificatory verdict of my explication as to whether a therapy whose characteristic factors comprise both efficacious and otiose members qualifies generically as a nonplacebo?

To answer this question, note that within the class of treatments for any given D, any member t will belong to the genus placebo exactly when *none* of its characteristic factors are remedial for D. Therefore any therapy whose characteristic factors include *at least one* that is therapeutic for D will pass muster as a nonplacebo. Evidently it is not necessary for being a nonplacebo that all of the F factors be remedial. It follows that, in the absence of further information, the designation of a given therapy—such as desensitization in the example above—as a nonplacebo does not tell us whether only

some of its characteristic factors are remedial or whether all of them are. But this fact hardly militates against either my explication or the usefulness of the concept of nonplacebo as rendered by it.

Upon recalling A. K. Shapiro and Morris's cited characterizations of "pure" and "impure" placebos (1978, p. 372), we see that my construal of the generic placebo notion explicates what they call a "pure placebo." Their "impure placebos" are, as they put it vaguely, "treatments that have specific components but exert their effects primarily through nonspecific mechanisms" (p. 372). This sort of treatment does count as a nonplacebo, according to my formulation. But my parlance can readily characterize their so-called impure placebos by saying the following. Although the characteristic ingredients of these therapies do make some therapeutic contribution, this remedial effect is exceeded by the therapeutic benefit deriving from the *incidental* treatment factors. This quantitative vagueness is, of course, not my problem but theirs.

(3) It must not be overlooked that my explication of "placebo" is relativized not only to a given target disorder D, but also to those characteristic factors that are singled out from a particular treatment process by a specified therapeutic theory ψ. It is therefore not my explication but a given theory ψ that determines which treatment factors are to be classified as the characteristic factors in any one case. And by the same token, as I illustrate presently, the given therapeutic theory ψ (in medicine or psychiatry) rather than my explication determines whether any factors in the physician-patient relationship are to count as only "incidental." Clearly, for example, a particular psychiatric theory might well designate some such factors as being characteristic. And just this sort of fact prompted A. K. Shapiro and Morris to disavow the common restriction of "specific activity" to "nonpsychological mechanisms of action," and to offer their "more general definition of specific activity" cited above.

An example given to me in a discussion at the Maudsley Hospital in London called my attention to allowing for the possible *time-dependence* of the effects of *incidental* treatment factors. In pharmacological research on rats, it was noticed that the effects of injected substances were enhanced after a while, via Pavlovian conditioning, by the continued presence of blue light. That light can be deemed an incidental treatment factor throughout, I claim, although its effects will vary as time goes on. Hence I reject the suggestion that once the blue light has begun to potentiate the effects of the injected substances, the light must be reclassified to become a characteristic treatment factor, after starting out as a merely incidental one.

The divergence between Jerome Frank's (1973) theory of healing as persuasion on the one hand, and such psychotherapeutic theories as Freud's or Hans Eysenck's on the other, will now serve to illustrate three important points as follows. (a) As is evident from my explication, it is the given therapeutic theory ψ rather than my explication of "placebo" that decides *which* treatment factors are to be respectively classified as "characteristic" and as "incidental." (b) Precisely because my analysis of the placebo concept does make explicit provision for the dependence of the memberships of these classes on the particular theory ψ at hand, it allows for the fact that rival therapeutic theories can *disagree* in regard to their classification of particular treatment factors as "characteristic," no less than in their attribution of significant therapeutic efficacy to such factors. (c) Hence, the relativization of the classification of treatment factors to a given theory ψ that is built into my explication prevents seeming inconsistencies and confusions, generated when investigators want to assess the generic placebo status of a therapy *t* across rival therapeutic theories, and without regard to whether these theories use different characteristic factors to identify *t*.

In language and notions of my explications, Jerome Frank's (1973, pp. xv–xx) view of the therapeutic status of the leading rival psychotherapies can now be outlined. For *each* of these treatment modalities *t* and its underlying theory ψ, he hypothesizes that *t* is as follows:

1. A generic placebo with respect to the characteristic treatment factors singled out by *its own* particular ψ.
2. An inadvertent placebo with respect to the beliefs of those dispensers of *t* who espouse ψ.
3. Therapeutically effective to the extent that the patient's hope is aroused by the doctor's healing symbols, which mobilize the patient's sense of mastery of his or her demoralization.

As is clear from the third item, Frank credits a treatment ingredient *common* to the rival psychotherapies with such therapeutic efficacy as they do possess. But his categorization of each of these therapies as a generic placebo rather than as a nonplacebo is now seen to derive just from the fact that he is tacitly classifying as "incidental," rather than as "characteristic," all those treatment factors that he deems to be therapeutic. In adopting this latter classification, he is speaking the classificatory language employed by the theories underlying the various therapies, although he denies their claim that the treatment ingredients they label "characteristic" are actually effective.

Yet in a language suited to Frank's own therapeutic tenets, it would, of course, be entirely natural to label as "characteristic" just those treatment factors that his own theory T deems remedial, even though these same ingredients count as merely incidental within each of the psychotherapeutic theories rejected by him. And if Frank were to couch his own T in that new classificatory language, then he would no longer label the leading psychotherapies as generic placebos, although he would be holding the same therapeutic beliefs as before.

It should now be clear that by explicitly relativizing to a given ψ the classification of particular treatment factors as "characteristic" or "incidental," no less than by relativizing their respective therapeutic efficacy to a particular D, my explication obviates the following sort of question, which is being asked across unspecified, tacitly presupposed therapeutic theories: If the effectiveness of a placebo modality depends on its symbolization of the physician's healing power, should this ingredient not be considered a *characteristic* treatment factor?

(4) In a paper devoted mainly to the ethical complexities of using placebo control groups in psychotherapy research, O'Leary and Borkovec (1978) write: "Because of problems in devising a theoretically and practically inert placebo, we recommend that the term *placebo* be abandoned in psychotherapy research" (p. 823). And they propose to "circumvent the ethical concerns inherent in placebo methodology" (p. 825) by devising alternative methods of research control. In this way, they hope to assure as well that "the confusion associated with the term *placebo* would be avoided" (p. 823).

But I hope it will become clear from my comparison of my explications above with the usual parlance in the literature that these confusions indeed can be avoided without abandoning the placebo concept in any sort of therapeutic research. Nor do I see why the theoretical identification of a particular incidental treatment factor that is effective for D rather than "inert" ever has to be detrimental to therapeutic research.

Logical Defects of Received Vocabulary

On the basis of my explications, I can now make two sets of comments on the logical defects of the key locutions commonly employed as technical terms throughout the medical and psychiatric literature on placebos.

(1) We are told that any effect that a placebo has on the target disorder D is "nonspecific." But a placebo can have an effect on D that is no less sharply defined and precisely known than the effect of a nonplacebo. To take a simple example, consider two patients A and B suffering from ordinary tension headaches of comparable severity. Suppose that A unwittingly swallows the proverbial sugar pill and gets no relief from it, because it is indeed pharmacologically "inert" or useless for such a headache *qua* mere sugar pill. A stoically endures his or her discomfort. Assume further that B consults his or her physician, who is very cautious. Mindful of the potential side effects of tranquillizers and analgesics, the doctor decides to employ a little benign deceit and gives B a few lactose pills, without disabusing B of his or her evident belief that he or she is receiving a physician's sample of analgesics. Posit that shortly after B takes the first of these sugar pills, the headache disappears altogether. Assume further that B's headache would not have disappeared just then from mere internal causes. Both of these conditions might well apply in a given case. Thus B assumedly received the same headache relief from the mere sugar pill as he or she would have received if a pharmacologically *noninert* drug had been slipped into his food without his knowledge.

Clearly, in some such situations, the therapeutic effect of the sugar pill placebo on the headache can have attributes fully as sharply defined or "specific" as the effect that would have been produced by a so-called active drug like aspirin (Frank, 1973). Moreover, this placebogenic effect can be just as precisely described or known as the nonplacebogenic effect of aspirin. In either case, the effect is complete headache relief, even though the sugar pill as such is, of course, pharmacologically inert for headaches whereas aspirin as such is pharmacologically efficacious. It is therefore at best very misleading to describe as "nonspecific" the *effect* that the placebo produces on the target disorder, while describing the at least qualitatively like effect of the nonplacebo as "specific." Yet just such a use of the terms "nonspecific" and "specific" as modifiers of the term "effect" is made in A. K. Shapiro's above-cited definition of "placebo," in a leading treatise on pharmacological therapeutics (Goodman and Gilman, 1975), in a German work on psychoanalysis (Möller, 1978), in a German survey article on placebos (Piechowiak, 1983), and in a fairly recent article on treatments to reduce high blood pressure (A. P. Shapiro et al. 1977). Equally infelicitously, Schwartz (1978, p. 83) speaks of a "nonspecific placebo response." Why describe a treatment effect as "nonspecific" in order to convey that the incidental treatment factors, rather than the characteristic elements, were the ones that produced it? Relatedly, Klein (1980) points out that when a placebo counteracts demoralization in a depressed person, it is wrong-headed to describe this therapeutic outcome as a "nonspecific" effect. After all, the demoralization and the effect on it are quite specific in the ordinary sense.

Worse, as it stands, the locution "specific effect" is quite ambiguous as between the following two very different senses: (a) the therapeutic effect on D is wrought by the characteristic ("specific") factors F of the therapy t; or (b) the remedial effectiveness of t is specific to a quite small number of disorders, to the exclusion of a far more multitudinous set of nosologically different afflictions and of their respective pathognomonic symptoms. Most writers on placebos, though not all, intend the first construal when speaking of "specific effect." But others use the term "specific" in the second of these senses. Thus, as we shall see in greater detail further on, according to whether the effects of a given therapy are or are not believed to be "specific" in the *second* sense above, H. Brody (1977, pp. 40–43) classifies that *therapy* as a "specific therapy" or as a "general therapy." And he wishes to allow for the fact that the placebogenic remedial efficacy of the proverbial sugar pill is presumed to range over a larger number of target ailments than the nonplacebogenic efficacy of widely used medications (e.g., penicillin). In an endeavour to make such an allowance, he uses the belief in the ability of a therapy to engender "specific effects" in the second sense above as the touchstone of its being a nonplacebo. In addition, Shepherd (1961) has pointed out yet another ambiguity in the loose use of "specific" and "non-specific" to designate treatment factors in psychopharmacology. And Wilkins (1985, p. 120) speaks of "non-specific events" not only to refer to treatment-factors *common* to rival therapies, but also to

denote life events outside the treatment process altogether. How much better it would be, therefore, if students of placebo phenomena banished the seriously ambiguous use of "specific" as a technical term altogether.

As if this degree of technical confusion were not enough, the misleading use of "specific" in the sense of "nonplacebo" is sometimes encountered alongside the use of "specific" in the usual literal sense of "precise" or "well-defined." Thus, when Miller (1980) writes that "placebo effects can be quite specific" (p. 476), the illustrations he goes on to give show that here "specific" has the force of "quantitatively precise." But in the very next paragraph, he uses the term "specific" as a synonym for "nonplacebo" when reporting that "it is only in the past 80 years that physicians have been able to use an appreciable number of treatments with specific therapeutic effects" (p. 476).

Indeed, the placebo research worker Beecher (1972), who is renowned for investigating the role of placebos in the reduction of pain, entitled one of his essays "The Placebo Effect as a Non-Specific Force Surrounding Disease and the Treatment of Disease." But even metaphorically and elliptically, it seems inappropriate to speak of the placebo effect as being a nonspecific *force*, as Beecher (1972) does repeatedly.

On the basis of the explications I have given, it is appropriate to speak of an *effect* as a "placebo effect" under two sorts of conditions: (a) even when the treatment t is a nonplacebo, effects on D—be they good, bad, or neutral—that are produced by t's *incidental* factors count as placebo effects, precisely because these factors wrought them; and (b) when t is a generic placebo whose characteristic factors have harmful or neutral effects on D, these effects as well count as placebo effects. Hence, if t is a placebo, then *all* of its effects qualify as placebo effects.

(2) A. K. Shapiro and Morris (1978) tell us in their definition that a placebo "is without specific activity for the condition being treated." And, as we recall, they contrast "active treatments" with placebos by saying that "active treatments may contain placebo components" (p. 371). Yet they also tell us that "in behavior therapy, some investigators have utilized 'active placebo' control groups" in which "some aspects of the therapy affect behavior but those aspects differ from the theoretically relevant ingredients of concern to the investigator" (p. 372). Furthermore, in the common parlance employed by two other investigators, even placebos that are acknowledged to be "potently therapeutic" or "effective" (for angina pectoris) are incongruously dubbed "inactive" just because they are placebos (Benson and McCallie, 1979). And Beecher (1972) emphasizes that some placebos are capable of "*powerful action*" (p. 178; italics in original), while contrasting them with treatments that he and others call "active" to convey that they are indeed nonplacebos.

By contrast to Beecher's use of "active," Bok (1974) tells us that any medical procedure, "whether it is active or inactive, can serve as a placebo whenever it has no specific effect on the condition for which it is prescribed" (p. 17). Thus, in

Bok's parlance, placebos may be said to be "active" (p. 17) and "placebos can be effective" (p. 18), but they must be devoid of so-called specific effect. Yet just what is it for a placebo to be "active"? Clearly, a placebo therapy as a whole might be productive of (remedial or deleterious) effects on the target disorder while being devoid of significant (negative or positive) side effects, or it may have only side effects. On the other hand, it might have both kinds of effects. And it matters therapeutically, of course, which of these effects—if either—is produced by any particular placebo. Hence clarity will be notably served by explicitly indicating the respect in which a given placebo intervention is being said to be "active." Yet such explicitness is lacking when Bok tells us, for example, that there is a clear-cut "potential for damage by an active drug given as a placebo" (p. 20). Thus it is only a conjecture just what she intends the term "active" to convey in the latter context. Is it that there are pharmacologically induced side effects in addition to placebogenic effects on the target disorder D? By the same token, her usage of "inactive" is unclear when she reports that "even inactive placebos can have toxic effects" (p. 20), even though she goes on to give what she takes to be an illustration. Bok's concern with placebos focuses, however, on ethically questionable dispensations of intentional placebos.

Evidently there are divergences among writers on placebos in regard to the usage of the term "active." But they tell us in one voice, as Bok does, that a placebo procedure "has no specific effect on the condition for which it is prescribed" (p. 17). To this conceptually dissonant discourse, I say: in the case of a placebo it is, of course, recognized that incidental treatment factors may be potently remedial for D, although the characteristic ones by definition are not. And if some of the incidental constituents are thus therapeutic, then the actual specificity of their activity—in the ordinary sense of "specificity"—clearly does not depend on whether the pertinent therapeutic theory ψ is able either to specify their particular identity or to afford understanding of their detailed mode of action. Hence if some of the incidental constituents of t are remedial but presently elude the grasp of ψ, the current inability of ψ to pick them out from the treatment process hardly lessens the objective specificity of their identity, mode of action, or efficacy. A theory's current inability to spell out certain causal factors and to articulate their mode of action because of ignorance is surely not tantamount to their being themselves objectively "nonspecific" as to their identity, over and above being unknown! At worst, the details of the operation of the incidental factors are left unspecified.

Hence, despite the assumed present inability of the pertinent theory ψ to spell out which particular incidental constituents render the given placebo remedial for D, it is at best needlessly obscure to say that these constituents are "without specific activity" for D and are "nonspecific." A fortiori, it is infelicitous to declare of any and every placebo treatment modality as a whole that, qua being a placebo, it must be devoid of "specific activity." It would seem that, when speaking generically of a placebo, the risk of confusion as well as outright unsound claims can be obviated by steadfast avoidance of the term "nonspecific activity." Instead, as I have argued earlier, the objective genus property of being a placebo should be codified as follows. With respect to the target disorder D, the treatment modality t belongs to the genus placebo just when its characteristic constituents fail to be remedial for D. Furthermore, clarity is served by using the term "incidental" rather than "nonspecific" when speaking of those treatment constituents that differ from the characteristic ones. In short, the generic distinction between placebos and nonplacebos has nothing whatever to do with the contrast between nonspecificity and specificity, but only with whether the characteristic treatment factors do play a therapeutic role for D or not. So much for my proposed rectifications of the misleading conceptualizations conveyed by the standard locutions whose confusion I have laid bare.

Clarifying Ramifications of My Explications

As is clear from my formulation, the genus property of being a placebo is altogether independent of the belief of the dispensing practitioner as to whether the treatment in question is a placebo. But, equally clearly, the species property of being an inadvertent placebo is explicitly relativized to this belief, no less than the species property of being an intentional one. Thus, a placebo treatment t that qualifies as inadvertent with respect to one school of therapeutic thought may be explicitly avowed to have intentional placebo status in the judgement of another school. By the same token, advocates of t who do not even entertain the possibility of its being a placebo will be preoccupied with its characteristic constituents, to the likely disregard of incidental factors in t that may turn out to be remedially potent for D. Consequently, if patients who received treatment t register gains, such advocates will erroneously discount any remedial efficacy actually possessed by these incidental factors. Moreover, these theoreticians will give undeserved credit to the characteristic factors for any successful results that issue from t. As recounted in Beecher's classic (1961) paper "Surgery as Placebo," which is summarized by Benson and McCallie (1979), the history of surgical treatment for angina pectoris in the United States during the mid-1950s furnishes a clear case in point.

Proponents of ligating the internal mammary artery claimed that this procedure facilitated increased coronary blood flow through collateral vessels near the point of ligation, thereby easing the ischemia of the heart muscle to which angina pectoris is due. And these enthusiasts then credited that ligation with the benefits exhibited by their surgical patients. But well-controlled, though ethically questionable, studies by sceptical surgeons in the late 1950s showed the following. When a mere sham bilateral skin incision was made on a comparison group of angina patients, then ligation of the internal mammary artery in randomly selected other angina patients yielded only equal or even less relief from angina than the sham surgery. Furthermore, the quality of the results achieved by the intentional placebo surgery was dramatic and sustained. Apart from subjective improvement, the deceived recipients of the sham surgery had increased exercise tolerance, registered less nitroglycerin usage, and improved electrocardiographically. Moreover, a similar lesson emerges from the use of a related surgical procedure due to Vineberg, in which the internal mammary artery was implanted into a tunnel burrowed into the myocardium. The results from this Vineberg operation (Benson and McCallie, 1979) suggest that placebogenic relief occurred even in a sizeable majority of angina patients who had angiographically verified coronary artery disease. This history has a sobering moral. It bears further monitoring to what extent the positive results from coronary artery bypass surgery are placebogenic (Detre et al., 1984).

Now consider those who allow that such beneficial efficacy as a therapy t has could well be placebogenic. This group may thereby be led to draw the true conclusion that the characteristic factors do not merit any therapeutic credit. On the other hand, the therapeutic efficacy of a nonplacebo is enhanced if its incidental factors *also* have a remedial effect of their own. Thus, it has been found (Gallimore and Turner, 1977) that the attitudes of physicians toward chemotherapy commonly contribute significantly to the effectiveness of nonplacebo drugs. Again, Wheatley (1967) reported that in the treatment of anxiety by one particular nonplacebo drug, enthusiastic physicians obtained better results than unenthusiastic ones, although enthusiasm did not enhance the positive effect of tricyclic antidepressants on depression. Indeed, there may be synergism between the characteristic and incidental treatment factors, such that they potentiate each other therapeutically with respect to the *same* target disorder.

On the other hand, one and the same treatment may be a placebo with respect to the target disorder and yet may function as a nonplacebo for a secondary ailment. For example, when a viral cold is complicated by the presence of a secondary bacterial infection, a suitable antibiotic may serve as an intentional placebo for the viral cold while also acting as a nonplacebo for the bacterial infection. This case highlights an important moral. It serves to discredit the prevalent stubborn refusal to relativize the placebo status of a medication or intervention to a stated target disorder, a relativization I have explicitly built into my definitions. For example, in the misguided effort to escape such relativization, Piechowiak (1983, p. 40) is driven to classify antibiotics as "false placebos." As he sees it, they are placebos because they are not pharmacologically effective for the typical sort of upper respiratory viral infection; but what makes them "false" placebos, in his view, is that they *are* pharmacologically potent (genuine medications, or, in the original German, *echte Pharmaka*) for other diseases (e.g., bacterial pneumonia).

But, according to this reasoning, "false" placebos are quite common. A telling illustration is provided by the following story reported by Jennifer Worrall, a British physician (personal communication, 1983). One of her patients, a middle aged woman, complained of a superficial varicose leg ulcer. As Worrall relates,

> [The patient] was very demanding and difficult to please and claimed to suffer continuous agony from her ulcer (although there were none of the objective signs of pain, such as sleep disturbance, increased heart rate and blood pressure, pallor and sweating). All of the many mild-to-moderate analgesics were "useless" [according to the patient] and I did not feel opiates were justified, so I asked the advice of my immediate superior. The superior [here referred to as "W."] saw the patient, discussed her pain and, with a grave face, said he wanted her to try a "completely different sort of treatment." She agreed. He disappeared into the office, to reappear a few minutes later, walking slowly down the ward and holding in front of him a pair of tweezers which grasped a large, white tablet, the size of [a] half-dollar. As he came nearer, it became clear (to me, at least) that the tablet was none other than effervescent vitamin C. He dropped the tablet into a glass of water which, of course, bubbled and fizzed, and told the patient to sip the water carefully when the fizzing had subsided. It worked—the new medicine completely abolished her pain! W. has used this method several times, apparently, and it always worked. He felt that the single most important aspect was holding the tablet with *tweezers*, thereby giving the impression that it was somehow too powerful to be touched with bare hands!

Some may find this episode amusing. Yet it has a devastating moral for the not uncommon claim that without regard to a *specified* target disorder, a pharmacological agent can qualify as a generic and even as an intentional placebo. Assume that, for the varicose leg ulcer that afflicted the given patient, vitamin C is a generic placebo even in high doses; this assumption allows that, in such large doses, it may have negative side effects. And furthermore, relying on W.'s findings, grant that for at least some patients suffering from a superficial leg ulcer, the administration of vitamin C as an intentional placebo in W.'s ceremonious manner ("with tweezers"!) is therapeutic for such an ulcer. Then surely such a placebo status for leg ulcer hardly detracts from the fact that, at least in sufficient doses, vitamin C is a potent nonplacebo for scurvy. And if Linus Pauling is to be believed, sufficiently high doses of this vitamin can even afford prophylaxis for certain cancers. In short, only conceptual mischief results from the supposition that the property of being a (generic) placebo is one that a treatment—be it pharmacological or psychiatric—can have *per se*, rather than only with respect to a stated target disorder.

Ironically, none other than the much-maligned proverbial sugar pill furnishes a *reductio ad absurdum* of the notion that a medication can be generically a placebo *simpliciter*, without relativization to a target disorder. For even a lay person knows that the glucose in the sugar pill is anything but a generic placebo if given to a victim of diabetes who is in a state of insulin shock, or to someone suffering from hypoglycemia. But if an antibiotic were a "false placebo" on the strength of the properties adduced by Piechowiak (1983), then—by parity with his reasoning—so also is the notorious sugar pill, the alleged paradigm of a "true" nonrelativized placebo. Even the diehards among the believers in intrinsic, nonrelativized placebos will presumably regard this consequence of their view as too high a price to pay. Nor would they ever think someone's Uncle Charlie to be a "false" uncle merely because Charlie is not also somebody else's uncle!

Suppose that, for specified types of diseases, a certain class of afflicted victims does derive placebogenic remedial gain from the use of a particular set of therapeutic interventions. Then it may become important, for one reason or another, to ascertain—*within* the classes of incidental treatment factors picked out by the pertinent set of therapeutic theories—which particular kinds of factors are thus remedial. And this quest for identification can proceed across various sorts of treatment modalities (e.g., chemotherapy, radiation therapy, surgery), or may be focused more narrowly on factors within such modalities (e.g., surgery). Research during the past three decades has envisioned (1) that such placebogenic treatment gain may require a so-called placebo reactor type of victim of disease, characterized by a specifiable (but as yet unspecified) personality trait or cluster of such traits; or (2) that the therapeutic success of placebos may depend on certain kinds of characteristics or attitudes possessed by the treating physician. It should be noted that my explications of both the intentional and inadvertent species of placebo have made provision for these two possibilities. Both explications are relativized to disease victims of a specifiable sort, as well as to therapists (practitioners) of certain kinds. As it turns out, for some two dozen or so of proposed patient-trait correlates of placebo responsiveness, the first hypothesis named above—that of placebo reactivity—has been largely unsuccessful empirically, except for the following: generalized chronic anxiety has been frequently and reliably found to correlate with placebo responsivity, notably in the treatment of pain (Gallimore and Turner, 1977). Yet in a 25-year series of studies of placebo responsiveness in psychotherapy, Frank (1974) found reason to discount the role of enduring personality factors in the patient (see also Liberman, 1964). As for the second hypothesis, which pertains to the therapeutic relevance of the physician's communicated attitudes, I have already commented on the demonstrated role of physician variables among incidental treatment factors in enhancing the therapeutic efficacy of nonplacebo drugs.

Having explicated the placebo concept by reference to A. K. Shapiro and Morris's proposed definition, I ought to comment on the divergences between theirs and the one offered by H. Brody (1977), which I have mentioned above. Shapiro and Morris's definition appeared in 1978 in the *second* edition of the Garfield and Bergin *Handbook of Psychotherapy and Behavior Change*. But in the first edition of this *Handbook*, which

appeared in 1971, Shapiro alone had published an only slightly different definition. This 1971 definition is not discussed by Brody (1977). But Brody claims rough consistency between Shapiro's (1968) definition of "placebo effect" and his own account of that notion. Hence I am concerned to point out that there are several important divergences between the construals of "placebo" given by Shapiro and Morris, on the one hand, and Brody, on the other. And these differences are such, I claim, that Shapiro and Morris render the generic placebo concept implicit in the medical and psychiatric literature far more adequately than Brody, notwithstanding the important respects in which I have found Shapiro and Morris's definition wanting.

The reader is now asked to recall my earlier remarks as to the consideration that seems to have prompted Brody's introduction of his notion of a "specific therapy": the putative fact that the placebogenic remedial efficacy of the proverbial sugar pill is presumed to range over a larger number of target ailments than the nonplacebogenic efficacy of widely used medications (e.g., of penicillin). Then the essence of his account becomes quite clear from his proposed definitions of the following terms: "therapy"; "specific therapy," which Brody avowedly contrasts with "general therapy" (1977, p. 41); and, finally, "placebo." Let me first cite these definitions and Brody's comment on them. (For the sake of consistency, I am substituting the abbreviations used up to this point in this article for Brody's here.)

(i) [t] is a therapy for condition [D] if and only if it is believed that administration of [t] to a person with [D] increases the empirical probability that [D] will be cured, relieved, or ameliorated, as compared to the probability that this will occur without [t]. (Brody, 1977, p. 38)

(ii) [t] is a specific therapy for condition [D] if and only if:
   (1) [t] is a therapy for [D].
   (2) There is a class A of conditions such that [D] is a subclass of A, and for all members of A, [t] is a therapy.
   (3) There is a class B of conditions such that for all members of B, [t] is not a therapy; and class B is much larger than class A.

For example, consider how the definition applies to penicillin used for pneumococcal pneumonia. Penicillin is a therapy for this disease, since it increases the empirical probability of recovery. Pneumococcal pneumonia is one of a class of diseases (infectious diseases caused by penicillin-sensitive organisms) for all of which penicillin is a therapy; but there is a much larger class of diseases (noninfectious diseases and infectious diseases caused by penicillin-resistant organisms) for which penicillin is not a therapy. (Brody, 1977, pp. 40–41)

It will be noted that Brody presumably intends the third requirement in the second definition to implement his stated objective of contrasting "specific therapy" with "general therapy"—an aim that, as we have seen, does *not* govern

Shapiro and Morris's construal of "specific." For Brody's third requirement here makes the following demand. The membership of the class B of disorders for which t is believed to be *ineffective* has to be numerically greater than the membership of the class A of target disorders for which t is deemed to be remedial. But clearly, Shapiro and Morris's cited account of what it is for t to possess "specific activity" for D does *not* entail logically Brody's third restriction on the relative number of disorders for which t is (believed to be) therapeutic! For example, just think of how Shapiro and Morris would analyse the claim that aspirin is not a placebo for arthritis or tension headaches and that it affords nonplacebogenic prophylaxis for blood clotting and embolisms. Nor would Brody's third restriction seem to be often implicit in the medical and psychiatric usage of "specific therapy."

Yet Brody does deserve credit for pointing out, in effect, that the placebogenic efficacy of intentional placebos is believed to range over a larger number of target ailments, as a matter of empirical fact, than the nonplacebogenic efficacy of such medications as penicillin. This is *much less significant*, though, than he thinks: after all, the old sugar pill and penicillin alike have *placebogenic* efficacy, such that the sugar pill does not excel in regard to the number of target disorders!

The third of Brody's definitions reads:

> (iii) A placebo is:
> (1) a form of medical therapy, or an intervention designed to simulate medical therapy, that at the time of use is *believed* not to be a specific therapy for the condition for which it is offered and that is used for its psychological effect or to eliminate observer bias in an experimental setting,
> (2) (by extension from 1) a form of medical therapy now believed to be inefficacious, though believed efficacious at the time of use.
> Clause 2 is added to make sense of a sentence such as, "Most of the medications used by physicians one hundred years ago were actually placebos." (Brody, 1977, p. 43; italics added)

A further major divergence between Brody's and Shapiro and Morris's definitions of "placebo" derives from the *multiple* dependence of Brody's generic placebo concept on therapeutic beliefs, in contrast to Shapiro and Morris's explicit repudiation of any such dependence of the generic notion of placebo. As shown by Brody's definition of "therapy" above, what renders a treatment a "therapy" in his construal is that "it is believed" to be remedial (by its advocates or recipients). Consequently, this dependence on therapeutic belief enters into Brody's definition of "specific therapy" via each of the three requirements that he lays down in his definition of that term above. On the other hand, no such belief-dependence is present in Shapiro and Morris's counterpart notion of "specific activity." As if this were not enough, Brody's definition of "placebo" invokes yet another layer of belief by requiring that "at the time of use," a placebo treatment be "believed not to be a specific therapy" for the target disorder, presumably by the doctor but not by the patient.

It is patent, therefore, that Shapiro and Morris's construal of the *generic* placebo notion, which we have seen to be objective rather than dependent on therapeutic beliefs, makes incomparably better sense than Brody's of such claims as "most of the medications used by physicians a century ago were actually placebos," a claim that Brody avowedly hopes to accommodate via the second requirement of his definition of "placebo." For on Shapiro and Morris's construal, physicians can in fact be *objectively* mistaken in deeming a treatment modality to be a nonplacebo. But on Brody's definition, it is merely a matter of a change in their therapeutic beliefs. For this reason alone, I have made Shapiro and Morris's definition rather than Brody's the focus of my explication.

Note that each of the two species of placebo therapy I have considered is defined by a *conjunction* of two sorts of statements: (1) an assertion of *objective fact* as to the therapeutic failure of t's characteristic constituents with respect to D; and (2) claims concerning the *beliefs* held by the therapist and/or the patient in regard to t. Clearly, the belief-content of (2) does not lessen the objectivity of (1). Yet, in a reply to me, Brody (1985, p. 45) runs afoul of this point. For he thinks incorrectly that the belief-content of (2) negates the greater objectivity I have claimed for my definitions *vis-à-vis* his own *entirely belief-ridden* renditions of the pertinent concepts.

I hope it is now apparent that the customary notions and terminology of placebo research foster conceptual confusion, and that the adoption of the conceptualizations and vocabulary I have proposed would obviate the perpetuation of such confusion.

REFERENCES

Beecher, H.K. (1961). Surgery as placebo. *Journal of the American Medical Association* **176**, 1102–1107.

Beecher, H.K. (1972). The placebo effect as a non-specific force surrounding disease and the treatment of disease. In *Pain: Basic Principles, Pharmacology, Therapy* (ed. R. Janzen, J.P. Payne, and R.A.T. Burt), pp. 176–178. Thieme: Stuttgart.

Benson, H. and McCallie, D.P. (1979). Angina pectoris and the placebo effect. *New England Journal of Medicine* **300**, 1424–1429.

Blakiston's Gould Medical Dictionary (3rd edn) (1972). McGraw-Hill: New York.

Bok, S. (1974). The ethics of giving placebos. *Scientific American* **231**, November, 17–23.

Brody, H. (1977). *Placebos and the Philosophy of Medicine*. University of Chicago Press: Chicago.

Brody, H. (1985). Placebo effect: an examination of Grünbaum's definition. In *Placebo: Theory, Research and Mechanisms* (ed. L. White, B. Tursky, and G.E. Schwartz), pp. 37–58. Guilford Press: New York.

Brody, J. (1979). Placebos work, but survey shows widespread misuse. *New York Times* 3 April, p. Cl.

Critelli, J.W. and Neumann, K.F. (1984). The placebo. *American Psychologist* **39**, 32–39.

Davis, J.M. and Cole, J.O. (1975a). Antipsychotic drugs. In *American Handbook of Psychiatry* (2nd edn), Vol. 5 (ed. S. Arieti), pp. 444–447. Basic Books: New York.

Davis, J.M. and Cole, J.O. (1975b). Antipsychotic drugs. In *Comprehensive Textbook of Psychiatry* (2nd edn), Vol. 2 (ed. A.M. Freedman, H.T. Kaplan, and B.J. Sadock), pp. 1922–1930. Williams and Wilkins: Baltimore.

Detre, K.M., Peduzzi, P., Takaro, T., *et al.* (1984). Eleven-year survival in the Veterans Administration randomized trial of coronary bypass surgery for stable angina. *New England Journal of Medicine* **311**, 1333–1339.

Frank, J.D. (1973). *Persuasion and Healing* (rev. edn). Johns Hopkins University Press: Baltimore.

Frank, J.D. (1974). Therapeutic components of psychotherapy: a 25-year progress report of research. *Journal of Nervous and Mental Disease* **159**, 325–342.

Gallimore, R.G. and Turner, J.L. (1977). Contemporary studies of placebo phenomenon. In *Psychopharmacology in the Practice of Medicine* (ed. M.E. Jarvik), pp. 47–57. Appleton-Century-Crofts: New York.

Goodman, L.S. and Gilman, A. (eds.) (1975). *The Pharmacological Basis of Therapeutics* (5th edn). Macmillan: London.

Grünbaum, A. (1981). The placebo concept. *Behaviour Research and Therapy* **19**, 157–167.

Grünbaum, A. (1984). *The Foundations of Psychoanalysis: A Philosophical Critique.* University of California Press: Berkeley.

Kazdin, A.E. and Wilson, G.T. (1978). *Evaluation of Behavior Therapy.* Ballinger: Cambridge, Mass.

Klein, D.V. (1980). *Diagnosis and Drug Treatment of Psychiatric Disorders* (2nd edn). Williams and Wilkins: Baltimore.

Kolata, G.B. (1979). New drugs and the brain. *Science* **205**, 774–776.

Levine, J.D., Gordon, N.C. and Fields, H.L. (1978). The mechanism of placebo analgesia. *Lancet* **312(8091)**, 654–657.

Levine, J.D., Gordon, N.C., Bornstein, J.C. and Fields, H.L. (1979). Role of pain in placebo analgesia. *Proceedings of the National Academy of Sciences USA* **76**, 3528–3531.

Liberman, R. (1964). An experimental study of the placebo response under three different situations of pain. *Journal of Psychiatric Research* **2**, 233–246.

Miller, N.E. (1980). Applications of learning and biofeedback to psychiatry and medicine. In *Comprehensive Textbook of Psychiatry* (3rd edn), Vol. 1 (ed. A.M. Freedman, H.T. Kaplan, and B.J. Sadock), pp. 468–484. Williams and Wilkins: Baltimore.

Möller, H.J. (1978). *Psychoanalyse.* Wilhelm Fink: München.

O'Leary, K.D. and Borkovec, T.D. (1978). Conceptual, methodological and ethical problems of placebo groups in psychotherapy research. *American Psychologist* **33**, 821–830.

Park, L.C. and Covi, L. (1965). Nonblind placebo trial. *Archives of General Psychiatry* **12**, 336–345.

Piechowiak, H. (1982). Die namenlose Pille. Über Wirkungen und Neben-wirkungen im therapeutischen Umgang mit Plazebopräparaten. *Internistische Praxis* **22**, 759–772.

Piechowiak, H. (1983). Die Schein-Heilung: welche Rolle spielt das Placebo in der ärztlichen Praxis? *Deutsches Ärzteblatt* 4 March, 39–50.

Schwartz, G.E. (1978). Psychobiological foundations of psychotherapy and behavior change. In *Handbook of Psychotherapy and Behavior Change* (2nd edn) (ed. S.L. Garfield and A.E. Bergin), pp. 63–99. Wiley: New York.

Shapiro, A.K. (1960). A contribution to a history of the placebo effect. *Behavioral Science* **5**, 109–135.

Shapiro, A.K. (1968). Semantics of the placebo. *Psychiatric Quarterly* **42**, 653–696.

Shapiro, A.K. and Morris, L.A. (1978). The placebo effect in medical and psychological therapies. In *Handbook of Psychotherapy and Behavior Change* (2nd edn) (ed. S.L. Garfield and A.E. Bergin), pp. 369–410. Wiley: New York.

Shapiro, A.P., Schwartz, G.E. and Ferguson, D.C. (1977). Behavioral methods in the treatment of hypertension. *Annals of Internal Medicine* **86**, 626–636.

Shepherd, M. (1961). Specific and non-specific factors in psychopharma-cology. In *Neuropsychopharmacology*, Vol. 2 (ed. E. Rothlin), pp. 117–129. Elsevier: Amsterdam.

Suedfeld, P. (1984). The subtractive expectancy placebo procedure: a measure of non-specific factors in behavioural interventions. *Behaviour Research and Therapy* **22**, 159–164.

Wheatley, D. (1967). Influence of doctors' and patients' attitudes in the treatment of neurotic illness. *Lancet* **290(7526)**, 1133–1135.

Wilkins, W. (1985). Therapy credibility is not a non-specific event. *Cognitive Therapy and Research* **9**, 119–125.

7

Deconstructing the Placebo Effect and Finding the Meaning Response

DANIEL E. MOERMAN AND WAYNE B. JONAS

Daniel E. Moerman and Wayne B. Jonas, "Deconstructing the Placebo Effect and Finding the Meaning Response," *Annals of Internal Medicine* 2002;136:471–476.

[The cure for the headache] was a kind of leaf, which required to be accompanied by a charm, and if a person would repeat the charm at the same time that he used the cure, he would be made whole; but that without the charm the leaf would be of no avail.

—Socrates, according to Plato (1)

There is a renewed interest in placebos and the placebo effect—on their reality, their ethics, their place in medicine, or not, both in and out of the clinic and academy. The U.S. National Institutes of Health recently sponsored a large conference called "Science of the Placebo" (2). At least five serious books on the subject (3–7) plus a book of poetry (8) and a novel (9)—each titled *Placebo Effect*—have been published since 1997. In the past 10 years, the National Library of Medicine has annually listed an average of 3972 scholarly papers with the keywords "placebo," "placebos," or "placebo effect," with a low of 3362 papers in 1992 and a high of 4814 in 2000. During the fall of 2000, a discussion of the effect of new "drag free" suits, which might give an edge to Olympic swimmers, appeared in US *News and World Report*: "[S]wimming officials aren't convinced this is anything more than the placebo effect. Swimmers excel because they *think* they've got an edge" (10). One widely reported study, which concluded that placebos were powerless (11), or represented the Wizard of Oz (12), occasioned a blizzard of criticism (13–26) and some support (27). It's in the papers (28,29). It's in the air.

Yet the most recent serious attempt to try logically to define the placebo effect failed utterly (30). Given the ways people have gone about it, this seems unsurprising. Arthur K. Shapiro, MD, who spent much of his career as a psychiatrist studying the placebo effect, recently wrote:

A placebo is a substance or procedure . . . that is objectively without specific activity for the condition being treated . . . The placebo effect is the . . . therapeutic effect produced by a placebo. (31)

If we replace the word "placebo" in the second sentence with its definition from the first, we get: "The placebo effect is the therapeutic effect produced by [things] objectively without specific activity for the condition being treated."

This makes no sense whatsoever. Indeed, it flies in the face of the obvious. The one thing of which we can be absolutely certain is that placebos do not cause placebo effects. Placebos are inert and don't cause anything.

Moreover, people frequently expand the concept of the placebo effect very broadly to include just about every conceivable sort of beneficial biological, social, or human interaction that doesn't involve some drug well-known to the pharmacopoeia. A narrower form of this expansion includes identifying "natural history" or "regression to the mean" (as we might observe them in a randomized, controlled trial) as part of the placebo effect. But natural history and regression occur not only in the control group. Nothing in the theory of regression to the mean (31) hints that when people are selected for being extreme on some measure (blood pressure or cholesterol, for example), they are immune to regression if they receive active treatment. Such recipients are as likely (or unlikely) to move toward homeostasis as are control group patients. So, regression to the mean is in no meaningful way a "placebo effect." Ernst and Resch (32) took an important step in trying to clarify this situation by differentiating the "true" from the "perceived" placebo effect. But "true placebo effect" hasn't really caught on as a viable concept.

The concept of the placebo effect has been expanded much more broadly than this. Some attribute the effects of various alternative medical systems, such as homeopathy (33) or chiropractic (34), to the placebo effect. Others have described studies that show the positive effects of enhanced communication, such as Egbert's (35), as "the placebo response without the placebo" (7).

No wonder things are confusing.

Meaning and Medicine

We suggest thinking about this issue in a new way. A group of medical students was asked to participate in a study of two new drugs, one a tranquilizer and the other a stimulant (36). Each student was given a packet containing either one or two blue or red tablets; the tablets were inert. The students' responses to a questionnaire indicated that 1) the red tablets acted as stimulants while the blue ones acted as depressants and 2) two tablets had more effect than one. The students were not responding to the inertness of the tablets. Moreover, these responses cannot be easily accounted for by natural history, regression to the mean, or physician enthusiasm (presumably the experimenters were as enthusiastic about the reds as the blues). Instead, they can be explained by the "meanings" in the experiment: 1) Red means "up," "hot," "danger," while blue means "down," "cool," "quiet" and 2) two means more than one. These effects of color (37–40) and number (41,42) have been widely replicated.

In a British study, 835 women who regularly used analgesics for headache were randomly assigned to one of four groups (43). One group received aspirin labeled with a widely advertised brand name ("one of the most popular" analgesics in the United Kingdom that had been "widely available

for many years and supported by extensive advertising"). The other groups received the same aspirin in a plain package, placebo marked with the same widely advertised brand name, or unmarked placebo. In this study, branded aspirin worked better than unbranded aspirin, which worked better than branded placebo, which worked better than unbranded placebo. Among 435 headaches reported by branded placebo users, 64% were reported as improved 1 hour after pill administration compared with only 45% of the 410 headaches reported as improved among the unbranded placebo users. Aspirin relieves headaches, but so does the knowledge that the pills you are taking are "good" ones.

In a study of the benefits of aerobic exercise, two groups participated in a 10-week exercise program. One group was told that the exercise would enhance their aerobic capacity, while the other group was told that the exercise would enhance aerobic capacity and psychological well-being. Both groups improved their aerobic capacity, but only the second group improved in psychological well-being (actually "self-esteem"). The researchers called this "strong evidence . . . that exercise may enhance psychological well-being via a strong placebo effect" (44).

In the red versus blue pill study, we can correctly (if not very helpfully) classify the responses of the students as "placebo effects" because they did indeed receive inert tablets; it seems clear, however, that they responded not to the pills but to their colors. In the second study, the presence of the brand name enhanced the effect of both the inert and the active drug. It doesn't seem reasonable to classify the "brand name effect" as a "placebo effect" because no placebos are necessarily involved. Meanwhile, calling the consequences of authoritative instruction to the exercisers a "placebo effect" could come only from someone who believes that words do not affect the world, someone who has never been told "I love you" or who has never read the reviews of a rejected grant proposal. It seems reasonable to label all these effects (except, of course, of the aspirin and the exercise) as "meaning responses," a term that seeks, among other things, to recall Dr. Herbert Benson's "relaxation response" (45). Ironically, although placebos clearly cannot do anything themselves, their meaning can.

We define the *meaning response* as the physiologic or psychological effects of meaning in the origins or treatment of illness; meaning responses elicited after the use of inert or sham treatment can be called the "placebo effect" when they are desirable and the "nocebo effect" (46) when they are undesirable. This is obviously a complex notion with several terms that would be challenging to unpack ("desirable," "effect," "meaning," "treatment," "illness")—an exercise that cannot be carried out here. Note that this definition excludes several elements that are usually included in our understanding of the placebo effect, such as natural history, regression, experimenter or subject bias, and error in measurement or reporting. Note as well that the definition is not phrased in terms of "nonspecific" effects; although many elements of the meaning response or placebo effect may seem nonspecific, they are often quite specific in principle after they are understood.

Meaning Permeates Medical Treatment

Insofar as medicine is meaningful, it can affect patients, and it can affect the outcome of treatment (47–49). Most elements of medicine are meaningful, even if practitioners do not intend them to be so. The physician's costume (the white coat with stethoscope hanging out of the pocket) (50), manner (enthusiastic or not), style (therapeutic or experimental), and language (51) are all meaningful and can be shown to affect the outcome; indeed, we argue that both diagnosis (52) and prognosis (53) can be important forms of treatment.

Many studies can be cited to document aspects of the therapeutic quality of the practitioner's manner (54). In one, a strong message of the effect of a drug (an inert capsule) substantially reduced the patients' report of the pain of mandibular block injection compared with the pain after a weak message. Patients who received the weak message reported less pain than a group that received no placebos and no message at all (55). In another study, 200 patients with symptoms but no abnormal physical signs were randomly assigned to a positive or a negative consultation. In a survey of patients 2 weeks later, 64% of patients in the positive consultation group said they were all better, while only 39% of those who had negative consultations thought they were better (56).

Although there is strong evidence for such "physician effects," little evidence shows that "patient effects" are very important. A mass of research in the 1970s designed to identify "placebo reactors" produced only inconsistent and contradictory findings (57–59).

Meaning Can Have Substantial Physiologic Action

Placebo analgesia can elicit the production of endogenous opiates. Analgesia elicited with an injection of saline solution can be reversed with the opiate antagonist naloxone and enhanced with the opiate agonist proglumide (60). Likewise, acupuncture analgesia can be reversed with naloxone in animals (61) and people (62). To say that a treatment such as acupuncture "isn't better than placebo" does not mean that it does nothing.

Meaning and Surgery

The classic example of the meaningful effects of surgery comes from two studies of ligation of the bilateral internal mammary arteries as a treatment for angina (63,64). Patients receiving sham surgery did as well—with 80% of patients substantially improving—as those receiving the active procedure in the trials or in general practice. Although the studies were small, the procedure was no longer performed after these reports were published. Of note, these effectiveness rates (and those reported by the proponents of the procedure at the time) are much the same as those achieved by contemporary treatments such as coronary artery bypass or β-blockers.

Some observers have suggested that the success of transmyocardial laser revascularization, a procedure without a clear mechanism, may be explained by what they call the placebo effect (65) but what we call the meaning response. This is a plausible interpretation of a recent trial showing dramatic improvement in very sick people in both participant groups of a control trial of transmyocardial laser revascularization ([65a]).

Surgery is particularly meaningful: Surgeons are among the elite of medical practitioners; the shedding of blood is inevitably meaningful in and of itself. In addition, surgical procedures usually have compelling rational explanations, which drug treatments often do not. The logic of arthroscopic surgery ("we will clean up a messy joint") is much more sensible and understandable (and even effective [66]), especially for people in a culture rich in machines and tools, than is the logic of nonsteroidal anti-inflammatory drugs (which "inhibit the production of prostaglandins which are involved in the inflammatory process," something no one would ever tell a patient). Surgery clearly induces a profound meaning response in modern medical practice (67–69).

Meaning, Culture, and Medicine

Anthropologists understand cultures as complex webs of meaning, rich skeins of connected understandings, metaphors, and signs. Insofar as 1) meaning has biological consequence and 2) meanings vary across cultures, we can anticipate that biology will differ in different places, not because of genetics but because of these entangled ideas; we can anticipate what Margaret Lock has called "local biologies" (70,71); Lock has shown dramatic cross-cultural variation in the existence and experience of "menopause" (70,71). Moreover, Phillips has shown that "Chinese Americans, but not whites, die significantly earlier than normal (1.3 to 4.9 y) if they have a combination of disease and birth year which Chinese astrology and medicine consider ill fated" (72). Among Chinese Americans whose deaths were attributed to lymphatic cancer (n = 3041), those who were born in "Earth years"—and consequently were deemed by Chinese medical theory to be especially susceptible to diseases involving lumps, nodules, or tumors—had an average age at death of 59.7 years. In contrast, among those born in other years, age at death of Chinese Americans with lymphatic cancer was 63.6 years—nearly 4 years longer. Similar differences were also found for various other serious diseases. No such differences were evident in a large series of "whites" who died of similar causes in the same period. The intensity of the effect was shown to be correlated with "the strength of commitment to traditional Chinese culture." These differences in longevity (up to 6% or 7% difference in length of life!) are not due to having Chinese genes but to having Chinese ideas, to knowing the world in Chinese ways. The effects of meaning on health and disease are not restricted to placebos or brand names but permeate life.

One of us has shown variation in the response of control groups to inert medication in diverse cultures for the same

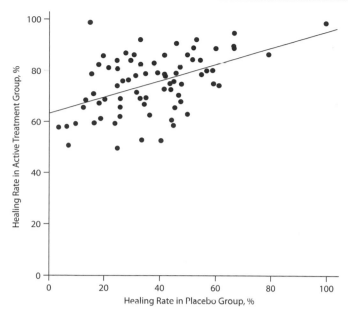

Figure 7.1. Data from 83 studies of the use of cimetidine or ranitidine for duodenal ulcer disease. In all cases, ulcers and ulcer healing were diagnosed endoscopically. Most studies lasted 4 weeks; a few were a bit shorter or longer. Sample sizes ranged from 12 to 210 participants (mean, 58). The quality of these studies was generally good for the era in which they were conducted (mostly between 1976 and 1986), although probably not fully adequate by contemporary standards. This analysis differs from the ordinary, in which placebo and active treatments are combined in an odds ratio, relative risk, or risk difference. The point of this analysis is not, however, to determine whether antisecretory medication is effective; clearly it is. The issue is the relationship between the pharmacologic and the meaningful dimensions of treatment. (A detailed account of these studies is available elsewhere [42].)

conditions (ulcers, hypertension, and anxiety) (42). Figure 7.1 shows the relationship between control group and active treatment group healing for endoscopically diagnosed duodenal ulcer treated with antisecretory medication. Control group healing and active treatment group healing seem functionally related in these studies. The correlation between control and active healing rates is 0.49; as the placebo group's healing rate increases, so does the rate of the active treatment group. Although the average control group healing rate in five German studies has been 62.4%, the healing rate was 16.7% in three studies from neighboring Denmark and the Netherlands. The number needed to treat for benefit (NNT_B), to obtain ulcer healing, can be calculated; for ulcer patients treated with placebo, the NNT_B for those who are German (not Danish or Dutch) is 2.

Conclusions

Practitioners can benefit clinically by conceptualizing this issue in terms of the meaning response rather than the placebo effect. Placebos are inert. You can't do anything about them. For human beings, meaning is everything that placebos are not, richly alive and powerful. However, we know little of this power, although all clinicians have experienced

it. One reason we are so ignorant is that, by focusing on placebos, we constantly have to address the moral and ethical issues of prescribing inert treatments (73,74), of lying (75), and the like. It seems possible to evade the entire issue by simply avoiding placebos. One cannot, however, avoid meaning while engaging human beings. Even the most distant objects—the planet Venus, the stars in the constellation Orion—are meaningful to us, as well as to others (76).

Yet, a huge puzzle remains: Obviously the meaning response is of great value to the sick and the lame. For example, eliciting the meaning response requires remarkably little effort ("You will be fine, Mr. Smith"). So why doesn't this happen all the time? And why can't you do it to yourself? Psychologist Nicholas Humphrey has suggested that this conundrum may have evolutionary roots: Healing has its benefits but also its costs (77). (For example, relieving pain may encourage premature activity, which could exacerbate the injury. Moreover, immune activity is metabolically very demanding on an injured system.) Perhaps only when a friend, relative, or healer indicates some level of social support (for example, by performing a ritual) is the individual's internal economy able to act. Moreover, as we have clarified, routinized, and rationalized our medicine, thereby relying on the salicylates and forgetting about the more meaningful birches, willows, and wintergreen from which they came—in essence, stripping away Plato's "charms"—we have impoverished the meaning of our medicine to a degree that it simply doesn't work as well as it might any more. Interesting ideas such as this are impossible to entertain when we discuss placebos; they spring readily to mind when we talk about meaning.

REFERENCES

1. Jowett B. Dialogues of Plato. Chicago: Univ Chicago Pr; 1952.
2. The Science of the Placebo: Toward an Interdisciplinary Research Agenda. National Institutes of Health, Bethesda, Maryland, 19–21 November 2000. Available at: placebo.nih.gov. [The proceedings from this conference were later published as a book: Guess HA, Kleinman A, Kusek JW, Engel LW (eds.). *The Science of the Placebo: Toward an Interdisciplinary Research Agenda.* London: BMJ Books, 2002—eds.]
3. Harrington A, ed. The Placebo Effect: An Interdisciplinary Exploration. Cambridge, Mass.: Harvard Univ Pr; 1997.
4. Shapiro AK, Shapiro E. The Powerful Placebo: From Ancient Priest to Modern Physician. Baltimore: Johns Hopkins Univ Pr; 1997.
5. Spiro HM. The Power of Hope: A Doctor's Perspective. New Haven: Yale Univ Pr; 1998.
6. Kirsch I, ed. How Expectancies Shape Experience. Washington, D.C.: American Psychological Association; 1999.
7. Brody H, Brody D. The Placebo Response: How You Can Release the Body's Inner Pharmacy for Better Health. New York: Cliff Street Books; 2000.
8. Beaumont JM. Placebo Effects: Poems. New York: W.W. Norton; 1997.
9. Russell G. Placebo Effect. New York: BBC Worldwide Americas; 1998.
10. Clark K, Milliken R. Today, it's "May the best swimsuit win." US News and World Report. 21 August 2000:55.
11. Hróbjartsson A, Gøtzsche PC. Is the placebo powerless? An analysis of clinical trials comparing placebo with no treatment. N Engl J Med. 2001; 344:1594–1602.
12. Bailar JC 3rd. The powerful placebo and the Wizard of Oz. N Engl J Med. 2001;344:1630–1632.

13. Beldoch M. Is the placebo powerless? N Engl J Med. 2001;345:1278.

14. DiNubile MJ. Is the placebo powerless? N Engl J Med. 2001;345:1278.

16. Kupers R. Is the placebo powerless? N Engl J Med. 2001;345:1278.

17. Einarson TE, Hemels M, Stolk P. Is the placebo powerless? N Engl J Med. 2001;345:1277.

18. Kaptchuk TJ. Is the placebo powerless? N Engl J Med. 2001;345:1277.

19. Miller FG. Is the placebo powerless? N Engl J Med. 2001;345:1277.

20. Lilford RJ, Braunholtz DA. Is the placebo powerless? N Engl J Med. 2001;345:1277–1278.

21. Spiegel D, Kraemer H, Carlson RW. Is the placebo powerless? N Engl J Med. 2001;345:1276.

22. Ader R. Much ado about nothing. Advances in Mind-Body Medicine. 2001;17:293–295.

23. Brody H, Weismantel D. A challenge to core beliefs. Advances in Mind-Body Medicine 2001;17:296–298.

24. Greene PJ, Wayne PM, Kerr CE, et al. The powerful placebo: doubting the doubters. Advances in Mind-Body Medicine. 2001;17:298–307.

25. Kirsch I, Scorboria A. Apples, oranges, and placebos: heterogeneity in a meta-analysis of placebo effects. Advances in Mind-Body Medicine. 2001;17:307–309.

26. Wickramasekera I. The placebo efficacy study: problems with the definition of the placebo and the mechanisms of placebo efficacy. Advances in Mind-Body Medicine. 2001;17:309–312.

27. McDonald CJ. Is the placebo powerless? N Engl J Med. 2001;345:1276–1277.

28. Talbot M. The placebo prescription. New York Times Magazine. 9 January 2001: 34–39, 44, 58–60.

29. Rubin R. "Eat one. You'll feel better." USA Today. 16 January 2001:D1.

30. Gøtzsche PC. Is there logic in the placebo? Lancet. 1994;344:925–926.

31. McDonald CJ, Mazzuca SA, McCabe GP Jr. How much of the placebo "effect" is really statistical regression? Stat Med. 1983;2:417–427.

32. Ernst E, Resch KL. Concept of true and perceived placebo effects. BMJ. 1995;311:551–553.

33. Ernst E, Pittler MH. Efficacy of homeopathic arnica: a systematic review of placebo-controlled clinical trials. Arch Surg. 1998;133:1187–1190.

34. Curtis P. Spinal manipulation: does it work? Occup Med. 1988;3:31–44.

35. Egbert LD, Battit GE, Welch CE, Bartlett MK. Reduction of postoperative pain by encouragement and instruction of patients. A study of doctor-patient rapport. N Engl J Med. 1964;270:825–827.

36. Blackwell B, Bloomfield SS, Buncher CR. Demonstration to medical students of placebo responses and non-drug factors. Lancet. 1972;1:1279–1282.

37. Schapira K, McClelland HA, Griffiths NR, Newell DJ. Study on the effects of tablet colour in the treatment of anxiety states. Br Med J. 1970;1:446–449.

38. Honzak R, Horackova E, Culik A. Our experience with the effect of placebo in some functional and psychosomatic disorders. Activa Nervosa Superior (Prague). 1971;13:190–191.

39. Cattaneo AD, Lucchilli PE, Filippucci G. Sedative effects of placebo treatment. Eur J Clin Pharmacol. 1970;3:43–45.

40. de Craen AJ, Roos PJ, Leonard de Vries A, Kleijnen J. Effect of colour of drugs: systematic review of perceived effect of drugs and of their effectiveness. BMJ. 1996;313:1624–1626.

41. de Craen AJ, Moerman DE, Heisterkamp SH, et al. Placebo effect in the treatment of duodenal ulcer. Br J Clin Pharmacol. 1999;48:853–860.

42. Moerman DE. Cultural variations in the placebo effect: ulcers, anxiety, and blood pressure. Med Anthropol Q. 2000;14:51–72.

43. Branthwaite A, Cooper P. Analgesic effects of branding in treatment of headaches. Br Med J (Clin Res Ed). 1981;282:1576–1578.

44. Desharnais R, Jobin J, Côté C, Lévesque L, Godin G. Aerobic exercise and the placebo effect: a controlled study. Psychosom Med. 1993;55:149–154.

45. Benson H, Klipper MZ. The Relaxation Response. New York: Wings Books; 1992.

46. Hahn RA. The nocebo phenomenon: concept, evidence, and implications for public health. Prev Med. 1997;26:607–611.

47. Levi-Strauss C. The Effectiveness of Symbols. In: Structural Anthropology. Garden City, N.Y.: Anchor Books; 1967:186–205.

48. Moerman DE. Anthropology of symbolic healing. Current Anthropology. 1979;20:59–80.

49. Kirmayer LJ. Healing and the invention of metaphor: the effectiveness of symbols revisited. Cult Med Psychiatry. 1993;17:161–195.

50. Blumhagen DW. The doctor's white coat. The image of the physician in modern America. Ann Intern Med. 1979;91:111–116.

51. Uhlenhuth EH, Rickels K, Fisher S, et al. Drug, doctor's verbal attitude and clinic setting in the symptomatic response to pharmacotherapy. Psychopharmacologia. 1966;9:392–418.

52. Brody H, Waters DB. Diagnosis is treatment. J Fam Pract. 1980;10:445–449.

53. Christakis NA. Death Foretold: Prophecy and Prognosis in Medical Care. Chicago: Univ Chicago Pr; 1999.

54. Gracely RH. Charisma and the art of healing: can nonspecific factors be enough? In: Devor M, Rowbotham MC, Wiesenfeld-Hallin Z, eds. Proceedings of the 9th World Congress on Pain. Seattle: IASP Pr; 2000:1045–1067.

55. Gryll SL, Katahn M. Situational factors contributing to the placebos effect. Psychopharmacology (Berl). 1978;57:253–261.

56. Thomas KB. General practice consultations: is there any point in being positive? Br Med J (Clin Res Ed). 1987;294:1200–1202.

57. Moerman DE. Edible symbols: the effectiveness of placebos. Ann N Y Acad Sci. 1981;364:256–268.

58. Fisher S. The placebo reactor: thesis, antithesis, synthesis, and hypothesis. Dis Nerv Syst. 1967;28:510–515.

59. Liberman RP. The elusive placebo reactor. In: Brill H, ed. Neuro-Psycho-Pharmacology: Proceedings of the Fifth International Congress of the Collegium Internationale Neuro-Psycho-Pharmacologicum. Amsterdam: Excerpta Medica Foundation. 1967:557–566.

60. Benedetti F, Amanzio M. The neurobiology of placebo analgesia: from endogenous opioids to cholecystokinin. Prog Neurobiol. 1997;52:109–125.

61. Pomeranz B, Chiu D. Naloxone blockade of acupuncture analgesia: endorphin implicated. Life Sci. 1976;19:1757–1762.

62. Mayer DJ, Price DD, Rafii A. Antagonism of acupuncture analgesia in man by the narcotic antagonist naloxone. Brain Res. 1977;121:368–372.

63. Cobb L, Thomas GI, Dillard DH, Merendino KA, Bruce RA. An evaluation of internal-mammary-artery ligation by a double-blind technic. N Engl J Med. 1959;260:1115–1118.

64. Dimond EG, Kittle CF, Crockett JE. Comparison of internal mammary ligation and sham operation for angina pectoris. Am J Cardiol. 1960;5:483–486.

65. Lange RA, Hillis LD. Transmyocardial laser revascularization. N Engl J Med. 1999;341:1075–1076.

[65a.Leon MB, Baim DS, Moses JW, Laham RJ, Knopf W. A randomized blinded clinical trial comparing percutaneous laser myocardial revascularization (using Biosense LV Mapping) vs. placebo in patients with refractory coronary ischemia. Presented at American Heart Association Scientific Session, 12–15 November 2000 (removed from main text and added as a reference—eds.)].

66. Moseley JB Jr, Wray NP, Kuykendall D, Willis K, Landon G. Arthroscopic treatment of osteoarthritis of the knee: a prospective, randomized, placebo-controlled trial. Results of a pilot study. Am J Sports Med. 1996;24:28–34.

67. Beecher HK. Surgery as placebo. A quantitative study of bias. JAMA. 1961;176:1102–1107.

68. Johnson AG. Surgery as a placebo. Lancet. 1994;344:1140–1142.

69. Kaptchuk TJ, Goldman P, Stone DA, Stason WB. Do medical devices have enhanced placebo effects? J Clin Epidemiol. 2000;53:786–792.

70. Lock MM. Encounters with Aging: Mythologies of Menopause in Japan and North America. Berkeley: Univ California Pr; 1993.

71. Lock M. Menopause: lessons from anthropology. Psychosom Med. 1998;60:410–419.

72. Phillips DP, Ruth TE, Wagner LM. Psychology and survival. Lancet. 1993;342:1142–1145.

73. Macklin R. The ethical problems with sham surgery in clinical research. N Engl J Med. 1999;341:992–996.

74. Reynolds T. The ethics of placebo-controlled trials. Ann Intern Med. 2000;133:491.

75. Evans M. Justified deception? The single blind placebo in drug research. J Med Ethics. 2000;26:188–193.

76. McCleary TP. The Stars We Know: Crow Indian Astronomy and Lifeways. Prospect Heights, Ill.: Waveland Pr; 1997.

77. Humphrey N. Great expectations: The evolutionary psychology of faith-healing and the placebo response. In: Humphrey N, ed. The Mind Made Flesh: Essays from the Frontiers of Evolution and Psychology. Oxford: Oxford Univ Pr; 2002: Chapter 19.

8

The Placebo Effect in Alternative Medicine

Can the Performance of a Healing Ritual Have Clinical Significance?

Ted J. Kaptchuk

Ted J. Kaptchuk, "The Placebo Effect in Alternative Medicine: Can the Performance of a Healing Ritual Have Clinical Significance?" *Annals of Internal Medicine* 2002;136:817–825.

Efficacious therapy, in one biomedical definition, is therapy that has positive effects greater than those of an indistinguishable dummy treatment in a randomized, controlled trial (RCT) (1–3). Such specific efficacy is actually a comparative measure: intervention contrasted with placebo. This relative effectiveness, which is estimated by statistical testing, is taken to indicate "authenticity." The clinical significance, that is, the outcome measured by using the patient's original condition as a baseline, is usually a secondary consideration for determining "legitimate" medical interventions. Any clinical impact due to the placebo, which is deemed to lack "truthfulness," is even less notable and is valued only as a comparison baseline for "genuine" effects (3). Specific effects are by definition superior to nonspecific effects. The clinical repercussions of the placebo are tolerated as necessary nuisance noise but are otherwise considered inconsequential or treated with contempt (4).

Given the privileged status of specific effects, it is not surprising that the clinical impact of alternative medicine's placebo effects are routinely ignored (5). The only serious question has been whether alternative medicine has more than a placebo effect. Discarding all placebo effects in a single trash basket of "untruthfulness," however, diminishes our knowledge of important dimensions of health care. This essay examines the neglected clinical significance of the placebo effect in alternative medicine and raises the possibility that some types of unconventional medicine may produce placebo outcomes that are dramatic and, from the patient's perspective, especially compelling. The term *placebo effect* is taken to mean not only the narrow effect of an imitation intervention but also the broad amalgam of nonspecific effects present in any patient-practitioner relationship, including attention; communication of concern; intense monitoring; diagnostic procedures; labeling of complaint; and alterations produced in a patient's expectancy, anxiety, and relationship to the illness. This essay asks whether alternative medicine can have an "enhanced" placebo effect. In some conditions, can any of alternative medicine's particular rituals have a greater impact than the rituals of conventional medicine or than a proven physiologically active treatment? After all, as many of the examples in this essay will demonstrate, "two interventions may have different effects on patient outcome even though both [are] equivalent to placebo in clinical trials" (6). Dismissing a treatment as "just a placebo" may not be enough.

Alternative medicine may be an especially successful placebo-generating health care system. Rather than specific biological consequences, which epidemiologists designate as "fastidious efficacy" (7), alternative medicine may administer an especially large dose of what anthropologists call "performative efficacy" (8). Performative efficacy relies on the power of belief, imagination, symbols, meaning, expectation, persuasion, and self-relationship. This essay takes five components of the placebo drama—patient, practitioner, patient-practitioner interaction, nature of the illness, and treatment and setting—and examines their "placebogenic" potentials in unconventional healing practices. Much of the evidence is derived from conventional research and is speculatively applied to alternative medicine. Also, it should be noted that most of the placebo research discussed in this essay does not represent an "artifactual" placebo effect explainable by natural history or regression to the mean. Rather, it usually involves comparative experiments with two different types of placebo or the same placebo delivered under different cognitive or emotional circumstances where two distinct placebo outcomes would not support the idea of placebo effect as only natural history. Finally, this essay argues mostly in generalities. Obviously, the placebo effect is likely to be at least as heterogeneous in alternative medicine as in conventional medicine, but it is hoped that raising these questions will encourage further discussion and research.

Patient Characteristics

Although the patient is the protagonist in the placebo drama, research has failed to find consistent placebo responders or to identify personality traits or other qualities of persons who frequently react to placebo (9–11). However, evidence shows that patient expectations influence outcomes of both placebo and active treatment. Asthmatic patients who believe that an inert substance is a bronchodilator or a bronchoconstrictor respond accordingly (12–14). In a small but classic crossover experiment, healthy volunteers received a placebo pill in which a magnet was embedded. In random order, at different times, they were told that they were receiving a relaxant, a stimulant, or a placebo. Subsequent gastric motility was significantly consistent with patients' expectations (15). Patient expectancies also significantly change or even reverse the actions of many potent pharmaceutical agents (16–19).

Adherence to placebo may also be a surrogate marker for a patient's own contribution to the activation of the placebo response (20,21). In RCTs, such "placebo adherence effects"—the post hoc differences observed in the placebo arm between those who comply with taking placebo and those who do not—are associated not only with symptom relief but also with concrete end points, including survival (22–24). Indeed, differences in adherence are associated with differences in outcomes that exceed the effects of many pharmaceutical agents (25). Patient preferences for one type of intervention, especially in participative interventions (for example, exercise or diet programs), may contribute significantly to outcomes, including increased placebo responses (26–28).

In contrast to conventional medicine, with its measured objectivity, alternative medicine offers a charged constellation of expectations. Alternative medicine's romantic vision is inhabited by benevolent and intentional forces (for example, the innate intelligence of chiropractic or the qi of acupuncture) that are unrestrained by the laws of normative physics (29). An exaggerated notion of the possible readily elicits patients' magical anticipation. These unconventional concepts do not require absolute belief "in the sense that their truth value is certified by logic or argument" but rather requires moderate openness "in the sense that they are taken into the imagination and lived with, if only for a time" (30).

Alternative medicine emphasizes personal responsibility, which can facilitate adherence. Indeed, the act of switching to another medical system and exhibiting preference by action demonstrates an openness to active participation and adherence and possibly enhances it. Paying out-of-pocket and other signs of commitment, such as following daily lifestyle regimens, undoubtedly marshal adherence effects. The reasons that patients choose alternative medicine may also potentiate a placebo response. Patients with chronic diseases often turn to unconventional healing after long-term negative conditioning with mainstream medicine (31). In this situation, patients' hope (based on no previous experience with alternative medicine) may provide an opportunity for "deconditioning" from previous unsuccessful medical experiences.

Practitioner Characteristics

The practitioner-healer must expertly play the role of heroic rescuer to facilitate a placebo effect (32). Numerous RCTs have compared optimistic or enthusiastic physician attitudes toward drug or placebo with neutral or doubtful physician attitudes. Practitioners have had significant impact on such clinical conditions as pain (33–36), psychiatric illness (37–41), hypertension (42,43), obesity (44), and perimenopause symptoms (45). Although some studies have shown no effect of physicians' expectations on clinical end points (46–48), a systematic review of 85 studies found that although more research is needed, provider-induced "expectancies are a mechanism for placebo effects, [which have] received support across a range of clinical areas in a variety of studies" (49). A second review, which used more stringent entry criteria, found 25 RCTs that examined the impact of randomly assigning patients with physical illnesses to different levels of expectancy and emotional support. Although researchers found inconsistent effects and determined that further research was needed, they also found that "enhancing patients' expectations through positive information about the treatment or illness, while providing support or reassurance, [seemed to] significantly influence health outcomes" (50).

Even in blinded RCTs, practitioner certitude seems to influence the magnitude of the placebo effect. In one RCT that simultaneously compared two double-blind RCTs, dental patients in one trial received placebo, narcotic analgesics, or narcotic antagonists and those in the other trial received only a placebo or a narcotic antagonist. Dentists knew the possible interventions in both trials but remained blinded to administration of medication. Pain in placebo recipients was significantly worse in the second trial, in which narcotic drugs were not an option, than in the first trial (51). An earlier RCT of the effect of physician expectations on hypertension drugs also found that practitioner belief can transform outcomes (52).

Practitioners of unconventional medicine are less restrained by scientific objectivity than practitioners of conventional medicine. The sensibilities of alternative practitioners are therefore often more optimistic and positive than those of their mainstream counterparts (53). The characteristics thought to enhance the placebo effect (and any active intervention) seem to be fully operational in the offices of alternative medicine.

Patient-Practitioner Interaction

The placebo drama is probably more successful if the patient and practitioner find each other's beliefs and actions mutually credible or at least intriguing. Reciprocal expectations need to be negotiated and joined in the patient-physician duet. Many studies indicate that the patient-practitioner encounter is a potent factor in health outcomes (54–56) and that for many non-life-threatening illnesses, clear diagnosis, assurance of recovery, opportunity for dialogue, and physician-patient agreement about the nature of the problem hasten recovery or relief (57,58). One study examined 200 patients who presented to general practitioners with symptoms but no abnormal physical signs and in whom no definite diagnosis could be made. Patients were randomly assigned in a 2×2 design to treatment or no treatment and to a positive consultation, in which they received "a firm diagnosis and [were] told confidently that [they] would be better in a few days," or a negative consultation, in which they were told that their condition was uncertain. Although provision of treatment made no difference, positive interaction produced significantly faster recovery (59). A similar experiment in 100 patients with acute tonsillitis had analogous results (60).

Consultation in unconventional medicine is more likely than its mainstream counterpart to produce a precise diagnosis that matches patients' perceptions. In unconventional medicine, patient experience is never devalued or brushed aside as unreliable (61). Inevitably, since the alternative world is not as constrained by the dichotomy of objectivity and subjectivity, the chiropractor will find the subluxation, the acupuncturist will detect the yin–yang disharmony, and the health food advocate will identify the transgression that makes sense of the patient's life-world. In addition, if a patient is new to alternative medicine, an opportunity for exchange is invariably offered, providing the patient with "theoretical explanations designed to take the mystery out of process and problems" (62). When it is considered that 40% to 60% of patients may never receive a firm diagnosis in conventional medicine (63,64), an alternative diagnosis may be a potent form of nonspecific healing that changes the circumstances under which the patient exists (65–67), including reducing the "dysphoria of uncertainty" (68).

Besides diagnosis, the healing encounter also establishes therapeutic goals. Paradoxically, while the alternative diagnosis tends to be precise, treatment aims can be diverse. Because of such notions as "holistic medicine" and "body, mind, spirit," alternative medicine can have extremely broad, indeterminate therapeutic targets and therefore, at least from a cultural view, "in some sense cannot fail" (69). Such amorphous goals can provide additional maneuvering room for positive progress, or at least incremental change (70). If the patient's symptoms do not directly improve, it is likely that something positive will happen and be attributed to the intervention (even if the change pertains only to alternative constructs, such as the homeopathic spiritual force or the acupuncture qi). Taken together, the alternative diagnosis, prognosis, and treatment aims serve "to regulate symptom intensity and distress" and "create enough certainty to diminish the threat of the inchoate while preserving enough ambiguity to allow for fresh improvisation" (71).

The Nature of the Illness

The placebo effect may benefit from the types of illnesses that alternative medicine commonly treats. Data indicate that the overwhelming majority of medical conditions treated by unconventional medicine fall into the following categories: highly subjective symptoms lacking identifiable physiologic correlates, chronic conditions with a fluctuating course often influenced by selective attention, and affective disorders (2,72). Not surprisingly, these conditions are precisely those that researchers believe are especially susceptible to inordinately strong placebo responses: back and chronic pain (73–75), fatigue (76,77), arthritis (78,79), headache (80,81), allergies (82,83), hypertension (in some situations) (84,85), insomnia (86,87), asthma (13,88), chronic digestive disorders (89,90), depression (91,92), and anxiety (93). Even researchers who question the existence or significance of a placebo effect—at least in the narrow sense of the outcome produced by a dummy intervention—concede its impact when outcomes are continuous and subjective (94). Also, persons with self-limiting diseases, such as the common cold and sprains and strains, also frequently use alternative medicine. In these cases, the natural course of the disease undoubtedly creates the appearance of treatment response and enhances the perception of unconventional medicine's effectiveness.

Treatment and Setting

Treatment paraphernalia and setting affect the impact of a placebo performance. For placebo pills, a regimen of four times per day seems more effective than a regimen of twice per day (95). A "brand-name" therapy that includes either active or inert ingredients may often yield better results than an identical treatment that is not as well known (96), and devices or elaborate procedures can have greater placebo effects than pills (97,98). Active placebos (placebos containing medications, such as atropine, that are ineffective for the condition being studied but produce recognizable drug-related side effects) seem to provide genuine treatment recognition that leads to heightened placebo effects (99,100). With good showmanship, a well-designed, totally inert stage prop can offer this kind of "feedback loop" and can produce exaggerated placebo effects.

Two RCTs—one of transcutaneous electrical nerve stimulation and one of "placebo electronic machines"—demonstrated that, with good staging, blank machines can provide feedback sensations. In the first study, all patients reported an electrical sensation after adjustment of the dummy apparatus, which was equipped with visual and sound feedback (101). In the second trial (which used only dummy machines under two different sets of expectations), a significant number of participants "felt" the nonexistent current, and some even volunteered that the sensation was "just amazing" (102).

Biomedicine and alternative medicine each have a special allure of mystery and exotic power; it would be hard to argue that one backdrop consistently provides a superior placebo effect. However, alternative medicine has the advantage of always having an intervention scenario. Therapeutic passivity is rarely an option, and practitioners can, at a minimum, offer something that is likely to have a placebo effect. In some situations, and at least for continuous subjective outcomes, an intervention presumably has a greater effect than no treatment (94,103). Also, to demonstrate "active" intervention, alternative medicine treatments have unique feedback loops that are likely to facilitate, if not heighten, substantial placebo responses. For example, chiropractic adjustment often triggers an audible "pop" so that the patient can hear the subluxation being fixed (104), acupuncturists propagate a sensation of vital energy coursing through invisible meridians (105), and psychic healers summon tingling vibrations (106).

Does Alternative Medicine Have Enhanced Placebo Effects?

Despite the arguments and speculations already presented, there is scant empirical evidence that any particular type of alternative medicine used for any particular condition has an augmented placebo effect. Even concerning the placebo effect in general, the evidence cited earlier is often methodologically weak and limited by small numbers and short follow-up periods. Some social scientists argue that "for the believer in science, medical care that appears to be scientific would provide a superior placebo; for the believer . . . of whatever other cultural system of meaning and values," alternative medicine may "provide a superior placebo" (107). Perhaps biomedicine's effort to eliminate ritual or placebo interventions itself produces an improved placebo effect.

Two examples from RCTs may help readers concretely envision an enhanced placebo effect. In a four-arm crossover RCT involving 44 patients with chronic cervical osteoarthritis of more than 6 months' duration, acupuncture, sham acupuncture, and diazepam were all equivalent and were superior to a placebo pill (108). In this study, the outcome of the ritual of acupuncture (real and sham acupuncture were not different) equaled the outcome of an effective drug. In a second RCT, which studied spinal manipulation, 256 patients with nonspecific back and neck disorders were randomly assigned to receive manual therapy (the Dutch equivalent of chiropractic), physical therapy, placebo-device therapy with a "detuned" ultrasonography machine and "detuned" short-wave diathermy that emitted sounds and lights, or treatment from a general practitioner (109). Six weeks of manual therapy and physical therapy were equally and significantly better than the sham machine, which significantly outperformed the general practitioner. It cannot be determined whether the manual and physical therapies had specific treatment effects or simply yielded better placebo effects than the inanimate gadget. Nonetheless, in this experiment, treatment with a sham machine surpassed treatment from a competent physician for relief of low back pain.

To more rigorously test these possible relative nonspecific effects, my colleagues and I are performing a National Institutes of Health–funded RCT that randomly assigns patients with chronic pain to one of two parallel run-in phases. Before entering two subsequent RCTs, one run-in group receives a conventional-appearing placebo pill and the other receives an alternative medicine sham procedure; the main goal of the run-in phases is to detect differing placebo effects (97). Any confident assertion about a placebo effect enhanced by alternative medicine would probably require many such experiments.

Some may dismiss these types of investigation as useless. After all, a placebo is just a placebo. Others would argue that such avoidance impoverishes and narrows the understanding of what patients receive from alternative medicine (and, by extension, conventional medicine). Even those who doubt the existence or significance of a "narrow" placebo effect seem open to the possibility of "broad" placebo effects embedded in the psychosocial context of the patient-practitioner relationship (110,111).

What Is Legitimate Healing?

Besides clinical and scientific value, the question of enhanced placebo effects raises complex ethical questions concerning what is "legitimate" healing. What should determine appropriate healing, a patient's improvement from his or her own baseline (clinical significance) or relative improvement compared with a placebo (fastidious efficacy)? As one philosopher of medicine has asked, are results less important than method (3)? Both performative and fastidious efficacy can be measured. Which measurement represents universal science? Which measurement embodies cultural judgment on what is "correct" healing? Are the concerns of the physician identical to those of the patient? Is denying patients with nonspecific back pain treatment with a sham machine an ethical judgment or a scientific judgment? Should a patient with chronic neck pain who cannot take diazepam because of unacceptable side effects be denied acupuncture that may have an "enhanced placebo effect" because such an effect is "bogus"? Who should decide?

Patients' attitudes toward placebo interventions (especially enhanced interventions) probably differ from physicians' attitudes (112). This distinction is probably most evident in surgery, another field in which a heightened placebo effect is possible (97,113), as illustrated by two RCTs that tested implantation of fetal dopaminergic cells for Parkinson disease. Patients with Parkinson disease seem to have a robust placebo response (114,115); the biochemical substrate of this response in relation to the release of dopamine in the striatum has recently been shown on positron emission tomography (116). At the conclusion of one of the two RCTs, patients were unblinded, and half were told they had received sham surgery that had performed the same as real surgery. In the early reports from this study, both groups experienced significant clinical improvement. (The subsequent full report, which included long-term data, reported a less durable placebo effect [117].) When patients who had received the sham surgery were told that they could not receive the real but now "discredited" surgery, as they had been promised in the informed consent form, 70% were disappointed or "outraged" because of the dramatic benefits they had already received from sham surgery (118–120). They wanted the "real" procedure even if it was equivalent to the sham. Of interest, the second RCT, which also found no difference between active and imitation surgery, demonstrated a stable and significant placebo effect after 18 months (121). For many patients, performative efficacy may be more critical than fastidious efficacy. Obviously, this illustration is not meant to advocate ritualistic surgery. Rather, it is meant to highlight the complex relationship among clinical, scientific, and ethical judgments.

Conclusion

Alternative medicine may be composed of healing rituals that have especially potent performative efficacy. Therapeutic characteristics that may enhance placebo effects seem especially prominent in unconventional healing. Although more research into this question is necessary before any such assertion can be made with confidence, an enhanced placebo effect raises complex questions about what is legitimate therapy, and who decides.

REFERENCES

1. Temple RJ. When are clinical trials of a given agent vs. placebo no longer appropriate or feasible? Control Clin Trials. 1997;18:613–620.
2. Kaptchuk TJ, Edwards RA, Eisenberg DM. Complementary medicine: efficacy beyond the placebo effect. In: Ernst E, ed. Complementary Medicine: An Objective Appraisal. Oxford: Butterworth-Heinemann; 1996.
3. Sullivan MD. Placebo controls and epistemic control in orthodox medicine. J Med Philos. 1993;18:213–231.
4. van Weel C. Examination of context of medicine. Lancet. 2001;357: 733–734.
5. Kaptchuk TJ. Powerful placebo: the dark side of the randomised controlled trial. Lancet. 1998;351:1722–1725.
6. Vickers AJ, de Craen AJ. Why use placebos in clinical trials? A narrative review of the methodological literature. J Clin Epidemiol. 2000;53:157–161.
7. Feinstein AR. Clinical Epidemiology. Philadelphia: WB Saunders; 1985.
8. Tambiah SJ. Magic, Science, Religion, and the Scope of Rationality. Cambridge, U.K.: Cambridge Univ Pr; 1990.
9. Shapiro AK, Shapiro E. The Powerful Placebo: From Ancient Priest to Modern Physician. Baltimore: Johns Hopkins Univ Pr; 1997.
10. Wolf S, Doering CR, Clark ML, Hagans JA. Chance distribution and the placebo "reactor." J Lab Clin Med. 1957;49:837–841.
11. Liberman RP. The elusive placebo reactor. Neuropsychopharmacology. 1967;5:557–566.
12. Luparello TJ, Leist N, Lourie CH, Sweet P. The interaction of psychologic stimuli and pharmacologic agents on airway reactivity in asthmatic subjects. Psychosom Med. 1970;32:509–513.
13. Butler C, Steptoe A. Placebo responses: an experimental study of psychophysiological processes in asthmatic volunteers. Br J Clin Psychol. 1986;25(Pt. 3):173–183.
14. Sodergren SC, Hyland ME. Expectancy and asthma. In: Kirsch I, ed. How Expectancies Shape Experience. Washington, D.C.: American Psychological Assoc; 1999.
15. Sternbach RA. The effects of instructional sets on autonomic responsivity. Psychophysiology. 1964;62:67–72.
16. Kaptchuk TJ. The double-blind, randomized, placebo-controlled trial. Gold standard or golden calf? J Clin Epidemiol. 2001;54:541–549.
17. Mitchell SH, Laurent CL, de Wit H. Interaction of expectancy and the pharmacological effects of d-amphetamine: subjective effects and self-administration. Psychopharmacology (Berl). 1996;125:371–378.
18. Flaten MG, Simonsen T, Olsen H. Drug-related information generates placebo and nocebo responses that modify the drug response. Psychosom Med. 1999;61:250–255.
19. Dworkin SF, Chen AC, Schubert MM, Clark DW. Cognitive modification of pain: information with N_2O. Pain. 1984;19:339–351.
20. Horwitz RI, Horwitz SM. Adherence to treatment and health outcomes. Arch Intern Med. 1993;153:1863–1868.
21. Czajkowski SM, Chesney MA. Adherence and the placebo effect. In: Shumaker SA, Schron EB, Ockene JK, eds. The Handbook of Health Behavior Change. New York: Springer; 1990.
22. The Coronary Drug Project Research Group. Influence of adherence to treatment and response of cholesterol on mortality in the coronary drug project. N Engl J Med. 1980;303:1038–1041.
23. Horwitz RI, Viscoli CM, Berkman L, et al. Treatment adherence and risk of death after a myocardial infarction. Lancet. 1990;336: 542–545.
24. Gallagher EJ, Viscoli CM, Horwitz RI. The relationship of treatment adherence to the risk of death after myocardial infarction in women. JAMA. 1993;270:742–744.
25. Mattocks KM, Horwitz RI. Placebos, active control groups, and the unpredictability paradox. Biol Psychiatry. 2000;47:693–698.
26. Wennberg JE. What is outcomes research? In: Gelijns AC, ed. Modern Methods of Clinical Investigation. Washington, D.C.: National Academy Pr; 1990.
27. McPherson K, Britton AR, Wennberg JE. Are randomized controlled trials controlled? Patient preferences and unblind trials. J R Soc Med. 1997;90:652–656.
28. Brewin CR, Bradley C. Patient preferences and randomised clinical trials. BMJ. 1989;299:313–315.
29. Kaptchuk TJ. History of vitalism. In: Micozzi MS, ed. Fundamentals of Complementary and Alternative Medicine. New York: Churchill Livingstone; 2001.
30. Kirmayer LJ. Healing and the invention of metaphor: the effectiveness of symbols revisited. Cult Med Psychiatry. 1993;17:161–195.
31. Zollman C, Vickers A. ABC of complementary medicine. Complementary medicine and the patient. BMJ. 1999;319:1486–1489.
32. Shapiro AK. Iatroplacebogenics. International Pharmacopsychiatry. 1969;2:215–248.
33. Gryll SL, Katahn M. Situational factors contributing to the placebos effect. Psychopharmacology (Berl). 1978;57:253–261.
34. Hashish I, Hai HK, Harvey W, Feinmann C, Harris M. Reduction of postoperative pain and swelling by ultrasound treatment: a placebo effect. Pain. 1988;33:303–311.
35. Ho KH, Hashish I, Salmon P, Freeman R, Harvey W. Reduction of postoperative swelling by a placebo effect. J Psychosom Res. 1988;32: 197–205.
36. Bergmann JF, Chassany O, Gandiol J, et al. A randomised clinical trial of the effect of informed consent on the analgesic activity of placebo and naproxen in cancer pain. Clin Trials Meta-Anal. 1994;29:41–47.
37. Uhlenhuth EH, Rickels K, Fisher S, et al. Drug, doctor's verbal attitude and clinic setting in the symptomatic response to pharmacotherapy. Psychopharmacologia. 1966;9:392–418.
38. Fisher S, Cole JO, Rickels K, Uhlenhuth EH. Drug-set interaction: the effect of expectations on drug response in outpatients. Neuropsychopharmacology. 1964;3:149–156.
39. Wheatley D. Influence of doctors' and patients' attitudes in the treatment of neurotic illness. Lancet. 1967;2:1133–1135.
40. Rabkin JG, McGrath PJ, Quitkin FM, et al. Effects of pill-giving on maintenance of placebo response in patients with chronic mild depression. Am J Psychiatry. 1990;147:1622–1626.
41. Affleck DC, Eaton MT, Mansfield E. The action of a medication and the physician's expectations. Nebr State Med J. 1966;51:331–334.
42. Agras WS, Horne M, Taylor CB. Expectation and the blood-pressure-lowering effects of relaxation. Psychosom Med. 1982;44:389–395.

43. Amigo I, Cuesta V, Fernández A, González A. The effect of verbal instructions on blood pressure measurement. J Hypertens. 1993;11: 293–296.

44. Freund J, Krupp G, Goodenough D, Preston LW. The doctor-patient relationship and drug effect. Clin Pharmacol Ther. 1972;13:172–180.

45. Wied GL. Über die Bedeutung der Suggestion in der Therapie klimakterischer Ausfallerscheinungen. ÄrztlicheArztliche Wochenschrift. 1953;8:623–625.

46. de Craen AJM. Impact of experimentally induced expectancy on the analgesic effect of tramadol in chronic pain patients: a 2 × 2 factorial, randomised, placebo-controlled, double-blind trial. In: Placebos and Placebo Effects in Clinical Trials [Dissertation]. Amsterdam: Univ of Amsterdam; 1998.

47. Cooper WD, Currie WJ, Vandenburg MJ. The influence of physicians' instructions on the outcome of antihypertensive therapy. Br J Clin Pract. 1983; 37:99–103.

48. Kincheloe JE, Mealiea WL Jr, Mattison GD, Seib K. Psychophysical measurement on pain perception after administration of a topical anesthetic. Quintessence Int. 1991;22:311–315.

49. Crow R, Gage H, Hampson S, Hart J, Kimber A, Thomas H. The role of expectancies in the placebo effect and their use in the delivery of health care: a systematic review. Health Technol Assess. 1999;3:1–96.

50. Di Blasi Z, Harkness E, Ernst E, Georgiou A, Kleijnen J. Influence of context effects on health outcomes: a systematic review. Lancet. 2001;357:757–762.

51. Gracely RH, Dubner R, Deeter WR, Wolskee PJ. Clinicians' expectations influence placebo analgesia. Lancet. 1985;1:43.

52. Shapiro AP, Myer T, Reiser MF, Ferris EB. Comparison of blood pressure response to Veriloid and to the doctor. Psychosom Med. 1954;16:478–488.

53. Kaptchuk TJ, Eisenberg DM. The persuasive appeal of alternative medicine. Ann Intern Med. 1998;129:1061–1065.

54. Stewart MA. Effective physician-patient communication and health outcomes: a review. CMAJ. 1995;152:1423–1433.

55. Ong LM, de Haes JC, Hoos AM, Lammes FB. Doctor-patient communication: a review of the literature. Soc Sci Med. 1995;40: 903–918.

56. Kaplan SH, Greenfield S, Ware JE Jr. Assessing the effects of physician-patient interactions on the outcomes of chronic disease. Med Care. 1989;27:S110–S127.

57. Finkler K, Correa M. Factors influencing patient perceived recovery in Mexico. Soc Sci Med. 1996;42:199–207.

58. Bass MJ, Buck C, Turner L, et al. The physician's actions and the outcome of illness in family practice. J Fam Pract. 1986;23:43–47.

59. Thomas KB. General practice consultations: is there any point in being positive? Br Med J (Clin Res Ed). 1987;294:1200–1202.

60. Olsson B, Olsson B, Tibblin G. Effect of patients' expectations on recovery from acute tonsillitis. Fam Pract. 1989;6:188–192.

61. Hahn RA. "Treat the patient, not the lab": internal medicine and the concept of 'person.' Cult Med Psychiatry. 1982;6:219–236.

62. Oths K. Communication in a chiropractic clinic: how a D.C. treats his patients. Cult Med Psychiatry. 1994;18:83–113.

63. Thomas KB. The placebo in general practice. Lancet. 1994;344: 1066–1067.

64. Adler HM, Hammett VB. The doctor-patient relationship revisited. An analysis of the placebo effect. Ann Intern Med. 1973;78:595–598.

65. Sox HC Jr, Margulies I, Sox CH. Psychologically mediated effects of diagnostic tests. Ann Intern Med. 1981;95:680–685.

66. Adler HM. The history of the present illness as treatment: who's listening, and why does it matter? J Am Board Fam Pract. 1997;10: 28–35.

67. Brody H, Waters DB. Diagnosis is treatment. J Fam Pract. 1980;10: 445–449.

68. Novack DH. Therapeutic aspects of the clinical encounter. J Gen Intern Med. 1987;2:346–355.

69. Csordas TJ. The rhetoric of transformation in ritual healing. Cult Med Psychiatry. 1983;7:333–375.

70. Csordas TJ. Elements of charismatic persuasion and healing. Med Anthropol Q. 1988;2:121–142.

71. Kirmayer LJ. Improvisation and authority in illness meaning. Cult Med Psychiatry. 1994;18:183–214.

72. Eisenberg DM, Davis RB, Ettner SL, et al. Trends in alternative medicine use in the United States, 1990–1997: results of a follow-up national survey. JAMA. 1998;280:1569–1575.

73. Turner JA, Deyo RA, Loeser JD, Von Korff M, Fordyce WE. The importance of placebo effects in pain treatment and research. JAMA. 1994;271:1609–1614.

74. Wall PD. Pain and the placebo response. In: Bock G, Marsh J, eds. Experimental and Theoretical Studies of Consciousness. Ciba Foundation Symposium 174. New York: J Wiley; 1993.

75. McQuay H, Carroll D, Moore A. Variation in the placebo effect in randomised controlled trials of analgesics: all is as blind as it seems. Pain. 1996;64:331–335.

76. Lasagna L, Laties VG, Dohan JL. Further studies on the "pharmacology" of placebo administration. J Clin Invest. 1958;37:533–537.

77. Brodeur DW. The effects of stimulant and tranquilizer placebos on healthy subjects in a real-life situation. Psychopharmacologia. 1965; 7:444–452.

78. Morison RA, Woodmansey A, Young AJ. Placebo responses in an arthritis trial. Ann Rheum Dis. 1961;20:178–185.

79. Pillemer SR, Fowler SE, Tilley BC, et al. Meaningful improvement criteria sets in a rheumatoid arthritis clinical trial. MIRA Trial Group. Minocycline in Rheumatoid Arthritis. Arthritis Rheum. 1997;40:419–425.

80. Couch JR Jr. Placebo effect and clinical trials in migraine therapy. Neuroepidemiology. 1987;6:178–185.

81. Diener HC, Dowson AJ, Ferrari M, Nappi G, Tfelt-Hansen P. Unbalanced randomization influences placebo response: scientific versus ethical issues around the use of placebo in migraine trials. Cephalalgia. 1999;19:699–700.

82. Kagan G, Dabrowicki E, Huddlestone L, Kapur TR, Wolstencroft P. A double blind trial of terfenadine and placebo in hay fever using a substitution technique for non-responders. J Int Med Res. 1980;8:404–407.

83. D'Souza MF, Emanuel MB, Gregg J, Charlton J, Goldschmidt J. A method for evaluating therapy for hay fever. A comparison of four treatments. Clin Allergy. 1983;13:329–335.

84. Preston RA, Materson BJ, Reda DJ, Williams DW. Placebo-associated blood pressure response and adverse effects in the treatment of hypertension: observations from a Department of Veterans Affairs Cooperative Study. Arch Intern Med. 2000;160: 1449–1454.

85. Suchman AL, Ader R. Classic conditioning and placebo effects in crossover studies. Clin Pharmacol Ther. 1992;52:372–377.

86. Storms MD, Nisbett RE. Insomnia and the attribution process. J Pers Soc Psychol. 1970;16:319–328.

87. Bootzin RR, Herman CP, Nicassio P. The power of suggestion: another examination of misattribution and insomnia. J Pers Soc Psychol. 1976;34:673–679.

88. Godfrey S, Silverman M. Demonstration by placebo response in asthma by means of exercise testing. J Psychosom Res. 1973;17: 293–297.

89. Moerman DE. Cultural variations in the placebo effect: ulcers, anxiety, and blood pressure. Med Anthropol Q. 2000;14:51–72.

90. Ilnyckyj A, Shanahan F, Anton PA, Cheang M, Bernstein CN. Quantification of the placebo response in ulcerative colitis. Gastroenterology. 1997;112:1854–1858.

91. Brown WA, Johnson MF, Chen MG. Clinical features of depressed patients who do and do not improve with placebo. Psychiatry Res. 1992;41:203–214.

92. Kirsch I, Sapirstein G. Listening to Prozac but hearing placebo: a meta-analysis of antidepressant medications. In: Kirsch I, ed. How Expectancies Shape Experience. Washington, D.C.: American Psychological Assoc; 1999.

93. Rosenberg NK, Mellergård M, Rosenberg R, Beck P, Ottosson JO. Characteristics of panic disorder patients responding to placebo. Acta Psychiatr Scand Suppl. 1991;365:33–38.

94. Hróbjartsson A, Gøtzsche PC. Is the placebo powerless? An analysis of clinical trials comparing placebo with no treatment. N Engl J Med. 2001;344:1594–1602.

95. de Craen AJ, Moerman DE, Heisterkamp SH, et al. Placebo effect in the treatment of duodenal ulcer. Br J Clin Pharmacol. 1999;48: 853–860.

96. Branthwaite A, Cooper P. Analgesic effects of branding in treatment of headaches. Br Med J (Clin Res Ed). 1981;282:1576–1578.

97. Kaptchuk TJ, Goldman P, Stone DA, Stason WB. Do medical devices have enhanced placebo effects? J Clin Epidemiol. 2000;53:786–792.

98. de Craen AJ, Tijssen JG, de Gans J, Kleijnen J. Placebo effect in the acute treatment of migraine: subcutaneous placebos are better than oral placebos. J Neurol. 2000;247:183–188.

99. Moncrieff J, Wessely S, Hardy R. Meta-analysis of trials comparing antidepressants with active placebos. Br J Psychiatry. 1998;172: 227–231.

100. Fisher S, Greenberg RP. How sound is the double-blind design for evaluating psychotropic drugs? J Nerv Ment Dis. 1993;181:345–350.

101. Marchand S, Charest J, Li J, et al. Is TENS purely a placebo effect? A controlled study on chronic low back pain. Pain. 1993;54:99–106.

102. Schwitzgebel RK, Traugott M. Initial note on the placebo effect of machines. Behav Sci. 1968;13:267–273.

103. Ernst E, Resch KL. Concept of true and perceived placebo effects. BMJ. 1995;311:551–553.

104. Kaptchuk TJ, Eisenberg DM. Chiropractic: origins, controversies, and contributions. Arch Intern Med. 1998;158:2215–2224.

105. Kaptchuk TJ. The Web That Has No Weaver: Understanding Chinese Medicine. Chicago: Contemporary; 2000.

106. McGuire MB. Ritual Healing in Suburban America. New Brunswick, N.J.: Rutgers Univ Pr; 1988.

107. Riley JN. Western medicine's attempt to become more scientific: examples from the United States and Thailand. Soc Sci Med. 1977; 11:549–560.

108. Thomas M, Eriksson SV, Lundeberg T. A comparative study of diazepam and acupuncture in patients with osteoarthritis pain: a placebo controlled study. Am J Chin Med. 1991;19:95–100.

109. Koes BW, Bouter LM, van Mameren H, et al. The effectiveness of manual therapy, physiotherapy, and treatment by the general practitioner for nonspecific back and neck complaints. A randomized clinical trial. Spine. 1992;17:28–35.

110. Hróbjartsson A, Gøtzsche PC. Is the placebo powerless? N Engl J Med. 2001;345:1278–1279.

111. Hróbjartsson A, Gøtzsche PC. Core belief in powerful effects of placebo interventions is in conflict with no evidence of important effects in a large systematic review. Advances in Mind-Body Medicine. 2001;17:312–318.

112. Lynöe N, Mattsson B, Sandlund M. The attitudes of patients and physicians towards placebo treatment—a comparative study. Soc Sci Med. 1993;36:767–774.

113. Johnson AG. Surgery as a placebo. Lancet. 1994;344:1140–1142.

114. Shetty N, Friedman JH, Kieburtz K, Marshall FJ, Oakes D. The placebo response in Parkinson's disease. Parkinson Study Group. Clin Neuropharmacol. 1999;22:207–212.

115. Goetz CG, Leurgans S, Raman R, Stebbins GT. Objective changes in motor function during placebo treatment in PD. Neurology. 2000;54: 710–714.

116. de la Fuente-Fernández R, Ruth TJ, Sossi V, et al. Expectation and dopamine release: mechanism of the placebo effect in Parkinson's disease. Science. 2001;293:1164–1166.

117. Freed CR, Greene PE, Breeze RE, et al. Transplantation of embryonic dopamine neurons for severe Parkinson's disease. N Engl J Med. 2001; 344:710–719.

118. Husten L. Fetal-cell-implantation trial yields mixed results. Lancet. 1999; 353:1501.

119. Macklin R. The ethical problems with sham surgery in clinical research. N Engl J Med. 1999;341:992–996.

120. Johannes L. Sham surgery is used to test effectiveness of novel operations. Wall Street Journal. 1998;11 December:A1, A8.

121. Watts RL, Freeman RA, Hauser RA, et al. A double-blind, randomized, controlled, multicenter clinical trial of the safety and efficacy of stereotaxic intrastriatal implantation of fetal porcine ventral mesencephalic tissue (Neurocell™-PD) vs. imitation surgery in patients with Parkinson's disease (PD). Parkinsonism and Related Disorders. 2001;7(Suppl.):S87.

PART II

Experimental Studies of the Placebo Effect

Placebo effects are complex phenomena with complex (and incompletely understood) causes. The existence of placebo effects has implications within a wide variety of scientific domains, including, for example, clinical trials methodology and the neurosciences. Within the context of clinical trials, placebo effects have been viewed merely as a source of bias in subjective symptom reporting, which needs to be factored out in order to assess the genuine therapeutic effects of study interventions. This view has been challenged by increasing evidence that placebo effects are mediated by specific physiological and neural mechanisms, thus making placebo effects themselves of scientific interest. Recent results in the neurosciences have demonstrated that responses to placebos are real and produced through specific mechanistic pathways. Such observed neurobiological changes are not attributable to the chemical properties of the drugs being studied; they are measurable, and they can be deliberately induced.

Many of the chapters in Part II of this anthology demonstrate such experimental findings. To begin, however, Section A of Part II opens with ten important historical studies on the psychobiological mechanisms—mostly conditioning and verbally induced placebo effects—that underlie placebo responses. Later sections of Part II focus on psychological and neurobiological mechanisms of the placebo response, along with contextual factors important in eliciting placebo effects. The overarching goal of Part II of this anthology is to introduce readers to the most important experimental results related to the placebo effect across a variety of disciplines. The chapters in Part II also collectively emphasize the importance of understanding the intricate and multifaceted nature of placebo responses in order to better understand their therapeutic value, thus setting the stage for the discussion in Part III concerning the value and use of placebos in clinical research and practice.

Section A. Pioneering Efforts

The pioneering experimental studies included in this section opened up new areas of thought, research, and theory into the placebo effect. Stewart Wolf, one of the first to research the mechanisms of the placebo effect, studied the effects of various agents (urogastrone, Benadryl, ipecac, prostigmine, atropine, lactose, and water) on gastric motility in five subjects in his classic 1950 study that leads off Part II, Section A, of this anthology. His results were surprising to researchers at the time. For example, he found that the emetic (nausea-

and vomit-inducing) action of ipecac varied under different verbal suggestions: whether a subject suffered from nausea and vomiting depended largely on what the subject was told they had ingested and what would happen to them as a result. In effect, the pattern of gastric inactivity typical of nausea was completely reversed when a patient received ipecac along with the (incorrect) information that it was a medicine used to abolish, not to cause, nausea. Considering all his results, Wolf reasoned that a number of factors played a role in the observations he recorded, including "1) the state of the end organ at the time of administration, i.e., the effect of forces already acting prior to administration of the agent; 2) the setting in which the agent was administered, including the route of administration, the presence of the experimenter and the effects of suggestions, implicit or expressed; [and] 3) conditioning circumstances and previously established habits of reaction" (Wolf 1950, 100). He concluded that "'placebo effects' which modify the pharmacologic action of drugs or endow inert agents with potency are not imaginary, but may be associated with measurable changes at the end organs. These effects are at times more potent than the pharmacologic action customarily attributed to the agent" (Wolf 1950, 108–109). Thus, contrary to earlier views about placebo effects, Wolf claimed not only that placebo effects were real but also that placebos may discernibly act on organs, often with greater effect than standard drugs. As many of the chapters collected in this anthology attest, Wolf was right about all of these claims.

Wolf's experimental results were important, and they raised other considerations for scientists at the time, including most pressingly whether placebo effects were idiosyncratic reactions or whether they were reproducible and predictable. Thus, the ipecac-induced nausea and vomiting model was applied to identify the occurrence of placebo responses (1) in one person through time and (2) between individuals. Wolf and his colleagues studied placebo responses across individuals in order to test the hypothesis of whether individuals could be divided into placebo responders (placebo "reactors," as they were called) and nonresponders (placebo "nonreactors") based on their propensity to react to placebos (Wolf et al. 1957). In their 1957 paper in this anthology, Wolf and his colleagues found no evidence that subjects could be divided into placebo "reactors" and "nonreactors," but for some today, this remains an open question.

Beyond any ability to predict particular placebo responses, it is obvious that if a study includes a large number of "placebo reactors," if indeed there are such individuals, then this would interfere with the slope of the dose-response curve of a standard drug, the validation of a drug as effective, and the search for optimal therapeutic dosages. These concerns are quite general for those who engage in clinical research; for, even if there are no "placebo reactors" as such, placebo effects can raise similar concerns. Based on this reasoning, Louis Lasagna and his collaborators investigated the response to morphine and placebos given under different sequential order and dosage number. In their 1954 paper in this anthology, Lasagna and his colleagues conclude that the proclivity to respond to inert substances is not an all-or-none phenomenon, but rather a graded one where different factors, psychological and nonpsychological, determine whether a patient is predisposed to anticipate pain relief and thus to respond to a placebo (Lasagna et al. 1954).

After these early experimental studies by Wolf (Wolf 1950; Wolf et al. 1957) and Lasagna (Lasagna et al. 1954), more systematic experimental evidence supported the idea that beliefs and expectations can markedly influence the response to pharmacological and nonpharmacological interventions. Although these claims were controversial at the time, and remain controversial to some, research from the 1950s encouraged others to further investigate the existence and mechanisms of the placebo effect. We include some of these investigations in the remainder of Part II, Section A, of this anthology.

Two important studies in rodents encouraged future investigators to treat placebo responses as drug-mimicking effects. We include them here. The first comes from Richard J. Herrnstein in his well-known 1962 study, "Placebo Effect in the Rat." After training rats to depress a lever by reinforcement with sweetened condensed milk, Herrnstein administered scopolamine, the unconditioned stimulus, a drug known to disrupt learned behaviors in the rat, along with injections of saline, the conditioned stimulus. As expected, the presentation of the conditioned stimulus alone (saline) caused scopolamine-like alteration of behavior; in other words, through conditioning reinforcement, saline predictably mimicked the effects of scopolamine (Herrnstein 1962). As Herrnstein concluded, the observed "depression of responding by saline may reasonably be termed a placebo effect," and although the study was carried out with rats, Herrnstein suggested that there appeared "to be no reason to suppose that the placebo effect in human patients differs in any way from that demonstrated here, other than in degree of complexity" (Herrnstein 1962, 678).

A second important demonstration of the ability of placebos to produce drug-mimicking effects comes from Robert Ader and Nicholas Cohen's study of the effects of conditioned immunosuppression on the development of the autoimmune disease systemic lupus erythematosus in mice (Ader and Cohen 1982). Ader and Cohen analyzed the rate of onset of lupus in four groups: two conditioned groups that received both an immunosuppressive chemotherapeutic regimen (cyclophosphamide—the unconditioned stimulus) paired with a saccharin solution (the conditioned stimulus); one nonconditioned cyclophosphamide-saccharin group; and a saccharin-only control group. Ader and Cohen showed that conditioned pairing of saccharin with the immunosuppressant cyclophosphamide enabled saccharin, acting as a conditioned stimulus, to suppress auto-immunological reactivity, thereby resulting in a significantly delayed onset of systemic lupus erythematosus.

While the repetitive associations of active drugs with conditioned stimuli were capable of producing robust drug-mimicking effects in animals, merely informing patients about the expected action of an intervention can impact therapeutic outcomes (Luparello et al. 1968; Luparello et al. 1970). These are so-called expectancy effects. For example, in one study by Thomas Luparello and colleagues, significant increases in airway resistance were observed in nearly half the asthmatic patients under investigation after they inhaled a nebulized saline solution which they were (wrongly) informed was an allergen with irritant properties. The same patients were able to reverse airway obstruction by inhaling the identical saline solution presented as a medicine with beneficial effects on asthma (Luparello et al. 1968). In another study by Luparello that we include here, the bronchoconstricting effect of the bronchoconstrictor carbachol were higher when administered with the information that it was a bronchoconstrictor than when subjects were told it was a bronchodilator. Similarly, the bronchodilating effect of isoproterenol (a bronchodilator) was greater in subjects told it was a bronchodilator than it was in those told it was a bronchoconstrictor (Luparello et al. 1970). Thus, under double-blind conditions, Luparello and his colleagues demonstrated that when instructions to subjects were concordant with the inhaled drug's pharmacological action, the observed effects were much greater than when those instructions were discordant.

One of the most important advances in placebo research was the discovery that placebo-induced behavior changes are related to the release of endogenous substances. The first important evidence was produced by Jon Levine, Newton Gordon, and Howard Fields who hypothesized that placebo-induced pain relief must be underpinned by the release of endogenous opioids (Levine et al. 1978). In their study included in this anthology, Levine, Gordon, and Fields looked at postoperative dental pain in subjects given combinations of placebo and naloxone (an opiate antagonist—i.e., a substance that will block opiate-mediated pain relief) using a randomized, double-blind design. Each subject received two postoperative doses of either (1) placebo followed by placebo, (2) placebo followed by naloxone, or (3) naloxone followed by placebo. Levine and his colleagues found that among placebo responders (those who experienced pain relief after the first dose of placebo), naloxone given as the second injection significantly increased pain, thus showing that placebo analgesia is naloxone-reversible. Moreover, when comparing the placebo–placebo group to the naloxone–placebo group, they found that giving naloxone first reduced the probability that a subject would experience pain relief from placebo. As Levine and his colleagues note, these results suggest, but do not directly show, that placebo analgesia is mediated by endogenous opioids (Levine et al. 1978).

Although little is currently known about the neural modulation of pain induced by social support, an early randomized study by Lawrence Egbert and his colleagues, which we include in this anthology, demonstrated that instruction, suggestion, and encouragement reduced the need for postoperative analgesics *by half* in a cohort of patients who underwent elective intra-abdominal surgery (Egbert et al. 1964). This study has clear implications regarding the value and use of placebo effects in clinical practice. The Egbert study depended on the fact that the possible (placebo) effects of suggestion were not disclosed to the patient. But, perhaps counter-intuitively, open-label placebos—that is, placebos described to recipients transparently *as placebos*—may also contribute to symptom management. While the general idea originated with Robert Liberman, who posited that therapeutic stimuli (for example, giving pills to patients) can mediate internal processes aimed at producing a placebo response (Liberman 1962), Lee C. Park and Lino Covi found that anxious and neurotic outpatients were willing to take placebos and, in fact, improved with placebos *despite* having the inert content of the pills disclosed to them. The study by Park and Covi was important because it showed that "unawareness of the inert nature of the placebo is not an indispensable condition for improvement on placebo" (Park and Covi 1965). (This study is not included in this anthology, but we encourage readers to consult it.)

The fact that placebos can exert effects in nonblind conditions is surprising, but also surprising is that different placebo preparations often exert, or can be expected to exert, very different effects, thus demonstrating the role of nondrug factors in the placebo response. Prior research had shown, for example, that two placebo capsules produced more changes than one capsule, that blue placebo capsules were significantly more effective than pink placebo capsules, and that placebos more frequently elicited sedative than stimulant effects (Blackwell et al. 1972; Buckalew and Ross 1981). In the study included here, Louis W. Buckalew and Kenneth E. Coffield demonstrated the effects of drug appearance on expectations of its effects. They asked their research subjects to rank capsules for perceived strength based on capsule *size*, to categorize capsules in terms of anticipated pharmacological effect based on capsule *color*, and to anticipate the strength of the drug based on preparation *form* (capsule vs. tablet). For instance, they found that most of the subjects ranked increasing capsule size with increasing perceived strength and that capsules were perceived to be superior to tablets (Buckalew and Coffield 1982). Although contrasting results concerning capsule color and expected drug effects are present in the literature, Buckalew and Coffield reported that white

is generally associated with analgesic effects, lavender with psychedelic or hallucinogenic effects, orange and yellow with stimulant or antidepressant action, and light blue with sedative effects.

Other nondrug factors have been found to influence placebo-induced analgesia in patients. For example, the method of drug administration (Levine and Gordon 1984) and the clinicians' knowledge of which drugs were *possibly* administered to patients (Gracely et al. 1985) can also impact analgesia following placebo administration. Among postoperative dental patients fitted with indwelling intravenous catheters, Jon Levine and Newton Gordon noted that postoperative pain changed in response to the way in which the placebo was delivered through the catheter. Different degrees of change in the intensity of pain were discovered in the three drug-administration groups: the "open infusion" group (delivery of drug with a person at the patient's bedside), the "machine infusion" group (delivery of drug by a preprogrammed infusion pump), and the "hidden infusion" group (delivery of drug by a person in an adjacent room; thus, the patient was presumably unaware that they were receiving any drug). Changes in pain intensity were greatest in the open infusion group, clearly showing that a placebo effect was elicited, but (surprisingly) similar changes in pain intensity were found in the hidden infusion group, suggesting that subtle, unintentional cues mediated a placebo response (Levine and Gordon 1984). (We encourage readers to consult the Levine and Gordon paper and to read it in conjunction with the Levine, Gordon, and Fields paper included here as chapter 15.)

Such subtle cues were investigated by Richard Gracely and his colleagues in their study of the effects of clinician expectation on placebo analgesia in patients. Patients who underwent unilateral extraction of two molars were informed that they might receive a placebo (saline solution), a narcotic analgesic (fentanyl), or a narcotic antagonist (naloxone), and that these drugs might increase, decrease, or have no effect on their pain. Clinicians who administered the drugs (in double-blind fashion) knew only that group "PN" would receive placebo or naloxone, while group "PNF" would receive placebo, naloxone, or fentanyl. Pain was assessed by patients 10 and 60 minutes after receiving their placebo injection, and the authors found that there was a significantly lower level of pain after placebo in group "PNF" than in group "PN." Because the only difference between these groups was the clinicians' knowledge of which injections they *might* receive, Gracely and his colleagues conclude that clinicians' expectations (as manifested in subtle, presumably unintentional, cues) can influence placebo analgesia in patients.

The pioneering research included in Part II, Section A, of this anthology resulted in a broader and deeper understanding of the initial interpretations of placebo effects. Expectations of benefit can impact a variety of physiological systems and alter clinical outcomes. However, it still remains to be seen to what extent placebo effects potentially interfere with the pathophysiological processes of diseases (Miller et al.

2009), thus suggesting the need for further investigation into the link between psychological and neurobiological mechanisms underlying the placebo effect.

Section B. Psychological Mechanisms

In terms of psychological mechanisms, placebo responses have typically been explained by appeals to expectancy and conditioning although any rigid distinction between the two might be hard to sustain. Conditioning may itself underlie the formation of expectancies, which in turn mediate placebo effects. Conditioning mechanisms are typically thought of as changes in physiological states that are not directly under a subject's conscious control. For example, endocrine changes can be produced by classical conditioning in which a neutral stimulus is paired with an agent with endocrine-modifying pharmacological properties; after such conditioning, exposure to the placebo stimulus alone can bring about the same effect as that brought about by the unconditioned stimulus. However, when subjects are told that an injection they receive will increase (or decrease) their growth hormone or cortisol levels, it has been shown that such verbal stimuli have no effect on the levels of these hormones (Benedetti et al. 2003). Such results suggest that placebo responses are mediated by conditioning when unconscious physiological functions are involved, whereas they are mediated by expectation when conscious physiological processes are involved; in short, conscious and unconscious processes may play a role in different contexts. Some have argued, moreover, that both classical and instrumental conditioning are best understood as processes generating expectations (Kirsch 2004). There are therefore still substantive issues to be resolved regarding the conceptual understanding of both conditioning and expectancy. Nevertheless, conscious and unconscious processes overlap to some extent, and expectations per se can be actively built up through various forms of learning, including verbal instructions, conditioning, and social observation (Colloca and Miller 2011a, 2011c). The articles collected in Section B of Part II should be read against the background of these concerns about the nature of conditioning and expectancy and their roles in the placebo effect. They stand as the first examples of support for the contribution of verbal suggestions, classical conditioning, and social observation in forming placebo responses.

In the first paper of this section, Nicholas Voudouris and his collaborators designed a study to analyze the role of verbal expectancy and conditioning manipulations (Voudouris et al. 1990). Subjects were exposed to iontophoretic pain stimulation (that is, skin pain caused by exposure to potassium ions) following the establishment of baseline pain tolerances. All subjects attended 4 sessions on 4 consecutive days. The experimental design consisted of verbal suggestion (the expectancy manipulation; session 1), pain-test 1 (session 2), pain stimulus change (for some) plus topical placebo cream (the conditioning manipulation; session 3), and pain-test 2 (session 4). In the first session, half of the subjects were informed that a topical cream was a powerful analgesic (it was, in fact, a placebo) and would provide pain relief (expectancy), while the other half was informed that the cream was neutral (no expectancy). In the second session, half of the subjects received a neutral cream (placebo) and the other half was given none. In the third session, half the subjects in each of the verbal suggestion and no verbal suggestion groups received conditioning in which the pain stimulus was reduced after the cream was applied, while the other half received the same pain stimulus. Therefore, group 1 received both expectancy and conditioning; group 2, expectancy alone; group 3, conditioning alone; and group 4 was the control. The results showed an enhancement of placebo response in groups 1 and 3, as compared to both groups 2 and 4. The authors concluded that conditioning based on direct experience of pain reduction is more powerful in eliciting placebo analgesia than are expectancies created by verbal suggestions (Voudouris et al. 1990). These findings have been extensively confirmed (Amanzio and Benedetti 1999; Colloca and Benedetti 2006; Colloca, Sigaudo, and Benedetti 2008; Klinger et al. 2007), and demonstrate the comparatively superior strength of conditioning over expectancy mechanisms in producing (at least, certain) placebo responses.

Conditioning responses, however, can be partially or completely reversed by instructions, that is, by expectancy (Montgomery and Kirsch 1997; Benedetti et al. 2003; Colloca and Benedetti 2006). In an experiment on placebo analgesia by Guy Montgomery and Irving Kirsch, subjects were randomly assigned to a conditioning (uninformed pairing) group or to an expectancy (informed pairing) group, received the same information about the effectiveness of a topical (placebo) cream, and experienced the same reduction of painful stimulus during manipulation trials. The subjects in the expectancy group were informed that the intensity of the pain stimulus was being reduced just before the manipulation trial, whereas the subjects in the conditioning group were not told about this reduction; both groups, however, received identical reductions in pain stimuli. Two other comparator groups were also included in the study. The results, which we include here, indicate that informing subjects that the pain stimulus would be reduced antagonized the effect of conditioning on placebo analgesia. It follows from these experiments that verbally induced expectancy responses can interact with conditioned responses, contributing to the formation of a placebo response. Indeed, Montgomery and Kirsch claim that their study demonstrates that the effects of conditioning on responses to placebos obtained by Voudouris et al. (1990) are "completely mediated by expectancy" (Montgomery and Kirsch 1997, 111).

The role of expectancy on placebo analgesia was investigated further in an experimental setting by Donald Price and his colleagues. We include their paper here. Price and colleagues applied pain stimuli and placebo cream to subjects under two experimental conditions—A (the "strong" placebo cream) and B (the "weak" placebo cream), although they were not told which analgesic was strong and which weak. A control substance, C (water), was also used. Prior to the conditioning phase, subjects were randomly assigned to two groups, those receiving instruction to elicit either a high desire for pain reduction or a low desire for pain reduction. During the conditioning procedure, the intensity of the stimulus was decreased from a baseline level by 67% in A and by 17% in B without informing participants that such reductions would take place. There was no pain reduction in C (control condition). This design allowed the researchers to measure both a within-subject factor (the expectancy effect related to being blind to the strength of the analgesic) and a between-subject factor (the impact of high versus low desire for pain reduction on placebo analgesia). Price and his colleagues found that expectancy, but not desire for pain reduction, was a causal factor in placebo analgesia, and further that the conditioning effect is mediated by expectancy (Price et al. 1999). This study may be read as, in part, a confirmation of the results of Montgomery and Kirsch (1997).

While the first three chapters in this section attend to the comparative contributions of psychological mechanisms (conditioning and expectancy) in the placebo response, the next chapter, by Martina Amanzio and Fabrizio Benedetti, looks into the pharmacological mechanisms that underlie these psychological mechanisms. In a model of experimentally induced human ischemic arm pain, Amanzio and Benedetti analyzed different kinds of placebo analgesia induced by different combinations of expectation cues and conditioning procedures in order to differentiate the neuropharmacology of expectancy and conditioning into opioid and nonopioid systems. They found that placebo analgesia, resulting from one verbal expectation (being told that they are going to receive a potent analgesic), was strong and totally blocked by the opioid antagonist naloxone, whereas placebo analgesia, resulting from another verbal expectation (being told that they are going to receive an antibiotic), was weak and only partially blocked by naloxone. In other words, because expectation-induced placebo analgesia was always sensitive to naloxone, they concluded that expectancy always triggers opioid systems. On the other hand, conditioning-induced placebo analgesia was more complicated. When placebo analgesia was obtained after conditioning exposure to an opioid such as morphine analgesia was completely blocked by naloxone, thus demonstrating the role of opioids in conditioning-induced placebo analgesia. However, if placebo analgesia was achieved after conditioning with a nonopioid (ketorolac tromethamine), then this response was naxolone insensitive; that is, it was not mediated by opioid systems. Furthermore, placebo responses following conditioning with ketorolac (naxolone insensitive) plus expectations (naloxone reversible) were partially reversed by naloxone, thus suggesting that expectations trigger endogenous opioids, independent of the other nonopioid systems in play (Amanzio and Benedetti 1999). These findings have been in part confirmed in mice by using a model of a hot plate test and pharmaco-

logical conditioning with morphine hydrochloride and aspirin (Guo et al. 2010). Conditioning with the opioid morphine produced placebo responses that were completely antagonized by naloxone. By contrast, conditioning with aspirin elicited placebo responses that were not blocked by naloxone, supporting the notion that the release of endogenous substances depends on the kind of pharmacological conditioning that is originally performed. In short, opioid conditioning produces opioid-mediated placebo responses, while nonopioid conditioning produces non-opioid-mediated placebo responses.

In general, the relation between prior therapeutic exposures and subsequent placebo responses is very important in pharmacotherapy (Colloca 2011). The same treatment or intervention, for example, can produce different outcomes, depending on the order of administration in sequential designs and on the effectiveness of the first exposure. A therapeutic exposure that has little effect on an outcome tends to reduce the effectiveness of subsequent identical treatment, while initially successful exposure to a substance often leads to enhanced outcomes on further exposure to the same substance (Colloca and Benedetti 2006).

Learning through prior first-person experience is not the only kind of process underpinning placebo analgesia. In fact, when subjects merely observe others experiencing analgesia, this can lead to robust placebo responses that are as robust as those elicited by the firsthand experience of a classical conditioning procedure. We close this section with a study by Luana Colloca and Fabrizio Benedetti who found that placebo analgesia responses from social observational learning were highly correlated with higher scores on the "empathic concern" component of an empathy trait questionnaire. The link between placebo responses and the ability to share the emotions of others (prosociality) emphasizes the fact that social observation is another form of learning that, along with conditioning and expectancy, can elicit placebo responses in an experimental setting (Colloca and Benedetti 2009).

Section C. Neurobiological Mechanisms

A growing body of research in neuroscience is exploring the central and peripheral processes that mediate the placebo effect, thus confirming earlier indirect pharmacological findings (Grevert et al. 1983; Levine et al. 1978; Levine and Gordon 1984). Following these pioneering findings, recent and carefully designed experiments have confirmed the effect of naloxone in antagonizing opioid-mediated placebo analgesia (Amanzio and Benedetti 1999; Eippert et al. 2009a). These pharmacological studies have been corroborated and extended by a number of brain imaging studies describing the functional neuroanatomy of placebo analgesia and other clinically relevant symptoms (Colloca, Benedetti, and Porro 2008). The chapters assembled in Section C investigate the neurobiological mechanisms involved in the placebo response. In a sense, these chapters attempt to look more deeply within the brains of those who experience placebo effects to determine which parts of the brain and which specific neurotransmitters are involved in placebo analgesia.

We open this section with the first brain imaging study of placebo and opioid analgesia by Predrag Petrovic and his collaborators (Petrovic et al. 2002). Petrovic and colleagues used positron emission tomography (PET) to show that a subset of brain regions are similarly affected either by a placebo or by the μ-opioid agonist remifentanil, thus supporting the hypothesis that placebo-induced analgesia (a psychological effect) and opioid-induced analgesia (a pharmacological effect) share an underlying mechanistic pathway via specific subsystems in the brain. In particular, they demonstrated that the administration of a placebo induces the activation of portions of the anterior cingulate cortex (ACC), the orbitofrontal cortex (OFC), and the anterior insula, three areas that had previously been shown to be active during pain processing. They further found a statistically significant covariation in brain activity between the rostral ACC (rACC) and the lower pons/medulla (parts of the brainstem) during both placebo and opioid analgesia, while the covariation between activity in the rACC and the periaqueductal gray (PAG; a region rostral to the pons) was statistically significant during opioid analgesia, but not during placebo analgesia. During the pain-only condition, activity was observed in the rACC, but not in the brainstem or the PAG. These and other findings indicate that the pain-modulating circuit that runs downstream from the frontal cortex (in particular, the rACC) into the PAG and brainstem is also involved in placebo analgesia (Petrovic et al. 2002; Fields 2004). Because placebo analgesia is often dependent on higher cognitive processes residing in the cortex (processes, that is, that are presented to the consciousness of the individual), one of the insights yielded by the study by Petrovic and his collaborators is that the cortex (via the ACC) may play a role in controlling parts of the brain that are below the level of the individual's consciousness (that is, the brainstem and the PAG) during placebo and opioid analgesia. The study is thus further evidence of the functional reach of the cortex.

The study by Petrovic and his colleagues indicated, in part, that a pain-responsive circuit traveling downstream from the cortex into the brainstem is also involved in placebo analgesia. The study we include by Falk Eippert and his colleagues shows that the circuit involved in placebo analgesia extends even further into the cervical (neck) segments of the spinal cord (Eippert et al. 2009b). Using functional magnetic resonance imaging (fMRI), which measures blood-flow changes caused by changes in metabolism that accompany neuronal activity, Eippert and his collaborators showed both that spinal cord activity (in the dorsal horn of C5-C6 segments) increased during painful stimulus, and decreased during a successful placebo analgesia response. This study was the first to provide direct evidence that a psychological factor—a placebo response—can influence pain perception processes within the upper spinal cord, well downstream from previously identified nociceptive locations.

Other elegantly designed fMRI studies have further clarified the neural mechanisms underlying placebo analgesia. In chapter 25, Tor Wager and his collaborators found that anticipation of analgesic benefit activates a cognitive-evaluative neural network that includes areas of the prefrontal cortex (PFC; in particular, the dorsolateral aspect [DLPFC] and the orbitofrontal cortex [OFC]); they also found increased activity during anticipation in the PAG region of the midbrain (Wager et al. 2004). Wager and his colleagues reasoned that, if placebo interventions reduce the experience of pain, then areas within pain-responsive regions of the brain (for example, the thalamus, somatosensory cortex, insula, and rACC) should show decreased metabolic activity during placebo analgesia. They also hypothesized that placebos work by creating expectations of pain relief that in turn modulate activity within pain-responsive brain regions; in particular, they hypothesized that an expectation of pain relief would be represented within the PFC (specifically, the DLPFC and the OFC), and that activity in the PFC would mediate placebo analgesia. In effect, Wager and his colleagues showed that placebo interventions reduce metabolic activity in pain-responsive areas of the brain, and they provided indirect (metabolic) evidence in support of a specific neural mechanism of placebo action.

In the next study, Jon-Kar Zubieta and his colleagues used a selective μ-opioid receptor agonist ([^{11}C]carfentanil) and PET imaging techniques to illustrate the specific role of μ-opioid receptors in pain and placebo analgesia (Zubieta et al. 2005). They compared the activation of the endogenous opioid system and μ-opioid receptors in two conditions—a sustained pain condition and a sustained pain condition during which time a placebo was administered; that is, research participants believed that they were receiving a strong painkiller, but in fact they were receiving saline solution. Zubieta and his collaborators found that significantly higher levels of endogenous opioid release occurred when pain was delivered under the expectation of pain relief (placebo manipulation). Moreover, the neurotransmitter activity during the placebo phase of the study occurred in associative, higher-order brain regions that are correlated with various aspects of the experience of pain. (The localization of neurotransmitter activity within the brain in this study was similar, but not identical, to that found in both Petrovic et al. [2002] and Wager et al. [2004].) This study represents the first direct neurochemical evidence that a placebo activates the endogenous opioid system. Combined with other results, the study by Zubieta and his collaborators demonstrates that the μ-opioid neurotransmitter system plays an important role in the neurobiology of pain and stress, and that it can be modulated by cognitive and emotional influences.

Endogenous opioids are not the only mediators of placebo analgesia, however. The study we include here by Fabrizio Benedetti and his collaborators (chapter 28) sheds light on the role of cholecystokinin (CCK), a hormone most active in the digestive system, and the so-called cholecystokininergic (CCKergic) system in placebo analgesia and nocebo hyperalgesia (that is, an expectancy induced increase in pain; Benedetti et al. 2006, 1995). They found that the oral administration of an inert talc pill along with verbal instructions that the pill was a potent vasoconstrictor, which would further increase their experimentally induced ischemic pain, induced hyperactivity of the hypothalamic-pituitary-adrenal (HPA) axis, as assessed by means of adrenocorticotropic hormone (ACTH) and cortisol plasma concentrations. Both nocebo-induced hyperalgesia and HPA hyperactivity were blocked by the benzodiazepine anxiolytic, diazepam (Valium), indicating that increased anxiety is involved in these effects. Conversely, the administration of the CCK antagonist, proglumide, blocked nocebo hyperalgesia completely but did not affect HPA hyperactivity. Taken together with the fact the both diazepam and proglumide had no effect on pain, the study by Benedetti and colleagues provides evidence for a specific involvement of the CCKergic system in the nocebo hyperalgesia; in particular, it suggests that CCK mediates the link between anxiety and pain. Placed in the context of the other studies in this anthology, Benedetti and his collaborators have pointed to the different mechanistic roles played by the opioidergic and CCKergic systems in the link between higher cognition and emotion, on one hand, and higher cognition and pain perception, on the other.

Although most of our knowledge about placebo effects derives from the study of pain and analgesia (Colloca and Benedetti 2005; Tracey 2010), the widespread interest in the placebo effect within the neuroscience community has led to studies of the neural mechanisms underlying placebo effects in other medical conditions (Benedetti et al. 2005), including Parkinson's disease (de la Fuente-Fernández et al. 2001, 2002; Lidstone et al. 2010; Strafella et al. 2006), depression (Mayberg et al. 2002), and drug addiction (Volkow et al. 2003; Volkow et al. 2006). By studying the placebo effect in those with other medical conditions, neuroscientists are using the placebo effect as a model to investigate the complex interaction between mental activities (such as expectancy) and various neuronal systems.

Our next study, by Raúl de la Fuente-Fernández and his colleagues, is an example of such an approach to the placebo effect (de la Fuente-Fernández et al. 2001). It had been established by others that the symptoms of Parkinson's disease can improve through a placebo effect. In their PET imaging study, de la Fuente-Fernández and his colleagues investigated the neural mechanism involved in such placebo-induced symptom improvement, in particular, whether the placebo effect activated the dopaminergic pathway in the nigrostriatal circuit (within the basal ganglia) that is damaged by degeneration in Parkinson's disease. De la Fuente-Fernández and his colleagues used a radiolabeled dopamine receptor antagonist ([¹¹C]raclopride, which binds to dopamine receptors without causing a biological response and measured its

binding potential in Parkinson's patients under placebo-controlled and open-study conditions. They found a significant decrease in [¹¹C]raclopride binding potential (indicating an increase in extracellular dopamine concentration) when patients received placebo as compared to their baseline state. This indicates that there is a placebo-induced release of dopamine in the striatum of Parkinson's patients. In addition to this, de la Fuente-Fernández and colleagues found that the magnitude of the placebo response was comparable to therapeutic doses of levodopa and apomorphine, drugs commonly prescribed to treat symptoms of Parkinson's disease, and that there was a dose-dependent relation between perceived placebo benefit and placebo-induced release of dopamine. One of the insights yielded by this study is that we now know that, in addition to the opioidergic and CCKergic systems, the dopaminergic system can also be a mediator of powerful (expectancy) placebo effects.

In chapter 30, Benedetti and his collaborators further investigate the neurobiology of the placebo response in placebo-responsive Parkinson's patients (Benedetti et al. 2004). They recorded the activity from single neurons in the subthalamic nucleus (STN, a functional part of the basal ganglia) before and after the administration of a placebo to test whether neuronal changes were linked to observed clinical placebo responses. A placebo (saline solution) was administered in the operating room after several preoperative administrations of apomorphine according to a conditioning procedure. Those patients who showed a clear-cut clinical placebo response—as assessed by means of a decrease in arm rigidity and a subjective report of well-being—also showed a significant decrease of neuronal discharge in the STN compared to the preplacebo condition, thus suggesting a placebo-induced increase in concentration of dopamine in the STN. None of the placebo nonresponders showed these differences. Moreover, the STN neurons of all the placebo responders shifted significantly from a pattern of bursting activity to a pattern of nonbursting discharge after placebo administration. In contrast, none of the placebo nonresponders showed any difference in the pattern of neuronal discharge before and after placebo injection. As Benedetti and colleagues note, this result also suggests that an increase concentration of dopamine in the striatum brought on by conditioning with apomorphine accounts for the observed pattern shift in STN bursting. Importantly, the study by Benedetti and his colleagues was the first to demonstrate a placebo effect at the single-neuron level.

The powerful modulating action of expectation is convincingly demonstrated by Nora Volkow and her colleagues in chapter 31 of Section C. Volkow and her collaborators investigated how expectancy effects modulated the response to methylphenidate (MP, a stimulant) in cocaine abusers (Volkow et al. 2003). They investigated the effects of MP on brain metabolism (using PET scans) and on reinforcing effects (via self-reports of drug effects) in four experimental conditions: (1) expect placebo, receive placebo; (2) expect placebo, receive MP; (3) expect MP, receive MP; and (4) expect MP, receive placebo. When subjects expected to receive MP, both the metabolic and subjective effects were about 50% greater than when the subjects expected placebo. This demonstrated that the reinforcement effects of certain drugs are a function both of expectancy and of their pharmacological properties. Similar results have been found in studies involving those without a history of drug abuse (Volkow et al. 2006). In their experimental paradigm, Volkow and her colleagues could both determine the magnitude of the expectation-induced reinforcing effects and localize the (anatomical and functional) areas of the brain that are in play during such effects. In doing so, they determined that the thalamus was particularly active in expectation-induced reinforcement effects, while the OFC was more active when MP was unexpected, thus suggesting a role for the OFC in unexpected rewards.

Section D. Contextual Factors

The placebo effect does not depend merely on the administration of a placebo intervention or treatment. The psychosocial context surrounding the patient during placebo administration is often a consistent and powerful causal determinant of the placebo response. The chapters in the last section of Part II deal with such contextual factors. As these chapters illustrate, such contextual factors include the words, attitudes, and behaviors of clinicians; the expectations of clinicians; the presence of and reassurance given by providers; the instructions and consent forms received; and the shape, smell, and costs of drugs. These factors taken individually or collectively form the ideal environment for studying the placebo phenomenon.

A particularly salient contextual factor is the research setting itself. In the first paper in Section D, Irving Kirsch and Michael Rosadino investigate the informational content of the informed consent process as one such contextual factor (Kirsch and Rosadino 1993). One of the important features of the randomized controlled trial methodology is its ability to produce externally valid—that is, generalizable—research results. Generalizability is a measure of the extent to which the results found during a study are applicable to (or can be generalized to) individuals who did not participate in the study. A number of factors can affect a study's generalizability, among which is the difference between procedures used in a study as compared to procedures used in clinical practice (Rothwell 2006). The informational content of the consent process is the procedure that Kirsch and Rosadino explore in their study. They note that informing patients that they will receive either placebo or active treatment in a research setting may produce a set of cognitive states (doubt, for example) in the patient that would not occur in a nonexperimental setting where patients have no reason to doubt the treatment they are going to receive. This is important, they note, because in the placebo-controlled research paradigm, the patient's cognitive set brought about by information given to them in a research setting ("You might receive placebo or you might receive active treatment") versus in a clinical setting ("You will receive active treatment") is assumed to be irrelevant to the active treatment outcomes; in other words, if outcome X is found for active treatment in a placebo-controlled trial, then it is assumed that outcome X should be expected in patients outside of the trial who receive the same active treatment and to whom the results of the trial are generalized.

With this in mind, Kirsch and Rosadino tested the external validity of a double-blind study by assessing the independent and interactive effects of instructions given to subjects on subjective changes (alertness, tension) and physiological changes (blood pressure, heart rate). They employed a $3 \times 2 \times 3$ design that contrasted instruction (told caffeine vs. told no caffeine vs. not told whether the beverage contained caffeine, i.e., double blind), drug content (caffeine vs. no caffeine), and time (15 vs. 30 vs. 45 minutes after ingestion). A significant drug-by-instruction effect in self-reported tension was observed as determined by comparing the tension outcomes of those in the told-caffeine group to those in the double-blind group. In other words, tension increased significantly only in those who knowingly took caffeine (told-caffeine/received-caffeine), and caffeine did not significantly affect tension in the double-blind group (double-blind/received-caffeine). As Kirsch and Rosadino note, the drug-by-instruction effect is a drug effect increased by the knowledge of what drug the subjects will receive, that is, by expectancy. This suggests both (1) that double-blind drug comparisons may fail to detect drug effects (because the "full" drug effect may only emerge in those who know that they are receiving the drug) and (2) that conditions in the told-drug group best approximate outcomes that would be discovered in clinical practice (where there is no doubt about what treatment one receives). However, there is no consensus on these points because drug effects and verbally induced expectations seem to be additive in some instances and interactive in others. For example, in another study comparing double-blind versus deceptive instructions on similar outcome measures, Kirsch and Lynne Weixel noted that the outcomes under deceptive instructions and those under double-blind instructions were in most instances opposite to each other and, when graphed, produced curves that were near mirror images of each other (Kirsch and Weixel 1988). The upshot of this, as Kirsch and Weixel and Kirsch and Rosadino note, is that one should assess whether, rather than assume that, the psychological and pharmacological effects of drug administration are additive.

Different verbal instructions can produce different sizes of placebo analgesic effects among healthy research subjects in an experimental context. In the next study in this anthology, Antonella Pollo and her colleagues investigate this effect among surgical patients in a clinical pharmacology setting

(Pollo et al. 2001). After an initial postsurgical run-in with buprenorphine, thoracotomized patients were given a basal intravenous infusion of a saline solution, and treated with buprenorphine only if they requested it over the span of three consecutive days. The analgesic effect of the basal infusion of saline was measured by recording the doses of buprenorphine requested over the three-day treatment period under three different verbal instructions. The first group was told nothing about any analgesic effects; rather, they were told that the basal infusion was a rehydrating solution (natural history). The second group was told that the basal infusion was either a powerful painkiller or a placebo; ten patients received placebo, four received buprenorphine (double-blind instruction). The third group was told that the basal infusion was a potent painkiller, but administration was identical to that in the double-blind condition; that is, ten received placebo and four received buprenorphine (deceptive administration). In both double-blind and deceptive administration groups, only the data from the ten placebo-administered patients in each group was used. Thus, the important difference to note between the double-blind and deceptive administration groups is that in the double-blind group they were told either placebo or painkiller but received placebo, while in the deceptive administration group, they were told painkiller but received placebo. They found that requests for buprenorphine decreased in the double-blind group by 20.8% compared with the natural history group, thus demonstrating an expectation-induced placebo effect and that such requests decreased by 33.8% in the deceptive administration group, thus demonstrating an even larger expectation-induced placebo effect. As with Kirsch and Rosadino (1993), the use of this methodology let Pollo and her colleagues determine the effects of knowledge of drug administration (analgesic is probable vs. analgesic is certain) on analgesia outcomes. Moreover, this study demonstrates that a more complete understanding of the way in which a placebo effect is elicited can be translated into the clinical setting and used to benefit patients.

Just as a placebo effect can be elicited in a clinical context to benefit patients, so too can expectation-induced nocebo effects be elicited in the clinical context, as the next study in this anthology demonstrates. Nicola Mondaini and her colleagues prospectively analyzed the impact of informing or not informing men with benign prostatic hyperplasia (BPH) of the expected sexual side effects of treatment with finasteride, a drug commonly used for both BPH and male pattern hair loss (Mondaini et al. 2007). After describing the treatment as a "compound of proven efficacy for the treatment of BPH," sexually active patients were randomly assigned to either one group, in which they were informed about possible adverse sexual effects ("it may cause erectile dysfunction, decreased libido, problems of ejaculation but these are uncommon"), or to another group, in which they were not given any information about sexual side effects. Follow-up questionnaires administered six and twelve months after the study began revealed that patients informed about the possibility of experiencing sexual dysfunction reported significantly greater sexual side effects (43.6%), as compared with those who were not informed (15.3%). Because patients in the clinic will be informed of likely side effects of finasteride, Mondaini and her colleagues rightly note that an awareness of the nocebo component of such side effects needs to be taken into account during the clinical encounter (Mondaini et al. 2007).

Although the mechanism of action is poorly understood and controversial, the action of merely taking pills (even if they are placebos) can induce improvement of clinical outcomes. This issue has recently been investigated in irritable bowel syndrome (IBS) patients in a study we include here that examined the efficacy of an open-label administration of sugar pills (Kaptchuk et al. 2010). Patients' improvement was assessed by the IBS Global Improvement Scale (IBS-GIS), the IBS Symptom Severity Scale (IBS-SSS), the IBS Adequate Relief (IBS-AR) questionnaire, and the IBS Quality of Life (IBS-QOL) questionnaire. IBS patients were randomized into two groups: those receiving placebo pills twice daily and those in a no-treatment control. Prior to randomization, eligible patients were told that, although placebos are inert, they have nonetheless been shown to cause significant improvements in IBS symptoms through mind-body self-healing processes (Kaptchuk et al. 2010). Receiving open-label (that is, nondeceptive and nonconcealed) placebos resulted in significantly improved IBS-GIS, IBS-SSS, and IBS-AR scores than receiving no treatment after both 11 and 21 days. A total of 59% of patients in the placebo group experienced "adequate relief" as measured by the binary (yes/no) IBS-AR measure, compared with 35% of those not receiving treatment. The observed effects were not related to the provider–patient interaction because both the placebo and no-treatment control groups met with a member of the health care team under similar conditions and with the same frequency. Thus, in this study Kaptchuk and his colleagues demonstrated that in the context of a supportive patient-provider relationship, and given a persuasive rationale for the placebo intervention, the symptoms of IBS patients improve over the course of three weeks after receiving a placebo without deception and without concealment. The implication of this study is that, at least for illnesses diagnosed by subjective symptoms and self-appraisals, open-label placebos may be appropriately prescribed in the clinic together with the prescription of active treatment.

As Luana Colloca and her colleagues discuss in their paper collected here (chapter 36), placebo responses can be observed by considering the different outcomes arising from expected (open) versus unexpected (hidden) administration of certain drugs (Colloca et al. 2004). A hidden treatment, of which the patient is completely unaware, is less effective than an identical treatment given overtly in accordance with routine medical practice. Across a number of conditions involving the nervous system, experimental evidence consistently supports the notion that expecting a therapeutic outcome may positively affect the outcome itself. For example, when a hidden treatment (morphine) is administered by a computerized infusion pump without the patient knowing when medication will be delivered, it is substantially less effective in reducing postoperative pain than the same dose of medication given overtly in the manner of routine medical practice. Similar results were found for hidden and overt interruption in exposure to anti-anxiety medication; when diazepam treatment was overtly interrupted, anxiety increased, whereas when it was interrupted without the patient's knowledge, no changes in anxiety were reported. More generally, the fact that patients who are given treatments along with verbal suggestions of benefit may experience enhanced improvement in a variety of symptoms indicates that the attempt to verbally induce expectations should be thought of as an element of, or a tool used in, clinical patient care.

Just as open administration of certain drugs is more powerful than their hidden administration, so too is a supportive provider–patient interaction *plus* a treatment ritual more powerful in relieving symptoms than comparable provider–patient interactions alone. In their paper collected here as chapter 37, Ted Kaptchuk and his collaborators demonstrated that a placebo effect could be elicited in IBS patients and, importantly, that this placebo effect could be dissected into (1) a placebo-related component and (2) a supportive provider–patient component (Kaptchuk et al. 2008). After initial assessment and observation, patients with IBS were randomized to one of three groups: (1) a waiting list (control) group that did not receive any intervention; (2) a limited interaction group that received a sham acupuncture intervention and limited contact (<5 minutes) with the health care team; and (3) an augmented interaction group that received a sham acupuncture intervention augmented by extended interactions (45 minutes) with warm and supportive members of the health care team instructed to promote positive expectations about acupuncture. At the end of three weeks, ordered comparisons (that is, waiting list vs. limited vs. augmented) between groups on all IBS-improvement outcomes were statistically significant for trend; moreover, comparisons between limited and augmented interaction groups showed the augmented interaction to be (statistically significantly) superior to the limited interaction on all outcome measures. The study by Kaptchuk and his colleagues shows that the elicited placebo effect (improved IBS outcomes) can be analyzed into its components parts (sham acupuncture, extended empathetic encounters with a provider) and can then be recombined to produce stepwise improvements in clinical outcomes. Importantly, this demonstrates the causal efficacy of both sham procedures used in the clinic and the clinical encounter itself, thus suggesting yet further tools for providers to use with their patients in order to improve clinical outcomes.

Yet another way that placebo effects can be harnessed to benefit patients in the clinic is demonstrated in the final chapter in this section by Robert Ader and his colleagues (Ader et al. 2010). In their study of pharmacological (corticosteroid) reinforcement in psoriasis patients, Ader and his colleagues demonstrated that placebos given after corticosteroid treatment mimic the effects of the corticosteroids, thus suggesting that placebos may be used in the clinic to *maintain* therapeutic outcomes without the side effects associated with active treatment. After an initial run-in period during which time all received corticosteroids, enrolled patients were randomized into three groups: (1) a standard therapy group that received 100% of the dose; (2) a partial reinforcement group that received 100% of the dose 25% to 50% of the time (and placebo the rest of the time); and (3) a dose control group that received 25% to 50% of the dose 100% of the time (partial reinforcement and dose control groups thus received identical cumulative amounts of drug). Using scores on the psoriasis severity scale as the primary outcome measure, Ader and his colleagues found that there were no differences between the standard therapy and partial reinforcement groups, even though those in the partial reinforcement group received between 25% and 50% less drug than those in the standard therapy group. This demonstrated a significant conditioning-induced placebo effect, one strong enough to maintain clinical outcomes among psoriasis patients. Other research has also shown that dose-extender placebo administration maintains drug efficacy under a conditioned schedule (Sandler et al. 2010). The strategy of giving placebos as dose extenders of standard treatments is one of several examples of harnessing placebo responses clinically to reduce side effects (and costs) of treatments while preserving therapeutic benefits (Colloca and Miller 2011b).

REFERENCES

Ader R, Cohen N. Behaviorally conditioned immunosuppression and murine systemic lupus erythematosus. *Science* 1982;215:1534–1536.

Ader R, Mercurio MG, Walton J, et al. Conditioned pharmacotherapeutic effects: A preliminary study. *Psychosomatic Medicine* 2010;72:192–197.

Amanzio M, Benedetti F. Neuropharmacological dissection of placebo analgesia: Expectation-activated opioid systems versus conditioning-activated specific subsystems. *Journal of Neuroscience* 1999;19:484–494.

Benedetti F, Amanzio M, Maggi M. Potentiation of placebo analgesia by proglumide. *Lancet* 1995;346:1231.

Benedetti F, Amanzio M, Vighetti S, Asteggiano G. The biochemical and neuroendocrine bases of the hyperalgesic nocebo effect. *Journal of Neuroscience* 2006;26:12014–12022.

Benedetti F, Colloca L, Torre E, et al. Placebo-responsive Parkinson patients show decreased activity in single neurons of subthalamic nucleus. *Nature Neuroscience* 2004;7:587–588.

Benedetti F, Mayberg HS, Wager T, et al. Neurobiological mechanisms of the placebo effect. *Journal of Neuroscience* 2005;25:10390–10402.

Benedetti F, Pollo A, Lopiano L, et al. Conscious expectation and unconscious conditioning in analgesic, motor, and hormonal placebo/nocebo responses. *Journal of Neuroscience* 2003;23:4315–4323.

Blackwell B, Bloomfield SS, Buncher CR. Demonstration to medical students of placebo responses and non-drug factors. *Lancet* 1972;299:1279–1282.

Buckalew LW, Coffield KE. An investigation of drug expectancy as a function of capsule color and size and preparation form. Journal of Clinical Psychopharmacology 1982;2:245–248.

Buckalew LW, Ross S. Relationship of perceptual characteristics to efficacy of placebos. Psychological Reports 1981;49:955–961.

Colloca L. Learned placebo analgesia in sequential trials: What are the pros and cons? Pain 2011;152:1215–1216.

Colloca L, Benedetti F. Placebos and painkillers: Is mind as real as matter? Nature Reviews Neuroscience 2005;6:545–552.

Colloca L, Benedetti F. How prior experience shapes placebo analgesia. Pain 2006;124:126–133.

Colloca L, Benedetti F. Placebo analgesia induced by social observational learning. Pain 2009;144:28–34.

Colloca L, Benedetti F, Porro CA. Experimental designs and brain mapping approaches for studying the placebo analgesic effect. European Journal of Applied Physiology 2008;102:371–380.

Colloca L, Lopiano L, Lanotte M, Benedetti F. Overt versus covert treatment for pain, anxiety, and Parkinson's disease. Lancet Neurology 2004;3:679–684.

Colloca L, Miller FG. How placebo responses are formed: A learning perspective. Philosophical Transactions of the Royal Society of London. Series B, Biological Sciences 2011a;366:1859–1869.

Colloca L, Miller FG. Harnessing the placebo effect: The need for translational research. Philosophical Transactions of the Royal Society of London. Series B, Biological Sciences 2011b;366:1922–1930.

Colloca L, Miller FG. Role of expectations in health. Current Opinion in Psychiatry 2011c;24:149–155.

Colloca L, Sigaudo M, Benedetti F. The role of learning in nocebo and placebo effects. Pain 2008;136:211–218.

de la Fuente-Fernández R, Phillips AG, Zamburlini M, et al. Dopamine release in human ventral striatum and expectation of reward. Behavioural Brain Research 2002;136:359–363.

de la Fuente-Fernández R, Ruth TJ, Sossi V, et al. Expectation and dopamine release: Mechanism of the placebo effect in Parkinson's disease. Science 2001;293:1164–1166.

Egbert LD, Battit GE, Welch CE, Bartlett MK. Reduction of postoperative pain by encouragement and instruction of patients—A study of doctor-patient rapport. New England Journal of Medicine 1964;270: 825–827.

Eippert F, Bingel U, Schoell ED, et al. Activation of the opioidergic descending pain control system underlies placebo analgesia. Neuron 2009a;63:533–543.

Eippert F, Finsterbusch J, Bingel U, Büchel C. Direct evidence for spinal cord involvement in placebo analgesia. Science 2009b;326:404.

Fields H. State-dependent opioid control of pain. Nature Reviews Neuroscience 2004;5:565–575.

Gracely RH, Dubner R, Deeter WR, Wolskee PJ. Clinicians' expectations influence placebo analgesia. Lancet 1985;325:43.

Grevert P, Albert LH, Goldstein A. Partial antagonism of placebo analgesia by naloxone. Pain 1983;16:129–143.

Guo J-Y, Wang J-Y, Luo F. Dissection of placebo analgesia in mice: The conditions for activation of opioid and non-opioid systems. Journal of Psychopharmacology 2010;24:1561–1567.

Herrnstein RJ. Placebo effect in the rat. Science 1962;138:677–678.

Kaptchuk TJ, Friedlander E, Kelley JM, et al. Placebos without deception: A randomized controlled trial in irritable bowel syndrome. PLoS ONE 2010;5(12):e15591.

Kaptchuk TJ, Kelley JM, Conboy LA, et al. Components of placebo effect: Randomised controlled trial in patients with irritable bowel syndrome. BMJ 2008;336:999–1003.

Kirsch I. Conditioning, expectancy, and the placebo effect: Comment on Stewart-Williams and Podd. Psychological Bulletin 2004;130:341–343.

Kirsch I, Rosadino MJ. Do double-blind studies with informed consent yield externally valid results? An empirical test. Psychopharmacology (Berl) 1993;110:437–442.

Kirsch I, Weixel LJ. Double-blind versus deceptive administration of a placebo. Behavioral Neuroscience 1988;102:319–323.

Klinger R, Soost S, Flor H, Worm M. Classical conditioning and expectancy in placebo hypoalgesia: A randomized controlled study in patients with atopic dermatitis and persons with healthy skin. Pain 2007;128:31–39.

Lasagna L, Mosteller F, von Felsinger JM, Beecher HK. A study of the placebo response. American Journal of Medicine 1954;16:770–779.

Levine JD, Gordon NC. Influence of the method of drug administration on analgesic response. Nature 1984;312:755–756.

Levine JD, Gordon NC, Fields HL. The mechanism of placebo analgesia. Lancet 1978;312:654–657.

Liberman R. An analysis of the placebo phenomenon. Journal of Chronic Diseases 1962;15:761–783.

Lidstone SC, Schulzer M, Dinelle K, et al. Effects of expectation on placebo-induced dopamine release in Parkinson disease. Archives of General Psychiatry 2010;67:857–865.

Luparello TJ, Leist N, Lourie CH, Sweet P. The interaction of psychologic stimuli and pharmacologic agents on airway reactivity in asthmatic subjects. Psychosomatic Medicine 1970;32:509–513.

Luparello TJ, Lyons HA, Bleecker ER, McFadden ER Jr. Influences of suggestion on airway reactivity in asthmatic subjects. Psychosomatic Medicine 1968;30:819–825.

Mayberg HS, Silva JA, Brannan SK, et al. The functional neuroanatomy of the placebo effect. American Journal of Psychiatry 2002;159:728–737.

Miller FG, Colloca L, Kaptchuk TJ. The placebo effect: Illness and interpersonal healing. Perspectives in Biology and Medicine 2009;52: 518–539.

Mondaini N, Gontero P, Giubilei G, et al. Finasteride 5 mg and sexual side effects: How many of these are related to a nocebo phenomenon? Journal of Sexual Medicine 2007;4:1708–1712.

Montgomery GH, Kirsch I. Classical conditioning and the placebo effect. Pain 1997;72:107–113.

Park LC, Covi L. Nonblind placebo trial: An exploration of neurotic patients' responses to placebo when its inert content is disclosed. Archives of General Psychiatry 1965;12:36–45.

Petrovic P, Kalso E, Petersson KM, Ingvar M. Placebo and opioid analgesia—imaging a shared neuronal network. Science 2002;295: 1737–1740.

Pollo A, Amanzio M, Arslanian A, et al. Response expectancies in placebo analgesia and their clinical relevance. Pain 2001;93:77–84.

Price DD, Milling LS, Kirsch I, et al. An analysis of factors that contribute to the magnitude of placebo analgesia in an experimental paradigm. Pain 1999;83:147–156.

Rothwell PM. Factors that can affect the external validity of randomised controlled trials. PLoS Clinical Trials 2006;1(1):e9.

Sandler AD, Glesne CE, Bodfish JW. Conditioned placebo dose reduction: A new treatment in attention-deficit hyperactivity disorder? Journal of Developmental and Behavioral Pediatrics 2010;31:369–375.

Strafella AP, Ko JH, Monchi O. Therapeutic application of transcranial magnetic stimulation in Parkinson's disease: The contribution of expectation. NeuroImage 2006;31:1666–1672.

Tracey I. Getting the pain you expect: Mechanisms of placebo, nocebo and reappraisal effects in humans. Nature Medicine 2010;16:1277–1283.

Volkow ND, Wang GJ, Ma Y, et al. Expectation enhances the regional brain metabolic and the reinforcing effects of stimulants in cocaine abusers. Journal of Neuroscience 2003;23:11461–11468.

Volkow ND, Wang GJ, Ma Y, et al. Effects of expectation on the brain metabolic responses to methylphenidate and to its placebo in non–drug abusing subjects. NeuroImage 2006;32:1782–1792.

Voudouris NJ, Peck C, Coleman G. The role of conditioning and verbal expectancy in the placebo response. Pain 1990;43:121–128.

Wager TD, Rilling JK, Smith EE, et al. Placebo-induced changes in fMRI in the anticipation and experience of pain. Science 2004;303:1162–1167.

Wager TD, Scott DJ, Zubieta J-K. Placebo effects on human μ-opioid activity during pain. *Proceedings of the National Academy of Sciences U.S.A.* 2007;104:11056–11061.

Wolf S. Effects of suggestion and conditioning on the action of chemical agents in human subjects—the pharmacology of placebos. *Journal of Clinical Investigation* 1950;29:100–109.

Wolf S, Doering CR, Clark ML, Hagans JA. Chance distribution and the placebo "reactor." *Journal of Laboratory and Clinical Medicine* 1957;49:837–841.

Zubieta J-K, Bueller JA, Jackson LR, et al. Placebo effects mediated by endogenous opioid activity on mu-opioid receptors. *Journal of Neuroscience* 2005;25:7754–7762.

9

Effects of Suggestion and Conditioning on the Action of Chemical Agents in Human Subjects

The Pharmacology of Placebos

STEWART WOLF

Stewart Wolf, "Effects of Suggestion and Conditioning on the Action of Chemical Agents in Human Subjects: The Pharmacology of Placebos," Journal of Clinical Investigation 1950;29:100–109.

The effect of administration of a drug or other chemical agent on a bit of muscle suspended in a standard solution is predictable and reproducible because it depends only on the pharmacologic action of the agent administered. The effect of administration of the same agent on an intact organism, however, is not necessarily predictable or reproducible because the pharmacologic action of the agent may either reinforce or run counter to other forces acting on the end organ at the same time. This is not a startling statement but a truism of which physicians and laymen have long been aware. Despite this awareness, drugs are often dealt with as if the intact organism were comparable to the water bath and little interest has been manifest in factors other than their pharmacologic action which may determine or modify the effects of chemical agents in the human body. The purpose of this communication is to describe some measurable "drug effects" which are not attributable to the chemical properties of the agents administered.

It is not intended here to elaborate the psychodynamic mechanisms which may be involved in such phenomena. Neither is it possible to identify with certainty or to distinguish between the various factors which modify in a given instance the action of a chemical agent. Therefore, this communication is not concerned with enumerating or weighing these various factors but with illustrating the magnitude of their effects, so that in the future drugs will be assessed not only with reference to their pharmacologic action but also to the other forces at play and to the circumstances surrounding their administration.

Method

Initial observations were made on Tom, a human subject with a large gastric fistula, in whom it was possible to observe directly the gastric mucous membrane, correlating changes in color and turgidity with simultaneous measurements of secretion and motor activity (1). Four other human subjects provided supplementary experimental opportunities.

The methods used in measuring and recording the indicators of gastric function are described in detail elsewhere (1). Acid secretion is designated not only in titratable units, but also as the quantity of 0.17 N HCl secreted by the stomach per 15-minute collection period. The figure for this quantity is derived from the volume of secretion and the total acidity with reference to a formula developed by Hollander (1). Under average circumstances the resting stomach secretion approximates 5 cc. 0.17 N HCl per hour.

Observations

Among the factors which appeared to be of leading importance in the experiments which follow are: 1) The state of the end organ at the time of administration, i.e., the effect of forces already acting prior to administration of the agent; 2) the setting in which the agent was administered, including the route of administration, the presence of the experimenter and the effects of suggestion, implicit or expressed; 3) conditioning circumstances and previously established habits of reaction.

Below are detailed examples of these phenomena observed following the administration of various agents.

1. Urogastrone

The literature reflects considerable divergence of opinion concerning the action of urogastrone and enterogastrone on the stomach. Inhibition of acid secretion has been reported, but this effect has not been consistently observed (2–5). In the published data, cognizance has not been taken of the relative state of activity of the stomach at the time of administration.

Dry powder containing an as yet unmeasured quantity of urogastrone was prepared from aqueous extract of pregnant mare's urine after the removal of the fat soluble fractions (courtesy Parke, Davis & Company). Page and Heffner (6) have reported the use of this same material in the treatment of peptic ulcer.

Eight experiments were performed with varying amounts of this preparation administered by mouth. The results are shown in Table 9.1. It will be noted that they are variable but correspond in general to the state of the gastric mucosa at the time of administration. That is, when the stomach was not hyperaemic and hypersecretive the agent induced an evident inhibition of secretion associated with pallor and diminution of turgidity. When, on the other hand, the agent was administered in the presence of gastric hyperfunction, little or no effect was noted. Two of the experiments are illustrated graphically in Figure 9.1. The first was performed at a time of relative relaxation and security when gastric function was average. The second was performed in a setting of intense feelings of frustration and resentment related to Tom's receipt of a dispossess notice from his landlord on the previous day. The stomach at the time of the experiment was turgid, hyperaemic and hypersecretive. This gastric hyperfunction was actually somewhat enhanced following ingestion of the drug.

Table 9.1.
The results of administration of capsules containing urogastrone directly into the stomach of Tom

	1	2	3	4	5	6	7	8
Dose	1 caps.	1 caps.	1 caps.	2 caps.	2 caps.	2 caps.	2 caps.	2 caps.
Maximum effect	45 min.	60 min.	75 min.	—	120 min.	—	75 min.	—
Color	55→45	50→40	55→55	65→70	60→50	65→65	55→40	60→60
Turgidity	3→2	2→1	3→3	4→4	3→1½	3½→3½	3→2	3→3
Free acid	50→12	26→0	60→55	70→85	12→0	58→56	36→12	45→50

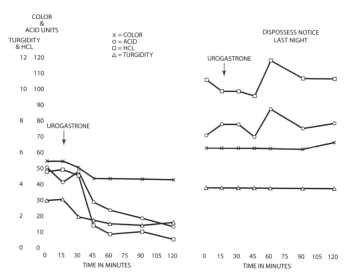

Figure 9.1. The effects of urogastrone on the stomach of Tom on two separate occasions. On the first occasion, the stomach was in a state of relative inactivity, and there resulted an evident depression of gastric function (left). On the second occasion, the agent administered during a phase of relative gastric hyperfunction showed no apparent effect (right).

COMMENT

The receipt of a dispossess notice was for Tom perhaps more of a traumatic experience than it would have been for the average person at a time of housing shortage because, as pointed out in detail elsewhere (1) performance as a competent family head was with him a prime value. The experience signified to him that he was losing his hold on the family destinies, and it provoked a reaction of insecurity, anxiety and resentment. As shown in Figure 9.1 gastric function on this occasion actually increased following urogastrone. As reported elsewhere (1) it has repeatedly been shown that gastric hyperfunction occurs in Tom in a setting of anxiety and resentment. It seems probable that the forces related to this reaction were more powerful than the pharmacologic action of urogastrone.

2. Benadryl

The effect on gastric acid secretion of the antihistaminic drug Benadryl has been similarly difficult to define (7,8). Figure 9.2 illustrates the depressing effect upon gastric

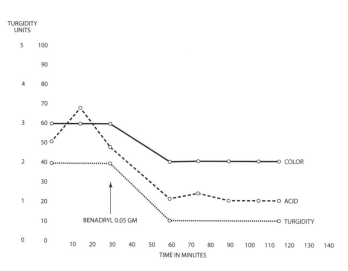

Figure 9.2. Depressing effect of Benadryl when administered at a time of average gastric function.

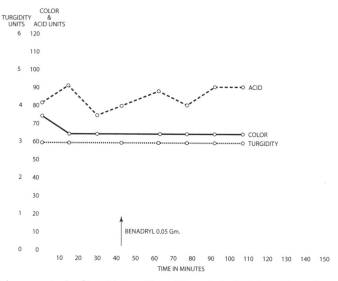

Figure 9.3. Lack of inhibiting effect of Benadryl administered to a hyperactive stomach.

blood flow and acidity exerted by 50 mg. of Benadryl when the stomach was in an average state and Tom was relatively relaxed and contented. Figure 9.3 illustrates the relative lack of effect observed upon another morning when Tom was tense and angry because of having had to run a fruitless errand for someone whom he particularly disliked. At the time of administration of the Benadryl his gastric mucosa was in-

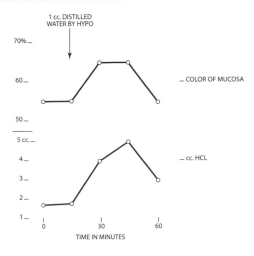

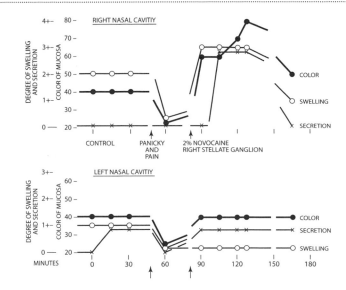

Figure 9.4. Increased gastric function following hypodermic injection of distilled water. Acid secretion in this figure is expressed as cc. of 0.17 N HCl per 15 min., as in Figures 9.1–9.3, 9.7–9.9. The recorded difference of 3 cc. is significant.

Figure 9.5. Unilateral nasal hyperfunction following temporary block of the stellate ganglion on that side. Note brief period of pallor and dryness in both nostrils during fright prior to injection.

tensely turgid and hyperaemic and acid values were high. Following ingestion of the same quantity of Benadryl as before there was no significant change in the measurable indicators of gastric function.

Similarly, pyribenzamine and posterior pituitary extract inhibited gastric function when the stomach was relatively inactive at the time of administration, but exerted no measurable effect when the stomach was in an episode of relative gastric hyperfunction.

COMMENT

The discrepancies in results in these experiments which correspond roughly to the state of the gastric mucosa at the time of administration may be attributed to modification of the effectiveness of an agent by other more powerful forces acting on the end organ at the same time.

3. Hypodermic of Sterile Water

Tom always resented being stuck by a needle. Accordingly, when he was given a hypodermic injection of sterile water the effect as shown in Figure 9.4 was to enhance gastric blood flow and secretion.

The same category of effect was observed in experiments on the nose when procaine hydrochloride was injected into the left stellate ganglion of a human subject. As reported elsewhere in detail, this interruption of sympathetic nerve fibers to the nose regularly results in hyperaemia and engorgement of the turbinates with increased mucus secretion (9). The injection procedure had its own effect, however, because it frightened the subject. The transitory fear reaction was accompanied by pallor and shrinkage of the turbinates and hyposecretion of mucus which preceded the sympathetic blocking effect of the procaine block as shown in Figure 9.5.

COMMENT

These effects which arise because the circumstances surrounding the administration of the agent constitute in themselves a stimulus may, of course, either reinforce or oppose the pharmacologic action of the agent administered.

4. Ipecac

The nausea which follows the ingestion of ipecac or indeed that induced by any nauseating stimulus is associated with interruption of contractile activity of the stomach and general relaxation and flaccidity of the organ as described in an earlier communication (10). In Figure 9.6A is shown the pattern observed in kymographic tracings during nausea after the ingestion of ipecac. An opposite effect attributable to a "placebo" action was experimentally induced in a 28-year-old female suffering from nausea and vomiting of pregnancy who had been continuously nauseated and vomiting for two days. She was intubated with a balloon attached to a recording manometer. In Figure 9.6B is shown the characteristic pattern of gastric inactivity which accompanies nausea (10). After a suitable control period the subject was given 10 cc. syrup of ipecac and told that it was medicine which would abolish her nausea. Within 20 minutes the nausea had subsided completely and did not recur until the following morning. As shown in Figure 9.6B the stomach began to display normal contractile activity coincident with the disappearance of nausea.

A second subject, also a 28-year-old female, had had recurrent nausea for several months associated with a reactive depression. A kymographic recording from her stomach revealed the characteristic absence of contractile activity during nausea. After a suitable control period she was given

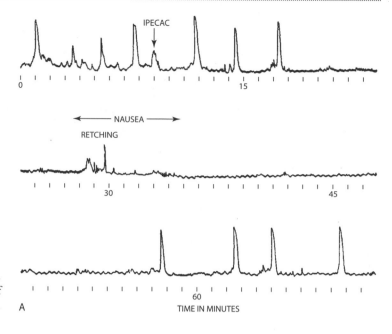

Figure 9.6A. Usual effect of ingestion of 10 cc. syrup of ipecac. Note interruption of contractile activity of the stomach during nausea.

A

TIME IN MINUTES

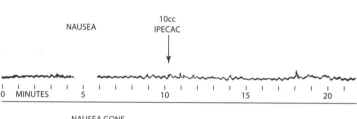

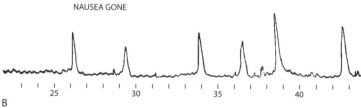

Figure 9.6B. Reversal of ipecac effect by suggestion. Note disappearance of nausea with resumption of gastric contractions at a time when ipecac is usually inducing nausea and interrupting contractions.

B

10 cc. syrup of ipecac directly into the stomach through a Levine tube. Repeatedly on previous occasions this amount of ipecac when swallowed had induced nausea and vomiting. On this occasion, however, not tasting and not knowing what she had been given, she was told that the agent would abolish her nausea; within 30 minutes nausea was gone and small waves of contraction were recorded from the stomach. Sixty minutes later when nausea had recurred with associated gastric hypomotility a second dose of ipecac was introduced into the Levine tube, this time with the reassurance that the nausea would be effectively abolished. Nausea disappeared again in 15 minutes and gastric contractions were resumed. No further nausea was experienced that day.

COMMENT

The above "placebo" actions depended for their force on the conviction of the patient that this or that effect would result.

It is likely that this mechanism is operative in part in any enthusiastically pursued therapeutic regime as well as in the successful cures of faith healers. It has even been shown experimentally that the threshold for pain perception may be greatly raised by suggestion (11).

5. Prostigmine, Tap Water, Lactose and Atropine

During a study of the effects of various pharmacologic agents on the stomach, Tom was repeatedly given prostigmine, an agent which predictably induced abdominal cramps and diarrhea as well as hyperaemia, hypersecretion and hypermotility in the stomach. Figure 9.7 shows the typical effect of the prostigmine on the stomach. Each day, following the prostigmine, regardless of what substance was administered to Tom he displayed gastric hyperfunction, abdominal cramps and diarrhea. Figure 9.8 illustrates the apparent stimulating effect of the ingestion of 20 cc. of ordinary tap

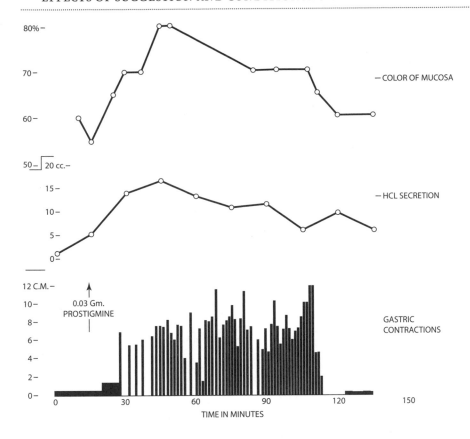

Figure 9.7. Usual effect of prostigmine 0.03 Gm. administered by mouth.

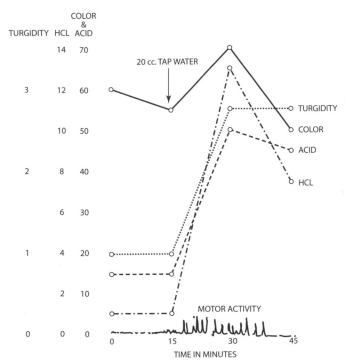

Figure 9.8. Apparent stimulating effect of tap water following suitable conditions of the stomach.

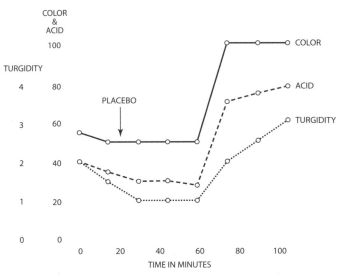

Figure 9.9. Marked increase in gastric function following ingestion of lactose placebo.

water, and in Figure 9.9 one sees, following administration of two large red lactose capsules, hyperaemia, engorgement and hyperacidity in the stomach exceeding in inten-sity the effect of prostigmine and associated with abdominal cramps and diarrhea. Finally, an attempt was made to interrupt this unsalutary chain of events by the administration of hypodermic of 0.0006 Gm. of atropine sulfate. The results are shown in Figure 9.10. Again hyperaemia, hypersecretion and hypermotility occurred. For comparison the usual inhibiting effect of atropine on gastric function is also illustrated.

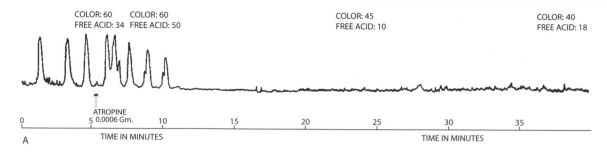

Figure 9.10A. Usual inhibiting effect on gastric motor activity of .0006 Gm. atropine hypodermically.

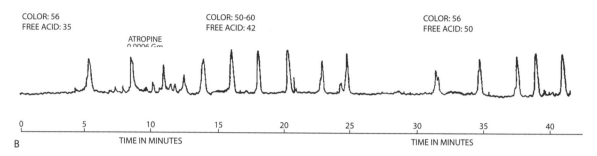

Figure 9.10B. Reversal of atropine effect on the stomach after suitable conditioning with increased contractile activity following injection of .0006 Gm.

COMMENT

Such a reversal of the usual effect of atropine has been also observed in the colon by Grace and reported in detail elsewhere (12). The experimental subject was a 28-year-old man with a large colonic fistula through which approximately 12 inches of cecum and ascending colon had evaginated and lay exposed on his abdominal wall. The administration of atropine was usually followed by pallor and dryness of the mucosa and interruption of contractile activity of the colon, but when the subject reacted to the experimental procedure with anger and hostility, as much as 0.012 Gm. of atropine administered intravenously was followed by hyperaemia, increased tone and hypermotility in the colon.

Discussion

The experiences related above encountered in the course of testing the pharmacologic action of various agents on various organs of the body could probably be reproduced in almost any organ system.

The fact that "placebo effects" occur depends, of course, on the generalization established repeatedly by numerous workers that the mechanisms of the human body are capable of reacting not only to direct physical and chemical stimulation but also to symbolic stimuli, words and events which have somehow acquired special meaning for the individual.

The frequency with which "placebo effects" would be expected and their magnitude probably vary from person to person and from time to time. Although in Tom more than 100 experiments have been performed with pharmacologic agents, it is not possible to state with certainty how frequently significant modification of the pharmacologic effect occurred by reason of situational factors, but in retrospect one can detect minor evidences of such in well over 50% of observations. Tom is a comparatively healthy, active and productive human subject, whose detailed personality study is available elsewhere (1).

Not only the frequency but also the magnitude of "placebo effects" is impressive and deserves attention in pharmacologic experimentation in animals and man. It is at present customary to control drug experiments on various clinical syndromes with placebos especially when the data to be evaluated are chiefly subjective but, when objective recording of indicators of the agents' effects are available, placebo control is not generally practiced. The need for such controls is suggested by the fact that "placebo effects" include objective changes at the end organ which may exceed those attributable to potent pharmacologic action. Indeed, the pharmacologic action of an agent may be outweighed and its effect thus reversed.

Conclusion

"Placebo effects" which modify the pharmacologic action of drugs or endow inert agents with potency are not imaginary, but may be associated with measurable changes at the end organs. These effects are at times more potent than the pharmacologic action customarily attributed to the agent.

Thus the familiar difficulty of evaluating in patients new therapeutic agents stems not only from inadequately curbed enthusiasm of the investigator, but also from the actual physiologic effects of their "placebo" action.

REFERENCES

1. Wolf, S., and Wolff, H.G., *Human Gastric Function: An Experimental Study of a Man and His Stomach.* Oxford Univ. Press, New York, 1947, Ed. 2.

2. Sandweiss, D.J., Anti-ulcer (anthelone) products in the treatment of peptic ulcer. *Gastroenterology*, 1946, **6**, 604.

3. Greengard, H., Atkinson, A.J., Grossman, M.I., and Ivy, A.C., The effectiveness of parenterally administered "enterogastrone" in the prophylaxis of recurrences of experimental and clinical peptic ulcer, with summary of 58 cases. *Gastroenterology*, 1946, **7**, 625.

4. Levin, E., Kirsner, J.B., and Palmer, W.L., Preliminary observations on histamine and insulin stimulated gastric secretion during the injection of an enterogastrone concentrate in man. *Gastroenterology*, 1948, **10**, 274.

5. Ferayorni, R.R., Code, C.F., and Morlock, C.G., The effect of enterogastrone concentrates on gastric secretion in human beings. *Gastroenterology*, 1948, **11**, 730.

6. Page, R.C., and Heffner, R.R., Oral treatment of chronic duodenal and jejunal ulcers with an extract of pregnant mare's urine. *Gastroenterology*, 1948, **11**, 842.

7. Moersch, R.U., Rivers, A.B., and Morlock, C.G., Some results of the gastric secretary response of patients having duodenal ulcer noted during the administration of benadryl. *Gastroenterology*, 1946, **7**, 91.

8. McElin, T.W., and Horton, B.T., Clinical observations on the use of benadryl: its effect on histamine-induced gastric acidity in man. *Gastroenterology*, 1946, **7**, 100.

9. Holmes, T.H., Goodell, H., Wolf, S., and Wolff, H.G., *The Nose: An Experimental Study of Reactions within the Nose in Human Subjects during Varying Life Experiences.* Charles C Thomas, Springfield, Ill., 1950.

10. Wolf, S., The relation of gastric function to nausea in man. *Journal of Clinical Investigation*, 1943, **22**, 877.

11. Wolff, H.G., and Goodell, H., The relation of attitude and suggestion to the perception of and reaction to pain. *Research Publications—Association for Research in Nervous and Mental Disease*, 1943, **23**, 434.

12. Grace, W.J., Wolf, S., and Wolff, H.G., *The Human Colon.* Paul Hoeber & Co., New York, 1951.

10

A Study of the Placebo Response

LOUIS LASAGNA, FREDERICK MOSTELLER, JOHN M. VON FELSINGER, AND HENRY K. BEECHER

Louis Lasagna, Frederick Mosteller, John M. von Felsinger, and Henry K. Beecher, "A Study of the Placebo Response," *American Journal of Medicine* 1954;16:770–779.

In 1945 Pepper wrote a paper on the use of the placebo.[1] In it he recorded his failure to find, up to that time, any references to the placebo phenomenon in the Index of the Surgeon General's Library and the Cumulative Index. With the increasing interest in properly controlled clinical trials in recent years the importance of the placebo in clinical medicine and investigation has been stressed by a number of authors.[2–7] The acknowledged power of inert substances to provide striking relief for a wide variety of symptoms and the frequent occurrence of "side-reactions" following their use indicate the need for detailed study of the placebo response.

The magnitude of the placebo effect in studies of postoperative pain has been repeatedly demonstrated in this laboratory. When surgical patients suffering from steady, severe wound pain are injected subcutaneously with 1 ml. of saline, three or four of every ten such patients report satisfactory relief of pain. Patients who are thus relieved by placebos are sometimes called "placebo reactors." Jellinek, on the basis of studies of patients with recurrent headache, has suggested that "placebo reactors" may mask real differences between drugs by their failure to discriminate potent from nonpotent agents.[6] Beecher, Keats, Mosteller and Lasagna,[7] in a study of oral analgesics in the treatment of postoperative pain, reported results similar to those of Jellinek.[6] Several considerations of importance are raised by these observations: (1) placebo reactors may change the slope of the dose-response curve and in consequence the sensitivity of the experiment; (2) an effective drug may be wrongly discarded because data have been diluted by inclusion within the test group of a large number of placebo reactors; and (3) the optimal dosage of a standard drug may be underestimated if the placebo reactor group within the population sample is large and readily relieved. Since most of the studies of analgesia in this laboratory have been concerned with subcutaneous medications and the use of morphine as a standard of reference, the present experiments were designed to investigate the placebo effect under these conditions, and also to inquire into the relationship of personality structure, past history, habits and attitudes to placebo reactivity.

Methods

Postoperative patients on the general surgical, urologic, orthopedic and gynecologic wards were employed. The time of observation was the period after surgery, starting as soon as relief of pain became necessary and ending with the cessation of need for narcotics. Postoperative pain for which morphine or similar narcotic was ordered by the house staff was considered satisfactory for study. Subjects under seventeen and over seventy-five (with one exception) were not employed. Pain relief was studied in two main categories: (1) steady wound pain on lying quietly in bed and (2) all other types of pain. A medication was considered to have produced relief when the patient indicated significant alleviation of pain ("over 50 per cent") at forty-five and again at ninety minutes after injection. The responses of the patients were elicited by technicians unaware of the nature of the medications employed. The study was conducted in two phases, sixty-nine patients being studied in phase I and ninety-three patients in phase II. In phase I, for every six medications each patient received one was a placebo (1 ml. of saline solution) and five were doses of morphine phosphate[A] (10 mg. of the salt per 70 kg. of body weight). The order of administration of the placebo was randomized so that some patients received the placebo first, some second, some third, some fourth and some fifth. In phase II, placebo and morphine doses were alternated in each patient, and the starting medication (placebo or morphine) was alternated from patient to patient. From the ninety-three patients in phase II twenty-four patients were chosen who had responded in consistent fashion to injections of placebo. Eleven of these patients were always relieved of pain by the placebo and thirteen always failed to obtain relief. In addition, three other patients were studied and considered non-reactors in view of their failure to obtain relief from placebos on most occasions (4 of 5, 5 of 6, and 7 of 8 responses, respectively). These twenty-seven patients represent a screened population since only responses to medications given for steady severe wound pain were considered, and for every placebo dose which produced relief it was required that pain return, to eliminate the possibility that the pain had subsided spontaneously. Consistent reactors and non-reactors were employed in the hope that such a procedure would heighten the contrast between the groups. Psychologic data were accumulated on these subjects by psychologists and technicians who were unaware of the nature of the placebo responses. The data consisted of (1) a standard interview with each patient designed to elicit past experiences and attitudes which might be pertinent to the study; (2) questionnaires filled out by the nurses on the wards evaluating the patients in regard to personality, staff-patient relationships and hospital course; (3) Rorschach psychodiagnostic test; (4) thematic apperception test; and (5) an estimation of the intelligence quotient based on the vocabulary sub test of the Wechsler-Bellevue Scale. These latter tests (items 3 to 5) and the interview were performed at the end of the hospital course, prior to discharge.

Results

Age and Sex

In phase I most patients received only one dose of placebo and were thus divided into "reactors" and "non-reactors" solely on the one response. Using this criterion there is no apparent difference between the two groups as far as sex distribution is concerned, but the mean age for the reactors is five years greater than that of the non-reactors:

	Sex	Age in Years		
		Range	Mean±S.E.	Median
Reactors.	14M, 13F	20–79	52±2.9	52
Non-reactors. . . .	20M, 22F	21–67	47±1.8	49

In phase II some patients received only one placebo dose, but the majority received two or more doses of saline solution. If one calculates the percentages of individuals of each sex that responded in the various possible ways, there is again no striking difference in the behavior of the two groups:

In regard to age, however, the mean values for the phase II reactors and non-reactors again showed a difference of five years:

	Age in Years		
	Range	Mean±S.E.	Median
Reactors.	35–64	52±1.6	54
Non-reactors. . . .	21–72	47±2.6	48
Inconsistent. . . .	17–74	46±2.5	44

If one pools the data from both phases, the results show a mean reactor age of 52±1.5 years and a mean non-reactor age of 47±1.8 years. This five-year difference is significant at the 5 per cent level.

Pain Relief from Morphine

The analgesic potency of morphine was analyzed by assigning an "average per cent relief" score to each person, based on the response to all doses of morphine administered to that person for steady wound pain. The average per cent relief for any *class* of subjects is thus the mean of the individual relief scores. In this way each person contributes equally to group scores, and the N for any sample is the number of individuals rather than the number of doses. In phase I all doses up to and including the sixth dose (of morphine) were counted. In phase II all doses of morphine up to and including the fourth dose (of morphine) were counted. (It should be recalled that in phase II morphine and placebo were alternated, whereas in phase I there was only one placebo dose out of every six medications.) Any dose given by the nursing staff whose outcome was not known to us or which was administered for reasons other than steady wound pain, is counted as a dose as far as order of administration is concerned, although the effect of such a dose does not enter into the calculations of analgesic potency.

The data from phase I reveal that morphine provided 79.4 per cent relief in the reactors and 66.0 per cent in the non-reactors. This difference of 13.4 per cent, while in the direction of greater effectiveness in the placebo-reactor group, is not statistically significant. In phase II the problem is somewhat more complicated because of the multiple doses of placebo. The data of phase II are presented in Table 10.1 for all patients receiving at least one dose each of placebo and morphine for steady wound pain. The patients are classified by

Sex (No.)	Reactors		Non-reactors		Inconsistent (%)
	One Dose (%)	Two or More Doses (%)	One Dose (%)	Two or More Doses (%)	
Male (41). . . .	14.6	9.8	7.4	24.3	43.9
Female (52). .	13.5	11.6	17.3	19.2	38.4

Table 10.1.

Phase II—Average per cent relief from early morphine doses for patients receiving at least one dose each of placebo and morphine for steady wound pain*

No. of Placebos	No. of Reported Placebo Reliefs					
	0	1	2	3	4	Average
1	100.0 (5)	85.7 (7)	—	—	—	91.7 (12)
2	47.9 (8)	91.9 (9)	91.7 (4)	—	—	75.0 (21)
3	43.8 (4)	61.1 (6)	72.2 (3)	75.0 (2)	—	60.6 (15)
4 (or more)	58.3 (9)	58.3 (3)	58.3 (3)	x	x	58.3 (15)

Note: * Numbers in parentheses represent numbers of cases. In the line for 4 (or more) placebos, reports of first four indicated placebos were used. Reports of first four morphine doses were used.

number of placebo doses and by the number of times such doses were effective. Such a procedure serves to locate a subject by his frequency of relief from placebo and approximately stratifies the sample according to total number of doses. (Only the first four placebo doses are used for purposes of classification.) Having classified an individual according to his placebo responses, the morphine responses for that person have been expressed as an average per cent for all morphine doses up to and including the fourth dose. The per cent relief scores in Table 10.1 are the mean scores for the individuals in the stratified groups. If one compares the per cent relief from morphine in patients never relieved by a placebo and in patients relieved one or more times by a placebo, there is a difference of 16.8 per cent (77.7 minus 60.9), the per cent relief being higher in the group obtaining at least occasional relief from the placebo. This difference is statistically significant and in keeping with the findings in phase I. Also evident in Table 10.1, in the extreme right-hand column, is the significant relationship of per cent relief from morphine and total number of placebo doses. As the latter (and therefore the total number of postoperative medications) increases, the average effectiveness of morphine decreases. This is in accord with earlier work in this laboratory[8] and presumably reflects the more frequent need for medication and the longer duration of pain in patients with more severe pain.

Pain Relief from a Placebo

Another analysis of the data in both phases of the study concerns the analgesic potency of the placebo when the total number of medications is controlled. In phase I seven of the fourteen patients who received four or fewer postoperative medications had relief from a placebo, averaging 50 per cent relief, whereas in those patients with five or more total doses twenty of fifty-four, or 37 per cent, were relieved. In phase II the analysis was based on total number of placebo doses, which in this instance is highly correlated with total number of doses of all kinds. For fifteen patients with one placebo dose 53 per cent of placebo

doses gave relief; for twenty-one patients with two placebo doses 40 per cent of placebo doses gave relief; for fifteen patients with three placebo doses 40 per cent gave relief; and for fifteen patients with four or more placebo doses 15 per cent gave relief. These results show a significant correlation between number of doses and per cent relief. The trend is thus similar in both phases and suggests that (like morphine) placebo doses are less effective in patients who receive many doses of medication and whose pain is of long duration.

Consistency of Response to Placebo

An interesting aspect of phase II was the opportunity to investigate the consistency of the placebo response. Sixty-nine patients received two or more doses of a placebo. Of these thirty-eight (55 per cent) behaved inconsistently, i.e., on some occasions placebos produced relief and on others they did not. Ten of the patients (14 per cent) were consistent reactors, i.e., all placebo doses were effective. Twenty-one of the patients (31 per cent) were consistent non-reactors, i.e., placebo doses were never effective. If one assumed uniformity of response and tried to predict the efficacy of subsequent placebos by the response to the initial dose of saline, one would thus have been wrong more frequently than right.

Psychologic Data

The duration of surgery and anesthesia, mean ages and summary of postoperative medications for the two groups of consistent reactors and non-reactors studied are given in Table 10.2. The reactors are (as in the unselected total group) some five years older than the non-reactors. The number of medications received during the postoperative period is greater for the non-reactors than for the reactors, and the pain relief obtained from morphine is less in the former group. These data are similar to the findings in the unselected population described previously. It will be seen that the duration of surgery and anesthesia are similar in the two

Table 10.2.

Mean age, medication data and duration of surgery and anesthesia for patients in psychologic study (with standard errors)

	Placebo Reactors (11)	Placebo Non-reactors (16)
Mean age, years	49.3±2.2	43.7±2.7
Mean no. of morphine doses per patient*	3.5±0.7	5.5±0.7
Mean no. of medications (morphine and placebo) per patient*	5.4±0.6	8.6±1.0
Mean pain relief from morphine*	95%±3.4%	54%±9.4%
Mean duration of anesthesia (minutes)	215±22	210±24
Mean duration of surgery (minutes)	181±21	177±24

Note: * Indicates significant difference (p<0.05) between reactors and non-reactors.

groups. The types of anesthesia and surgery also were similar in both groups. For example, all of the reactors and all but two of the non-reactors received nitrous oxide–oxygen–ether for anesthesia. Ten of the reactors had abdominal operations (gastrectomy, cholecystectomy, hysterectomy, bowel surgery) and one had a thoracotomy. Ten of the non-reactors underwent abdominal surgery (gastrectomy, cholecystectomy, hysterectomy, appendectomy) and one had a thoracotomy. The other six non-reactors had the following operations: prostatectomy, sympathectomy, herniorrhaphy, arthroplasty and spinal fusion. The easier postoperative course of the reactor group, which is evident in the decreased frequency and increased efficacy of medications and in the subjective reports of the nurses and the patients themselves (vide infra), thus cannot be attributed to obvious major differences in surgery or anesthesia. It should be noted that in no instance can the surgery in the reactor group be described as "minor."

While the two groups of patients could not be differentiated by the examiners on the basis of superficial observation or intelligence as measured by the vocabulary subtest of the Wechsler-Bellevue scale, the data from the interviews and the Rorschach testing revealed definite and consistent personality differences between the two groups.[B]

Table 10.3 presents the pertinent interview material. For all data dealing with discrete variables, Fisher's exact test of independence for contingency tables was used. When continuous variables were involved, "Student's" t-test was employed. Several aspects of these data deserve comment. It appears that the placebo reactors found the discomfort and pain of the postoperative period less severe than the non-reactors did. From an objective standpoint, the nurses reported that fewer of the reactors seemed to have severe pain. These statements by the reactors and nurses are thus in accord with each other and with the objective data described above. The reactors all considered the hospital care "wonderful," whereas only four of the sixteen non-reactors felt this way. The reactors tended to ask less frequently for medications and to be more cooperative with the nursing staff. The female reactors, judging from their case histories, tended to have more menstrual pain (and to take medications for such pain). The reactors also tended to have more somatic symptoms ("nervous stomach," diarrhea, headache) during periods of stress. In regard to use of drugs there was a definitely greater use of cathartics in the reactor group, and a tendency to use more medications of the "aspirin" type. In the testing situation the reactors tended to be more emotionally expressive, and there was more tendency to speak freely, most frequently of themselves and their problems. In answer to the question, "What sort of people do you like best?" reactors were more likely to respond with, "Oh, I like everyone." The placebo reactors were more frequently active church-goers than the non-reactors and had less formal education.

Table 10.3 also summarizes the Rorschach data for the two groups. While for many of the individual categories the groups differ significantly, this is of less importance than the total pattern of "signs," which is more easily interpretable and of greater practical significance. Thus, the responses have been grouped to discover the largest combination that adequately differentiates the two groups. We find that six signs are common to 60 per cent of the reactor group while none of the non-reactors is so characterized, only one non-reactor having as many as four signs. The six signs[C] are: (1) more than one "insides" response; (2) $\Sigma C > M$; (3) A % below 50%; (4) CF > FC; (5) more than two "anxiety" responses; and (6) less than two "hostility" responses.

Submitting the differential distribution of the reactors and non-reactors who have all six signs to Fisher's exact test yields a $p < .01$. A test of the distribution of our groups based on any four of the six signs also gives a $p < .01$. In contrast to the non-reactors the reactors were more productive of responses, more anxious, more self-centered and preoccupied with internal bodily processes, and more emotionally labile. They are individuals who seem more dependent on outside stimulation than on their own mental processes. These processes tend to be less mature than in the case of the non-reactors. The reactors are in general individuals whose instinctual needs are greater and whose control over the social expression of these needs is less strongly defined and developed than in the non-reactors. While more anxious and dependent, the fact that they are also more labile and outwardly oriented may enable them to relieve this anxiety and tension more easily than the non-reactors. Over a period of time they may appear less anxious by reason of their ability to, as it were, "drain off the tension." The finding in the interviews of more "talkers" in the reactor group is probably the expression of one such mechanism.

The most striking Rorschach record characteristic of the reactors is the great frequency of responses dealing with the abdominal and pelvic viscera. The high incidence of these responses and their extremely poor form level would be considered definitely pathologic were it not that a certain amount of preoccupation with one's bodily processes may be expected in a hospital setting.[12] Our reactor group, however, produced many more such responses than the non-reactors.

We find that the non-reactors as a group do not by contrast present a "normal" picture. While showing less deviation from the normal than the reactors, they are far more rigid and emotionally controlled than the "average" for their age and background. Since the pressures and tensions of the hospital situation presumably accentuate the protective and defensive mechanisms of the personality, the rigidity of the non-reactors may well be an expression of their defense mechanism in a stressful situation.

Comment

An impairment of ability to discriminate between active drugs and inert substances is implicit in the phrase "the placebo reactor." It is obvious that a population composed exclusively of such individuals would be unsatisfactory for the

Table 10.3.
Psychologic data*

Interview Material			
	Percentage of Patients Giving Response		p
	Reactors (11) %	Non-reactors (16) %	
Postoperative pain minimized by patient	72	19	.01–.02
Seemed to have severe pain (nurses)	9	50	.02–.05
Asked for medication frequently (nurses)	27	62	>.10
Cooperative (nurses)	81	50	>.10
Concerned about self (nurses)	36	19	>.10
Likes "everyone"	54	12	.02–.05
Hospital care "wonderful"	100	25	.001–.01
Somatic symptoms under stress	66	25	.05–.10
"Bad" menstrual pain	71 (N=7)	25 (N=8)	>.10
Uses medication for menstrual pain	71 (N=7)	25 (N=8)	>.10
Frequency of drug use:			
"Aspirin" (and related drugs)	45	12	>.10
Sedatives	9	6	>.10
Cathartics	54	6	.001–.01
Behavior during interview:			
Apprehensive	45	44	>.10
Weepy	36	6	>.10
"Talkers"	54	6	.001–.01
Years of education	8.73	10.57	.02–.05
Regular church-goers, interested in church affairs	100	44	.001–.01
Rorschach "Signs"*			
No. of responses (median)	13.5	7.0	
No. of responses (average)	13.5	10.1	.05–.10
No. of "anxiety" responses (average)	4.8	1.7	<.05
No. of "hostility" responses (average)	0.9	1.9	>.10
F per cent (average)	41.6	64.0	<.001
F + per cent (average)	51.3	90.7	<.001
No color responses	30	63	>.10
CF > FC	80	27	.02–.05
ΣC > M	70	18	.02–.05
A per cent	40.8	75.1	<.01
FM > M	90	45	.06
Per cent giving "insides" responses	80	18	<.001
Number of "insides" responses (average)	3.5	0.27	<.01
Intelligence Quotient			
Average	109.3	110.7	—

Note: * For definition of symbols, see [endnote [C]—eds.].

evaluation of certain kinds of drugs. Experimental populations probably vary considerably in the number and degree of placebo responses exhibited. For example, 60 per cent of the 199 subjects with chronic headache studied by Jellinek[6] received relief from a placebo on one or more occasions, whereas only 30 to 40 per cent of postoperative patients studied in this laboratory obtain relief of pain from an injection of saline. The uniformity of response is also greater in Jellinek's data since 69 per cent of a special group of 121 subjects each receiving five placebo doses gave consistent responses (either positive or negative), whereas only 45 per cent of the group reported in this paper (considering those who received at least two placebo doses) gave consistent responses. Because the present patients had fewer placebo doses on the average, they should have been more consistent than Jellinek's, whereas in fact they were less so.[D]

Jellinek thus had a U-shaped distribution for his frequency of relief, with a piling up of consistent never-relieved or always-relieved patients. Our distribution looks like most frequency distributions with a mode in the middle. This makes it more difficult for us to divide our patient group into placebo reactors and placebo non-reactors.

The importance of the placebo effect is demonstrated by the work of Jellinek[6] and Beecher et al.[7] The former author was able to differentiate between three active agents and lactose without classifying his patients into reactors and non-reactors. Inter-drug differences, however, were revealed only by separate analysis of the responses of the non-reactor group. Beecher et al. were able, under the conditions of their study, to show that oral "aspirin" was superior to a placebo, whereas oral morphine and codeine were not. The comparison of "aspirin" and the two narcotic agents by standard technics revealed "aspirin" to be superior at only a 0.06 level, whereas separate analysis of the non-reactor data showed significance at a 0.028 level. Thus, in both studies a sharpening of focus was accomplished by elimination of the placebo reactor data. The reactors in Jellinek's study obtained a fairly constant relief rate from all three drugs (82 to 87 per cent), which, taken in conjunction with the "success rate" for all placebo administrations in this group (86 per cent), points up the striking lack of discriminatory ability of his subjects. The 58 per cent relief obtained with both "aspirin" and morphine-codeine in the reactor groups of Beecher et al. is probably also merely a reflection of the mean "success rate" of repeated placebo doses in the reactor population studied by these authors, since the figure for the placebo reactor group of roughly similar subjects described in the present report is 67 per cent. The higher success rate (79 and 78 per cent) of morphine in the reactor group in both phases of the current study suggests that within this group the lack of power to discriminate between drugs is relative rather than absolute, at least when an analgesic of the potency of morphine is being compared with a placebo.

There are two other factors which might conceivably contribute to the difference in performance of morphine in the reactor and non-reactor groups. One is suggested by the apparent relationship of pain severity to placebo reactivity. It is possible that (despite the stratification attempted in Table 10.1) the non-reactor group had on the average more severe pain than the reactor group. In such a situation morphine would be expected to be somewhat less effective in the non-reactors. The other factor is the possible existence of "negative reactors," i.e., people who are psychologically predisposed to resist relief from drugs. Such traits are probably present in some of those individuals in clinical studies who "get worse" while on a placebo. There were a number of patients studied in phase II who failed to obtain relief from anything administered to them. It is possible that some of these people had pain of such great severity, or decreased sensitivity to morphine of such magnitude, as to preclude relief from the doses of morphine employed. However, the possibility must also be entertained that some of them may have been so psychologically oriented as to be unable to discriminate between the active and the inactive agents. Either or both of the factors mentioned would tend to diminish the contribution of placebo reactivity to the observed differences in morphine relief.

It is thus apparent that an awareness of this general methodological problem is important for investigators concerned with the evaluation of drug effects. It must be appreciated that the placebo effect can be one of the reasons for failure to recognize a useful drug in a therapeutic trial, as pointed out originally by Jellinek.[6] The application of available technics for dissecting out this effect presupposes an awareness of its existence and importance. In preliminary investigations on a population which is to serve as a source of material for drug trials, it is desirable that an evaluation be made of the magnitude of the placebo response likely to be encountered. Such data may be helpful in deciding how much attention is to be devoted to the phenomenon. It appears reasonable to assume that the higher the incidence of placebo responses, the greater the dilution of the desired data, and the more important the screening of subjects. (In the studies of Jellinek and Beecher et al. it is obvious that for some situations standard controls are quite adequate for demonstrating differences.) The employment of single doses of placebo to "label" subjects as "reactors" or "non-reactors" is at best only a partial solution to the problem. Our data on consistency of response show that persons who fail to respond initially to a placebo may get satisfactory relief from a subsequent dose, so that for increasing the accuracy of classification of subjects multiple placebo responses should be observed.

There are a number of arguments which may be raised against the routine inclusion of multiple placebo doses in an experimental design. From an ethical standpoint it is difficult to rationalize such a procedure when a standard agent of known potency is available to serve as a yardstick of performance. A further consideration regarding the use of placebos is that if one is studying a drug which turns out to be inactive, patients will be lacking effective treatment for a large proportion of the time. Such a situation may be deleterious to the patient and will certainly arouse antagonism and promote a spirit of uncooperativeness among hospital resident and nursing staffs. In a situation such as postoperative pain, where there is a limit on the amount of time available for accumulating data, inclusion of multiple placebo doses will also prolong the duration and increase the expense of the study.

One possible solution to these problems is suggested by our data on the relationship of placebo response to number of doses required in the postoperative period. If this relationship is real, and it seems to be, it might be of advantage to compare the performance of two agents in the patients who get few doses and in those who get many doses. If the data of the latter group are less diluted with placebo responses, it might serve to sharpen the focus sufficiently to bring out differences not evident in the pooled data.

Despite the common recognition of the frequency of placebo reactions there has been no detailed study of the psychologic aspects of the problem and no previous attempt to investigate the distinguishing personality characteristics of the placebo reactor. One possible explanation for this may lie in the confidence of many physicians and nurses in their ability to pick out "the reactor type" with ease. Part of this lack of interest in the placebo reactor may also be due to the general reluctance to accept the pain that is relieved by a placebo as "real" and the temptation to consider relief from a placebo as proof of the "imaginary" nature of the complaint. That the incidence of placebo relief may bear a relation to the psychologic components of the illness seems reasonable. On the other hand, relief by an analgesic need not prove the "non-psychologic" nature of the pain. One portion of the pain experience, sometimes described as "reaction to pain," is that elaboration, including anxiety and fear, provided at the cortical level. It is not possible at present to say how much of the analgesic action of various drugs is due to an effect at this level.

Our psychologic studies were oriented around two main questions: (1) Is the placebo reactor a recognizable type of person? (2) What are the outstanding psychologic characteristics of the reactor?

The Rorschach and interview data indicate that consistent reactors and non-reactors possess certain different psychologic characteristics. Thus, the reactor is a recognizable type but only in the sense that intensive interview and psychologic testing can differentiate him from a non-reactor. Off-the-cuff impressions by the interviewers as to which patients were reactors were more often wrong than right. The reactors, e.g., were not "whiners" or "nuisances," not typically male or female, young or old, and had the same average intelligence as the non-reactors.

The reported data suggest that, should it be desirable to exclude consistent reactors from a study, this might be accomplished in advance by excluding those patients who showed a preponderance of the Rorschach signs noted above under "Results." Because of our focus on the consistent reactor and non-reactor, we should not necessarily expect by these signs to identify the occasional reactor, since it is likely that the personality factors predisposing to placebo relief are present to varying degree in different people.

Considered in the light of defensive patterns to stress the Rorschach differences may contribute to our understanding of the individual's reaction to pain and medication. It may be postulated, for example, that in the stressful postoperative situation placebo reactors behave in immature, dependent, and yet more outwardly responsive fashion, and thus receive considerable relief of pain through comfort received from attentive nursing care and from their confidence in the effectiveness of drugs. On the other hand, the non-reactors, withdrawn and rigidly clinging to critical intellectual processes, are less comforted by the care received and evidently more critical of drug effects.

It is theoretically possible that the Rorschach pattern obtained in the convalescent period and the placebo responses exhibited in the immediate postoperative period are not reflections of the basic personality type but are both determined in some way by the severity of the postoperative course. This seems unlikely, since it would necessitate the postulation of major modifications of the basic personality pattern by the hospital experience. In addition, there is evidence in the interview data of differences in attitudes and habits of reactors and non-reactors antedating surgery. Another possibility is that the severity of the subjective postoperative course and the placebo responses are both predetermined by the basic neuropsychiatric structure of the patient. Consistent with this hypothesis is the failure to find sufficient explanation in the anesthesia and surgery for differences in the severity of course of the two groups. There is certainly considerable variability possible, however, in the amount of operative trauma in patients undergoing the same operation, and it is not difficult to visualize differences in the intensity of pain stimuli being presented to the higher centers of the various individuals. Nor is there a necessary correlation between type of course and placebo response, since even in patients having an "easy" postoperative course (in that only a few medications were required for pain) there were many who did not get relief from a placebo. Also, an occasional patient receiving six or more doses of medication postoperatively did receive consistent relief from placebos.

Part of the explanation for the complaints of the phase II non-reactors about their hospital course is certainly due to the failure to obtain consistent relief from alternate medications (i.e., the placebo doses) since this is inherent in their selection as non-reactors. That they received more morphine doses and more total medications than the reactors might possibly be due in part to a "reinforcement" of painful stimuli by reason of failure to relieve pain early and consistently. On the other hand, the reactors in the special group studied had almost complete relief of pain from all medications and were thus in an optimal position to benefit from any such effect.

The considerable number of inconsistent reactors suggests the operation of multiple factors in determining the placebo response, since it is not likely that the basic personality was altering rapidly in such individuals. In addition to chance factors, one parameter which we know is changing rapidly is that of severity of pain, since even severe, steady postoperative wound pain usually disappears in two or three days. Another possible factor contributing to the inconsistency of the placebo response is the development of what might be called "pharmacologic sophistication," i.e., learning to distinguish between placebo and morphine after repeated alternate exposure to both agents. In other work in this laboratory we have observed a tendency for subjects to exhibit less frequent and less marked placebo responses after they have experienced definite effects from a potent drug.

A reasonable working hypothesis based on our data is the following: There is a certain psychologic set which predisposes to anticipation of pain relief and thus to a positive placebo response. The presence of the traits making this set is probably not an all-or-none phenomenon but rather a graded one. Other factors (such as severity of pain) also affect the response to inert agents, and the resultant of these factors, psychologic and non-psychologic, known and unknown, determines whether or not a particular dose of placebo produces an effect in a given patient.

Summary

1. A group of 162 postoperative patients was observed for the ability of such patients to receive significant relief of pain from subcutaneous injections of placebo and of morphine.

2. There was a significantly higher incidence of relief from morphine in the placebo reactors than in the non-reactors.

3. Morphine and placebo are less effective analgesics in patients with persistent pain than in those with pain of short duration.

4. Less than half of the patients who received multiple doses of a placebo responded consistently to the placebo.

5. There was no sex difference and no difference in intelligence between reactors and non-reactors.

6. Significant differences in attitudes, habits, educational background and personality structure were demonstrated between consistent reactors and non-reactors.

7. The complexities of placebo controls in clinical trials are discussed and suggestions made for dealing with this important methodological problem.

8. A hypothesis to explain the placebo response is postulated.

REFERENCES

1. Pepper, O.H.P. A note on the placebo. Tr. & Stud., Coll. Physicians, Philadelphia, 13: 81, 1945.

2. Conferences on Therapy. The use of placebos in therapy. New York State J. Med., 46: 1718, 1946.

3. Wolf, S. Effects of suggestion and conditioning on the action of chemical agents in human subjects—the pharmacology of placebos. J. Clin. Investigation, 29: 100, 1950.

4. Beecher, H.K. Experimental pharmacology and measurement of the subjective response. Science, 116: 157, 1952.

5. Wolf, S. and Pinsky, R. Toxic effects following placebo administration. J. Clin. Investigation, 32: 613, 1953.

6. Jellinek, E.M. Clinical tests on comparative effectiveness of analgesic drugs. Biometrics Bull., 2: 87, 1946.

7. Beecher, H.K., Keats, A.S., Mosteller, F. and Lasagna, L. The effectiveness of oral analgesics (morphine, codeine, acetylsalicylic acid) and the problem of placebo "reactors" and "non-reactors." J. Pharmacol. & Exper. Therap., 109: 393, 1953.

8. Beecher, H.K. A method for quantifying the intensity of pain. Science, 118: 322, 1953.

9. Klopfer, B. and Kelley, D.M. The Rorschach Technique. Yonkers-on-Hudson, 1946. World Book Co.

10. Beck, S.J. Rorschach's Test. I. Basic Processes. New York, 1949. Grune and Stratton.

11. Elizur, A. Content analysis of the Rorschach with regard to anxiety and hostility. Rorschach Research Exchange and J. Projective Techniques, 13: 247, 1949.

12. Klatskin, E. An analysis of the effect of the test situation upon the Rorschach record: formal scoring characteristics. J. Projective Techniques, 16: 193, 1952.

[A]. "Morphine" will be used throughout this paper to indicate this salt.

[B]. The thematic apperception test protocols were too brief to warrant a standard thematic analysis.

[C]. Rorschach scoring and interpretation used here is standard procedure based primarily on Klopfer and Kelley.[9] Scoring is in terms of determinants of the response: form (F), movement, human and animal (M and FM), color (C), more or less integrated with form (FC, CF), and content of the responses—animals (A), objects, anatomy, etc. F + per cent is the percentage of form-determined responses

occurring with great frequency in an "average" group.[10] The "insides" category used here is our own designation for responses related to the internal anatomy, chosen because of the particular frequency of patient usage of the term for such responses. The "hostility" and "anxiety" categories are responses so classified because of fairly obvious content, according to Elizur.[11] For another example of Rorschach analysis in a hospital population see Klatskin.[12]

[D]. Possible explanations for these differences between the groups include: the nature of the pain, the dose-to-dose variation in severity of the pain, and the personality make-up of the patients involved.

[Note: references [A]—[D] were originally in-text footnotes that we have converted to endnotes—eds.]

II

Chance Distribution and the Placebo "Reactor"

STEWART WOLF, CARL R. DOERING, MERVIN L. CLARK, AND JAMES A. HAGANS

Stewart Wolf, Carl R. Doering, Mervin L. Clark, and James A. Hagans, "Chance Distribution and the Placebo 'Reactor,'" Journal of Laboratory and Clinical Medicine 1957;49:837–841.

It has been proposed that experimental subjects may be separated according to their proclivity for reacting to placebo medication.[1–5] The present study was undertaken to test the consistency with which placebo responses occurred from individual to individual and in the same individual from time to time.

Methods

Data from an earlier study of agents tested for their ability to prevent ipecac-induced nausea and vomiting showed that none was more effective or more consistent in its effect than a placebo.[6] Since none of the agents showed evidence of pharmacodynamic activity, they were all regarded as placebos. The experimental group consisted of 21 volunteers who had consistently exhibited nausea upon the ingestion of ipecac alone on two separate occasions and 14 who had consistently exhibited vomiting. Each underwent 7 additional trials with ipecac preceded by oral administration of the above agents according to a double-blind systematized randomization technique. Both the subjects and the investigator were aware that an antiemetic effect was being sought. Following each of their 7 trials, a subject's failure to develop the anticipated nausea and/or vomiting was designated as a placebo response. Those who consistently displayed placebo responses or consistently failed to do so were called pure reactors or nonreactors, respectively; those who displayed placebo responses on exactly half the trials were called half-reactors; and those who had more placebo responses than nonresponses, but were not totally consistent, were termed impure reactors (or impure nonreactors, if they demonstrated more nonresponses than responses).

These data were particularly suitable for testing the concept of the placebo reactor because both a subjective response (nausea) and an objective response (vomiting) were observed. Accordingly, the distribution of complete "protection" against nausea in the 21 subjects and of complete "protection" against vomiting in the 14 subjects, as well as the distribution of partial "protection" against either nausea or vomiting, was recorded and compared to the theoretical distribution attributable to chance as derived from the binomial expansion equation. Further, the total of all placebo responses in the 35 subjects were compiled and compared again to the appropriate chance curve. Finally, the variation in the occurrence of placebo responses from time to time in the same individual was compared with that observed from person to person. Since the number of tests performed on each subject was 7, the subjects were divided into groups of 7, and each was analyzed from the standpoint of the variations described above.

Results

In Figs. 11.1 and 11.2, the interindividual and intraindividual variations in the incidence of placebo responses with respect to nausea are compared with the appropriate chance curve derived from the binomial expansion equation. Fig. 11.1 gives data for complete "protection" against nausea, and Fig. 11.2 gives data for partial "protection." It will be seen that the curves for variation in placebo response, both inter- and intraindividual, did not differ from each other or from chance. Figs. 11.3 and 11.4 illustrate, in the same manner, the data on complete and partial "protection" against vomiting. Again there is no significant difference between the observed results and chance. Fig. 11.5 shows the combined data compared to its binomial expansion curve and again there are no significant differences. In each instance, the data were subjected to chi-square analysis by which the lack of any significant differences was established mathematically.

The next question involved an attempt to establish whether or not the occurrence of a placebo reaction had predictive value with respect to the likelihood of that individual displaying further placebo reactions in the future. The incidence of placebo reactors and nonreactors, pure and impure, and half-reactors on the basis of the first test alone, the first 2 tests, and so on up to and including all 7 tests, is illustrated in Fig. 11.6. There was essentially a 50:50 distribution of reactors and nonreactors when an odd number of tests were analyzed and a 33:33:33 distribution of reactors, nonreactors, and half-reactors when an even number of tests were analyzed. The pure placebo reactor virtually disappeared from the group after the sixth successive test. The observed variations are well within the range of chance, and none differed significantly from the theoretical expected values (Fisher's Exact Method of analysis).

It was not possible on the basis of 1, 2, 3, 4, 5, or 6 tests to predict whether or not an individual would display a placebo response on subsequent testing (Fig. 11.7). Further, the pure reactors, even when defined on the basis of 5 previous successive placebo tests, showed no greater incidence of subsequent positive responses than when defined on the basis of 1, 2, 3, or 4 previous tests (Fig. 11.8).

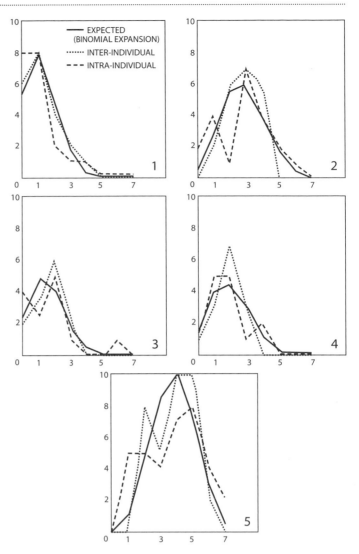

Figs. 11.1 to 11.5. All figures represent the interindividual and the intraindividual variation in response to a placebo compared to the theoretical variation due to chance as derived from the binomial expansion equation. The abscissa represents the number of placebo responses possible in 7 trials on different subjects (for interindividual) and in 7 trials on the same subject (for intraindividual). The ordinate indicates the number of occasions on which the placebo responses were observed among the groups in each category. Fig. 11.1 (top left) represents the data for complete "protection" against nausea and Fig. 11.2 (top right) represents the data for partial "protection" (21 subjects, each with 7 successive placebo tests). Fig. 11.3 (middle left) represents the data for complete "protection" against vomiting and Fig. 11.4 (middle right) the data for partial "protection" (14 subjects, each with 7 successive placebo tests). Fig. 11.5 (bottom) represents the combined data for both complete and partial "protection" against both nausea and vomiting (35 subjects, 7 successive placebo tests each).

The incidence of reactors, nonreactors, and half-reactors was examined on the basis of the first test compared to the last test, the first 2 tests compared to the last 2 tests, and then the first 3 tests compared to the last 3 tests (Table 11.1). The individual consistency was also examined for each of these groups, comparing the first to the last tests as above. No significant differences occurred and the consistency of re-

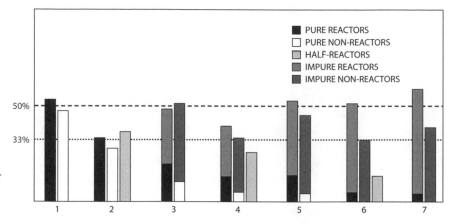

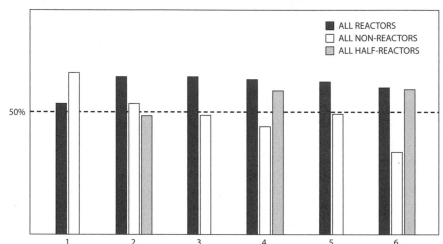

Fig. 11.6. The incidence of reactors and nonreactors, pure and impure, and of half-reactors on the basis of 1, 2, 3, 4, 5, 6, and 7 successive placebo tests.

Fig. 11.7. The incidence of subsequent placebo responses in the reactor, nonreactor, and half-reactor groups as defined on the basis of 1, 2, 3, 4, 5, or 6 successive placebo tests.

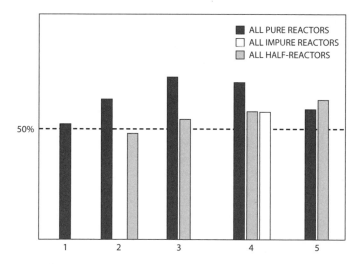

Fig. 11.8. The incidence of subsequent placebo responses in the pure reactor, impure reactor, and half-reactor groups as defined on the basis of 1, 2, 3, 4, and 5 subsequent placebo tests.

Table 11.1.

	First Test Compared to Last Test			
	Reactors	Nonreactors	Half-Reactors	Consistent Response
First	19 (54%)	16 (46%)	0	18 (51%)
Last	18 (51%)	17 (49%)	0	

	First Two Tests Compared to Last Two Tests			
	Reactors	Nonreactors	Half-Reactors	Consistent Response
First 2	12 (34%)	10 (29%)	13 (37%)	11 (31%)
Last 2	15 (43%)	10 (29%)	10 (29%)	

	First Three Tests Compared to Last Three Tests			
	Reactors	Nonreactors	Half-Reactors	Consistent Response
First 3	17 (49%)	18 (51%)	0	20 (57%)
Last 3	22 (63%)	13 (37%)	0	

sponses was nowhere greater than would be expected to occur by chance.

Summary

These data do not support the concept that either a placebo reactor or a nonreactor really exists as a separate or distinct entity in an experiment measuring an objective phenomenon (vomiting) and a subjective phenomenon (nausea) or even with respect to the potentially more highly suggestible partial relief of nausea and/or vomiting. Since the intraindividual variation in response to a placebo was found to be as great as the interindividual variation, the likelihood of predicting placebo responses was not enhanced by increasing the number of placebo tests performed on any individual.

REFERENCES

1. Jellinek, E.M.: Clinical Tests on Comparative Effectiveness of Analgesic Drugs, Biometrics **2**: 87, 1946.
2. Beecher, H.K.: Clinical Studies of Analgesic Drugs. I. Experimental Pharmacology and Measurement of the Subjective Response, Biometrics **8**: 218, 1952.
3. Mosteller, F.: Clinical Studies of Analgesic Drugs. II. Some Statistical Problems in Measuring the Subjective Response to Drugs, Biometrics **8**: 220, 1952.
4. Lasagna, L., Mosteller, F., von Felsinger, J.M., Beecher, H.K.: A Study of the Placebo Response, Am. J. Med. **16**: 770, 1954.
5. Beecher, H.K., Keats, A.S., Mosteller, F., and Lasagna, L.: The Effectiveness of Oral Analgesics (Morphine, Codeine, Acetylsalicylic Acid) and the Problem of Placebo "Reactors" and "Non-Reactors," J. Pharmacol. and Exper. Therap. **109**: 393, 1953.
6. Hagans, J.A., Doering, C.R., Ashley, F., Clark, M.L., and Wolf, S.: The Therapeutic Experiment: Observations on the Meaning of Controls and on Biologic Variation Resulting from the Treatment Situation, J. Lab. and Clin. Med. **49**: 282, 1957.

12

Placebo Effect in the Rat

RICHARD J. HERRNSTEIN

Richard J. Herrnstein, "Placebo Effect in the Rat," *Science* 1962;138:677–678.

A human patient may react strongly to a drug that is pharmacologically inert. Such reactions, called placebo effects, figure prominently in both therapy and research. Each generation of medical practitioners acknowledges the power of the placebo by rejecting as inert (or worse!) many of the chemical agents believed in by its predecessors. The placebo effect is usually attributed to some kind of "suggestion" that operates, even if temporarily, to fulfill the patient's expectations about a treatment. Viewed as suggestion, the placebo effect derives from the human capacity to react to symbols. The physician, the hypodermic syringe or the tablet, the verbal interchange with the patient—all symbolic of a therapeutic effect—may produce a result that would otherwise have required some specific chemical agent.

The placebo effect can, however, be viewed in a different way. The elicitation of a specific reaction by arbitrary agents, such as the abatement of a symptom after the mere sight of a physician and his medicines, may be nothing more than simple conditioning of the sort originally demonstrated by Pavlov with animals. Pavlov showed that one stimulus may come to elicit responses ordinarily appropriate to a second stimulus after the two stimuli are presented together. Viewed as conditioning, the placebo effect is merely a particular instance of a phylogenetically widespread behavioral phenomenon, and not a manifestation of man's special symbolic capacities. Since we are disposed to speak of nonverbal animals as conditionable rather than suggestible, it may be with animals that the two views are most profitably tested.

Pavlov and others (1) have reported the conditioning of some of the effects of morphine on animals. Vomiting and sleep are often caused by morphine, and these reactions sometimes occur while the experimenter is preparing an experienced animal for an injection. Presumably, events associated with the administration of morphine become the conditioned stimuli for some of the reactions that are characteristically induced by the drug. The parallel to the placebo effect is clear, but past research has been restricted to morphine, and there have not been enough controls to exclude other interpretations.

The present experiment (2) is an attempt to obtain a placebo effect simulating the known effect of scopolamine on the learned behavior of rats (3). A rat was placed daily in a chamber that was insulated for light and sound and contained a lever and a feeding device. The rat was hungry and was trained to depress the lever by reinforcement with sweetened condensed milk. After initial training, it was arranged to have the operation of the lever produce milk intermittently according to the following schedule, which constitutes one cycle: (i) 5 minutes: chamber illuminated; no reinforcement; (ii) 2 minutes or less: chamber illuminated; terminated by first response, which is reinforced with 0.3 ml of milk, or, if no response, no reinforcement, and period terminated after 2 minutes; (iii) 5 minutes: chamber dark; no reinforcement; an occasional intraperitoneal injection during this period, after eighth or ninth cycle.

This cycle was repeated 13 or 14 times every day, and preliminary experimentation continued for 4 months to accommodate the rat to this intermittent schedule of reinforcement and also to the accompanying injections of small quantities of physiological saline into the peritoneal cavity. These injections were made at the end of the eighth or ninth cycle during the first 30 seconds of the period of darkness, after which the session continued for five more cycles.

By the end of this preliminary period of four months, the schedule of reinforcement had established a characteristic pattern of responding, one whose primary feature is that at the beginning of each cycle there is little or no pressing of the lever, whereas, as the time for reinforcement approaches, the rate of lever-pressing increases continuously but quite gradually. The effect of scopolamine on this behavior is to depress the overall frequency of response and to abolish the orderly progression of rates (3). At this time, there was no detectable effect on behavior of the saline administrations.

The scopolamine hydrobromide was administered intraperitoneally 14 times in dosages of 1 mg/kg. Its injection was, like the saline, given at the end of the eighth or ninth cycle and was always followed by five more cycles. These injections were spread over 3 months of daily experimental sessions and were interspersed among an equal number of injections of physiological saline. The two kinds of injections differed in volume by less than 0.03 ml, and they followed each other in an irregular order.

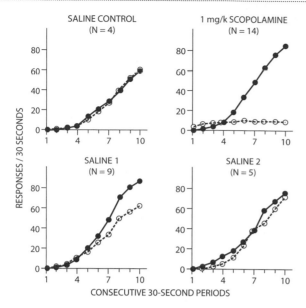

Fig. 12.1. Rates of lever-pressing during the 5-minute period prior to reinforcement. The filled circles (●) plot average rates during the eight or nine preinjection periods; the open circles (○), those during the five postinjection periods. The curves labeled "saline control" were obtained before any administrations of scopolamine. Those labeled "saline 1" show the average effect of a saline injection that followed a scopolamine injection. Those labeled "saline 2" show the average effect following a saline injection. N refers to the number of injections contributing to these average curves.

The major findings of this experiment are summarized in Fig. 12.1 with data from a single rat. Entirely analogous results were obtained from a second rat with an earlier version of the present procedure. The abscissa in Fig. 12.1 covers the 5-minute interval prior to the priming of the apparatus for reinforcement, and is broken down into ten consecutive 30-second periods. The ordinate plots the mean rates of responding during these 30-second periods. The increasing rate of responding that typifies behavior on this schedule of reinforcement results in increasing monotonic curves. The curves drawn through filled circles show the preinjection rates; those through open circles, the postinjection rates. Each pair of curves is an average of the data from the indicated number of sessions. The saline-control curves, being for four sessions prior to any administration of scopolamine, demonstrate that saline causes no disruption. The scopolamine curve shows the typical effect of this drug. In it, responding is depressed, having lost the increasing monotonic pattern normal for this schedule of reinforcement. The curves labeled "saline 1" are for the sessions in which saline was administered after a prior injection of scopolamine,

whereas the curves labeled "saline 2" are from sessions with saline when the prior injection had been saline.

The curves show that when saline is administered after scopolamine (saline 1), there is considerable depression of responding, whereas with two consecutive administrations of saline (saline 2) this effect is diminished, although not quite obliterated (4). Such a depression of responding by saline may reasonably be termed a placebo effect. This placebo effect does not involve a loss of the monotonic increase in rate during the 5-minute interval. The characteristics of the depression and the manner in which it was brought about suggest, moreover, that it is an example of Pavlovian conditioning. It seems probable that the conditioned stimulus includes the injection of a hypodermic needle into the peritoneal cavity, for mere handling of the animal in several "mock" injections did not result in any noticeable change in responding. The effectiveness of this conditioned stimulus disappeared rapidly (see saline 2 in Fig. 12.1). In the parlance of classical conditioning, it would be said that extinction of the conditioned response (that is, the depression of responding) was rapid. Conditioning itself appears also to have been rapid in this situation, for the depression of responding by saline was evident after the first administration of scopolamine. Finally, it may be said, further analysis of the data showed that saline depressed responding more after two consecutive scopolamine injections than it did after just one.

It appears, then, that an injection of saline can come to depress the responding of a rat that is occasionally given scopolamine, which is a genuinely suppressive drug. This placebo effect is based on the animal's experience and can be eliminated by withholding the drug, in conformity with the traditional paradigm of simple Pavlovian conditioning. There appears to be no reason to suppose that the placebo effect in human patients differs in any way from that demonstrated here, other than in degree of complexity.

REFERENCES AND NOTES

1. I.P. Pavlov, *Conditioned Reflexes* (Oxford Univ. Press, London, 1927), pp. 35ff.; K.H. Collins and A.L. Tatum, Am. J. Physiol. **74**, 14 (1925); N. Kleitman and G. Crisler, Am. J. Physiol. **79**, 571 (1927).
2. Supported by grants from the National Science Foundation and by a gift from the Ciba Pharmaceutical Co., Inc., to Harvard University.
3. R.J. Herrnstein, J. Exptl. Anal. Behavior **1**, 351 (1958).
4. For the saline-control injections, the average rate of responding was higher during the postinjection than during the preinjection periods in three of the four cases. For the curves "saline 1" (Fig. 12.1), the postinjection rates were lower than the preinjection rates in all nine cases. For the curves "saline 2," the postinjection rates were lower in four of the five cases. By the sign test for matched pairs (based on the binomial theorem), the results for "saline 1" alone achieve statistical significance (1-percent level of confidence).

13

Reduction of Postoperative Pain by Encouragement and Instruction of Patients

A Study of Doctor-Patient Rapport

LAWRENCE D. EGBERT, GEORGE E. BATTIT, CLAUDE E. WELCH, AND MARSHALL K. BARTLETT

Lawrence D. Egbert, George E. Battit, Claude E. Welch, and Marshall K. Bartlett, "Reduction of Postoperative Pain by Encouragement and Instruction of Patients: A Study of Doctor-Patient Rapport," *New England Journal of Medicine* 1964;270:825–827.

Many reports have discussed the treatment of patients suffering after operation. Narcotics are not without danger; they also vary considerably in effectiveness. Hypnosis will reduce pain but is difficult to achieve and requires special training for the operator. Despite considerable effort the problems of treating postoperative pain remain.

Janis[1] has shown that patients who were told about their operations before the procedure remembered the operation and its sequelae more favorably than those who were not well informed. We have determined the effects of instruction, suggestion and encouragement upon the severity of postoperative pain.

Method

We studied 97 patients after elective intra-abdominal operations (Table 13.1). All patients were visited the night before operation by the anesthetist, who told them about the preparation for anesthesia, as well as the time and approximate duration of the operation, and warned them that they would wake up in the recovery room. Preanesthetic medication, consisting of pentobarbital sodium, 2 mg. per kilogram of body weight, and atropine, 0.6 mg., was administered intramuscularly approximately one hour before operation. Induction of anesthesia was accomplished with thiopental sodium; intubation of the trachea was performed on all patients. Anesthesia was maintained with ether and cyclopropane or nitrous oxide and curare.

The patients were divided into two groups by random order; 51 patients (control group) were not told about postoperative pain by the anesthetist. The "special-care" group consisted of 46 patients who were told about postoperative pain. They were informed where they would feel pain, how severe it would be and how long it would last and reassured that having pain was normal after abdominal operations. As soon as the patients appeared aware of the nature of the suffering that would begin on the following day, they were told what would be done about the pain. They were advised that pain is caused by spasm of the muscles under the incision and that they could relieve most of the pain themselves by relaxing these muscles. They could achieve relaxation by slowly taking a deep breath and consciously allowing the abdominal wall to relax. Also, they were shown the use of a trapeze that was hanging over the middle of the bed (control patients also had the trapeze but were not instructed by the anesthetist). Special-care patients were taught how to turn onto one side by using their arms and legs while relaxing their abdominal muscles. Finally, they were told that at first they would find it difficult to relax completely. If they could not achieve a reasonable level of comfort, they should request medication. The presentation was given in a manner of enthusiasm and confidence; the patients were not informed that we were conducting a study. The surgeons, not knowing which patients were receiving special care, continued their practices as usual.

After the operations, narcotics were ordered by the surgical residents; these were later administered by the ward nurses, who were also unaware that we were studying these patients. After the patients were discharged we tabulated the total dose of morphine in milligrams for the first five twenty-four-hour periods after the operation. When meperidine had been administered, we assumed 100 mg. of meperidine to be equal to 10 mg. of morphine (Lasagna and Beecher[2] indicated that "meperidine, in parenteral doses of 50 to 100 mg., was at least as good as 10 mg. of morphine in incidence and duration of pain relief"); 60 mg. of codeine was assumed to be nearly equal to 10 mg. of morphine.[2]

During the afternoon after operation (day zero) the anesthetist visited his patients receiving special care. He reiterated what he had taught the patients the night before and reassured them that the pain they were experiencing was normal; they were again told to request pain medication whenever they could not make themselves tolerably comfortable. The anesthetist listened to their breathing and encouraged them to

Table 13.1.
Types of operations and anesthetics*

Procedure	Control Group (No. of Patients)	Special-Care Group (No. of Patients)
Operation:		
Cholecystectomy	15	17
Hiatus hernia	4	1
Gastrectomy	9	8
Bowel resection	9	6
Colectomy	6	9
Hysterectomy	6	4
Ventral hernia	2	1
Totals	51	46
Anesthesia:		
Cyclopropane & ether	31	27
Nitrous oxide & curare	20	19

Note: *Differences not statistically significant.

take a deep breath and relax. All this was repeated on the morning after operation and once or twice a day until they had no further need of narcotics.

On the first and second postoperative days, 57 of the patients were visited by an anesthetist whom the patients had not met and who was not aware of the type of treatment being received. This independent observer attempted to record without bias the patients' evaluations about their pain as well as his own impressions from their appearance.

Comparisons of differences between the two groups were made with the use of the t test.

Results

Table 13.1 shows the types of operations done and the anesthetics given. The average age of the patients in the control group was fifty-two and two-tenths years; in the special-care group the average age of the patients was fifty-two years. There were 17 men in each group. Randomization in the selection of patients seems to have been satisfactory.

Figure 13.1 compares the narcotic requirements of the patients. On the day of operation the difference was not statistically significant. For the next five days, however, patients receiving special care requested less narcotics (p less than 0.01).

All the suggestions given the special-care patients favored a reduction in postoperative narcotics. Table 13.2 shows that these patients did not suffer through the postoperative course just to please the doctor. The independent observer recorded that the special-care patients appeared to be more comfortable and in better physical and emotional condition than the control group. This was emphasized by the surgeons, who, although unaware of the care each patient received, sent the special-care patients home an average of two and seven-tenths days earlier than the control group (p less than 0.01).

Discussion

Approximately 9 out of every 10 patients will respond at some time to placebo therapy for postoperative pain;[3] this type of

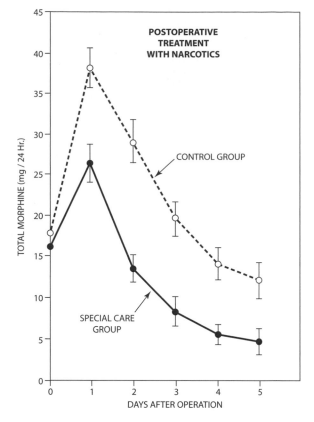

Figure 13.1. Postoperative treatment with narcotics (means for each day ± standard error of the mean).

emotional stress is readily modified by psychotherapy.[1,4,5] Placebo effect may be defined as one that is not attributable to a specific pharmacologic property of the treatment;[6] the effects of placebos are readily modified by suggestion[4,5] and depend upon the symbolic implications of the physician and his ministrations.[5] We believe that our discussions with patients have changed the meaning of the postoperative situation for these patients. By utilizing an active placebo action, we have been able to reduce their postoperative pain.

Others have shown that talking out anxieties and understanding the source of anxiety helps patients.[1] Our data demonstrate that anesthetists, untrained in hypnotism or formal psychiatry, may nevertheless have a very powerful effect on their patients. We have previously shown[7] that this reassurance (we call it "superficial psychotherapy") can be started during the preoperative visit; it should be continued into the postoperative period.

It should be pointed out that a great deal more work is involved in this practice of anesthesia than in the customary practice of anesthesia. We found that our methods of talking to patients changed during the study—for example, one of our early patients became hysterical during the discussion about postoperative pain, and we now know it is wise to build up the discussion slowly in patients who become too frightened. Nevertheless, retreating from the frightened pa-

Table 13.2.
Pain on the first and second days after operation (averages ± standard errors)

Postoperative Day	Severity of Pain*	
	Control Group (30 Patients)	Special-Care Group (27 Patients)
1st:		
Subjective report	1.768 ± 0.200	1.594 ± 0.205
Objective report	1.735 ± 0.191	1.187 ± 0.192[†]
2d:		
Subjective report	1.333 ± 0.188	0.966 ± 0.195
Objective report	1.333 ± 0.216	0.827 ± 0.172[‡]

* Pain graded as follows: severe, + + +; moderate, + +; mild, +; and almost none, 0.
[†] Difference statistically significant (p < 0.05).
[‡] Approaches significance (p < 0.1).

tient before operation exposes that patient to greater psychic stress during the postoperative period.[1] The patient who persistently avoids discussing these problems before he is operated on is a particularly troublesome patient later. Another error was of interest: one patient was seen before operation and anesthetized, and then the anesthetist went on vacation without notifying the patient or surgeon. Upon seeing the patient five days later, the anesthetist was greeted with great annoyance ("Where the hell have you been?") by the patient. To balance these errors, we found that almost none of the patients in the special-care group had the complaint, "Why didn't you tell me it was going to be like this?"—which was not uncommon in the control group. Each patient has his own personal psychologic makeup; each patient needs "special" treatment, tailored to meet his own particular psychologic needs.

The specialty of anesthesia has been criticized sharply as lacking in involvement with patient care and responsibility.[8] Our data show that an anesthetist is able to establish rapport with surgical patients and that a useful purpose is served by this contact. Since the sole purpose of the anesthetist in administering anesthesia is to reduce pain associated with operations, it appears reasonable for him to consider the whole job. The anesthetist who understands his patient and who believes that each patient is "his" patient ceases to be merely a clever technician in the operating room.

Summary and Conclusions

The effect of encouragement and education on 97 surgical patients was studied. "Special-care" patients were told what to expect during the postoperative period; they were then taught how to relax, how to take deep breaths and how to move so that they would remain more comfortable after operation. Comparing these patients with a control group of patients, we were able to reduce the postoperative narcotic requirements by half. Patients who were encouraged during the immediate postoperative period by their anesthetists were considered by their surgeons ready for discharge from the hospital two and seven-tenths days before the control patients. We believe that if an anesthetist considers himself a doctor who alleviates pain associated with operations, he must realize that only part of his work is in the operating rooms; the patients need ward care by their anesthetists as well.

REFERENCES

1. Janis, I.L. *Psychological Stress: Psychoanalytical and behavioral studies of surgical patients.* New York: Wiley, 1958.
2. Lasagna, L., and Beecher, H.K. Analgesic effectiveness of codeine and meperidine (Demerol). *J. Pharmacol. and Exper. Therap.* **112**: 306–311, 1954.
3. Houde, R.W., Wallenstein, S.L., and Rogers, A. Clinical pharmacology of analgesics. 1. Method of assaying analgesic effect. *Clin. Pharmacol. and Therap.* **1**: 163–174, 1960.
4. Keats, A.S. Postoperative pain: research and treatment. *J. Chronic Dis.* **4**: 72–83, 1956.
5. Modell, W., and Houde, R.W. Factors influencing clinical evaluation of drugs: with special reference to the double-blind technique. *J.A.M.A.* **167**: 2190–2199, 1958.
6. Wolf, S. Pharmacology of placebos. *Pharmacol. Rev.* **11**: 689–704, 1959.
7. Egbert, L.D., Battit, G.E., Turndorf, H., and Beecher, H.K. Value of preoperative visit by anesthetist: study of doctor-patient rapport. *J.A.M.A.* **185**: 553–555, 1963.
8. Dripps, R.D., et al. Special report to American Society of Anesthesiologists. *A.S.A. Newsletter*, August, 1963.

14

The Interaction of Psychologic Stimuli and Pharmacologic Agents on Airway Reactivity in Asthmatic Subjects

THOMAS J. LUPARELLO, NANCY LEIST, CARY H. LOURIE, AND PAULINE SWEET

Thomas J. Luparello, Nancy Leist, Cary H. Lourie, and Pauline Sweet, "The Interaction of Psychologic Stimuli and Pharmacologic Agents on Airway Reactivity in Asthmatic Subjects," *Psychosomatic Medicine* 1970;32:509–513.

It is a commonplace observation, especially in large emergency treatment centers, that the expectation of an asthmatic patient often plays an important role in that patient's response to treatment. House staff officers will joke about the dramatic recovery of a given asthmatic after an injection of sterile water, and patients will state spontaneously that at times they can begin to feel their chest "loosening up" as soon as the doctor walks into the room. Experimental evidence has supported the impression that psychologic stimuli, including expectation, can markedly influence airway reactivity (1–3). When given nebulized saline to inhale, but told that it was an allergen or irritant, nearly half the asthmatic subjects studied reacted with significant increases in airway resistance (1). These same subjects were able to reverse airway obstruction by inhaling the identical saline when it was presented as medicine to help the asthma. In a follow-up study (2), it was shown that subjects who reacted to a suggested allergen had a therapeutic response to placebo, but not to isoproterenol when they were told that the latter was an allergen. In contrast, asthmatics who did not react to sham allergen, responded with increased airway conductance to the inhalation of isoproterenol even though it was presented to them as an allergen or irritant. However, in that study, reactors were given isoproterenol during a time when they had marked airway obstruction, while nonreactors were given the drug at a time when airway conductance was normal. In addition, those previous studies were conducted single blind so that subtle, unintentional influences, reflecting the experimenter's expectation, may have contributed to the differences obtained.

The present study was conducted in an effort to better delineate the influence of expectation on the airway response of asthmatics to the inhalation of bronchoactive pharmacologic agents. In an effort to deal with some of the problems encountered in prior studies, all inhalations were given to subjects under double-blind conditions and at a time when baseline airway conductance levels were at or near normal.

Subjects

Twenty asthmatics, 13 females and 7 males, whose ages ranged from 16 to 56 years, were referred from the emergency service of a large county hospital. The diagnosis of asthma was based on a characteristic history of episodic attacks of reversible airway obstruction and an absence of irreversible mechanical defects within the lungs. In all instances, the diagnosis was clinically confirmed by the referring source. These subjects had not been used in previous experiments.

Methods

The bronchodilator used was an isoproterenol aerosol, packaged as the hydrochloride, in a standard 15-ml vial with a nebulizer and metered valve designed to deliver a measured dose of approximately 125 μg isoproterenol in mist form. Inert propellants, aromatic flavors, 33% ethyl alcohol (as solvent) and 0.1% ascorbic acid as preservative were also contained in the vial. The bronchoconstrictor was 0.1% carbachol, packaged with the same components and in the same manner as the isoproterenol with the metered valve delivering approximately 50 μg carbachol/dose.

All aerosol containers were covered and coded so that only one experimenter was aware of the contents of each vial. Using a random table, this experimenter assigned the coded containers and informed the second experimenter as to which instructions the subject was to receive. The second experimenter gave instructions to the subject and operated the plethysmograph, unaware of which substance the subject was inhaling. At each session, the subject inhaled a single self-administered dose of whichever material was presented to him.

The subject was told that he would be inhaling one of two substances: one, a bronchodilator which would open up his airways and make it easier to breathe; the other, a bronchoconstrictor which would tighten up the airways and make it more difficult to breathe. The rationale presented to the subject was that by studying the manner in which his airways reacted to these substances, more information could be gained about his asthma and this in turn might lead to more effective treatment.

Each subject was tested four times with at least 24 hr between sessions. At each session, baseline measures of airway resistance (Ra) and thoracic gas volume (TGV) were obtained by means of a Collins body plethysmograph. Ra and TGV were calculated as the mean of five successive measures of each variable. Resistance was converted to its reciprocal or conductance (Ga) and was expressed as a conductance-thoracic gas volume ratio (Ga/TGV) in order to correct for variation in lung volume during testing (4). More specifically, after baseline data were obtained at each test session, one of the following four conditions was met: (1) The subject was told he would be inhaling a bronchodilator[A] and was actually given a bronchodilator (isoproterenol). (2) The subject was told he would be inhaling a bronchoconstrictor[B] but was actually given a bronchodilator (isoproterenol). (3) The subject was told he would be inhaling a bronchoconstrictor and was actually given a bronchoconstrictor (carbachol). (4) The subject was told he would be inhaling a bronchodilator but was actually given a bronchoconstrictor (carbachol). Ra and TGV were then remeasured during the 5 min after inhalation. The postinhalation values were recorded as the mean of five successive measures of each variable (as had been done with baseline values).

Conditions 1, 2, 3 and 4 were randomized in order to preserve the double blind and as a control for order effects. Subjects were instructed to avoid medication after midnight if they were to be studied the following day. In the event that a subject developed an asthmatic attack and required treatment, the experimental session was postponed. This was done to avoid possibly confusing effects brought about by prior medication.

Since each sitting took place on a separate day (in order to allow sufficient time for the effects of the previously given drug to wear off completely) baseline Ga/TGV was never the same for all four experimental conditions. Analysis of responses under the different experimental conditions was accomplished by first expressing postinhalation changes in Ga/TGV as percent change from the baseline value obtained at that session:

$$\frac{\text{Baseline value} - \text{Postdrug value}}{\text{Baseline value}} = \text{present change}$$

Statistical comparisons of the effect of each drug as a function of the instruction conditions (i.e., Conditions 1 vs. 2, Conditions 3 vs. 4) were carried out by means of the Wilcoxon Matched-Pairs Signed-Ranks test (5).

Results

As seen in Table 14.1, the expectation of the subject significantly influenced airway responses to inhalation of isoproterenol and carbachol. The bronchodilator effect of isoproterenol was greater when the subject was told it was a dilator (Condition 1, mean change +39.6%) than when told it was a constrictor (Condition 2, mean change +20.1%). Similarly, the bronchoconstricting effect of carbachol was greater when the subject was told it was a constrictor (Condition 3, mean change −22.3%) than when told it was a dilator (Condition 4, mean change −12.8%). In four instances, the Ga/TGV fell or remained the same under Condition 2, whereas it rose in all cases under Condition 1. In five instances, the Ga/TGV rose or remained unchanged under Condition 4, although it fell in all instances under Condition 3. In one subject, Ga/TGV fell under Condition 2 and rose under Condition 4;

Table 14.1.

Airway reactivity following inhalation of pharmacologic agents: influence of expectation

Condition	Percent change	Condition	N	T value*	p (two-tailed)
1	+39.6				
2	+20.1	12	20	43[‡]	0.02
3	−22.3				
4	−12.8	34	19[†]	39[§]	0.05

Mean change in Ga/TVG from baseline — Comparison of conditions

* Wilcoxon Matched-Pairs Signed-Ranks Test.

[†] One score was the same in both conditions and therefore not included.

[‡] In 16 of the 20 matched comparisons, a greater percent increase in Ga/TGV from baseline values was noted in Condition 1.

[§] In 15 of the 20 matched comparisons, a greater percent decrease in Ga/TGV from baseline values was noted in Condition 3.

however, in the other instances, a fall of Ga/TGV under Condition 2 was not accompanied by a rise under Condition 4, or vice versa.

In most instances, upon inhaling isoproterenol, the subjects were unaware of changes taking place in their lungs. This was especially so under Condition 1. Six subjects reported feeling chest tightness under Condition 2. Two of these subjects showed plethysmographic evidence of decreased Ga/TGV, one showed a minimal decrease, and the other three showed an actual increase in Ga/TGV. Seven subjects reported feeling tightness when inhaling carbachol; five, under Condition 3; and two, under Condition 4. In each of these instances, Ga/TGV fell. Treatment with nebulized isoproterenol immediately reversed these changes; within 5 min all Ga/TGV values were above 0.13 liter/sec/cm H_2O/liter which is considered the cutoff point for pathologic airway obstruction in this laboratory. All other subjects reported no awareness of change following carbachol inhalation.

Discussion

Previous experiments have shown that inhalation of an inert substance (saline), when presented as an allergen or irritant, is capable of inducing significant changes in airway reactivity (1,2). Results of the present study demonstrate that psychologic factors can also influence airway responses of asthmatics to inhalation of pharmacologically active substances. When instructions to subjects are consonant with the pharmacologic action of the inhalant, the airway reaction to that substance is greater than when instructions are dissonant. In a few instances, instructions to a subject exerted an influence of sufficient magnitude to completely reverse the airway response so that it was opposite in direction from that expected on the basis of the pharmacologic action of the drug alone.

Previous studies cited (1,2) were conducted single blind so that a variety of influences could be brought to bear on the subject's airway responses. It is possible that the expectations of the experimenters were subtly transmitted to subjects, thereby enhancing the results of those experiments.

The present data, which were obtained under double-blind conditions, indicate that verbal instructions to subjects with a minimum of other types of communications can alter airway reactivity. This is not to preclude the possibility that subtle communications between experimenter and subject can influence airway response. It may be that these two variables actually complement one another, thereby enhancing the subject's response. However, available information is insufficient to permit a factor analysis of the relative impact that each of these variables (i.e., verbal instructions vis-à-vis other nonverbal communications) would exert upon a subject's airway reactivity.

In previous studies, saline was presented as a series of dilutions of allergen or irritant with a cumulative effect being noted in certain subjects (i.e., some subjects showed more of a change in Ga/TGV to each successive inhalation, and some subjects did not begin to react until the fourth or fifth inhalation). The design of the present experiment precluded such cumulative effects. It is possible that with a design more nearly like that of previous experiments, it may be possible to induce even greater differences among conditions than those seen in the present study.

Bronchomotor tone is regulated by interaction of stimulation provided by the sympathetic and parasympathetic segments of the autonomic nervous system (6). When viewed from the standpoint of autonomic balance, bronchodilation can be induced by increasing adrenergic stimulation or by decreasing cholinergic stimulation. Conversely, bronchoconstriction can be brought about by increasing cholinergic stimulation or by decreasing adrenergic stimulation. The peripheral mechanism by which a subject's expectation can influence the response of the bronchi to pharmacologic agents used in this study is not clear. It would appear, on the basis of the previous work cited, that vagal stimulation probably plays a key role. The administration of atropine (1–2 mg, intravenously) was found to block the airway response to inhalation of bogus allergens (2). However, more data will be necessary before this question can be addressed adequately.

It should be noted that these studies were conducted at times when the baseline Ga/TGV values of all subjects were within or near normal limits (in this laboratory, a Ga/TGV of 0.13 liter/sec/cm H_2O/liter is considered the lowest limit of normal). Therefore, these findings may not necessarily pertain to conditions in which abnormal airway obstruction is present.

Summary

Twenty asthmatic subjects were used in a double-blind study of the influence of expectation on airway reaction to bronchoactive drugs. There were four parts to the experiment, with at least a 24-hr interval between each. At each session, baseline measures of the conductance/thoracic gas volume ratio (Ga/TGV) were obtained after which one of the four following conditions was met: (1) The subject was told he would inhale a bronchodilator and was given isoproterenol. (2) The subject was told he would inhale a bronchoconstrictor but was given isoproterenol. (3) The subject was told he would inhale a bronchoconstrictor and was given carbachol. (4) The subject was told he would inhale a bronchodilator but was given carbachol.

Following inhalation, Ga/TGV measures were again made. It was found that greater airway reactivity occurred when the instructions were consonant with the pharmacologic action of the drugs than when the instructions were dissonant.

In 16 of 20 matched comparisons, a greater percent increase in Ga/TGV was found in Condition 1 as compared to Condition 2. In 15 of 20 matched comparisons, a greater percent decrease in Ga/TGV was noted in Condition 3 as compared to Condition 4. (In one instance, the score was the same in Conditions 3 and 4.)

REFERENCES

1. Luparello T, Lyons HA, Bleecker ER, McFadden ER Jr.: Influences of suggestion on airway reactivity in asthmatic subjects. Psychosom Med 30:819, 1968.
2. McFadden ER Jr., Luparello T, Lyons HA, Bleecker ER: The mechanism of action of suggestion in the induction of acute asthma attacks. Psychosom Med 31:134, 1969.
3. Dekker E, Groen J: Reproducible psychogenic attacks of asthma. J Psychosom Res 1:58, 1956.
4. Briscoe WA, DuBois AB: The relationship between airway resistance, airway conductance and lung volume in subjects of different age and body size. J Clin Invest 37:1279, 1958.
5. Siegel S: Nonparametric Statistics for the Behavioral Sciences. New York, McGraw-Hill, 1956, pp. 75–83.
6. Widdicombe JG: Regulation of tracheobronchial smooth muscle. Physiol Rev 43:1, 1963.
[A]. The actual instructions to the subject were: "This is a bronchodilator, a substance that will open up your airways and make it easier for you to breathe."
[B]. In this case, the instructions were: "This is a bronchoconstrictor, a substance that will tighten up your airways and make it harder for you to breathe."
[Note: references [A] and [B] were originally in-text footnotes that we have converted to endnotes—eds.]

15
The Mechanism of Placebo Analgesia

JON D. LEVINE, NEWTON C. GORDON, AND HOWARD L. FIELDS

Jon D. Levine, Newton C. Gordon, and Howard L. Fields, "The Mechanism of Placebo Analgesia," Lancet 1978;312(8091):654–657.

Introduction

In a variety of painful conditions a remarkably constant proportion (about one third) of patients obtain significant relief from a placebo.[1] Almost nothing is known about what causes placebo effects, but the recently discovered endogenous opiate-like substances (endorphins) seem likely to be involved. The analgesic placebo effect and narcotic analgesia appear to have a similar mechanism. With repeated use over longer periods placebo analgesia becomes less effective (tolerance), there is a compulsion to continue taking placebo with a tendency to increase "dose" over time, and an abstinence syndrome appears when placebo is suddenly withdrawn.[2–4] Placebo may partially reverse withdrawal symptoms in narcotic addicts,[5] and people who respond to placebos get significantly more relief from postoperative pain with narcotic analgesics.[1,6–9]

If placebo-induced analgesia is mediated by endorphins, then naloxone, a pure opiate antagonist, would be expected to block it. The early observation by Lasagna that 8 mg of naloxone produced less analgesia than placebo[10] supports this hypothesis. In this study we investigated the direct effect of naloxone upon placebo-induced analgesia.

Patients

The patients were 27 males and 24 females with ages ranging from the late teens to early thirties. Forty-seven patients were from the private practice and 4 from the clinic of the Department of Oral Surgery. Subjects were healthy except for impacted wisdom teeth. Oral consent and written consent on forms following the guidelines of our campus committee on human experimentation were obtained. Patients were told that they might receive either morphine, placebo, or naloxone (an agent that might increase their pain). In previous double-blind studies, telling patients that they might receive placebo did not inhibit the placebo response.[11–13]

Methods

Patients received 10–20 mg intravenous diazepam. Nitrous oxide (N_2O) (15–40%) was inhaled and mepivacaine (3% without vasoconstrictor), a local anaesthetic effective for 45–75 min, was used to block the mandibular and long buccal nerves.[1–4] Impacted mandibular third molars were removed with a standardised technique and all surgery was done by N.C.G. After surgery, N_2O was stopped, and after 100% oxygen for 10 min, patients were transferred to a nearby recovery room for continued observation, where they were given experimental drugs and pain was measured. Patients were randomly placed in experimental groups by selecting a coded envelope. Experimental drugs were delivered in equal volumes as a bolus via an intravenous catheter and were given double blind. No codes were broken during any experiment.

Two pain-rating scales were used:[14] the visual analogue scale, a 10 cm horizontal line on 8 × 10 in (203 × 254 mm) white paper, had "no pain" printed at the left end and "worst pain ever" at the right end. Patients were asked to make a mark crossing this line at a point representing the intensity of their pain. A separate card was given for each rating and patients could not refer back to their previous ratings. Beginning at the second pain rating, a second, verbal rating was requested in order to check the reliability of the first. On the verbal scale, patients indicated whether their pain had increased, decreased, or remained the same since the last time they rated their pain level. For more than 95% of measurements, the change in the visual analogue scale correlated with the verbal scale. When the pain was rated as unchanged on the verbal scale, 50% of the visual analogue scale ratings were within ±2 mm of the previous score and 92% were within ±10 mm.

The times when pain was rated and drugs were given are shown by the data points in the figures. Drugs were given at 2 h (drug 1, D_1) and 3 h (drug 2, D_2), respectively, after the start of anaesthesia (zero time) as determined by paraesthesiae and sensory testing of analgesia. All patients were given 10 mg naloxone (Endo Laboratories) or an identical volume of naloxone vehicle (placebo) or morphine sulphate (7.5 mg) each time. Seventeen patients received placebo as D_1 and D_2; 23 patients received placebo as D_1 and naloxone as D_2; and 11 patients received naloxone as D_1 and placebo as D_2. Five patients dropped out of the study.

Results

The patients were randomly given morphine, placebo, or naloxone (the combination of morphine followed by naloxone being excluded) so that patients could expect a powerful analgesic as well as something which might make pain worse. Patients given morphine were excluded from the subsequent analysis of the results.

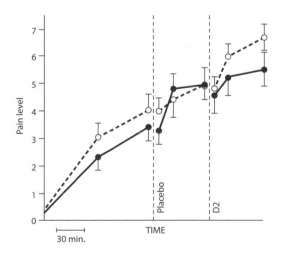

Figure 15.1. The effect of naloxone on pain. Time was measured from the start of anaesthesia. Both patient groups were given placebo as their first drug. The administration of the second drug is denoted by D_2. ● – mean (±S.E.) pain ratings for patients given placebo as a second drug (n = 17); ○ – mean pain ratings for patients given 10 mg naloxone as a second drug (n = 23). Difference during the three immediately postoperative hours was insignificant. The group given naloxone had significantly greater mean pain ratings 1 h after its administration (p < 0.05 by t test).

As part of the consent form, patients were permitted to withdraw from the experiment. Five did so before the final pain determination, presumably because they had reached the limit of pain tolerance, although analysis of the 8 data points (out of a possible 9) does not suggest that these patients differed from those who completed the study.

Naloxone Enhancement of Pain

We compared the effect of naloxone and placebo in patients given placebo as D_1 and either naloxone or placebo as D_2. Five minutes before and 1 h after giving of placebo as D_1, the pain ratings of patients in each group did not differ significantly (fig. 15.1). Throughout the measurement period, there was a rise in the mean pain level reported. However, 1 h after D_2 was given, the group given naloxone reported significantly more pain than the group given a second placebo.

Comparison of Placebo Responders and Nonresponders

In this study, placebo responders were defined as patients whose pain rating 1 h after taking placebo remained constant or decreased compared with their rating 5 min before they took it. Placebo nonresponders were those whose pain was greater 1 h after placebo. By this definition, when placebo was given as D_1, 39% of patients were responders. The bimodal distribution of change in pain observed 1 h after placebo as D_1 indicates that this distinction between responders and nonresponders is not arbitrary (fig. 15.2).

Patients receiving placebo as D_1 were divided into responders and nonresponders in order to compare naloxone's differential effect on the two patient groups. Naloxone enhanced pain ratings much more in placebo responders (fig. 15.3), bringing their mean pain rating to the same level as that of nonresponders. This convergence suggested that most, if not all, the analgesic effect of placebo is naloxone-reversible, a conclusion supported by the observation that naloxone had no obvious effect upon placebo nonresponders.

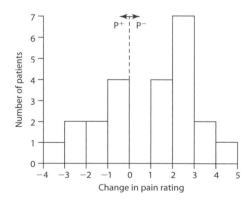

Figure 15.2. Change in pain 1 h after placebo compared with pain rating 5 min before placebo. P^+ and P^- indicate the placebo responders and nonresponders, respectively. A bimodal distribution is apparent.

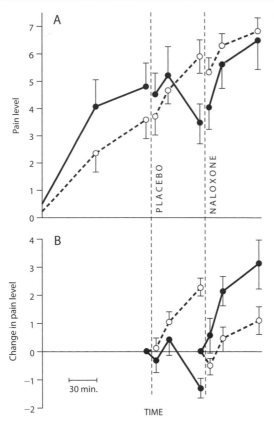

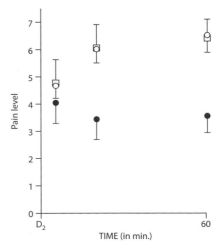

Figure 15.4. Absence of naloxone effect in placebo nonresponders: pain ratings during the hour after the second drug was given. ○ – patients given placebo followed by naloxone (n = 23); ■ – patients given placebo followed by a second placebo to which they did not respond (n = 6); ● – patients given placebo followed by a second placebo to which they did respond (n = 11).

Figure 15.3. Differential effect of naloxone on placebo responders and nonresponders. All patients received placebo as the first drug and naloxone as the second. *Upper graph:* mean pain levels for placebo responders (●) (n = 9) and nonresponders (○) (n = 14) are plotted. After naloxone, the difference in mean pain level for these two groups becomes insignificant. *Lower graph:* cumulative change in pain level compared with 5 min before the drug was given (data from upper curve). After naloxone the change in pain level is greater in positive placebo responders. A significant difference is apparent 5 min after naloxone (p < 0.05 by t test), and is greater 20 and 60 min after naloxone (p < 0.125). The latency of the placebo effect seems to be less than 5 min.

Fig. 15.4 shows that the time course and final pain level were the same for placebo nonresponders and patients receiving naloxone.

Magnitude and Time Course of Effect

Except during the recovery period, mean pain ratings during the experiment were well within ±2 cm of the middle of the visual analogue scale (fig. 15.3), which suggests that the scale was appropriate to the pain levels experienced. The difference in final mean levels between placebo responders (3.5) and nonresponders (6.5) (fig. 15.4) is almost the full range of mean pain levels in fig. 15.3. The mean pain rating for nonresponders was almost double that of responders, indicating that the placebo effect, when present, was quite large. The increase in pain caused by naloxone was also quite large.

Enhancement of pain ratings in placebo responders was significantly greater than in nonresponders as early as 5 min after naloxone was given (p < 0.05) (fig. 15.3, lower graph). This naloxone enhancement was greater after 20 min but appeared to level off at 60 min (fig. 15.4). Thus the peak of the placebo effect was later than 20 min, and its duration was greater than 1 h, a time course consistent with that observed by others for analgesic placebo.[15]

Five of 14 patients given placebo as both D_1 and D_2 responded to the second placebo. If naloxone was given first, the number of responders dropped to 2 of 11. This difference, although not statistically significant, suggested that giving naloxone first reduced the probability that a patient would be a positive placebo responder.

Discussion

This study supports the hypothesis that endorphin activity accounts for placebo analgesia, first because naloxone causes a significantly greater increase in pain ratings in placebo responders than in nonresponders, and second because prior administration of naloxone reduces the probability of a positive placebo response.

The observation that placebo nonresponders have almost the same postoperative pain levels as those receiving naloxone suggests that the enhancement of pain by naloxone can be completely accounted for by an action on placebo responders. If naloxone had had a pain-enhancing action independent of the placebo response naloxone would have increased pain even in placebo responders. That it did not, even with the large dose of naloxone (10 mg) employed, supports the conclusion that the placebo effect is endorphin mediated.

Four of the five patients who prematurely dropped out of the study had received naloxone as the second drug, and they dropped out between the 20- and 60-min pain ratings after naloxone. In this group the pain rating at the time of termination (mean 6.4) was almost identical to the 60-min rating of the patients who continued in the experiment and who had either received naloxone or were placebo nonresponders to the second drug. This preliminary observation suggests that a patient's ability to tolerate pain is, to some degree, separable from his own perception of its intensity.

Naloxone is a specific opiate antagonist and, in the dose employed in this study, has no known effect when administered to opiate-naive subjects.[16,17] Although no patient received narcotics before participation in the experiment, diazepam and N_2O were given before surgery. Naloxone reverses the effect of 67% N_2O on tail flick in the rat,[18] but in this study measurements were made 1–3 h after N_2O, when the amount left in the body is minimal. Diazepam is not an effective analgesic, although it may work synergistically with narcotics to enhance analgesia. In animals diazepam and opiates act upon independent neural systems.[19,20] More important, all patients received diazepam and N_2O so that the difference in naloxone effects between placebo responders and nonresponders could not be explained simply by a selective antagonism of naloxone towards these two drugs or to systemically absorbed local anaesthetic. Furthermore, the N_2O, diazepam, and mepivacaine levels fell during the measurement period while the effect of naloxone increased with time, being greatest 1 h after being given. Although this is relatively late compared with the reversal of narcotic overdose (which occurs within 2 min of intravenous administration), the peak for naloxone blockade of stimulation-produced analgesia in cats is 30–40 min after injection and may last several hours.[20] This prolonged time course is also consistent with our observation that the proportion of positive responders is reduced when placebo is given an hour after naloxone.

In our experiments, a relatively homogenous group of patients were operated upon with a standardised procedure. Interestingly, the mean pain ratings were almost identical in patients given naloxone and those who did not respond to placebo (figs. 15.3 and 15.4), which may mean that part of the variability in pain intensity reported by patients who all have similar lesions may be due to differences in endorphin activity.

In contrast to our previous results,[14] investigators using experimental noxious stimulation have either failed to find pain enhancement with naloxone[21,22] or have shown mixed effects in unselected subjects.[23] It is not clear why our clinical paradigm revealed naloxone hyperalgesia while experimental paradigms did not. Perhaps the prolonged duration of the pain or the added stress of the clinical situation accounts for this difference. That stress may be a factor is indicated by the strong positive correlation between plasma levels of adrenocorticotrophin (a stress indicator) and endorphins.[24] Recently, an endogenous pain-suppression system has been described which can be activated by electrical stimulation of the brain or by systemically administered opiates.[25,26] In patients with chronically implanted electrodes, naloxone-reversible relief of clinical pain has been produced with only minimal effects on experimental pain thresholds.[27]

Conceivably, the analgesic effect of placebo upon clinical pain results from activation of the same pain-suppression system.

If, as the present study suggests, the analgesic effect of placebo is based on the action of endorphins, future research can proceed with an analysis of variables affecting endorphin activity rather than simply recording behavioural manifestations of placebo effects. Greater understanding of endogenous mechanisms of analgesia should lead to more effective management of clinical pain with a combination of pharmacological, behavioural, and physical methods.

REFERENCES

1. Beecher, H.K. J. Am. Med. Ass., 1955, 159, 1602.
2. Vinar, O. Brit. J. Psychiatry, 1969, 115, 1189.
3. Tyler, D.B. Am. J. Physiol., 1947, 150, 253.
4. Wagner, W.A., Hubbell, A.O. J. Oral Surg., 1959, 17, 14.
5. Leslie, A. Am. J. Med., 1954, 16, 854.
6. Beecher, H.K. J. Pharmacol. Exp. Therap., 1953, 109, 393.
7. Glick, B.S. Dis. Nerv. Syst., 1967, 28, 737.
8. Lasagna, L., et al. Am. J. Med., 1954, 16, 770.
9. Shapiro, A.K. Am. J. Psychother., 1964, 18, suppl., 73.
10. Lasagna, L. Proc. R. Soc. Med., 1965, 58, 978.
11. Park, L.C., Covi, L. Arch. Gen. Psychiatry, 1965, 12, 336.
12. Park. L.C., Slaughter, R., Covi, L., Kniffin, H.G., Jr. J. Nerv. Ment. Dis., 1966, 143, 199.
13. Park, L.C., Covi, L., Uhlenhuth, E.H. J. Nerv. Ment. Dis., 1967, 145, 349.
14. Levine, J.D., et al. Nature, 1978, 272, 826.
15. Houde, R.W., Wallenstein, S.L., Rogers, A. Clin. Pharmac. Ther., 1966, 1, 163.
16. Zaks, A., Jones, T., Fink, M. J. Am. Med. Ass., 1971, 215, 2108.
17. Jaffe, J.H., Martin, W.R. in The Pharmacological Basis of Therapeutics (edited by L.S. Goodman and A. Gilman); New York, 1975.
18. Berkowitz, B., Finck, A.D., Ngai, S.H. Neurosci. Abst., 1977, 3, 286.
19. Hayes, R.L., et al. Neurosci. Abst., 1977, 3, 483.
20. Oliveras, J.L., et al. Brain Res., 1977, 120, 221.
21. El-Sobky, A., Dostrovsky, J.O., Wall, P.D. Nature, 1976, 263, 783.
22. Grevert, P., Goldstein, G. Proc. Natn. Acad. Sci. U.S.A., 1977, 74, 1291.
23. Buchsbaum, M.S., Davis, G.C., Bunney, W.E., Jr. Nature, 1977, 270, 620.
24. Guillemin, R., et al. Science, 1977, 197, 1367.
25. Mayer, D.J., Price, D.D. Pain, 1977, 2, 379.
26. Fields, H.L., Basbaum, A.I. Ann. Rev. Physiol., 1977, 40, 193.
27. Hosobuchi, Y., Adams, J.E., Linchitz, R. Science, 1977, 197, 183.

16
Behaviorally Conditioned Immunosuppression and Murine Systemic Lupus Erythematosus

ROBERT ADER AND NICHOLAS COHEN

Robert Ader and Nicholas Cohen, "Behaviorally Conditioned Immunosuppression and Murine Systemic Lupus Erythematosus," Science 1982;215:1534–1536.

Several converging lines of evidence implicate the central nervous system in the regulation of immune processes (1). Of relevance here is that behavioral conditioning procedures

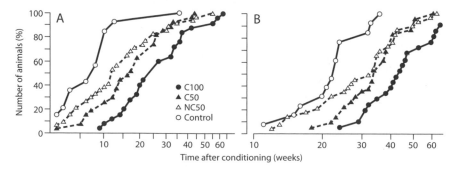

Fig. 16.1. (A) Rate of development of an unremitting proteinuria in NZF$_1$ female mice under different chemotherapeutic regimens. Group C100 (N = 25) received weekly a saccharin drinking solution (SAC) followed by an injection of cyclophosphamide (30 mg/kg); group C50 (N = 27) received weekly the SAC followed by an injection of cyclophosphamide (30 mg/kg) two times in each 4 weeks or an injection of saline; group NC50 (N = 34) received weekly the SAC and an injection of cyclophosphamide (two times in each 4 weeks) but the SAC and the drug were not paired; control mice (N = 14) received SAC weekly but no cyclophosphamide. (B) Cumulative mortality rate in NZF$_1$ female mice maintained on different chemotherapeutic regimens. Symbols as in (A).

can be used to suppress humoral and cell-mediated immune responses (2). Conditioned immunosuppression is accomplished by pairing consumption of a novel drinking solution— the conditioned stimulus (CS)—with an immunosuppressive drug, for example, cyclophosphamide—the unconditioned stimulus (US). When subsequently treated with antigen, conditioned animals that are reexposed to the CS show attenuated immune responses. The present study was designed to examine the impact of conditioned immunosuppression on the development of systemic lupus erythematosus (SLE) in New Zealand mice, an autoimmune disease for which the female (NZB × NZW)F$_1$ (NZF$_1$) mouse has become a standard experimental model (3). Treatment of NZF$_1$ mice with cyclophosphamide prolongs survival of animals that would otherwise develop a lethal glomerulonephritis between approximately 8 and 14 months of age (4). On the basis of observations that immune responses can be suppressed by conditioning procedures, we hypothesized that, in conditioned mice, the substitution of conditioned stimuli (placebo treatment) for the immunosuppressive drug would delay the development of proteinuria and mortality relative to nonconditioned animals treated with the same dose of drug.

Individually caged female NZF$_1$ mice were maintained under a 12-hour light-dark cycle and given free access to food and water. A chemotherapeutic regimen was initiated when the animals were 4 months of age. Once each week for 8 weeks all the animals were administered a 0.15 percent solution of sodium saccharin (SAC) by pipette (up to 1.0 ml). Cyclophosphamide (5) was injected according to the following schedule.

The standard treatment group (C100) received, once weekly, an intraperitoneal injection of cyclophosphamide (30 mg/kg) immediately after they received the SAC solution. These stimuli were presented at the same time on the same day of each week. Results derived from this conditioned group defined the effects of traditional immunosuppressive therapy administered for 8 weeks. The dosage and duration of treatment

prolonged survival but was insufficient to prevent the ultimate development of SLE.

Another conditioned group (C50) received, two times (in random sequence) in each 4 weeks, an intraperitoneal injection of cyclophosphamide (30 mg/kg) after they received the SAC solution. For the two times in each 4 weeks that they did not receive the drug, they received an intraperitoneal injection of saline following SAC.

A nonconditioned group (NC50) also received cyclophosphamide injections after the SAC presentations two times in each 4 weeks, but these stimuli were administered on a noncontingent basis (that is, on different days of the same week).

Control animals received no immunosuppressive therapy. They did, however, receive the weekly dose of SAC solution and injections of saline on a noncontingent basis.

Group NC50, since they received only 50 percent of the cyclophosphamide that group C100 received, were expected to manifest symptoms of SLE and die sooner than animals treated weekly. Group C50 also received only 50 percent of the drug given to group C100. However, to the extent that reexposure to SAC (the CS paired with cyclophosphamide) is capable of eliciting a conditioned immunosuppressive response, it was predicted that the animals in group C50 would show a greater resistance to the development of SLE than the animals in group NC50.

At weekly intervals, proteinuria was measured on freshly expressed urine samples with tetrabromphenol paper ("Albustix") (6). When autolysis was not extreme or when moribund animals were killed, glomerulonephritis was examined histologically (and, in all instances, verified). Ten animals died without showing proteinuria and were eliminated from the experiment.

As expected, the weekly cyclophosphamide treatment delayed the onset of proteinuria and prolonged the survival of NZF$_1$ mice in group C100. Considering the total population of animals that developed SLE, there was a significant difference in the onset of proteinuria (values consistently ≥ 100 mg/100 ml) (F[3,96] = 8.28; P < .001). Since the mice in all groups were likely to develop proteinuria and die, the longer the disease was monitored, the less likely it would be to discern treatment effects. Differences among the groups (Fig. 16.1A) become striking when one uses as a reference point the rate of development of proteinuria for the initial 50 percent of the population developing the disease ($F[3,47] = 18.29$; $P < .001$). Animals in group C100 developed proteinuria later than any of the other groups ($P < .001$ in each instance). The nonconditioned animals (group NC50) did not differ from the untreated controls ($t = 1.78$), whereas the conditioned animals in group C50 developed proteinuria significantly more slowly than the untreated controls ($t = 3.86$, $P < .001$). The critical comparison between groups C50 and NC50 revealed that group C50 developed proteinuria significantly more slowly than group NC50 ($t = 2.38$, $P < .05$).

There were also group differences in mortality ($F[3,85] = 10.49$; $P < .001$) that were especially dramatic when one considers the rate at which the first half of each group died ($F[3,44] = 15.67$; $P < .001$) (Fig. 16.1B). Nonconditioned animals (group NC50) did not differ from untreated controls ($t = 1.62$). In contrast, group C50 survived significantly longer than untreated controls ($t = 4.24$, $P < .001$) and did not differ statistically from group C100 ($t = 1.28$), animals that received twice as much drug. Again, the critical comparison is between groups C50 and NC50, which received the same amount of drug: group C50 survived significantly longer (27.6 ± 1.5 weeks) than group NC50 (22.1 ± 1.7 weeks) ($t = 2.42$, $P < .05$).

Differences in both the rate of development of proteinuria and mortality can be traced to the variable onset of disease among the groups. Within-group correlations between the development of proteinuria and mortality ranged from .66 to .84 and were statistically significant in all instances. The interval between the development of proteinuria and death was also relatively constant (ranging from 14.4 ± 1.2 to 16.7 ± 1.2 weeks). Therefore, although the progression of SLE followed a similar course in all groups, there was a clear difference in the onset of disease that could be attributed to the differential treatment of the groups. These differences were consistent with the effects of cyclophosphamide in retarding the development of SLE. The results were also consistent with previous observations of conditioned immunosuppression (2) and with predictions that follow from the application of such conditioning within this biologic model.

The mechanisms mediating these conditioning effects are unknown. There are, however, several possibilities. An elevation in adrenocortical steroid levels, for example, might be invoked to explain the observed differences. Novel stimuli (saccharin) can elicit an adrenocortical response, as can an injection of saline or cyclophosphamide (7). Conditioned and nonconditioned animals, however, received the same number of such stimuli. Moreover, since combined environmental stimuli are not additive (8), it could be argued that the nonconditioned animals (group NC50) exposed to SAC and intraperitoneal injections at different times received twice as many "stressful" experiences as the conditioned animals (group C50). A differential adrenal response (that is, a conditioned elevation in corticosterone level) is possible but unlikely. It is possible to condition an elevation in steroid level in fluid-deprived rats (7), but 30 mg of cyclophosphamide is insufficient to induce an aversion to a flavored drinking solution in NZF$_1$ or C57BL/6 mice (9). Several other endocrine- and neuroendocrine-immune system interactions have been described (1), and these physiologic processes may be subject to or influenced by conditioning.

The present study does not provide direct evidence of conditioned immunosuppression per se (for example, depressed autoantibody titers). Nonetheless, the results are consistent with previous data (2), indicating that the pairing of saccharin and cyclophosphamide enables saccharin, acting as a CS, to suppress immunologic reactivity; they are also consistent with the hypothesis that such conditioning might thereby delay the onset of autoimmune disease under a regimen of chemotherapy that was not, in itself, sufficient to influence the development of SLE in comparison with an untreated control group. As such, these findings constitute an elaboration of the biologic impact of conditioned immune-pharmacologic responses. The present study suggests, further, that there is some heuristic value in analyzing a pharmacotherapeutic regimen in terms of conditioning operations. Based on the present paradigm in which conditioned stimulus presentations (placebo treatments) were substituted for some active immunosuppressive therapy, it may be hypothesized that the prescription of a noncontinuous schedule of pharmacologic treatment in contrast to an analysis of the effects of continuous regimens of drug (or placebo) would be applicable in the pharmacotherapeutic control and regulation of a variety of physiologic systems.

REFERENCES AND NOTES

1. R. Ader, Ed., *Psychoneuroimmunology* (Behavioral Medicine Series) (Academic Press, New York, 1981).
2. R. Ader and N. Cohen, *Psychosom. Med.* **37**, 333 (1975); R. Ader, N. Cohen, L.J. Grota, *Int. J. Immunopharmacol.* **1**, 141 (1979); D. Bovbjerg, N. Cohen, R. Ader, *Proc. Natl. Acad. Sci. U.S.A.* **79**, 583 (1982); N. Cohen, R. Ader, N. Green, D. Bovbjerg, *Psychosom. Med.* **41**, 487 (1979); M. P. Rogers, P. Reich, T.B. Strom, C.B. Carpenter, *Psychosom. Med.* **38**, 447 (1976); E.A. Wayner, G.R. Flannery, G. Singer, *Physiol. Behav.* **21**, 995 (1978).
3. A.D. Steinberg, D.P. Huston, J.D. Taurog, J.S. Cowdery, E.S. Raveché, *Immunol. Rev.* **55**, 121 (1981); A.N. Theofilopoulos and F. Dixon, *Immunol. Rev.* **55**, 179 (1981); N. Talal, *Transplant. Rev.* **31**, 240 (1976).
4. T.P. Casey, *Blood* **32**, 436 (1968); B.H. Hahn, L. Knotts, M. Ng, T.R. Hamilton, *Arthritis Rheum.* **18**, 145 (1975); D.H. Lehman, C.B. Wilson, F.J. Dixon, *Clin. Exp. Immunol.* **25**, 297 (1976); A.D. Morris, J. Esterly, G. Chase, G.C. Sharp, *Arthritis Rheum.* **19**, 49 (1976); P.J. Russell and J.D. Hicks, *Lancet* **1**, 440 (1968); A.D. Steinberg, M.C. Gelfand, J.A. Hardin, D.T. Lowenthal, *Arthritis Rheum.* **18**, 9 (1975).
5. Cyclophosphamide was generously supplied by the Mead Johnson Research Center, Evansville, Ind.
6. There is a correlation between proteinuria and immunologic and histologic manifestations of disease (3, 4). Therefore, in order to minimize extraneous manipulations of the animals, we obtained no additional measures.
7. R. Ader, *J. Comp. Physiol. Psychol.* **90**, 1156 (1976).
8. S.B. Friedman and R. Ader, *Neuroendocrinology* **2**, 209 (1967).
9. R. Ader, unpublished observations.

17

An Investigation of Drug Expectancy as a Function of Capsule Color and Size and Preparation Form

Louis W. Buckalew and Kenneth E. Coffield

Louis W. Buckalew and Kenneth E. Coffield, "An Investigation of Drug Expectancy as a Function of Capsule Color and Size and Preparation Form," *Journal of Clinical Psychopharmacology* 1982;2:245–248.

Preparations of no medicinal value can produce powerful and wide-ranging effects.[1,2] Shapiro[3] placed the placebo in perspective by tracing its history and assigned importance. Effort in the last 25 years has been devoted to a more comprehensive understanding and appreciation of the placebo and mechanisms of action. What is still needed is a more comprehensive analysis of the placebo, facilitating accurate conceptualization and effective use of its properties.[2] Shapiro and associates[4] believed that the stimulus nature of the placebo was a crucial factor in effects, as supported by Buckalew and Ross.[5] Years ago, Lasagna[6] stipulated that drug response, to a variable extent, was a product of color, name, origin, appearance, and avenue of administration. Drug manufacturers have been aware that perceptual characteristics constitute relevant stimuli to responsivity to a drug.[7]

Buckalew and colleagues[8] reviewed attempts to relate placebo responsivity to personality variables, concluding that there was little merit to claims of any substantial relationship. Furthermore, Buckalew and Ross[5] provided an extensive consideration of drug efficacy and perceptual characteristics, finding little evidence relating to such meaningful characteristics as preparation size and color. They did offer several guarded conclusions: (1) capsules are slightly better than pills; (2) the larger the dose or number of pills, the more effective the placebo; and (3) blue preparations seem more tranquilizing, while red, pink, and yellow are associated with stimulating effects.

Few studies have investigated the role of quantity, color, or form on drug perception. Blackwell and coworkers[9] determined that two capsules produced more pronounced changes than one. Significant effect differences between blue and pink capsules were reported, and sedative responses to placebos were found more frequently than stimulant responses. Perceptual consequences of color as influencing affect has been well researched, as noted in the review by Adams and Osgood.[10] Buckalew and Ross[5] acknowledged limited research on color and placebo efficacy and found it difficult to consolidate due to few replications and diversity of colors employed. A study by Jacobs and Nordan[11] did reflect an effort to evaluate placebo classification based on color. With capsule size controlled, blue was associated with a depressant–tranquilizer effect, red and yellow were associated with a stimulant–antidepressant effect, and white was not attributed to any specific effect. Although the study represented a solid effort at clarifying the role of color in determining placebo perception, it was restricted to six colors and three classifications and failed to consider sex.

The present study sought to determine the effects of preparation color, size, and form on expectations of drug action. Of specific concern was the effect of capsule color on drug classification, the effect of capsule size on perceived drug strength, and the comparison of preparation forms on perceived efficacy. In accord with Buckalew and Ross,[5] such physical variables were suggested as important to drug efficacy. Also, this study sought to reveal potential sex differences in the use of physical factors.

Methods

Subjects

Volunteers were recruited from undergraduate psychology classes: 34 women (mean age, 25.0 years) and 34 men (mean age, 20.2 years). A blind condition was used in which subjects were unaware that capsules were placebos.

Materials

One capsule of each of six sizes (nos. 00 to 4) was painted orange, placed on cotton, and sealed in a small petri dish with a cover. These capsules were used in the drug strength task. Twenty-four no. 1 capsules were painted 12 different colors, with two capsules per color: white, black, brown, dark blue, light blue, gray, dark green, light green, yellow, dark red, orange, and lavender. All except light colors were saturated hues obtained with Testors Pla Enamel. Light colors were made by diluting a saturated hue with white. Two capsules of each color were placed on cotton, sealed in a petri dish with a cover, and used in the drug classification task. A single no. 1 white capsule and a white tablet of an equivalent amount of acetaminophen were sealed in a petri dish with a cover and used in the drug form task.

Two chartboards were used, with stenciled information about tasks 1 and 2. The drug strength (task 1) chart had six categories: (1) very powerful, (2) strong, (3) moderate, (4) weak, (5) minimal, and (6) very weak. The drug classification (task 2) had five parts: (S–A) stimulant–antidepressant, (A–N) analgesic–narcotic, (P–H) psychedelic–hallucinogenic, (D–S) depressant–sedative, and (U) unknown. For each classification there was a brief description of general effects associated with drugs of that type. Individual data sheets were used to record results of the classification and ordering tasks.

Procedure

All persons were individually tested in a small laboratory room and informed that the study involved only drug classification. Instructions for each task, printed on data record sheets, were read to participants. Subjects were seated and given each task's capsules, as a group, and chartboard. Task

1 (drug strength) involved six different-sized capsules, with color held constant, and required arrangement of capsules in order of perceived strength. Ranking was done by placing each capsule container in a chartboard category, with one container per category. Task 2 (drug classification) involved 12 containers of capsules, each with a different color of capsule, with size held constant. The task was to place each container in the drug category thought most appropriate in describing the action or type of drug it contained. All capsules had to be categorized, with no restriction on the number of containers in any single category. Task 3 (preparation comparison) required indication of whether the tablet or capsule was stronger or more powerful, with a response of "equal strength" available. Individual testing time averaged about 4 min, with no performance feedback.

Results

Task 1 required rank-ordering six capsules for perceived strength. Kendall's coefficient of concordance was computed, by sex, resulting in a W of 0.157 ($p > 0.05$) for men, a W of 0.130 ($p > 0.05$) for women, and a W of 0.130 ($p > 0.05$) for combined rankings. This indicated poor intersubject agreement in ranking. However, if for each capsule size mean ranks of strength were computed and ordered from 1 to 6, correlation for capsule size rank and capsule strength rank would be $\rho = +1.00$ for each sex and combined data. This suggests that the larger the capsule, the greater the perceived strength, with this specific ranking system reflected in 59% of women and 56% of men. Data showed the opposite ranking ($\rho = -1.00$) for capsule size versus strength in 19% of men and 21% of women.

Task 2 involved nominal classification of 12 sets of colored capsules into five categories. Frequency counts of how often each color capsule was placed in a specific classification were noted, and chi-square was computed for male, female, and combined distributions of each capsule color. Data, converted to percentage, are shown in Table 17.1. Nine capsule colors yielded significant chi-square values ($df = 4$, $p < 0.05$) for combined data, with four colors (white, lavender, orange, and yellow) having specific classification significance as determined by the critical observed frequencies technique.[12] Sex differences in the distribution of capsules by color may be seen in the data in Table 17.1.

For task 3, a frequency count was obtained for each possible response (tablet, capsule, and equal weight). Table 17.2 shows the application of chi-square to these data, converted to percentages to aid interpretation. The resulting values for data on men and women, separate and combined, were significant ($df = 2$, $p < 0.05$). Data indicated that the male subjects made a more definitive choice than the female subjects as to which preparation was "stronger."

Discussion

Blackwell and colleagues[9] suggested that two capsules are more effective than one, and Evans[13] indicated that higher

Table 17.1.
Placebo classifications[a] in percentages as a function of color[b]

Color	Group	S–A	A–N	P–H	D–S	U	χ^2	p
White	Male	15	38	6	12	29	12.18	<0.05
	Female	9	35	18	12	26	5.94	
	Combined	12	37	12	12	28	18.63	<0.01
Black	Male	38	15	6	15	26	10.71	<0.05
	Female	23	6	18	26	26	5.11	
	Combined	31	10	12	21	26	10.97	<0.05
Lavender	Male	6	12	62	9	12	37.46	<0.01
	Female	26	15	35	21	3	10.13	<0.05
	Combined	16	13	49	15	7	36.12	<0.01
Light blue	Male	12	26	29	26	6	7.47	
	Female	21	26	9	38	6	11.38	<0.05
	Combined	16	26	19	32	6	12.76	<0.05
Light green	Male	15	29	18	9	29	5.71	
	Female	12	26	15	32	15	4.91	
	Combined	13	28	16	21	22	4.35	
Gray	Male	0	12	12	29	47	23.06	<0.01
	Female	12	21	15	29	23	3.36	
	Combined	6	16	13	29	35	19.80	<0.01
Orange	Male	47	24	24	6	0	23.06	<0.01
	Female	47	15	29	6	3	22.78	<0.01
	Combined	47	19	26	6	1	44.79	<0.01
Dark blue	Male	18	29	12	38	3	13.35	<0.01
	Female	15	21	32	18	15	3.65	
	Combined	16	25	22	28	9	8.75	
Dark red	Male	3	32	12	38	15	14.84	<0.01
	Female	18	18	18	23	23	.69	
	Combined	10	25	15	31	19	9.06	
Dark green	Male	29	24	21	15	12	3.36	
	Female	21	38	23	12	6	10041	<0.05
	Combined	25	31	22	13	9	10.83	<0.05
Brown	Male	3	18	15	35	29	11.01	<0.05
	Female	15	21	15	21	29	2.49	
	Combined	9	19	15	28	29	10.38	<0.05
Yellow	Male	68	15	6	12	0	50.41	<0.01
	Female	44	21	21	9	6	15.42	<0.01
	Combined	56	18	13	10	3	58.62	<0.01

Note: [a] S–A = stimulant–antidepressant; A–N = analgesic–narcotic; P–H = psychedelic–hallucinogenic; D–S = depressant–sedative; U = unknown. [b] Underlined values were determined as significant using the technique developed by Buckalew and Pearson.[12]

doses are clinically more effective. Buckalew and Ross[5] concluded that the larger the dose is, the more powerful it is likely to be perceived to be. Results of task 1, investigating comparative strengths of six capsule sizes, showed little concordance between subjects in rankings based on capsule size. However, 57% employed a ranking system of increases in perceived strength associated with increases in capsule size. A conclusion of "bigger is better" seems warranted, although appreciable variability in the specificity of this relationship was noted.

There is appreciable evidence that color is a meaningful and consequential perceptual characteristic. For example,

Table 17.2.
Strength comparison in percentages as a function of preparation form[a]

Group	N	Capsule	Tablet	Equal weight	χ^2	p
Male	34	<u>59</u>	15	26	10.65	<0.01
Female	34	44	12	44	7.12	<0.05
Combined	68	<u>51</u>	14	35	15.03	<0.001

[a] Underlined values were determined as significant using the technique developed by Buckalew and Pearson.[12]

Adams and Osgood[10] found fairly universal meanings ascribed to red, black, gray, white, yellow, blue, and green. Knowledge of constancies in the ascribed meanings of specific colors, particularly those associated with expected pharmacological actions, should be valuable in enhancing or supporting drug efficacy. It is logical to assume that certain drug effects based on preparation color may be expected.[5]

Task 2 investigated capsule classification based on preparation color. When the combined data on male and female subjects were considered, significant differences from chance were found for 9 of the 12 capsule colors in their distribution over five classification categories. Light green, dark blue, and dark red capsules were distributed in chance fashion, although the male subjects tended to classify the latter two as depressant–sedative. Blackwell and co-workers[9] and Jacobs and Nordan[11] found blue associated with sedative action, a finding only weakly supported by present data and primarily for light as opposed to dark blue. Both Jacobs and Nordan[11] and Berg[7] suggested that red capsules are typically classified as stimulants. Present data reflect that dark red is more commonly classified as a depressant–sedative, although not with significant frequency. Also, the red-based lavender capsules in our study were clearly, and at significant levels, categorized as psychedelic–hallucinogenic.

Clear agreement exists between Jacobs and Nordan,[11] Schapira and associates,[14] and the present study in the perception of a yellow capsule as stimulant–antidepressant. Jacobs and Nordan[11] found black capsules typically classified as depressants among students, although they were most frequently categorized as stimulant–antidepressant in the present study. Both Berg[7] and Jacobs and Nordan[11] suggested white as a weak and indistinct preparation color, although white capsules were significantly categorized as analgesic–narcotic in the present data. This perceptual change may be a function of increasing exposure to the white, pain-killing association made in television drug advertising. Jacobs and Nordan[11] also reported green capsules as undifferentiated, a finding supported for light green capsules. Schapira and associates[14] suggested green as associated with an antianxiety effect, although present data show green most commonly classified as analgesic–narcotic.

Our study confirms the hypothesis of Buckalew and Ross[5] that conclusions of anticipated drug action based on preparation color are difficult due to the infinite number of stimuli available. Subtle differences in saturation appear particularly important. Of the few studies attempting to assess color effects of drug preparations, the range of colors and classifications has been appreciably restricted, compared to the present effort.

Data in Table 17.1 show the associations of white with analgesic action, lavender with hallucinogenic effect, and both orange and yellow with stimulant–antidepressant action. Dark red, dark blue, and light green appeared to have undifferentiated associations and, therefore, are unlikely to enhance drug efficacy. Gray capsules were typically related to unknown effects and should also detract from drug efficacy. Dark green had a weak analgesic association, black had a weak stimulant association, and light blue had a weak depressant–sedative association. If only the four active classifications are considered, and if the 12 capsule colors are condensed to a single group, no response bias would be evident, enhancing the reliability of these findings.

Advertising often suggests the greater "power" of a capsule compared to a tablet due to time-release potentials. An early effort noted by Haas and co-workers[15] found capsules superior to tablets, although Nash[16] noted only slight differences between the two. Task 3 specifically compared a capsule and tablet, controlling for quantity, in terms of perceived strength. Potential distortion in a forced-choice situation was reduced by allowing a judgment of equal strength. Table 17.2 data indicate a clear choice of the capsule as more powerful. These data suggest that the capsule form of a preparation should enhance the efficacy of a drug.

REFERENCES

1. Rachman J, Philips C. A new medical psychology. New Scientist 1975;65(938):518–520.
2. Ross S, Buckalew LW. On the agentry of placebos. Am Psychol 1979;34:277–278.
3. Shapiro AK. Semantics of the placebo. Psychiatr Q 1968;42:653–695.
4. Shapiro AK, Wilensky H, Struening EL. Study of the placebo effect with a placebo test. Compr Psychiatry 1968;9:118–137.
5. Buckalew LW, Ross S. Relationship of perceptual characteristics to efficacy of placebos. Psychol Rep 1981;49:955–961.
6. Lasagna L. Placebos. Sci Am 1955;193(2):68–71.
7. Berg AO. Placebos: a brief review for family physicians. J Fam Pract 1977;5:97–100.
8. Buckalew LW, Ross S, Starr BJ. Nonspecific factors in drug effects: placebo personality. Psychol Rep 1981;48:3–8.
9. Blackwell B, Bloomfield SS, Buncher CR. Demonstration to medical students of placebo responses and non-drug factors. Lancet 1972;1:1279–1282.
10. Adams FM, Osgood CE. A cross-cultural study of the affective meanings of color. J Cross-Cult Psychol 1973;4:135–156.
11. Jacobs KW, Nordan FM. Classification of placebo drugs: effect of color. Percept Mot Skills 1979;49:367–372.
12. Buckalew LW, Pearson WH. Determination of critical observed frequencies in chi-square. Bull Psychon Soc 1981;18(5):289–290.
13. Evans FJ. The placebo response in pain reduction. Adv Neurol 1974;4:289–295.

14. Schapira K, McClelland HA, Griffiths NR, Newell DJ. Study on the effects of tablet colour in the treatment of anxiety states. Br Med J 1970;2:446–449.

15. Haas H, Fink H, Härtfelder G. Das Placeboproblem. Fortschr Arzneimittelforsch 1959;1:279–454 ([English version in:] Psychopharmacol Serv Cent Bull 1963;2:1–65).

16. Nash H. Psychologic effects of amphetamines and barbiturates. J Nerv Ment Dis 1962;134(3):203–217.

18

Clinicians' Expectations Influence Placebo Analgesia

RICHARD H. GRACELY, RONALD DUBNER, WILLIAM R. DEETER, AND PATRICIA J. WOLSKEE

Richard H. Gracely, Ronald Dubner, William R. Deeter, and Patricia J. Wolskee, "Clinicians' Expectations Influence Placebo Analgesia," Lancet 1985;325(8419):43.

Administration of an inert substance may produce potent analgesia. The magnitude of this placebo effect depends on several factors, including the probability and potency of the expected analgesia.[1] However, few studies have examined the influence of the placebo administrator. We show here that the clinician's knowledge of the range of possible treatments may be transmitted to the patient and influence placebo efficacy in a conventional double-blind study.

Sixty dental patients took part in this study after signing a consent form approved by a clinical research review committee at the National Institutes of Health. After unilateral extraction of an upper and lower third molar under 2% lignocaine anaesthesia without a vasoconstrictor, patients assessed their pain with the McGill pain questionnaire at 1 hour and at 10 min, before and after an intravenous injection or no treatment (n = 14).[2] The patients were told that they might receive a placebo (saline), a narcotic analgesic (fentanyl, 1.1 µg/kg), or a narcotic antagonist (naloxone, 10 mg) and that these medications might decrease their pain, increase it, or have no effect. The clinicians administering the drugs and questionnaire knew that group PN would receive only placebo (n = 8) or naloxone (n = 5) and not fentanyl and that group PNF would receive fentanyl (n = 18) as well as placebo (n = 18) or naloxone (n = 11). All drugs were administered double blind.

The figure shows the effects of placebo in groups PN and PNF after 10 and 60 min. Pain after placebo administration in group PNF was significantly less than pain after placebo in group PN at 60 min (t[23 df] = 3.56, p < 0.01).

The two placebo groups differed only in the clinicians' knowledge of the range of possible double-blind treatments. This knowledge may result in subtle behaviours that influence patient responsiveness to a possible analgesic manipulation. This experiment supports previous findings that

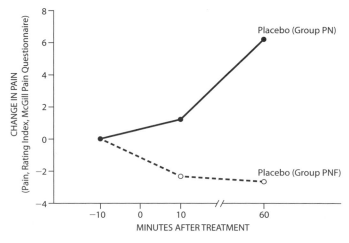

Figure 18.1. Change in pain rating index between baseline (10 min before injection) and 10 and 60 min after administration of placebo. PN = group that could have received either placebo or naloxone; PNF = group that could have received placebo, naloxone, or fentanyl.

clinical analgesia depends not only on the physiological action of the treatment administered but also on the expectations of patient and clinician.

REFERENCES

1. Evans FJ. Expectancy, therapeutic instructions, and the placebo response. In: White L, Tursky B, Schwartz GE, eds. Placebo: Theory, Research, and Mechanisms. New York: The Guilford Press, 1985, pp. 215–228.

2. Melzack R, ed. Pain Measurement and Assessment. New York: Raven Press, 1983.

SECTION B. PSYCHOLOGICAL MECHANISM

19

The Role of Conditioning and Verbal Expectancy in the Placebo Response

NICHOLAS J. VOUDOURIS, CONNIE L. PECK, AND GRAHAME COLEMAN

Nicholas J. Voudouris, Connie L. Peck, and Grahame Coleman, "The Role of Conditioning and Verbal Expectancy in the Placebo Response," Pain 1990;43:121–128.

Introduction

Although the placebo effect has been described for centuries in clinical practice and has been demonstrated in numerous studies, it is still not well understood theoretically. As a result, placebos continue to be considered "non-specific" in their effect. This gap in our knowledge means that the considerable promise which the placebo effect holds for pain control remains unfulfilled. Without an adequate understanding of exactly how and why placebo phenomena occur, we cannot appropriately use placebos on their own or increase the efficacy of treatments by enhancing their placebo components. Indeed, until the underlying mechanisms of the placebo response are better understood, our potential for maximizing the effectiveness of all therapies will remain underutilized.

Over the past 20 years, various models have been proposed to explain the placebo effect. Two that have received attention in recent years are the conditioning model [27] and the expectancy model [11]. As will be discussed below, these two models overlap to some extent; their main difference is one of emphasis—the conditioning model gives priority to the importance of learning through direct experience and the expectancy model places greater emphasis on the importance of verbal expectancy.

The idea that placebo responses are conditioned through classical conditioning has been suggested by a number of authors [7,8,12,24], but the concept was most fully developed by Wickramasekera [27]. The model is based on Pavlov's [16] classic discoveries during his work on digestive secretion in dogs. Pavlov noticed that his dogs were salivating *before* they saw their food, for example, as soon as they saw the food container. He reasoned that neutral stimuli must be acquiring the ability to elicit a specific response through repeated pairing with a stimulus which naturally elicited the response. Pavlov then presented the dogs with a new neutral stimulus (the sound of a bell) just before their food was presented. As he anticipated, after a number of pairings, the dogs began to salivate to the sound of the bell. Pavlov concluded that classical conditioning occurs through the temporal association of a neutral stimulus, such as a bell, with an unconditioned stimulus, such as food.

When applied to the placebo phenomenon, neutral, non-active stimuli may acquire an ameliorative effect through repeated association with stimuli which have a proven ameliorative effect. For example, a headache sufferer who regularly takes aspirin to obtain pain relief may eventually begin to respond to a neutral stimulus which has similar characteristics to aspirin. In other words, white pills which look like aspirin and which taste like aspirin (but which are pharmacologically neutral) might act to provide pain relief through classical conditioning. Thus, Wickramasekera [27] argues that placebo responses are conditioned through the association of neutral places, persons or things (for example, the hospital, the doctor, pills, injections) with effective treatment. After repeated association, these places, persons or things may themselves take on an ameliorative effect, as they become conditioned.

Evidence for the applicability of the classical conditioning model to the placebo effect comes primarily from work with animals [7,8,13,16,17,19,20,21,28]. Indeed, Pavlov was again the first to report this when he conditioned a tone with apomorphine and, after a number of associations, was able to produce the active symptoms of the drug to the sound of the tone. Other studies have reported drug-mimicking responses to saline following the repeated administration of anticholinergic drugs [13], insulin [17,21], scopolamine hydrobromide [8], and morphine [16].

A few studies have also reported successful attempts to condition placebo responses in humans [12,14,25,26]. Our own studies [25,26] have shown that subjects can be conditioned to give a placebo response after the repeated pairing of a placebo cream with reduced pain stimulation using an experimental pain paradigm.

In contrast to the conditioning model, the expectancy model is derived from expectancy theory [4,5,10,11,18,22,23] in which a person's specific expectations for what will happen in a given situation are a primary determinant of what he or she will experience. Kirsch [11] argues that placebo effects are based on the individual's response expectancies for automatic responses, such as pain.

The two models, however, are not mutually exclusive. They have some degree of overlap since response expectancies can be developed through conditioning. Nonetheless, Kirsch [11] argues in favour of the expectancy model by pointing out that response expectancies can also be learned in other ways, through verbal persuasion, modelling, self-observation or attributional processes. He presents a number of studies in which response expectancy effects are inconsistent with a conditioning hypothesis. While acknowledging the overlap between conditioning and expectancy and recognizing that expectancies may enhance the acquisition or credibility of a conditioned response, Wickramasekera [27] argues that learning is more effective through direct experience without such expectancies. As evidence, he cites a number of studies in which learning occurred without awareness.

This debate, however, is more than a theoretical one and has important clinical implications for the use of placebos on their own or as controls in evaluations of therapeutic agents. If, indeed, verbal expectancy and direct experience affect the placebo response differently, this would have implications for how placebos are administered or how experiments involving placebo controls are set up and interpreted.

This study, therefore, undertakes to examine the relative contribution of direct experience and verbal expectancy in creating a placebo response. The current study manipulated these variables, alone and in combination, using four experimental groups. The first group received both expectancy and conditioning. The second group was given expectancy alone. The third group experienced conditioning alone. The fourth group served as a control.

To examine the placebo effects, all four groups were subsequently tested on their responses to experimental pain stimulation, administered with and without the neutral placebo cream. An experimental analogue similar to the one used in our previous studies [25,26] was employed.

Methods

Subjects

Forty subjects, 21 females and 19 males, participated in this study. The subjects were predominantly university students who responded to an advertisement in the campus newsletter. Their ages ranged from 18 to 46 years. Before participating, all subjects completed a consent form which explained the nature of the noxious stimulation and warned people with heart conditions, hypertension or those on medication, not to take part. Subjects were told that they could withdraw from the experiment at any time should they wish to do so.

Apparatus

IONTOPHORETIC PAIN

Noxious stimulation was administered using a modified iontophoretic pain generator. Iontophoresis, by the repulsion of positive potassium ions from the positive pole of an electric (DC) current, drives these ions into the skin, causing a prickling sensation at lower levels of stimulation and a cramping sensation at higher levels. The degree of noxious stimulation is dependent on the amount of current and the duration of administration and is independent of skin resistance [3].

The apparatus consisted of a plastic clamp, which was attached to the flexor surface of the forearm and which incorporates a small bowl on the upper surface. The bowl uses the surface of the arm as its base and is filled with a 3% solution of potassium chloride (the contact medium between the electrode and skin). Enclosed within the bowl is a metal anode plate. A gauze pad saturated with a 9% solution of sodium chloride wrapped around a silver-silver chloride cathode plate is placed on the surface of the arm. This gauze base acts as an insulator. The DC current is increased or decreased to the desired level by manipulating a potentiometer on the console. An electronic display gives a constant readout on the level of stimulation, measured in milliampere (mA). The duration of each stimulus is preset via a built-in timer (set at 1 sec in this study).

VISUAL ANALOG SCALE

Subjects were provided with a series of standard 100 mm graphic visual analog scales (VAS) and a fine-point pencil to mark the scales with their judgement of pain intensity. The end points of the VAS were labelled "no pain" (left) and "extreme pain" (right).

PLACEBO

The placebo analgesic was in the form of a cream. Simple cold cream was mixed with linalol, which contained rubdown cream in the ratio of 8:1 to give the cream a distinct smell. It was pink in colour. The cream was removed with cotton, soaked in a 70% alcohol solution.

Table 19.1.
Experimental design

Session 1 (expectancy manipulation)	Session 2 (pain test 1)*	Session 3 (conditioning manipulation)	Session 4 (pain test 2)*
Expectancy		Conditioning (group 1)	
		No conditioning (group 2)	
No Expectancy		Conditioning (group 3)	
		No conditioning (group 4)	

Note: * Pain tests 1 and 2: 5 trials × mA = 50 mm VAS (with placebo cream); 5 trials × mA = 50 mm VAS (without placebo cream). [VAS = visual analog scales—eds.]

Experimental Design

Table 19.1 shows the experimental design which compared four groups. All subjects attended four sessions on four consecutive days. In the first session, half of the subjects were informed that the cream was a powerful analgesic and would provide pain relief (expectancy) and the other half were informed that the cream was neutral (no expectancy). On the second session, the subjects received a neutral cream (placebo) on half the trials and the other half were given none (no placebo). All subjects were then tested for a placebo response using the experimental pain stimulus. On the third session, half the subjects in each of the Expectancy and No Expectancy groups received conditioning in which the pain stimulus was reduced after the cream was applied (conditioned placebo), while the other half received the same pain stimulus (no conditioning). This manipulation yielded four groups varying in expectancy and conditioning.

Procedure

All subjects were seen at the same time of day. At the beginning of each session, the subject was seated in a comfortable chair in a testing chamber divided by a one-way mirror. This allowed the experimenter to keep direct contact with the subject to an absolute minimum, and to view the subject without being visible. An intercom with a headset permitted conversation between the experimenter and subject when necessary; otherwise the experimenter made contact with the subject only during the administration or removal of the cream, or at the request of the subject. The experimenter wore a white lab coat at all times to enhance credibility. Next, the apparatus was attached and the subject read a set of instructions while listening to an explanatory audio tape. Each session was structured as follows:

SESSION 1: VERBAL MANIPULATION AND CALIBRATION OF VAS LEVELS

Prior to the commencement of testing, each subject completed a consent form which contained the verbal manipulation as part of the instructions about the nature of the experiment. There were two versions of the form, one for subjects in groups 1 and 2 (which instructed them to expect that the cream was a powerful analgesic which would provide pain relief) and one for subjects in groups 3 and 4 (which told them that they were in a control group which was using a neutral cream and that they should expect no relief).

This was followed by a questionnaire which asked subjects to rate how often they have used analgesics, how effective analgesics have been for them, their past use of commercially available analgesic cream, whether they have found analgesic creams to be effective and whether they expected this cream to be effective. The purpose of this question was as a manipulation check to determine whether the expectancy manipulation had been effective. The question assessing their expectancy was embedded in a series of other questions to enhance the validity of the experiment and to disguise the purpose of the questionnaire.

Because of the large individual differences in pain responsivity to the same stimuli, we decided to follow our previous practice [25] of using equivalent pain-rating levels for each subject rather than equivalent intensity of stimulation. This ensures that each subject is receiving a subjectively similar level of pain stimulation and a subjectively similar reduction in pain stimulation and the procedure allows a more meaningful interpretation of the data. Stimulation levels were calculated in session 1 and mA levels equivalent to each subject's 25 mm and 50 mm position on the visual analog scale were used in all subsequent sessions. Further, to enhance the reliability of each subject's pain ratings from session to session, end anchors were determined and presented at the beginning of subsequent sessions to familiarize subjects with their own previous ratings [1].

Thus, the rest of session 1 was devoted to calibration of the subject's use of the VAS against the equipment's range of possible stimulus intensities. A stepwise judgement procedure was undertaken in order to establish the subject's sensitivity and range. Stimuli were administered beginning at an intensity of 1 mA and each subsequent stimulus was incremented in intensity by 5 mA until the subject recorded a judgement of 95 mm or greater. Subjects were instructed to complete a VAS for each pain stimulus and to place it in a slotted box after each trial to avoid comparison between trials. When the subject recorded 95 mm on the VAS, the experimenter collected the VAS sheets from the slotted response box and made calculations of the subject's range while the subject rested.

A second step in the calibration method involved a procedure described by Anderson [1] to maximize the reliability of subjects' VAS judgements and to minimize "end effects" in the use of the VAS. The end anchors consisted of two stimuli. The first, 0 mA, was administered with the instruction that it would be the least painful stimulus received and that the subject should consider it to be the bottom anchor (0 mm) on the VAS. An additional 4 mA was arbitrarily added to the stimulus at which the subject had previously signalled a VAS judgement of 95 mm to establish the top anchor (at 100 mm) and to compensate for any possible downward shift which

might occur in subsequent trials. Subjects were told that this should be considered to be the top anchor (100 mm) on the VAS. The range of stimulation intensity across subjects for this anchor ranged from 22 to 37 mA.

As a final step in determining the iontophoretic settings which would with most reliability correspond to the two VAS intensities that were to be used for the rest of the experiment (i.e., 25 mm and 50 mm), a set of fifteen stimuli were randomly chosen from within the range of intensities established by the stepwise trials and bounded by the end anchors of each subject. These stimuli were then administered twice in randomized order and subjects were asked to record a judgement of painfulness for each. The resulting pain judgements were plotted against the record of stimulation intensities, to allow an approximate line of best fit to be calculated for each subject. From this function, the stimulation intensities most closely corresponding to 25 mm and 50 mm VAS judgements were recorded for use in subsequent sessions. These individual levels were used for each subject during all further sessions. The between-subject range for the 25 mm VAS was 8–14 mA; the range for the 50 mm VAS was 16–26 mA.

SESSION 2: TEST 1

Session 2 involved testing the subject's pain responses with and without the placebo cream to determine the effect of the expectancy manipulation. Although subjects had experienced the noxious stimulation in session 1 as part of the calibration process, this represented their first experience with the placebo cream. The subject was seated, made comfortable and the apparatus prepared as previously described. The subject was asked to read a set of instructions in conjunction with an explanatory audio tape. End anchors determined in session 1 were administered to refer the subject to his previous anchor points in order to increase the intersession reliability.

The main part of the session involved five pain trials with the placebo cream and five pain trials without the placebo cream. Each pain trial consisted of one iontophoretic stimulus at the mA value which matched the subject's 50 mm VAS score. The order of no-placebo and placebo trials was randomized within each group to protect against order effects in the data.

The iontophoretic pain trials were separated by a gap of 20 sec, with the exception of trials where the cream was applied or removed. On these occasions, there was a break of 5 min duration, to allow time for the cream to "take effect" or in the case of removal, for its effect to "wear off."

SESSION 3: CONDITIONING

In this session subjects were prepared as above, instructions were given and end anchors administered. Each subject received ten pain trials under each of the placebo and the no-placebo conditions. Ten trials were used because repeated pairings are necessary for conditioning to occur. All subjects received an intensity that corresponded to their VAS judgement of 50 mm during the no-placebo (no cream) trials. For subjects in groups 1 and 3, the intensity of stimulation during placebo trials was reduced to their 25 mm VAS level. These stimulation intensities were manipulated without the subject's knowledge. Groups 2 and 4 continued to receive a stimulation level equal to their 50 mm VAS judgement during both placebo and no-placebo trials.

SESSION 4: TEST 2

Session 4 involved a second test of the subject's pain response with and without the placebo cream in order to assess the effects of the conditioning manipulation. The procedures for test 2 were identical to those in test 1. Following refamiliarization with their end anchors, subjects were given five trials with and five trials without the placebo cream; these were presented in random order. As in test 1, pain stimulation was set at the value which corresponded to the subject's 50 mm VAS for all trials.

A final meeting, at which the actual purpose of the experiment was explained, was held at the end of the study to debrief subjects.

Results

The pre-test measure of expectancy, intended as a manipulation check, suggested that the expectancy manipulation included in the instructions had the effect of creating the desired expectancies. Those who were told that the cream was a powerful analgesic (groups 1 and 2) reported an expectancy that it would be effective and those who were told that they were in a control group (groups 3 and 4) reported expecting little or no effect. This difference was significant (t = 10.67, df = 38, P < 0.001).

Means for the four groups are shown in Fig. 19.1. For the purpose of data analysis, the design was reduced to a 2-factor design by using placebo minus no placebo difference scores in pain ratings as the dependent variable. The data were analyzed using six a priori comparisons based on these difference scores. The comparisons were chosen to explore the hypotheses of interest. The repeated factor error term was used for comparisons within tests. For comparisons between tests for particular groups, the within cell error terms were pooled [9]. Although the actual power of the tests varied with each contrast, the obtained power for the overall group by placebo condition interaction was 1−β = 0.97. The power for the overall group effect was 1−β = 0.90 [9].

The first planned contrast was between the expectancy manipulation (groups 1 and 2 at test 1) and the no expectancy manipulation (groups 3 and 4 at test 1) and showed no difference (F_{1,35} = 2.15). The second comparison between the Conditioning group (group 3 at test 2) and the control group (group 4 at test 2) showed an effect in favour of the Conditioning group (F_{1,35} = 19.70, P < 0.001). The third comparison between the Combined group (group 1 at test 2) and the control group (group 4 at test 2) also showed a significant result in favour of the Combined group (F_{1,35} = 25.18, P < 0.001). The fourth test

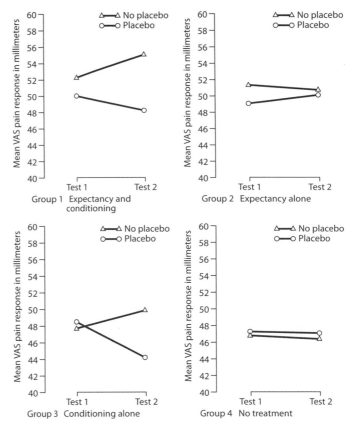

Fig. 19.1. Mean VAS score between placebo and no-placebo conditions for each group.

compared the expectancy manipulation (group 2 at test 1) and the conditioning manipulation (group 3 at test 2) and found that conditioning was significantly better than expectancy (F_{1,35} = 14.03, P < 0.001). The fifth contrast compared the Combined group (group 1 and test 2) with the Expectancy group (group 2 as test 1) and found that the Combined group was significantly better than the Expectancy group (F_{1,35} = 7.70, P < 0.01). The last contrast between the Combined group (group 1 at test 2) and the Conditioning group (group 3 at test 2) showed no significant difference (F_{1,35} = 0.34).

In summary, the Conditioning group (group 3) and the Combined group (group 1) showed a placebo effect, but the Expectancy group (group 2) did not. The Combined group (group 1) and the Conditioning group (group 3) were both superior to the Expectancy group (group 2), but not different from each other.

Discussion

This study replicated our previous finding that placebo responses can be conditioned in the laboratory [25,26]. In attempting to assess the relative contributions of expectancy and conditioning, results from the design used in this study suggest that the direct experience of conditioning appears to be more powerful than verbal expectancy formed through verbal persuasion, at least within the paradigm used here.

While it is tempting to enter into the debate between the two models, the distinctions may be overdrawn. Even in the case of group 3, conditioning probably created a response expectancy which may have enhanced the effect of future trials. Indeed, as Bandura [2] has suggested in other contexts, it may be the case that expectations are shaped more strongly by experience than by verbal persuasion. In retrospect, it would have been interesting and perhaps revealing to have repeated the expectancy questionnaire at the end of session 3 to determine the effects of direct experience on expectancy for all groups, both for those whose expectancy was matched by direct experience and those whose expectancy was violated.

The most important implications of this study, however, pertain to the classical conditioning model proposed by Wickramasekera [27] which predicts that interventions which use "active" ingredients will be more potent in inducing placebo responses than those which do not. During the conditioning sessions in groups 1 and 3, the placebo cream was repeatedly paired with reduction in pain stimulation to produce the association needed for conditioning. When this situation was compared with that of the group 2 subjects where the cream was not paired with pain reduction, the prediction was supported.

The importance of this association was also found by Laska and Sunshine [15] in a clinical setting with patients suffering from moderate to severe post-operative, fracture and somatic pain. In this study varying doses of analgesic were followed by a placebo. The time-effect curves for the placebo show that patients' placebo responses corresponded in degree of pain relief to their original dosage of analgesic (although as conditioning theory would predict, they were slightly less than their responses to the analgesic itself). What these authors termed a "psychological carryover effect" seems to be the result of classical conditioning. The poor response of subjects who were given a placebo on both administrations suggests that expectancy alone did not play as significant a part as direct experience.

These results have some important implications for within-subject crossover designs involving placebos. The data suggest that subjects receiving placebos before the administration of an analgesic might not be equivalent to subjects receiving placebos after the administration of an analgesic, since subjects receiving placebos first would be responding to verbal expectation, whereas subjects receiving placebos second would be likely to be responding to both verbal expectation and conditioning.

This issue also has relevance to the administration of placebos on their own for a therapeutic purpose. These findings suggest that the best way to administer placebo treatment (if it is to be used) is to pair it (in the first instance) with an active treatment which reduces the patient's symptoms. Such a procedure would seem to be more effective than merely telling the patient that a given placebo treatment will be beneficial. What we did not test, however, is how long such an effect might last and what the optimum parameters of the conditioning paradigm might be. Presumably, the extensive literature on classical conditioning would be able to offer some useful ideas which could be used to design an optimum combination of "active" and placebo treatments. Indeed, the success of the widely used pain cocktail [6] may, in part, be attributable to this operation.

An unexplained finding, which has also occurred in our two previous studies [25,26] was a corresponding, but opposite change in subjects' responses under the no-placebo condition, with pain report increasing from pre-test to post-test in the no-placebo condition for groups 1 and 3 (the two groups which received conditioning). This effect does not occur in groups 2 and 4 (the groups with no conditioning) where the no-placebo conditions seem to decrease slightly in the direction of the mean. Although the planned contrasts chosen for this design did not allow an analysis of the statistical significance of these data, the trend which is evident in all three studies suggests that conditioned placebo responses seem to be having an effect on pain report when the placebo is not administered, as well as when it is. If this finding generalizes to the clinical situation, this apparent adverse effect may have some interesting implications for short-term symptomatic treatment and may even help to explain the worsening symptoms that are sometimes observed in stable chronic disorders (e.g., chronic pain) when multiple short-term palliative treatments are tried and then abandoned.

Conclusion

Our data confirm that placebo responses can be conditioned and suggest that conditioning based on direct experience with pain reduction may be more powerful in establishing a placebo response than expectancies created by verbal instruction. While conditioning may also operate through expectancies, it seems that direct experience with pain relief is more powerful than an expectancy conveyed verbally. These results have important implications for maximizing placebo effects.

REFERENCES

1. Anderson, N.H., Methods of Information Integration Theory, Academic Press, New York, 1982.
2. Bandura, A., Self-efficacy: toward a unifying theory of behavioral change, Psychol. Rev., 84 (1977) 191–215.
3. Benjamin, F.B. and Helvey, W.M., Iontophoresis of potassium for experimental determination of pain endurance in man, Proc. Soc. Exp. Biol. Med., 113 (1963) 566–588.
4. Bootzin, R.R., The role of expectancy in behavior change. In: L. White, B. Tursky and G.E. Schwartz (Eds.), Placebo: Theory, Research and Mechanisms, Guilford Press, New York, 1985, pp. 196–211.
5. Evans, F.J., Expectancy, therapeutic instructions and the placebo response. In: L. White, B. Tursky and G.E. Schwartz (Eds.), Placebo: Theory, Research and Mechanisms, Guilford Press, New York, 1985, pp. 215–229.
6. Fordyce, W.E., Behavioral Methods for Chronic Pain and Illness, Mosby, St. Louis, Mo., 1976.
7. Gliedman, L.H., Gantt, W.H. and Teitlebaum, H.A., Some implications of conditioned reflex studies for placebo research, Am. J. Psychiatry, 113 (1957) 1103–1107.
8. Herrnstein, R.J., Placebo effect in the rat, Science, 139 (1962) 677–678.
9. Kirk, R., Experimental Design: Procedures for the Behavioral Sciences, Brooks/Cole, Belmont, Calif., 1968.

10. Kirsch, I., The placebo effect and the cognitive-behavioural revolution, Cogn. Ther. Res., 2 (1978) 255–264.
11. Kirsch, I., Response expectancy as a determinant of experience and behavior, Am. Psychol., 40 (1985) 1189–1202.
12. Knowles, J.B., Conditioning and the placebo effect, Behav. Res. Ther., 1 (1963) 151–157.
13. Lang, W.J., Brown, M.L., Gershon, S. and Korol, B., Classical and physiologic adaptive conditioned responses to anticholinergic drugs in conscious dogs, Int. J. Neuropharmacol., 5 (1986) 311–315.
14. Lang, W. and Rand, M., A placebo response as a conditioned reflex to glyceryl trinitrate, Med. J. Aust., 1 (1969) 912–914.
15. Laska, E. and Sunshine, A., Anticipation of analgesia: a placebo effect, Headache, 13 (1973) 1–11.
16. Pavlov, I.P., Conditioned Reflexes (G.V. Anrep, Trans.), Oxford Univ. Press, London, 1927.
17. Reiss, W.J., Conditioning of a hyperinsulin type of behaviour in the white rat, Science, 51 (1958) 301–303.
18. Ross, M. and Olson, J., An expectancy-attribution model of the effects of placebos, Psychol. Rev., 88 (1981) 408–437.
19. Sherman. J.E., Proctor, C. and Strub, H., Prior hot plate exposure enhances morphine analgesia in tolerant and drug-naive rats, Pharmacol. Biochem. Behav., 17 (1982) 229–232.
20. Siegel. S., Evidence from rats that morphine tolerance is a learned response, J. Comp. Physiol. Psychol., 89 (1975) 498–506.
21. Siegel, S., Drug-anticipatory responses in animals. In: L. White, B. Tursky and G.E. Schwartz (Eds.), Placebo: Theory, Research and Mechanisms, Guilford Press, New York, 1985, pp. 288–305.
22. Stotland, E., The Psychology of Hope, Jossey-Bass, San Francisco, Calif., 1969.
23. Suedfeld, P., The subtractive expectancy placebo procedure: a measure of non-specific factors in behavioural interventions, Behav. Res. Ther., 22 (1984) 159–164.
24. Ullman, L.P. and Krasner, F., Cognitions and behavior, Behav. Ther., 1 (1969) 201–204.
25. Voudouris, N.J., Peck, C.L. and Coleman, G.J., Conditioned placebo responses, J. Pers. Soc. Psychol., 48 (1985) 47–53.
26. Voudouris, N.J., Peck, C.L. and Coleman, G.J., Conditioned response models of placebo phenomena: further support, Pain, 38 (1989) 109–116.
27. Wickramasekera, I., A conditioned response model of the placebo effect: predictions from the model, Biofeedback Self-Regul., 5 (1980) 5–18.
28. Wikler, A., Pescor, F.T., Miller, D. and Norrell, H., Persistent potency of a secondary (conditioned) reinforcer following withdrawal of morphine from physically dependent rats, Psychopharmacologia (Berl.), 20 (1971) 103–117.

20

Classical Conditioning and the Placebo Effect

GUY H. MONTGOMERY AND IRVING KIRSCH

Guy H. Montgomery and Irving Kirsch, "Classical Conditioning and the Placebo Effect," Pain 1997;72:107–113.

1. Classical Conditioning and the Placebo Effect

Although effects of placebos are well established (Kirsch, 1997), the mechanisms by which those effects are produced have only recently been seriously investigated. Hypothesized mechanisms include enhanced endorphin release (Levine et al., 1978), reduced anxiety (Sternbach, 1968), classical conditioning (Wickramasekera, 1980), and response expectancy (Kirsch, 1985, 1990). Montgomery and Kirsch (1996) reported data that are difficult to reconcile with the hypothesis that placebo responses are mediated by such global mechanisms as anxiety reduction or the release of endogenous opioids. They obtained a placebo effect by administering the placebo in the guise of a local anesthetic and applying a pain stimulus to treated and untreated parts of the body. Because the pain stimulus was applied simultaneously to both the treated (by placebo) and untreated locations, the differences in reported pain could not have been due to any global changes in sensitivity, perception, or affect. Conversely, this placebo effect can be explained both by classical conditioning and response expectancy hypotheses.

According to stimulus substitution models of placebo effects (Herrnstein, 1962; Ader, 1988; Wickramasekera, 1980; Turkkan, 1989), active treatments are unconditional stimuli (USs) and the vehicles in which they are delivered (i.e., pills, capsules, syringes, etc.) are conditional stimuli (CSs). The medical treatments that people experience during their lives constitute conditioning trials, during which the vehicles are paired with their active ingredients. These pairings endow the pills, capsules, and injections with the capacity to evoke therapeutic effects as conditional responses (CRs).

Note that these models are based on a Pavlovian, stimulus substitution conception of conditioning. Research in the broader field of classical conditioning has led to the replacement of stimulus substitution models by a conception of conditioning phenomena that is consistent with expectancy theory (Rescorla, 1988). An example of the kind of data leading to the rejection of stimulus substitution models is the finding that under certain circumstances, the pairing of a CS with a US does not lead to associative learning. The common feature of these circumstances is the fact that the information value of the CS as a predictor of the US is masked. For example, if the US has a high base rate of occurrence in the absence of the CS, the effect of US-CS pairings can be negligible. Data of this sort have led contemporary theorists to describe conditioning as the learning of relations between events. Conditioning leads to the acquisition of expectancies that certain events will follow other events, and its occurrence depends on "the information that the CS provides about the US" (Rescorla, 1988, p. 153), rather than on contiguity. The unconditional response (UR) can be viewed as an anticipatory response that prepares the organism for the occurrence of the anticipated US (Siegel, 1983). The response may be compensatory (e.g., when performance inhibition is anticipated) or preparatory (e.g., when food is anticipated).

The informational view of classical conditioning can be applied to placebo phenomena (see Kirsch, 1990, 1997). Doing so begins with the premise that for a stimulus to function as a US, it has to be perceived. But the active nature of a drug, with which its vehicle is paired, is perceived only by its effects. Therefore, in terms of information value, the drug response is the US, rather than the UR. What is learned during conditioning is that active drugs produce particular effects. Thus, classical conditioning is one means by which the response expectancies are acquired (Kirsch, 1990).

The question that is not answered by a cognitive interpretation of classical conditioning is how expectancies produce the expected responses. Kirsch has hypothesized that response expectancies, defined as the anticipation of non-volitional responses, are capable of eliciting the expected response in much the same way that intentions elicit voluntary behaviors (cf. Ajzen and Fishbein, 1980). Because conscious thoughts and feelings are covert stimuli and responses (Hull, 1930), response expectancies can be thought of as unconditional stimuli for corresponding subjective experiences (covert responses). The effect of placebos depends on the strength of the person's expectancies, not on how those expectations were formed. The neurobiology of the effects of expectancies and intentions remains to be established.

Conditioned enhancement of placebo pain responses has been demonstrated in a series of studies by Voudouris et al. (1985, 1989, 1990). In each of these studies, Voudouris et al. reported enhanced placebo effects following a series of conditioning trials, during which the intensity of a pain stimulus was surreptitiously lowered when paired with placebo administration, and in one of the studies (Voudouris et al., 1990), they reported that this conditioning effect was greater than that of a verbal expectancy manipulation. From a cognitive perspective, conditioning trials are themselves expectancy manipulations. So what was demonstrated by Voudouris et al. (1990) can be interpreted as indicating that conditioning trials are more effective than at least some verbal manipulations in altering expectancies, a finding that had previously been reported by expectancy theorists (Wickless and Kirsch, 1989).

The purpose of the present study was to provide a test of conflicting predictions derived from stimulus substitution and expectancy models of conditioned placebo effects. We did this in two ways. Firstly, in addition to replicating the conditioning procedure used by Voudouris et al., we added an informed pairing condition, in which participants were told that the stimulus intensity was being lowered during conditioning trials. If the conditioning effect demonstrated by Voudouris et al. (1985, 1989, 1990) is a direct consequence of CS-US pairings, it should not be hindered by informing participants of the manipulation. Conversely, if the conditioning effect is mediated by expectancy, non-deceptive pairings should fail to produce conditioning. We also included an extinction condition. According to the stimulus substitution model of placebo effects, repeated administration of a placebo should weaken its effects (Wickramasekera, 1980). In contrast, from an informational perspective, the effect of a treatment is the US that reinforces expectancies. Thus, placebo effects should confirm the expectancies that generate them, thereby preventing extinction. Unlike Voudouris et al. (1985, 1989, 1990), we also assessed pain response expectancies after the experimental manipulations, so as to evaluate the extent to which changes in reported pain were preceded by changes in expected pain.

2. Method

2.1. Participants

Participants were 24 female and 24 male undergraduate students, ranging in age from 18 to 26 years old, who volunteered to participate in exchange for partial course credit and who reported an absence of medical conditions and medication use that might interfere with pain sensitivity or pose an increased risk of resultant tissue damage. These conditions and medications were: high blood pressure, circulatory problems (e.g., Reynaud's disease or family history of the same), diabetes, heart disease or any other heart problems, asthma, seizures, frostbite, past trauma to hands, lupus erythematosus, arthritis, other large or small joint disease or injury, or use of psychoactive drugs, analgesics, antihistamines, and anti-inflammatory medications. Participants were randomly assigned to groups with the restriction that there would be the same proportions of males and females in each condition.

2.2. Setting and Materials

Pain was generated by an iontophoretic pain stimulator modeled closely after the apparatus used by Voudouris et al. (1985, 1990). Iontophoresis is the driving of ions into a participant's skin with electric current. The intensity of the pain stimulus is dependent on the amount and duration of electric current utilized. Iontophoresis of potassium ions causes a prickling sensation at lower intensities and a cramping sensation at higher intensities (Voudouris et al., 1985, 1989, 1990). The effect has been shown to be independent of skin resistance (Benjamin and Helvey, 1963).

Our iontophoretic pain stimulator was powered by a series of 12-volt direct current (DC) batteries. The console was separate from the battery pack to provide increased maneuverability of the apparatus. The console contained controls for intensity and duration of electric current and a battery monitor to provide an easy check on battery levels. A cylinder was attached to participants' arms with Velcro strips, such that the skin on the ventral side of the forearm formed the bottom of a cup. The interior of the cylinder (cup) contained a platinum anode. When filled with 3% potassium chloride solution, the solution formed the contact between skin and anode. On the dorsal side of the middle forearm, a metal cathode was covered by a 0.9% sodium chloride saturated gauze to complete the circuit. Wires attached the anode and cathode to the console. The apparatus could deliver a range of 0–50 mA of current.

The placebo was a mix of iodine, oil of thyme, and water which produced a brownish, medicinal-smelling effect when applied topically. The placebo was placed in a medicinal-looking bottle and labeled, "Trivaricane: approved for research purposes only." Placebo was applied to areas on the ventral part of the forearm surrounding the cylinder. A constant current source was incorporated in the apparatus to control for changes in skin conductance due to use of placebo and to ensure that differences in skin conductance would not be confounded with placebo treatment (Voudouris et al., 1985). An office in the University Health Center was used as the setting for the experiment to alleviate skepticism on the part of participants that might have been caused by prior associations with the psychology department.

2.3. Measures

2.3.1. PAIN INTENSITY SCALE

Participants were asked to rate the intensity of their pain on a visually presented, 11-point, analog scale, anchored with the captions "no pain" and "intolerable pain," for 0 and 10, respectively. Participants were shown the scale and responded by verbally stating the number on the scale corresponding to their experienced intensity of the pain.

2.3.2. PAIN EXPECTANCY MEASURE

Participants were asked, "What do you expect the pain intensity to be with the Trivaricane?" and "What do you expect the pain intensity to be without the Trivaricane?" Pain expectancy ratings were on an 11-point intensity scale with the same anchors as those on the pain intensity scale.

2.4. Procedure

Participants were greeted in the lobby of the University Health Center, escorted to an office by a research assistant, and introduced to the experimenter, who wore a white lab coat and was described as a "Behavioral Medicine Researcher." Participants were told that a new, topical local anesthetic was being tested for its pain-reducing effects. They were told

the drug's name was "Trivaricane," and that it had been proven effective in reducing pain in preliminary studies at other universities. The number of pain trials was described to each participant as part of the informed consent procedure. Participants were told they could discontinue participation at any time, without negative consequences. Those agreeing to participate then completed the medical screening form. Acceptable participants were randomly assigned to one of four groups: extinction, no treatment, informed pairing, or uninformed pairing.

The design of the study is depicted in Table 20.1. Participants in the informed pairing, uninformed pairing, and extinction groups experienced four blocks of pain trials (calibration trials, pretest trials, manipulation trials, and posttest trials). Participants in the no-treatment group did not participate in the block of manipulation trials. Calibration, pretest, and posttest trials were identical for all groups. Order of administration (placebo trials first or second) was counterbalanced during pretest, manipulation, and posttest trials.

2.4.1. CALIBRATION TRIALS

To control for individual differences in pain perception, a calibration procedure adapted from Voudouris et al. (1985) was utilized. In order to lessen the overall aversiveness of study participation, we decreased the number and intensity of calibration trials. Voudouris et al. (1985) increased ascending calibration trials until a subjective "10" on a 0–10 scale was reported by participants, and descending trials were followed by fifteen trials of randomly chosen stimulus intensity values sampled from each of their participant's 0 (no pain) to 10 (intolerable pain) range. In the present study, all participants were given an ascending series of pain stimulation trials, beginning at 1 mA and then increasing by 3 mA until the participant rated the pain intensity as 7 or higher. The highest mA level was then repeated and followed by a descending series of trials, each 3 mA less until reaching 1 mA. Pain trials were separated by approximately 5 s, and participants verbally rated pain intensity immediately following each trial. At the conclusion of calibration trials, a separate regression equation was calculated for each participant by imputing the verbal intensity ratings and their corresponding stimulus intensity levels in milliamperes. This was used to calculate the stimulus intensity level corresponding to each individual's rating of 6 and 3, as predicted by the regression equation. For brevity, these numbers will be used to indicate the corresponding stimulus intensity level, although this level differs between individual participants according to their personal perceptions of pain.

2.4.2. PRETEST

The pretest consisted of two trials with placebo and two trials without placebo. The mA setting during pretest was always equivalent to each participant's 6 for all trials. The medication was allowed at least 1 min to take effect and at least 1 min to wear off following cleaning of the skin with

Table 20.1.
Stimulation intensity as a function of experimental condition and trial block

Group	Pretest	Manipulation	Posttest
		Trial block	
No treatment			
Placebo trials	6	—	6
No-placebo trials	6	—	6
Extinction			
Placebo trials	6	6	6
No-placebo trials	6	6	6
Informed pairing			
Placebo trials	6	3	6
No-placebo trials	6	6	6
Uninformed pairing			
Placebo trials	6	3	6
No-placebo trials	6	6	6

Note: During the manipulation block, the intensity reduction on placebo trials was made explicit to the informed pairing group but not to the uninformed pairing group.

70% rubbing alcohol. Placebo was applied liberally with a cotton swab to areas on the forearm surrounding the cup.

2.4.3. MANIPULATION TRIALS

Three minutes after the conclusion of the pretest, manipulation trials were commenced. All participants in the extinction, informed pairing, and uninformed pairing groups received ten pain trials with placebo and ten without placebo. No-treatment participants waited for 5 min, following which, the posttest trials were administered. Stimulus intensity levels depended on group assignment. The uninformed pairing group replicated the conditioning groups of Voudouris et al. (1985, 1990). Participants received stimulation corresponding to their level 3 ratings on placebo trials and to their level 6 ratings on no-placebo trials. They were not informed that stimulus intensity levels were being altered. The informed pairing group was designed to test the importance of verbal information and expectancies in establishing placebo analgesia. Stimulus intensity levels were identical to those in the uninformed pairing group. However, unlike the uninformed pairing group, the informed pairing group was advised of the intensity reduction on placebo trials prior to the administration of the manipulation trials. The experimenter stated that the intensity would be reduced on medication trials to examine the effectiveness of Trivaricane at lower intensities. For the extinction group, both placebo and no-placebo trials had an intensity level corresponding to their rating of 6. Following completion of the manipulation trials, the expectancy measure was administered. Prior to its administration, informed pairing participants were told that the intensity level during medication trials would be raised to its original setting.

2.4.4. POSTTEST

Posttesting was begun 3 min after the conclusion of the manipulation trials. Procedurally, the posttest was identical to the pretest. For all participants, the intensity level remained at 6 for placebo and no-placebo trials. Participants were debriefed following completion of data collection.

3. Results

Following the procedures used by Voudouris et al. (1985, 1989, 1990), pain intensity ratings on trials with placebo were subtracted from pain intensity ratings on trials without placebo. The resulting placebo response score is the change in pain intensity rating due to placebo administration. Expected placebo response was calculated similarly (expected no-placebo pain ratings minus expected placebo pain ratings). Means and standard deviations of placebo responses and expected placebo responses as a function of group membership are presented in Table 20.2.

A t-test on pretest placebo response scores (mean = 0.29, SD = 1.02) indicated that these scores were significantly different than 0, $t_{(47)} = 1.97$, $P < .05$. This indicates that the creme produced a small but significant effect even prior to conditioning. A one-way analysis of variance on pretest placebo response scores failed to reveal any significant differences as a function of group assignment, $F_{(3,44)} = 0.20$, $P < 0.90$.

One-way analysis of covariance, with pretest placebo response as the covariate, revealed significant group differences for placebo response, $F_{(3,43)} = 5.62$, $P < 0.01$, and expected placebo response, $F_{(3,43)} = 17.95$, $P < 0.01$. Mean scores, adjusted for pretest placebo responses, are presented in Table 20.3. Tukey's HSD tests indicated that posttest placebo responses and expected placebo responses were significantly greater in the uninformed pairing group than in each of the other three groups, $P < 0.05$. No other comparisons between groups were significant.

Differences in posttest adjusted means could be due to improvement in some conditions or deterioration in others. Therefore, it was important to analyze within group changes as well as between group differences. Paired comparison t-tests revealed that the uninformed pairing group had greater placebo responses at posttest than at pretest, to $t_{(11)} = 2.81$, $P < 0.02$. Placebo responses did not change significantly in the extinction group, $t_{(11)} = -0.18$, $P < 0.86$, informed pairing group $t_{(11)} = -0.23$, $P < 0.83$, or no-treatment group $t_{(11)} = 0.77$, $P < 0.46$.

To test the hypothesis that changes in placebo response were mediated by expectancy, we added expectancy scores to the regression equation in the analysis of covariance of posttest placebo response scores. This analysis indicated that expectancy was significantly related to changes in placebo response, $F_{(1,42)} = 20.35$, $P < 0.001$, and with expectancy controlled, between group differences in posttest placebo response were not significant, $F_{(3,42)} = 1.93$, $P < 0.17$. Mean posttest placebo response scores, adjusted for pretest scores and expectancy, are reported in Table 20.4. The correlation between posttest placebo response and expectancy was highly significant, $r = 0.70$, $P < 0.001$.

The pain response scores of participants in the extinction condition during the ten extinction trials are depicted in Fig. 20.1. A 10×2 (trial by placebo) repeated measures analysis of variance revealed significant effects for trial, $F_{(9,99)} = 4.20$, $P < 0.001$, placebo, $F_{(1,11)} = 11.09$, $P < 0.01$, and the trial by placebo interaction, $F_{(9,99)} = 2.07$, $P < 0.04$. Trend analysis revealed significant linear effects for trial, $F_{(1,11)} = 8.43$, $P < 0.02$, and the linear trial by placebo interaction, $F_{(1,11)} = 5.29$, $P < 0.04$. Analyses of simple effects revealed a significant linear effect across no-placebo trials, $F_{(1,11)} = 22.71$, $P < 0.001$, but not across placebo trials, $F_{(1,11)} = 1.24$, $P < 0.29$. Interpreted in conjunction with Fig. 20.1, these data indicate a significant increase in pain when the placebo was not administered, which was inhibited by the administration of placebo, thus resulting in an increase in the placebo effect across the ten extinction trials. (The trial by placebo interaction is mathematically equivalent to a main effect on placebo response scores—no-placebo pain ratings minus placebo pain ratings for each pair of trials.) [Parenthetic remark was originally an in-text footnote—eds.]

Table 20.2.

Means and standard deviations for pain ratings, expected pain ratings, placebo effect, and expected placebo effect as a function of placebo administration and experimental condition

Variable	Group			
	Extinction	No treatment	Informed pairing	Uninformed pairing
Pain ratings				
Pretest				
Placebo				
Mean	4.83	5.50	5.71	5.75
SD	1.34	1.48	1.42	1.73
No-placebo				
Mean	5.13	5.79	6.17	5.88
SD	1.17	1.16	1.54	1.13
Placebo effect				
Mean	0.29	0.29	0.46	0.13
SD	0.84	0.99	1.08	1.26
Posttest				
Placebo				
Mean	5.42	5.38	5.96	4.71
SD	1.33	1.15	1.05	1.27
No-placebo				
Mean	5.63	5.96	6.33	6.75
SD	1.45	1.16	1.23	1.48
Placebo effect				
Mean	0.21	0.58	0.38	2.04
SD	1.12	1.02	1.03	1.54
Expected pain ratings				
Placebo				
Mean	5.50	5.33	4.92	2.75
SD	1.51	1.07	0.67	1.22
No-placebo				
Mean	6.42	6.58	6.83	6.92
SD	1.31	1.08	1.40	1.16
Expected placebo effect				
Mean	0.92	1.25	1.92	4.17
SD	0.79	1.22	1.16	1.47

Table 20.3.

Mean posttest placebo response and expected placebo response adjusted for pretest placebo response

Variable	Group			
	Extinction	No treatment	Informed pairing	Uninformed pairing
Placebo response	0.21[a]	0.58[a]	0.40[a]	2.01[b]
Expected placebo response	0.92[a]	1.25[a]	1.91[a]	4.18[b]

Note: Adjusted means sharing a common superscript do not differ significantly from each other.

Table 20.4.

Mean posttest placebo response adjusted for pretest scores and expectancy

Group			
Extinction	No treatment	Informed pairing	Uninformed pairing
0.86	1.05	0.49	0.81

4. Discussion

According to Baron and Kenny (1986): "To establish mediation, the following conditions must hold: First, the independent variable must affect the mediator . . . second, the independent variable must be shown to affect the dependent variable . . . and third, the mediator must affect the dependent variable . . . Perfect mediation holds if the independent variable has no effect when the mediator is controlled" (p. 1177).

By these criteria, we have established that the effect of the Voudouris et al. (1985, 1989, 1990) conditioning procedure on responses to placebo is completely mediated by expectancy. Conditioning trials in the uninformed pairing group altered participants' placebo response expectancies. They also altered their pain reports. Expectancy was highly predictive of pain reports, and conditioning had no effect when expectancy was controlled.

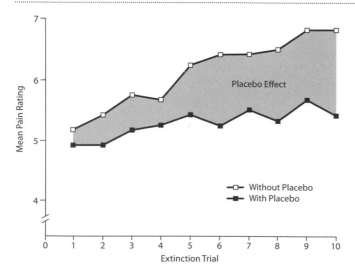

Fig. 20.1. Increases in the magnitude of the placebo effect during extinction trials.

The mediating role of expectancy was further supported by the ability of expectancy-altering verbal information to obstruct the effect of conditioning trials. Our verbal manipulation was designed to alter participants' interpretations of their experience during conditioning trials. Participants in the uninformed pairing condition were led to attribute pain reduction on placebo trials to the effect of the ointment. Those in the informed pairing condition were led to attribute pain reduction to changes in stimulus intensity. Because significant enhancement of the placebo effect was limited to participants in the uninformed pairing group, we conclude that it is the interpretation of conditioning trials, rather than the trials themselves, that affects placebo responding.

Contemporary interpretations of conditioning phenomena stress cognitive functions (Rescorla, 1988). Conditioning is a means by which representations of the environment are acquired. With respect to placebo phenomena, they are one way in which expectancies about the effect of treatments are acquired. However, they do not explain how these expectancies elicit the expected responses. This stands in marked contrast to stimulus substitution conceptions of classical conditioning, upon which conditioning models of placebo effects have been based (e.g., Herrnstein, 1962; Wickramasekera, 1980; Ader, 1988; Turkkan, 1989). According to stimulus substitution formulations, expectancies are epiphenomenal, at best, and conditioning trials are directly responsible for the production of placebo responses. This model of conditioned placebo effects is not supported by the data of the study reported here.

A final aspect of the data worth noting is the failure of the initial pain reduction response to extinguish. Although this is inconsistent with the report of Fedele et al. (1989) of a gradual decrease in the effectiveness of placebo treatment of dysmenorrhea over three consecutive menstrual cycles, it is consistent with most other clinical data. For example, eight weeks of daily placebo administration failed to reduce the effectiveness of placebo treatment for panic disorder (Coryell and Noyes, 1988); placebos retained their effectiveness in the treatment of angina over a 6-month period (Boissel et al., 1986); and continued placebo treatment of rheumatoid arthritis was shown to be effective for as long as 30 months (Traut and Passarelli, 1957). These data are inconsistent with a stimulus substitution model (Wickramasekera, 1980), but not with an informational model of conditioned placebo responses (Kirsch, 1997). According to the stimulus substitution formulation, the active ingredients of medications are USs. From an informational perspective, it is the effect of treatment, rather than the active ingredients of treatment, that constitute the US. Extinction fails to occur because by mimicking the effects of drugs, placebos produce the US that confirms expectancies of the drug responses.

We not only failed to obtain evidence of extinction over ten extinction trials, we found a significant increase in the placebo effect over these trials. Pain stimulation trials without placebo produced an increase in reported pain. Increases in reported pain across repeated administration of nociceptive stimulation have been reported previously (Baker and Kirsch, 1993). Surprisingly, in the present study, placebo administration inhibited this increase in pain reports over trials, resulting in an increase in the placebo effect, which returned to baseline levels, however, after the 3-min rest period. The reason for this temporary enhancement of the placebo effect remains to be determined. One possibility is that the magnitude of the placebo effect is proportional to the magnitude of experienced pain without the placebo. In any case, the finding of a significant increase in the placebo effect during extinction trials is inconsistent with the stimulus substitution hypothesis (see Wickramasekera, 1980).

Some caution in interpreting these extinction data is warranted. The apparent preconditioning effect of the creme was very small and may not have been a placebo effect. Conversely, an expectancy interpretation is supported by the finding that the posttreatment placebo effect in the extinction group was highly correlated with the expected placebo response ($r = 0.79$, $P < 0.002$). The extinction hypothesis should be tested in future studies by conducting extinction trials following conditioning trials.

Besides their theoretical significance, the questions of whether and how conditioning affects placebo analgesia have important implications for clinical practice. Placebo effects and drug effects are often additive, and drug expectancies can potentiate drug effects (Kirsch, 1990; Kirsch and Rosadino, 1993). For this reason, placebo factors can be used to enhance the effectiveness of active treatments. Our data are consistent with those of previous studies in indicating that direct experience is a potent means of enhancing the effects of a pain reduction intervention. For example, large initial doses of a pain medication should increase the efficacy of subsequent smaller doses. However, our data also suggest that this effect might be blocked if patients were aware of the subsequent reduction in dosage. Based on our data, it is reasonable to suspect that pain reduction experiences have an impact on subsequent pain reduction only to the extent that they are provided in such a way as to impact patient's expectations.

REFERENCES

Ader, R., The placebo effect as a conditioned response. In: R. Ader, H. Weiner and A. Baum (Eds.), Experimental Foundations of Behavioral Medicine: Conditioning Approaches, Lawrence Erlbaum, Hillside, N.J., 1988, 47–66.

Ajzen, I. and Fishbein, M., Understanding Attitudes and Predicting Social Behavior, Prentice-Hall, Englewood Cliffs, N.J., 1980.

Baker, S.L. and Kirsch, I., Hypnotic and placebo analgesia: order effects and the placebo label, Contemp. Hypnosis, 10 (1993) 117–126.

Baron, R.M. and Kenny, D.A, The moderator-mediator variable distinction in social psychological research: conceptual, strategic arid statistical considerations, J. Pers. Soc. Psychol., 51 (1986) 1173–1182.

Benjamin, F.B. and Helvey, W.M., Iontophoresis of potassium for experimental determination of pain endurance in man, Proc. Soc. Exp. Biol. Med., 113 (1963) 566–568.

Boissel, J.P., Philippon, A.M., Gauthier, E., Schbath, J., Destors, J.M. and the B.I.S. Research Group, Time course of long-term placebo therapy effects in angina pectoris, Eur. Heart J., 7 (1986) 1030–1036.

Coryell, W. and Noyes, R., Placebo response in panic disorder, Am. J. Psychiatry, 145 (1988) 1138–1140.

Fedele, L., Maurizio, M., Acaia, B., Garagiola, U. and Tiengo, M., Dynamics and significance of placebo response in primary dysmenorrhea, Pain, 36 (1989) 43–47.

Herrnstein, R., Placebo effect in the rat, Science, 138 (1962) 677–678.

Hull, C.L., Knowledge and purpose as habit mechanisms, Psychol. Rev., 37 (1930) 511–525.

Kirsch, I., Response expectancy as a determinant of experience and behavior, Am. Psychol., 40 (1985) 1189–1202.

Kirsch, I., Changing Expectations: A Key to Effective Psychotherapy, Brooks/Cole, Pacific Grove, Calif., 1990.

Kirsch, I., Specifying nonspecifics: psychological mechanisms of placebo effects. In: A. Harrington (Ed.), The Placebo Effect, Harvard University Press, Cambridge, Mass., 1997, 166–186.

Kirsch, I. and Rosadino, M.J., Do double-blind studies with informed consent yield externally valid results? An empirical test, Psychopharmacology, 110 (1993) 437–442.

Levine, J.D., Gordon, N.C. and Fields, H.L., The mechanism of placebo analgesia, Lancet, 312 (1978) 654–657.

Montgomery, G. and Kirsch, I., Mechanisms of placebo pain reduction: an empirical investigation, Psychol. Sci., 7 (1996) 174–176.

Rescorla, R.A., Pavlovian conditioning: it's not what you think it is, Am. Psychol., 43 (1988) 151–160.

Siegel, S., Classical conditioning, drug tolerance and drug dependence. In: Y. Israel, F.B. Glaser, H. Kalant, R.E. Popham, W. Schmidt and R.G. Smart (Eds.), Research Advances in Alcohol and Drug Problems (Vol. 7), Plenum Press, New York, N.Y., 1983, 207–246.

Sternbach, R.A, Pain: A Psychological Analysis, Academic Press, New York, N.Y., 1968.

Traut, E.F. and Passarelli, E.W., Placebos in the treatment of rheumatoid arthritis and other rheumatic conditions, Ann. Rheum. Dis., 16 (1957) 18–22.

Turkkan, J.S., Classical conditioning: the new hegemony, Behav. Brain Sci., 12 (1989) 121–179.

Voudouris, N.J., Peck, C.L. and Coleman, G., Conditioned placebo responses, J. Pers. Soc. Psychol., 48 (1985) 47–53.

Voudouris, N.J., Peck, C.L. and Coleman, G., Conditioned response models of placebo phenomena: further support, Pain, 38 (1989) 109–116.

Voudouris, N.J., Peck, C.L. and Coleman, G., The role of conditioning and verbal expectancy in the placebo response, Pain, 43 (1990) 121–128.

Wickless, C. and Kirsch, I., The effects of verbal and experiential expectancy manipulations on hypnotic susceptibility, J. Pers. Soc. Psychol., 57 (1989) 762–768.

Wickramasekera, I., A conditioned response model of the placebo effect: predictions from the model, Biofeedback Self-Regul., 5 (1980) 5–18.

21

An Analysis of Factors That Contribute to the Magnitude of Placebo Analgesia in an Experimental Paradigm

DONALD D. PRICE, LEONARD S. MILLING, IRVING KIRSCH, ANN DUFF, GUY H. MONTGOMERY, AND SARAH S. NICHOLLS

Donald D. Price, Leonard S. Milling, Irving Kirsch, Ann Duff, Guy H. Montgomery, and Sarah S. Nicholls, "An Analysis of Factors That Contribute to the Magnitude of Placebo Analgesia in an Experimental Paradigm," Pain 1999;83:147–156.

1. Introduction

Nearly all studies that have sought to explain the psychological basis of the placebo effect have focused on either a classical conditioning model or a single psychological factor such as anxiety, expectancy, hope, or faith in the treatment. Recently, the possibility that multiple or alternative psychological factors mediate placebo effects has been recognized (Price and Barrell, 1984; Bootzin, 1985; Evans, 1985; White et al., 1985; Montgomery and Kirsch, 1996, 1997; Fields and Price, 1997; Price and Fields, 1997). For example, Montgomery and Kirsch (1997) introduced an experimental manipulation that dissociated expectancy from conditioning to determine which mechanism best accounted for variance in placebo response. In this paradigm, a placebo cream is applied to the skin under the guise of a local analgesic, and the painful stimulus strength is surreptitiously lowered only during conditioning trials. The placebo response is obtained during post-conditioning trials wherein the painful stimulus strength is applied at the same baseline levels prior to conditioning.

Montgomery and Kirsch modified this paradigm by informing one group of subjects about the lowering of painful stimulus intensity and not informing the other group. The uninformed group was thereby provided with an experience of placebo-induced analgesia during conditioning and, as expected, demonstrated placebo analgesia in the subsequent test trials. In contrast, expectations of analgesia were lowered in the informed group and no overall placebo analgesic effect occurred in this group. Furthermore, although conditioning trials significantly enhanced placebo responding, this effect was eliminated by adding participant's expectancy ratings to the regression equation, further indicating that the effect of pairing trials on placebo response was mediated by expectancy (Baron and Kenny, 1986). This study demonstrated that conditioning is not sufficient for placebo effects, and it provided evidence that expectation of a therapeutic effect is necessary for placebo effects. The results of this study constituted multiple lines of evidence against the Pavlovian conditioning model and supported the mediating role of expectancy.

These findings are consistent with response expectancy theory (Kirsch, 1990). Response expectancy theory hypothesizes that (1) expectations for non-volitional outcomes are sufficient to cause the expected outcome, (2) response expectancy effects are not mediated by other psychological variables, and (3) effects of response expectancies are self-confirming and seemingly automatic. For example, an expectation that one will be depressed for a long period of time is quite depressing and an expectation of being anxious before an exam can evoke anxiety. In the same way, expectations for pain reduction following placebo administration are hypothesized to directly cause subsequent pain relief.

Although expectancy appears to have a critical mediating role in producing placebo analgesia, it is unlikely to operate alone. Placebo analgesia often occurs under conditions wherein subjects want a therapeutic agent to provide pain relief. That is, an individual's desire for reduction in pain may also directly contribute to subsequent pain relief by providing a need to experience a treatment as effective. Similar to response expectation theory, the need to experience an effective analgesic treatment could have a direct effect on pain. The possible mediating role of motivation or desire for relief could account for several observations. It could indirectly account for the increase in placebo response with the severity of clinical pain (Beecher, 1955, 1959; Jospe, 1978; Levine et al., 1978). It might also account for the greater placebo response for clinical pain versus experimental pain and for the observation that placebo responses in experimental pain increase as a function of its duration and severity (Jospe, 1978). In other words, greater and more open-ended threats may lead to greater needs for relief and placebo responses.

Unfortunately, the role of desire for a specific symptom change has yet to be tested for placebo analgesia and it has only rarely been tested for placebo effects in general. In one exceptional study of placebo manipulations suggesting possible sedative or stimulant effects, Jensen and Karoly (1991) assessed the separate contributions of motivation and expectancy to placebo effects. According to the authors, motivation was "the degree to which subjects desire to experience a symptom change," and expectancy was considered the subjects' expectation of a symptom change. They found that motivation but not expectancy contributed a significant amount of variance to placebo responses that included perceived sedation or perceived stimulant effects. However, limitations of their study were that desire and expectancy manipulations and not direct measures of these factors constituted the independent variables of the study, and the authors questioned the effectiveness of their expectancy manipulation.

One purpose of this study was to evaluate two factors for their possible contribution to placebo analgesia: (1) a desire for treatment to significantly relieve pain and (2) the level of expectation that pain will be significantly relieved. Based on the literature reviewed above, one would anticipate direct effects of both response expectancy and desire for pain reduction on the magnitude of placebo analgesia. Thus, we sought to determine the extent to which either of these two factors predicts placebo-induced reductions in ratings of sensory and unpleasantness dimensions of experimental pain. The evaluation of expectancy also represents an extension and replication of the study by Montgomery and Kirsch (1997).

A second major purpose of the present study was to compare the magnitudes of placebo effects based on concurrent and retrospective ratings of pain and to determine whether the same factors of desire and expectation also influence placebo effects based on remembered pain. Concurrent placebo effects were based on ratings of pain that had just been evoked from heat stimuli applied within baseline control and placebo-treated areas of skin and were assessed during placebo treatments. "Remembered placebo effects" were based on retrospective ratings of these same evoked pains approximately 2 min afterwards. The rationale for the evaluation of "remembered placebo effects" is based on results of previous studies that show that memory distortion of pretreatment pain contributes to an exaggeration of self-reports of pain relief (Linton and Melin, 1982; Jamison et al., 1989; Mathias et al., 1995; Feine et al., 1998). This exaggeration was shown to result from inaccurate memory of pretreatment baseline pain as being more intense than it actually was (Feine et al., 1998). Since reports of pain relief rely on memory of pretreatment pain intensity, exaggerations of pretreatment pain ratings and hence magnitudes of self-reported pain relief may occur among numerous studies that use self-reports of pain relief, including those resulting from placebo treatments. However, the possible enhancement of placebo analgesia by this memory mechanism has yet to be explicitly tested. Furthermore, mechanisms of such enhancement, such as mediation by expectancy or desire for relief, are also of interest.

In this report, we compare concurrent placebo analgesic effects with those based on remembered pain, both of which were produced by a placebo manipulation similar to that used previously (Voudouris et al., 1990; Montgomery and Kirsch, 1997), as described above. Both types of placebo effects are analyzed with regard to their possible mediation by expectancy and desire for pain reduction.

2. Methods

2.1. Participants

Participants consisted of 40 undergraduate students (24 female and 16 male; mean age = 19.3, range = 18–22 years; 34

Caucasian, 1 African-American, 1 Asian, and 4 Hispanic). They volunteered to participate in exchange for partial course credit and reported an absence of medical conditions and medication use that might interfere with pain sensitivity or pose an increased risk of resultant tissue damage. These conditions and medications included high blood pressure, circulatory problems (e.g., Raynaud's syndrome or family history of the same), diabetes mellitus, heart disease or any other heart problems, asthma, seizures, frostbite, past trauma to hands, lupus erythematosus, arthritis, other large or small joint disease or injury, or use of psychoactive drugs, analgesics, antihistamines, and anti-inflammatory medications. Participants were randomly assigned to two groups (see below) with the restriction that there were the same proportions of males and females in each condition. Forty participants successfully completed all phases of the study protocol. Six participants were excluded from participation in the study because of medical reasons or because their calibrated pain stimulus levels would have been higher than 50°C.

2.2. Setting and Materials

Pain was induced by means of a Peltier thermal probe. This device provides brief skin temperature increases within the noxious range (45–51°C) with up to a 10°C/s rise time from a 35°C adapting temperature. It employs a feedback-controlled contact thermode whose contact surface (to skin) is 3 cm². An attractive feature of this device is that it provides a quick return to the adapting temperature via a water-circulating cooling mechanism. This prevents progressive warming of the skin. The controlling temperature of the thermal probe allows the experimenter or computer control of the temperature at the thermode-skin interface. Nociceptive thermal stimuli of 5 s duration were applied to the skin by means of the contact thermal probe. The thermode-skin temperatures rose rapidly (10°C/s) from a baseline of 35°C to a peak temperature preset on the stimulator and held at peak temperature for the remainder of the 5-s stimulus. All stimuli were 5 s in duration in order to minimize cues to participants that would lead them to expect differences in pain intensity based on stimulus duration. This was especially important for post-manipulation trials in which participants received the identical stimulus intensity and duration for all three areas (i.e., A, B, and C).

The placebo cream was a mixture of iodine, oil of thyme, and water that produced a brownish, medicinal-smelling effect when applied topically. The placebo was placed in two medicinal-looking bottles labeled "Trivaricaine-A: Approved for research purposes only" and "Trivaricaine-B: Approved for research purposes only." These placebo agents were applied to areas on the ventral part of the forearm, which had corresponding labels of A and B. A third area, labelled C, was used for control trials in which water from a bottle labelled C was applied. This procedure provided a baseline control, which included effects of vehicle solution on pain stimuli. An office in the University Health Center infirmary was used as the setting for the experiment to alleviate skepticism on the part of participants that might have been caused by prior associations with the psychology department.

2.3. Response Measures

In each experimental session, well-validated visual analogue scales (M-VAS) were used to measure pain sensation intensity and degree of unpleasantness evoked by the nociceptive thermal stimuli described above (Price et al., 1994). Subjects were instructed how to rate both pain sensation intensity and unpleasantness according to standardized written statements described in detail elsewhere (Price et al., 1985, 1994). As in previous applications of these scaling methods, verbal anchors served to establish the distinction between these two pain dimensions. The VAS sensory scale was anchored at the left by the descriptors "no pain sensation" and at the right by "the most intense pain sensation imaginable." Likewise, the VAS-unpleasantness was anchored by the descriptors "not at all unpleasant" and "the most unpleasantness imaginable." Expectancy measures were obtained by asking participants, "What do you expect the pain intensity to be with the Trivaricaine-A?" in area A, and "What do you expect the pain intensity to be with the Trivaricaine-B?" in area B, and "What do you expect the pain intensity to be without the Trivaricaine in area C where only the wetting agent is applied?" Pain expectancy ratings were made on the same VAS as those on the pain intensity scale. Participants rated desire for relief on VAS just after they were instructed about the number of trials they would endure during the post-manipulation trials. This VAS was anchored as "no desire for relief" at the left and as "the most intense desire for relief imaginable" at the right.

2.4. Procedure

Participants were greeted in the lobby of the University Health Center, escorted to an office by a research assistant, and introduced to the experimenter, who wore a white lab coat and was described as a "Behavioral Medicine Researcher." Although the experimenter was not blind with respect to procedures and treatments given, all instructions to participants that are described below followed a standardized script given to all participants. Participants were told that a new, topical, local anesthetic was being tested for its pain-reducing effects. They were told the drug's name was "Trivaricaine," and that it had been proven effective in reducing pain in preliminary studies at other universities. The number of pain trials was described to each participant as part of the informed consent procedure, and they were told that they could discontinue participation at any time, without negative consequences. Those participants agreeing to participate then completed the medical screening form. Acceptable participants were randomly assigned to one of two experimental manipulation groups (see Section 2.8): (1) those receiving instructions presumed to elicit high desire for pain reduction (n = 20) and (2) those receiving instructions presumed to elicit low desire for pain reduction (n = 20).

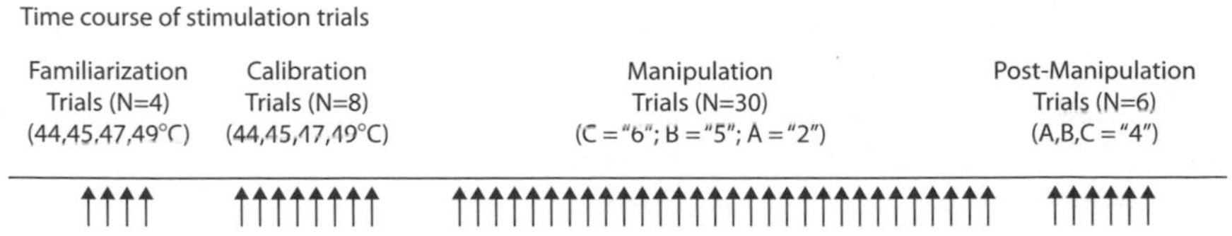

Time course of stimulation trials

Familiarization Trials (N=4) (44,45,47,49°C)	Calibration Trials (N=8) (44,45,47,49°C)	Manipulation Trials (N=30) (C = "6"; B = "5"; A = "2")	Post-Manipulation Trials (N=6) (A,B,C = "4")
↑↑↑↑	↑↑↑↑↑↑↑↑	↑↑↑↑↑↑↑↑↑↑↑↑↑↑↑↑↑↑↑↑↑↑↑↑↑↑↑↑↑↑	↑↑↑↑↑↑

Fig. 21.1. Time course of experimental conditions and experimental design.

Participants in the two groups were given four blocks of pain trials that included: (1) familiarization trials (n = 4), (2) calibration trials (n = 8), (3) manipulation trials (n = 30), and (4) posttest trials (n = 6) identical for both groups, as shown in Fig. 21.1. Order of administration of baseline and placebo trials was randomized during manipulation and post-manipulation trials.

2.5. Familiarization Trials

One trial each of 44, 45, 47, and 49°C stimuli were given in ascending order to familiarize participants with the range of stimulus intensities to be used in the experiment and to quickly identify those few participants unwilling to participate in the study.

2.6. Calibration Trials

To control for individual differences in pain perception, a calibration procedure similar to that of Montgomery and Kirsch (1997) was utilized. Two trials each of 44, 45, 47, or 49°C stimuli were randomly presented during the calibration session to establish a stimulus-response curve (based on linear regression analysis). Care was taken to ensure that subjects could not determine which of the four temperatures would be presented on a given trial. Nociceptive thermal stimuli, extending from 44 to 49°C, were chosen because the stimuli spanned a broad range of intensity, extending from a level close to pain threshold (44°C) to a level that is close to but nearly always less than pain tolerance (> 50°C [Price et al., 1980, 1994]). Pain trials were separated by approximately 15–20 s and participants rated pain intensity and unpleasantness immediately on VAS following each trial. At the conclusion of calibration trials, a separate regression equation was calculated for each participant by inputting the VAS ratings and their corresponding stimulus intensity levels in °C. This was used to calculate the stimulus intensity levels corresponding to each individual's ratings of "6" (applied to area C, control solution), "5" (applied to area B, "weak" placebo), and "2" (applied to area A, "strong" placebo) as predicted by the regression equation. For brevity, this number was used to indicate the corresponding stimulus intensity level, although this level differs between individual participants according to their personal perceptions of pain.

2.7. Manipulation Trials

Manipulation trials began after the conclusion of the pretest calibration trials. All participants in high and low desire groups received ten stimulus trials with "strong" placebo (Trivaricaine A), ten stimulus trials with "weak" placebo,

and ten stimulus trials with the vehicle solution (C). These three agents corresponded to bottles labelled A, B, and C, respectively, and were applied to three corresponding forearm regions also labelled A, B, and C (marked with labels/bandaids). The locations of the three forearm regions were randomly selected across the 40 participants. Participants were informed that bottle C was a control wetting solution and that bottles A and B contain different strengths of the local analgesic Trivaricaine. They were further informed that the study was double blind with neither the participants nor the investigators knowing whether bottle A or B contained the highest-strength local analgesic. The conditioning procedure represents an extension of that used by Voudouris et al. (1990) and Montgomery and Kirsch (1997). Participants were given the stimulus strength corresponding to levels 5 and 6 (based on individual regression equations) for areas B and C, respectively. They were given a stimulus strength corresponding to level 2 for area A in order to provide participants with an experience of pain reduction associated with a strong local analgesic (A) in comparison to baseline control (C). In effect, trials in areas B and A provided a basis for evaluation of effects of weak and strong placebo manipulations, respectively. Similar to previous use of this type of paradigm, participants were not informed that stimulus intensity levels were being altered on placebo trials in which stimuli were presented to areas A and B. The assessment of expectancy and desire for pain reduction was made just prior to the postmanipulation trials.

2.8. Instructions Designed to Alter Desire for Relief

After the manipulation trials and just prior to postmanipulation trials, all participants were informed about the level of pain they would receive and the maximum number of trials they would be given in the posttest trial condition. Participants in the high desire group were instructed that they would receive thirty trials of the heat stimulus at the highest pain level they had experienced thus far and that this may be difficult to endure if the local analgesic was not working. Further, they were told that they would receive ten trials applied to area A, ten trials to area B, and ten trials to area C. Participants in the low desire group were instructed that they would receive six trials at a stimulation level that may be at the highest level they had experienced so far, but since there were only six trials, most participants had found this easy to endure. They were then told that two trials each would be applied to areas A, B, and C. All participants received six post-manipulation trials, two trials each for areas A, B, and C. Those in high desire groups knew this only at the end of the six trials. Post-manipulation testing began 3 min after the conclusion of the manipulation trials and after the instructions for the number of trials to be endured. For all participants, the procedures for the post-manipulation trials were similar to that of the manipulation trials except that the intensity level remained at the same level (i.e., 4) for all three areas (A, B, and C). Stimulus trials applied to areas A, B, and C were delivered in random order (two trials/area = six trials). Desire for relief and expected pain levels for each of these three agents were assessed prospectively just prior to the beginning of the post-manipulation condition.

2.9. Post-Experimental Ratings of Pain

Approximately 2 min after the posttest trials, participants rated pain they remembered experiencing during these trials. The following instructions were given and questions were asked: "We are very interested in your experience during the last six trials in which you received the test stimuli. Please take a few minutes and answer the following questions to the best of your ability." A VAS was provided for each of the following questions.

1. What was the pain sensation intensity without the Trivaricaine-A or -B?
2. What was the pain sensation intensity with Trivaricaine-A? Trivaricaine-B? (2 ratings).
3. What was the pain unpleasantness without Trivaricaine-A? Trivaricaine-B? (2 ratings).
4. What was the pain unpleasantness with Trivaricaine-A? Trivaricaine-B? (2 ratings).

3. Results

The experimental paradigm employed herein represents a mixed model containing a within-subjects repeated measures factor (i.e., an expectancy manipulation in the form of control, "weak" placebo, and "strong" placebo analgesic solutions provided to each participant) and a between-subjects factor (i.e., a desire manipulation in which participants were assigned to either high desire or low desire conditions). Therefore, the main analytic strategy consisted of 2 × 3 (desire by expectancy) mixed model analyses of variance (ANOVAs) on expected, concurrent, and retrospective ratings of pain intensity and unpleasantness. Parametric analyses were utilized because the specific VAS used has been shown to have ratio scale properties (Price et al., 1994).

3.1. Effects of Experimental Manipulations on Ratings of Pain During Manipulation Trials

Based on the regression analysis of calibration trials, the stimulus intensities chosen were predicted to evoke pain intensity ratings of "6," "5," and "2" for areas C, B, and A, respectively.

The overall mean ratings of pain intensity collapsed across the ten manipulation trials for areas C, B, and A were 6.2 (SD = 1.3), 4.5 (SD = 1.1), and 2.5 (SD = 0.9), respectively, and

reasonably close to levels predicted on the basis of participants' regression analysis of calibration trials.

3.2. Effects of Experimental Manipulations on Expectations and Desires for Pain Reduction

The experimental manipulations that were designed to produce differences in expectation and desire for pain reduction succeeded in doing so. Means and standard deviations of expected pain and desire for pain reduction are presented in Table 21.1 and Fig. 21.2. A series of 2 × 3 (desire by expectancy) mixed model ANOVAs on expectancy scores indicated a significant main effect for the conditioning manipulation on both expected intensity, $F_{(2,76)} = 168.94$, $P < 0.001$, and expected unpleasantness, $F_{(2,76)} = 128.31$, $P < 0.001$. Post-hoc contrast tests, with alpha set at $P < 0.05$ indicated that participants expected less intense pain at area A (mean = 2.95, SD = 1.38) than at area B (mean = 4.30, SD = 1.18), and less intense pain at area B than at area C (mean = 7.25, SD = 1.37).

Table 21.1.
Mean expected pain ratings as a function of desire/expectation

	Low desire (N=20) Mean (SD)	High desire (N=20) Mean (SD)	Overall group (N=40) Mean (SD)
Expected intensity			
C: No placebo	6.9 (1.0)	7.6 (1.6)	7.3 (1.4)
B: Weak placebo	4.0 (1.2)	4.6 (1.1)	4.3 (1.2)
A: Strong placebo	2.8 (1.4)	3.1 (1.4)	3.0 (1.4)
Expected unpleasantness			
C: No placebo	6.7 (1.4)	7.5 (2.0)	7.1 (1.7)
B: Weak placebo	3.7 (1.2)	4.5 (1.4)	4.1 (1.3)
A: Strong placebo	2.3 (1.1)	2.9 (1.8)	2.6 (1.5)

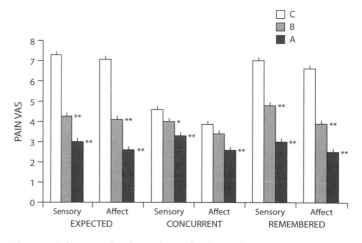

Fig. 21.2. Pain sensation intensity and pain unpleasantness ratings of 40 participants for three areas of skin (A, B, and C). Area C was untreated with conditioning trials, area B was treated with weak placebo conditioning trials, and area A was treated with strong placebo conditioning trials. These ratings are for: (1) expected pain within areas C, B, and A; (2) pain just after placebo conditioning trials for these same areas, that is, concurrent pain; and (3) remembered pain about 2 min after post-test trials for these same areas.

Table 21.2.
Mean pain ratings during placebo treatment and during post-trial questioning

| | Concurrent ratings | | | Post-manipulation questionnaire ratings |
	Low desire	High desire	Overall group	Overall group
Resulting intensity				
C: No placebo	4.7 (1.7)	4.5 (1.7)	4.6 (1.7)	6.8 (1.5)
B: Weak placebo	3.7 (1.3)	4.3 (2.0)	4.0 (1.5)	4.7 (1.6)
A: Strong placebo	3.0 (1.2)	3.6 (1.7)	3.3 (1.5)	3.0 (1.6)
Resulting unpleasantness				
C: No placebo	3.8 (1.5)	3.8 (2.0)	3.8 (1.7)	6.4 (1.6)
B: Weak placebo	3.0 (0.9)	3.8 (1.9)	3.4 (1.5)	3.8 (1.7)
A: Strong placebo	2.2 (1.0)	2.9 (1.6)	2.5 (1.3)	2.5 (1.3)

Similarly, post-hoc contrast tests revealed that participants expected less unpleasant pain at area A (mean = 2.57, SD = 1.48) than at area B (mean = 4.06, SD = 1.33), and less unpleasant pain at area B than at area C (mean = 7.13, SD = 1.71). The analysis also revealed a significant effect of the desire manipulation on desire ratings, $t(38) = 2.65$, $P < 0.05$. Participants who were told that they would have to endure thirty more trials at a high intensity level had a mean desire rating of 6.5 (SD = 2.4), whereas those who were told that they would receive only six more trials had a mean desire rating of 4.5 (SD = 2.4).

3.3. Effects of Manipulations on Ratings of Pain in Placebo-Treated and Untreated Areas

Means and standard deviations of concurrent ratings of pain sensation and pain unpleasantness are displayed in Table 21.2. Similar to pain ratings during manipulation trials, the mean rating of pain intensity within the control area C (mean = 4.56, SD = 1.7) was reasonably close to actual stimulus intensity (4). A series of mixed model ANOVAs on concurrent pain ratings did not yield a significant effect of the desire manipulation or the interaction of the desire and expectancy manipulations. However, these analyses indicated a significant effect for the conditioning manipulation on both intensity, $F(2,76) = 14.65$, $P < 0.001$, and unpleasantness, $F(2,76) = 17.20$, $P < 0.001$. Post-hoc contrast tests, with alpha set at $P < 0.05$, showed that the mean rating of stimulus intensity in area A (mean = 3.32, SD = 1.46) was significantly lower than that for area B (mean = 4.00, SD = 1.68) and that the mean rating for area B was significantly lower than that for area C (mean = 4.56, SD = 1.70). Therefore, a definite placebo effect was obtained in the case of pain sensation intensity for areas A and B. In contrast, post-hoc contrast tests revealed that the mean rating of unpleasantness at area A (mean = 2.52, SD = 1.33) was lower than that for area B (mean = 3.43, SD = 1.51) and for area C (mean = 3.81, SD = 1.74). However, the difference in unpleasantness between areas B and C was not significant. Thus, a placebo effect on ratings of unpleasantness occurred only for area A.

3.4. Effects of Manipulations on Remembered Pain Levels in Placebo-Treated and Untreated Areas

Means and standard deviations of remembered pain intensity and unpleasantness are displayed in Table 21.2. A series of 2 × 3 (desire by expectancy) mixed model ANOVAs on ratings of remembered pain failed to yield a significant effect for desire or interaction of desire and expectancy but did indicate significant effects for the conditioning manipulation on both intensity, $F(2,74) = 55.62$, $P < 0.001$, and unpleasantness, $F(2,74) = 69.10$, $P < 0.001$. Post-hoc contrast tests, with alpha set at $P < 0.05$, indicated that participants remembered less intense pain at area A (mean = 3.02, SD = 1.60) than at area B (mean = 4.72, SD = 1.60), and less intense pain at area B than at area C (mean = 6.82, SD = 1.52). Thus, definite placebo effects were obtained in the case of remembered pain intensity for areas A and B. Similarly, post-hoc contrast tests revealed that participants remembered less unpleasant pain at area A (mean = 2.46, SD = 1.44) than at area B (mean = 3.84, SD = 1.67), and less unpleasant pain at area B than at area C (mean = 6.44, SD = 1.65). Thus, unlike concurrent ratings of pain intensity and unpleasantness, strong placebo effects on ratings of remembered pain intensity and of unpleasantness occurred for both areas A and B.

3.5. Associations among Ratings of Desire and Expected, Concurrent, and Remembered Ratings of Pain in Placebo-Treated and Untreated Areas

Consistent with the ANOVAs and post-hoc tests for possible group one (high desire) and group two (low desire) effects on pain ratings, none of the correlations of desire ratings with expected, concurrent, and remembered ratings of pain intensity and unpleasantness for areas A, B, and C were significant. Table 21.3 shows correlations among expected, concurrent and remembered ratings of intensity and unpleasantness by experimental area. Consistent with ANOVA analyses of the experimental manipulations designed to induce differences in expectancy, correlations between expected and concurrent ratings of intensity were highly significant for areas

Table 21.3.

Correlations among expected, concurrent, and remembered pain intensity and unpleasantness ratings for placebo and control solutions

	Concurrent pain		Remembered pain	
	Intensity	Unpleasantness	Intensity	Unpleasantness
Area A				
(strong placebo)				
Expected pain				
Intensity	0.51[a]	0.48[b]	0.52[a]	0.47[b]
Unpleasantness	0.29	0.40[b]	0.62[a]	0.62[a]
Concurrent pain				
Intensity	—	—	0.14	0.29
Unpleasantness	—	—	0.10	0.34[c]
Area B				
(weak placebo)				
Expected pain				
Intensity	0.54[a]	0.36[c]	0.11	0.21
Unpleasantness	0.39[c]	0.37[c]	0.26	0.38[c]
Concurrent pain				
Intensity	—	—	0.29	0.32[c]
Unpleasantness	—	—	0.28	0.38[c]
Area C				
(control solution)				
Expected pain				
Intensity	0.28	0.32[c]	0.51[a]	0.45[b]
Unpleasantness	0.09	0.21	0.62[a]	0.55[b]
Concurrent pain				
Intensity	—	—	0.26	0.17
Unpleasantness	—	—	0.35[c]	0.32[c]

[a] $P < 0.001$.
[b] $P < 0.01$.
[c] $P < 0.05$.

A and B, but not for area C. Likewise, correlations between expected and concurrent ratings of unpleasantness were significant for areas A and area B, but not area C.

Associations between expected and ratings of remembered pain evidenced a slightly different pattern. Expected and remembered ratings of intensity were highly correlated for areas A and C, but not for area B. Corresponding ratings of unpleasantness were significantly correlated for A and C, but not for B. Finally, concurrent and remembered ratings of pain intensity and unpleasantness for areas A, B, and C were inconsistently correlated at no more than modest levels of strength.

3.6. Comparisons between Concurrent and Remembered Placebo Effects

Table 21.4 compares concurrent and remembered placebo effects across areas A and B and across pain intensity and pain unpleasantness dimensions. Whereas concurrent placebo effects for areas A and B were small (0.37 to 1.28 VAS units), those of remembered placebo effects were consistently over three times larger (2.10 to 3.98). A series of one-way repeated measures ANOVAs on the four arithmetic

Table 21.4.

Concurrent and remembered placebo effects

	Concurrent	Remembered
Pain sensation intensity		
Strong (C–A)	1.24	3.81
Weak (C–B)	0.56	2.60
Pain unpleasantness		
Strong (C–A)	1.28	3.98
Weak (C–B)	0.37	2.60

difference scores (i.e., area C minus area A; area C minus area B) for intensity and unpleasantness ratings, thereby representing the placebo effect for concurrent and remembered pain, indicated a significant effect of time (i.e., concurrent versus remembered) for intensity, $F(3,114) = 35.10$, $P < 0.001$, and unpleasantness, $F(3,114) = 43.95$, $P < 0.001$. Post-hoc contrast tests, with alpha set at $P < 0.05$ revealed that at area A, participants obtained a significantly larger placebo effect for the remembered intensity of pain (delta = 3.81) than concurrent pain (delta = 1.24), as well as for the remembered unpleasantness of pain (delta = 3.98) than concurrent pain (delta = 1.28). Likewise, post-hoc contrast tests showed that at area B, participants experienced a significantly larger placebo effect for intensity of remembered (delta = 2.10) versus concurrent pain (delta = 0.56), as well as for the unpleasantness of remembered (delta = 2.60) versus concurrent pain (delta = 0.37). This appears to result mainly from the fact that remembered baseline levels of pain intensity and unpleasantness were much larger than concurrent ratings of these dimensions, as shown in Fig. 21.1.

4. Discussion

Expectancy but not desire for relief was confirmed as contributing to the magnitude of placebo analgesia. A placebo effect was shown by statistically reliable reductions in pain ratings after conditioning trials had taken place. This result indicates that the pairing of surreptitiously lowered pain stimulus intensity with placebo administration results in subsequent placebo analgesia. The effect was graded according to the extent of surreptitious lowering of stimulus strength during the manipulation trials, a result that also is consistent with conditioning. This placebo effect also was manifested both within sensory and affective dimensions of pain. However, expectancy contributed to a large proportion of the variance in sensory and affective pain ratings within areas treated with placebo cream, providing further evidence that the conditioning effect is mediated by expectancy. The results did not confirm the hypothesized factor of desire for relief as having a mediating role in placebo analgesia.

Placebo effects assessed by ratings of remembered pain intensity and unpleasantness were over three times greater than concurrent placebo effects assessed during the posttest stimulation trials. Although placebo effects based on ratings of remembered pain were much greater than concurrent placebo effects, they were also strongly associated with expectancy ratings (Table 21.3). These combined results further establish expectancy as a causal factor in placebo analgesia and extend previous work by showing that expectancy has a role in both placebo effects based on concurrent and remembered pain.

4.1. Further Evidence That Placebo Analgesic Effects Are Mediated by Expectancy

Similar to Montgomery and Kirsch (1997), a strong association occurred between expectancy levels and pain ratings of stimuli presented to areas treated with placebo cream (i.e., placebo-treated areas B and A). These results further support Montgomery and Kirsch's conclusion that classical conditioning may occur, but that the proximal mediator of placebo analgesia is that of expectancy. The present study further extends their conclusions in three ways. First, it demonstrates that the expectancy hypothesis is confirmed across different types of experimental pain, iontophoretically induced pain in their study and heat-evoked pain in the present one. Second, it demonstrates that increasing the strength of the conditioning manipulation, the degree of surreptitious lowering of stimulus intensity during manipulation trials, produces increasing levels of expectation of pain reduction and increasing magnitudes of placebo analgesia. Third, it provides evidence in support of the hypothesis that placebo effects based on actual pain as well as placebo effects based on remembered pain are both mediated by expectancy.

The results also confirm those of a second study by Montgomery and Kirsch (1996) that provided evidence that psychological mediation of placebo analgesic effects involves much more specific mechanisms than the simple reduction of anxiety or other global effects on emotions. They demonstrated that the application of a placebo in the guise of a topical anesthetic-produced reduction in pain at a body site at which the placebo anesthetic agent was administered but not at a control body site. Controlled mechanical pain stimuli were administered simultaneously to treated and untreated fingers for one group of participants and sequentially for another. For both groups, reduction in pain occurred on the finger that was treated with the placebo analgesic but not on the untreated finger, thereby indicating a spatially restricted mechanism. Similarly, the present study showed placebo effects for skin areas treated with "strong" placebo cream (A) and not nearby skin areas (C). Results of both studies suggest that not all placebo effects are mediated by such global mechanisms as anxiety reduction or hormonal release of endogenous opioids. Such specificity in response would be consistent with a highly specific response expectancy on the part of the participant (Kirsch, 1990).

It is interesting that the magnitude of the placebo effect was consistent with the experimental pairings. Trials in which the placebo was paired with a large decrease in pain stimulus intensity (i.e., the strong placebo condition) resulted in a greater placebo analgesic effect than trials in which the placebo was paired with a small decrease in pain stimulus intensity (i.e., the weak placebo condition). This finding is consistent with both response expectancy theory (Kirsch, 1990) and stimulus substitution models of classical conditioning. Although it was not the purpose of this study to compare the relative contribution of classical conditioning factors and response expectancies to the gradient in placebo effectiveness, relations between the placebo conditions and participants' expectations established are consistent with a response expectancy mechanism. Based on our previous work (Montgomery and Kirsch, 1997), it seems likely that nature of the pairings (i.e., strong and weak placebo) contribute to participants' expectations which in turn determine the resulting placebo analgesic effect. Simply put, it appears that greater expectations resulted in greater placebo pain reduction. However, one must acknowledge that a stimulus substitution explanation of the magnitude gradient found in placebo analgesia cannot be formally ruled out.

Another possible limitation of this study is that the noxious stimuli, instructions to participants, and placebo manipulations were not given in a fashion unknown to the experimenter. Thus, it is possible that the experimenter's expectations could have been communicated to the participants. We attempted to control for this possibility by having the experimenter follow standardized experimental procedures (including a script) when giving instructions to the participants (see Methods). Although it is still possible that subtle cues were at least partly responsible for the expectancy effects, this does not critically influence the major conclusions drawn from this study. The purpose of the study was not to establish how expectancies are changed, but rather to investigate the effect of altered expectancies on concurrent and retrospective pain reports. In a sense, it doesn't matter whether the expectancies were changed by the manipulation or by the subtle cues from a non-blind experimenter, as also would be the case for placebo effects that occur under many clinical circumstances. Regardless of how expectancies were generated, evidence is provided that expectancy mediates placebo analgesia.

4.2. The Possible Role of "Desire for Relief" in Placebo Effects

One of the major hypotheses, that desire for pain reduction contributes to the magnitude of placebo analgesia, was not supported by the results nor was there a trend in the direction of a direct positive influence of this factor. The manipulation designed to modulate desire for pain reduction resulted in two groups of participants with significantly different magnitudes of desire for pain reduction. Despite the effectiveness of this approach, a difference in placebo effect did not occur between the two groups nor was there a significant association between this factor and magnitude of placebo analgesia. Taken together, these results indicate that desire for pain reduction is not a contributing factor in placebo analgesia under these experimental conditions.

Although these results cast doubt on the possible contribution of desire for pain reduction to placebo analgesia, there are reasons that the hypothesis should not be completely rejected at this point. First, nearly all participants had some degree of desire for pain reduction and so it is possible that some minimal level of desire for pain relief may be necessary for placebo analgesia. Second, desire for reduction in pain may be a more critical factor in placebo effects during clinical pain studies and have much less application to placebo effects in experimental pain. This issue may be particularly relevant when the test stimulus is brief, as in the present study. Desire for relief may be much more of a factor when the pain is threatening or has a more uncertain duration and therefore likely to induce fear or anxiety, as would be present in many instances of clinical pain. It has been suggested that the generally larger placebo analgesic effects in clinical as compared to experimental pain studies may reflect a stronger desire for pain relief in the former (Price, 1988; Price and Fields, 1997). This possibility needs to be evaluated in clinical studies that use measures of expectancy and desire for pain relief and that provide both placebo and natural history control conditions.

The lack of effects from our desire manipulation contrasts with Jensen and Karoly (1991) findings that desire to experience sedative effects from a drug resulted in greater placebo sedative effects. However, their desire manipulation was that of providing instructions to the effect that response to the drug meant that the participants had more favorable personality characteristics, whereas that of the present study relied more on participants' intrinsic desire for pain relief. It may be that some types of motivations or desires are more effective than others and/or that "desire for pain relief" has limited applicability to our experimental paradigm.

4.3. Placebo Effects Based on Remembered versus Actual Pain

When participants were asked to remember and rate pain intensities and unpleasantness levels within each of the three areas during the last six trials, these ratings closely followed their expected but not actual pain levels associated with post-manipulation trials (Fig. 21.2). As shown in Fig. 21.2, participants remembered the untreated pain within control area C as being much more intense and unpleasant than it actually was. This distortion was less for area B and minimal for area A. Selective distortions, in turn, resulted in large placebo effects for remembered pain, effects that were over three times larger than that of concurrent placebo effects (Fig. 21.2; Table 21.4). Moreover, these large placebo effects occurred for both areas A and B and for both sensory and affective dimensions. However, similar to concurrent placebo effects, they were strongly associated with expectancy ratings. Another line of evidence that placebo effects based on remembered pain follow participants expectations of pain more closely than actual pain intensities is that systematically higher correlation coefficients were found between expected and remembered pain than between actual and remembered pain (Table 21.3).

The selective exaggeration of remembered pain intensity within untreated area C and the consequent enhancement of placebo analgesia are consistent with previous studies that show that memory distortion of pretreatment pain contributes to an exaggeration of self-reports of pain relief (Feine et al., 1998; Mathias et al., 1995). Feine et al. (1998) found that pain relief scores based on memory were over three times higher than those based on pre-treatment minus present pain VAS ratings, consistent with the results of the present study of placebo analgesia. This similarity exists despite the facts that the former study was based on data obtained from temporomandibular dysfunction (TMD) patients who received active treatments for ten weeks and the present study was based on pain free volunteers exposed to brief experimental pain stimuli for about one hour. Feine et al. also found that overestimation of pretreatment pain was largest for patients whose pretreatment pain was low to moderate (<50 mm on 100 mm VAS). They point out that since pain associated with many chronic pain conditions is often low to moderate, it seems likely that most patients will report high levels of relief for small actual changes in pain intensity. Since the mean baseline pain rating of post-manipulation trials was about four on a scale of ten in the present study, a large distortion in remembered baseline pain would be consistent with conclusions of Feine et al. The present results extend their observations by providing evidence that their explanation for exaggerated estimates of pain relief apply to placebo treatments and in showing that, similar to concurrent placebo effects, remembered placebo effects are predicted by participants' expected pain levels (Fig. 21.2, Table 21.3). Based on the combination of present and previous results (Montgomery and Kirsch, 1997), it is likely that expectancy mediates both placebo effects based on actual pain as well as those based on remembered pain intensities.

As pointed out by Feine et al. (1998), patients' reports of relief following treatment are often used to establish the effectiveness of treatments. To the extent that such measures are used in clinical studies of pain treatments, estimates of magnitudes of analgesic effects from both placebo and active treatments are likely to be significantly enhanced when reports are made retrospectively. One has to openly wonder about the extent to which commonly quoted magnitudes of placebo analgesia (Beecher, 1955, 1959; Turner et al., 1994) as well as reported magnitudes of analgesia from active treatments have been based on retrospective judgments of pain relief. To take a relevant example, decisions as to whether and to what extent patients with chronic nonmalignant pain should rely on opioid analgesics are likely to be critically determined by whether their efficacy is assessed concurrently or retrospectively by clinicians who prescribe them and by researchers who study them.

The present study demonstrates the importance of response expectancies in determining both concurrent placebo analgesic effects as well as placebo analgesic effects based on remembered pain and provides further evidence that retrospective measurement of any treatment effect may exaggerate estimates of treatment efficacy. These findings are consistent with the growing literature on expectancy effects in clinical medicine (Montgomery et al., 1998) and future research should determine whether the findings of the present study generalize to treatments of other clinical problems (e.g., nausea, distress, fatigue).

REFERENCES

Beecher HK. The powerful placebo. J Am Med Assoc 1955;159:1602–1606.

Beecher HK. Measurement of Subjective Responses: Quantitative Effects of Drugs. New York: Oxford University Press, 1959.

Bootzin RR. The role of expectancy in behavior change. In: White L, Tursky B, Schwartz GE, editors. Placebo: Theory, Research, and Mechanisms. New York: The Guilford Press, 1985. pp. 196–210.

Baron RM, Kenny DA. The moderator-mediator variable distinction in social psychological research: conceptual, strategic, and statistical considerations. J Pers Soc Psych 1986;51:1173–1182.

Evans FJ. Expectancy, therapeutic instructions, and the placebo response. In: White L, Tursky B, Schwartz GE, editors. Placebo: Theory, Research, and Mechanisms. New York: The Guilford Press, 1985. pp. 215–228.

Feine JS, Lavigne GJ, Dao TTT, Morin C, Lund J. Memories of chronic pain and perceptions of relief. Pain 1998;77:137–141.

Fields HL, Price D. Toward a neurobiology of placebo analgesia. In: Harrington A, editor. The Placebo Effect: An Interdisciplinary Exploration. Cambridge, Mass.: Harvard University Press, 1997. pp. 93–116.

Jamison RN, Sbrocco T, Parris WCV. The influence of physical and psychological factors and accuracy for memory for pain in chronic pain patients. Pain 1989;37:289–294.

Jensen MP, Karoly P. Motivation and expectancy factors in symptom perception: a laboratory study of the placebo effect. Psych Med 1991;53:144–152.

Jospe M. The Placebo Effect in Healing. Lexington, Mass.: Lexington Books, 1978.

Kirsch I. Changing Expectations: A Key to Effective Psychotherapy. Pacific Grove, Calif.: Brooks/Cole, 1990.

Linton SJ, Melin L. The accuracy of remembering chronic pain. Pain 1982;13:281–285.

Levine JD, Gordon NC, Fields HL. The mechanism of placebo analgesia. Lancet 1978;2:654–657.

Mathias BJ, Dillingham TR, Zeiger DN, Chang AS, Belandres PV. Topical capsaicin for neck pain: a pilot study. Am J Phys Med Rehabil 1995;74:39–44.

Montgomery GH, Kirsch I. Mechanisms of placebo pain reduction: an empirical investigation. Psych Sci 1996;7:174–176.

Montgomery GH, Kirsch I. Classical conditioning and the placebo effect. Pain 1997;72:107–113.

Montgomery GH, Tomoyasu N, Bovbjerg DH, et al. Patients' pretreatment expectations of chemotherapy-related nausea are an independent predictor of anticipatory nausea. Ann Behav Med 1998;20(2):104–109.

Price DD. Psychological and Neural Mechanisms of Pain. New York: Raven Press, 1988.

Price DD, Barrell JJ. Some general laws of human emotion: interrelationships between intensities of desire, expectation, and emotional feeling. J Personality 1984;52:389–409.

Price DD, Barrell JE, Barrell JJ. A quantitative-experiential analysis of human emotions. Motiv Emot 1985;9:19–38.

Price DD, Barrell JJ, Gracely RH. A psychophysical analysis of experiential factors that selectively influence the affective dimension of pain. Pain 1980;8:137–179.

Price DD, Bush FM, Long S, Harkins SW. A comparison of pain measurement characteristics of mechanical visual analogue and simple numerical rating scales. Pain 1994;56:217–226.

Price DD, Fields HL. The contribution of desire and expectation to placebo analgesia: implications for new research strategies. In: Harrington A, editor. The Placebo Effect: An Interdisciplinary Exploration. Cambridge, Mass.: Harvard University Press, 1997. pp. 117–135.

Turner JA, Deyo RA, Loeser JD, Von Korff M, Fordyce WE. The importance of placebo effects in pain treatment and research. J Am Med Assoc 1994;271:1609–1614.

Voudouris NJ, Peck CL, Coleman G. The role of conditioning and expectancy in the placebo response. Pain 1990;43:121–128.

White L, Tursky B, Schwartz GE, editors. Placebo: Theory, Research, and Mechanisms. New York: The Guilford Press, 1985.

22

Neuropharmacological Dissection of Placebo Analgesia

Expectation-Activated Opioid Systems versus Conditioning-Activated Specific Subsystems

MARTINA AMANZIO AND FABRIZIO BENEDETTI

Martina Amanzio and Fabrizio Benedetti, "Neuropharmacological Dissection of Placebo Analgesia: Expectation-Activated Opioid Systems versus Conditioning-Activated Specific Subsystems," *Journal of Neuroscience* 1999;19:484–494.

The neurobiology of placebo was born when Levine et al. (1978) discovered that the opioid antagonist naloxone inhibits the placebo analgesic response. There are now several lines of evidence indicating that placebos activate endogenous opioid systems, thus producing placebo analgesia (Grevert et al., 1983; Fields and Levine, 1984; Levine and Gordon, 1984; Benedetti et al., 1995; Benedetti, 1996; Benedetti and Amanzio, 1997; Fields and Price, 1997). However, Gracely et al. (1983) showed that placebo analgesia may also occur without the involvement of endogenous opioid systems. In addition, in the study by Grevert et al. (1983) naloxone blocked placebo analgesia only partially, suggesting that both opioid and nonopioid components play an important role.

The activation of opioid or nonopioid systems represents only the final pathway of a complex mechanism that is poorly understood. In the typical paradigm used to produce placebo analgesia, a substance known to be nonanalgesic (e.g., saline solution) is administered, and the subject is told that it is a powerful painkiller. At least two theories have been proposed to explain this phenomenon as the basis for the activation of endogenous opioids. First, cognitive factors, like expectation of pain relief, are supposed to trigger the release of opioids in the CNS (for review, see Benedetti and Amanzio, 1997; Fields and Price, 1997). Second, a classical conditioning mechanism has been proposed, in which repeated associations between active analgesics, pain relief, and therapeutic surroundings produce a conditioned placebo analgesic response (Wickramasekera, 1985; Voudouris et al., 1989, 1990; Benedetti and Amanzio, 1997; Fields and Price, 1997; Price and Fields, 1997). In addition, the anxiety theory postulates that placebo analgesia is caused by a reduction of anxiety (Evans, 1985), whereas the response-appropriate sensation theory proposes that the global experience of pain results from a complex internal analysis of different brain states (Wall, 1993). These theories are not necessarily in conflict because each of them may represent a different aspect of the same phenomenon (Wall, 1992).

Therefore, although there is now a general agreement on the involvement of endogenous opioids in some types of placebo analgesia (ter Riet et al., 1998), the mechanisms of their activation is not known. As stressed by Fields and Levine (1984), it is necessary to understand the conditions and the mechanisms capable to produce naloxone-reversible and naloxone-insensitive placebo responses. On the basis of Fields and Levine's considerations, we analyzed different types of placebo analgesia that were induced by different combinations of expectation cues and conditioning procedures, and by different opioid and nonopioid conditioning drugs. In such a way, we could perform a true neuropharmacological dissection of placebo analgesia into opioid and nonopioid components and could identify how these neurochemical systems are related to cognitive and conditioning mechanisms.

Part of this study has been published in abstract form (Amanzio et al., 1998).

Materials and Methods

Subjects

A total of 229 subjects participated in the study after they signed a written informed consent in which the experimental procedure was described, and the use of morphine, ketorolac, and naloxone was explained in detail. In particular, they were told that these drugs were not dangerous and did not produce side effects at the doses used in the study. Each subject underwent a clinical examination in which blood pressure and electrocardiogram were recorded. All subjects with heart problems were not allowed to participate in the study. Most of the subjects referred to a previous experience with analgesics, either opioids or nonopioids, for different types of pathological conditions (e.g., headache or previous surgery). All the experimental procedures were conducted in conformance with the policies and principles contained in the Declaration of Helsinki. The 229 subjects were subdivided into 12 groups, whose characteristics are shown in Table 22.1. It should be noted that the ratio of males to females, age, and weight did not differ among the different groups.

Table 22.1.
Characteristics of the groups

Group	Number of subjects	Sex (male/female)	Age (years)	Weight (kg)
1	56	31/25	47.3±7.6	61.2±10.5
2	25	15/10	49.9±8.3	63.5±12.4
3	16	9/7	45.1±9.9	58.2±9.7
4	15	9/6	50.5±8.7	57.6±9.3
5	13	8/5	51.1±11.4	59.8±10.4
6	14	7/7	47.7±9.2	60.6±10.8
7	14	8/6	46.3±11.8	60.1±8.5
8	16	10/6	47.5±7.9	60.9±9.0
9	17	10/7	48.2±9.5	58.8±9.7
10	15	9/6	50.0±8.8	59.5±10.6
11	14	9/5	45.9±10.0	62.4±11.1
12	14	7/7	49.2±7.8	61.0±8.9

Pain Stimulus

Pain was induced experimentally by means of the tourniquet technique. This test produces ischemic pain of the arm that increases over time (Smith et al., 1966, 1972; Benedetti, 1996). To avoid variability among different subjects, we induced a quick increase of pain according to the following procedure. The subject reclined on a bed, his or her nondominant forearm was extended vertically, and venous blood was drained by means of an Esmarch bandage. A sphygmomanometer was placed around the upper arm and inflated to a pressure of 300 mmHg. The Esmarch bandage was maintained around the forearm, which was lowered on the subject's side. After this, the subject started squeezing a hand spring exerciser twelve times while his or her arm rested on the bed. Each squeeze was timed to last 2 sec, followed by a 2 sec rest. The force necessary to bring the handles together was 7.2 kg. This type of ischemic pain increases over time very quickly, and the pain becomes unbearable after about 13–14 min (Table 22.2). A timer was started after the last squeeze, and the subject stopped the timer when the pain became unbearable. At this point, the experiment was discontinued, and the time was recorded. Thus, pain tolerance was defined as the time from the last squeeze to unbearable pain.

Drug Administration

All drugs used in the present study were administered through an intravenous line. Before starting the experimental procedure, a needle was inserted into a vein of the dominant forearm. The needle was connected to a line, 1 m long, through which a slow infusion of 5% glucose solution was administered. The intravenous line reached a screen behind the subject's bed. In such a way, hidden injections could be performed by the experimenter. Naloxone (Crinos, Italy) was administered at a dose of 0.14 mg/kg in sterile solution of NaCl 0.9%. The infusion rate (controlled by an infusion pump) was 0.1 ml/sec for a total infusion time ranging from 180 to 250 sec. The conditioning drugs were morphine hydrochloride and ketorolac tromethamine. Morphine hydrochloride is an opioid agonist and was administered at a dose of 0.12 mg/kg in sterile solution of NaCl 0.9%, with an infusion rate of 0.1 ml/sec (total infusion time ranging from 70 to 100 sec). Ketorolac tromethamine (Formit, Italy) is a nonsteroidal anti-inflammatory drug (NSAID) with no activity on opioid receptors, and was administered at a dose of 0.43 mg/kg in sterile solution of NaCl 0.9%, with an infusion rate of 0.1 ml/sec (total infusion time ranging from 70 to 110 sec).

Experimental Procedure

The experiments were performed according to a randomized double-blind design in which neither the subject nor the experimenter knew what drug was administered. To do this, either morphine or saline were given on days 2 and 3. Similarly, either ketorolac or saline were given on days 2 and 3. On day 4, either morphine or naloxone or saline were administered. To avoid a large number of subjects, only two or three subjects per group received saline on days 2 and 3 and morphine or ketorolac on day 4. These subjects were not included in the study because they were used only to allow the double-blind design. By using this experimental approach, we were completely blind to morphine, ketorolac, and naloxone. All drugs were administered 10 min before inflating the sphygmomanometer cuff, and the time interval from cuff inflation to the last squeeze was 1 min. Thus, the time interval from drug administration to last squeeze was the same in all subjects (11 min). The complete experimental procedure is shown in Figure 22.1.

Group 1 (natural history) was tested with the tourniquet technique for four consecutive days without receiving any treatment. Group 2 received a hidden injection of naloxone performed through the intravenous line behind the screen on days 2 and 4, to ascertain whether naloxone per se af-

Table 22.2.
Pain tolerance comparisons

Group	Pain tolerance baseline on day 1 (min)	Comparison with natural history on day 1 (ANOVA)	Pain tolerance on the day after experimental test (min)	Comparison with day 1 (ANOVA)
2	13.32±4.2	$F_{(1,79)}=0.26; p=0.612$	(day 3) 13.24±3.03	$F_{(1,24)}=0.01; p=0.910$
3	14.12±4.38	$F_{(1,70)}=0.04; p=0.838$	(day 3) 13.87±3.83	$F_{(1,15)}=0.33; p=0.572$
4	13.33±4.25	$F_{(1,69)}=0.17; p=0.683$	(day 3) 12.53±3.64	$F_{(1,14)}=2.09; p=0.171$
5	12.77±4.13	$F_{(1,67)}=0.64; p=0.427$	(day 5) 12.92±2.9	$F_{(1,12)}=0.03; p=0.862$
6	12.14±4.49	$F_{(1,68)}=1.64; p=0.204$	(day 5) 11.71±4.43	$F_{(1,13)}=0.40; p=0.538$
7	13.57±3.72	$F_{(1,68)}=0.05; p=0.824$	(day 5) 13.43±3.11	$F_{(1,13)}=0.04; p=0.842$
8	13.69±4.27	$F_{(1,70)}=0.02; p=0.893$	(day 5) 13.19±4.02	$F_{(1,15)}=0.48; p=0.497$
9	14.35±4.14	$F_{(1,71)}=0.16; p=0.690$	(day 5) 13.71±3.33	$F_{(1,16)}=1.39; p=0.256$
10	13.27±3.77	$F_{(1,69)}=0.22; p=0.643$	(day 5) 12.67±3.29	$F_{(1,14)}=0.93; p=0.352$
11	13.86±4.07	$F_{(1,68)}=0.00; p=0.999$	(day 5) 13.21±3.72	$F_{(1,13)}=0.84; p=0.375$
12	12.86±4.24	$F_{(1,68)}=0.57; p=0.454$	(day 5) 12.29±3.22	$F_{(1,13)}=0.55; p=0.470$

Note: The left columns show the pain tolerance baseline on day 1 in all experimental groups and the comparisons with the natural history group on day 1 (p levels). The right columns show the pain tolerance on the day after drug administration and its comparison with pain tolerance on day 1.

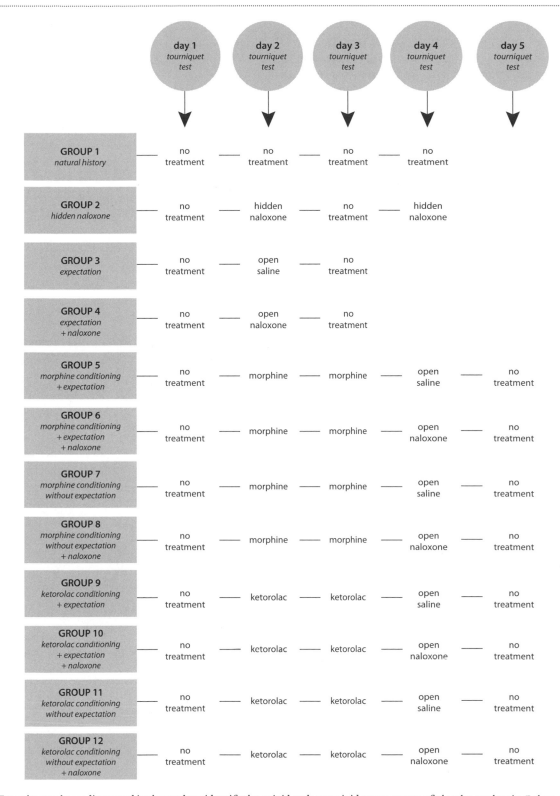

Figure 22.1. Experimental paradigm used in the study to identify the opioid and nonopioid components of placebo analgesia. Below each group the experimental condition is specified. *No treatment* means that the tourniquet test was performed without infusion of any drug.

fected the ischemic pain. It is important to emphasize that this group did not know that any injection was performed. Group 3 received an open injection (in full view of the subject) of saline (NaCl 0.9% solution) on day 2 and was told that it was a powerful painkiller (placebo with expectation of pain relief). Group 4 received an open injection of naloxone on day 2 and was told that it was a potent painkiller (placebo with expectation plus naloxone). Group 5 was treated with morphine (open injection) on days 2 and 3 (conditioning) and received an open injection of saline on day 4, believing that it was morphine (placebo with expectation). Group 6 was treated with morphine (open injection) on days 2 and 3 (conditioning) and received an open injection of naloxone on day 4, believing that it was morphine (placebo with expectation plus naloxone). Groups 7 and 8 received the same treatment as groups 5 and 6. However, the open injections of saline or naloxone on day 4 were believed to be a neutral nonanalgesic solution (antibiotic) used for sterility purposes; in this case, subjects did not expect any pain relief (placebo without expectation but with previous conditioning). Groups 9–12 were treated as groups 5–8, with the exception that conditioning on days 2 and 3 was performed with the nonopioid ketorolac.

The verbal instructions used in the different experimental conditions are reported below. In the conditioning procedures with either morphine or ketorolac on days 2 and 3, subjects were told that the drugs were potent analgesics producing a quick pain reduction and, therefore, an increase of tolerance. On day 4, in the expectation procedure (groups 5, 6, 9, and 10), subjects were told that the drug was the same potent analgesic used on days 2 and 3. By contrast, in the no-expectation procedure (groups 7, 8, 11, and 12), subjects were told that the drug was an antibiotic used "to clean the blood" for the sake of sterility; thus, these subjects believed that day 4 was not used for analgesic tests.

It should be noted that the tourniquet test was performed without any treatment on the first and last days in all groups, and it was used as a control.

Statistical Analysis

The differences between and within treatments were tested by means of the ANOVA followed by the Newman-Keuls multiple range test for multiple comparisons. In addition, linear regression analysis was performed by considering the data from single subjects. Therefore, data are presented as mean ± SD or for single subjects. Differences were considered to be statistically significant at $p < 0.05$.

Results

The Natural History of Ischemic Arm Pain

The natural history group showed no variation of pain tolerance when the tourniquet test was repeated for four consecutive days ($F_{(3,165)} = 1.5$; $p = 0.216$), indicating that the tourniquet technique produces pain tolerances that remain constant for several days (Fig. 22.2A). In all groups, the pain tolerance baseline on day 1 did not differ from the mean value of the natural history group (Fig. 22.2B). It can also be seen in Table 22.2 that no significant difference was found between each group and the natural history on day 1. In addition, the post-treatment control test (either day 3 for groups 2–4 or day 5 for the other groups) did not differ from the pretreatment control test of day 1 (Table 22.2). In conclusion, when the tourniquet test was performed without any treatment (controls), it always produced constant and consistent results in a range of time of at least 5 d. Therefore, any depar-

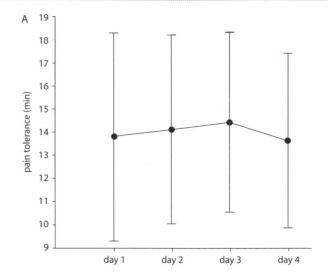

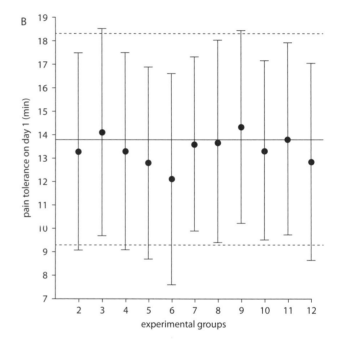

Figure 22.2. Analysis of the natural history of ischemic pain. A, Means and SDs of the natural history are shown for group 1 on 4 consecutive days. B, Pain baseline (mean ± SD) on day 1 in all groups and comparison with the natural history group on day 1. The *horizontal bold line* represents the mean of day 1 shown in A, the *broken lines* represent the SD. The statistical analysis of the natural history is shown in Table 22.2.

ture from this pain tolerance baseline (natural history) can be viewed as a true placebo effect.

Opioid-Mediated Placebo Analgesia

Before starting the conditioning procedures, we wanted to test whether a placebo effect and its reversal by naloxone could be adequately observed in these experimental conditions. First of all, we tested whether naloxone per se affects this type of experimental pain. A hidden injection of naloxone (group 2) on days 2 and 4 did not produce any variation of pain tolerance compared with days 1 and 3 ($F_{(3,72)} = 0.01$; $p = 0.991$) (Fig. 22.3A). Then we evoked a placebo response by

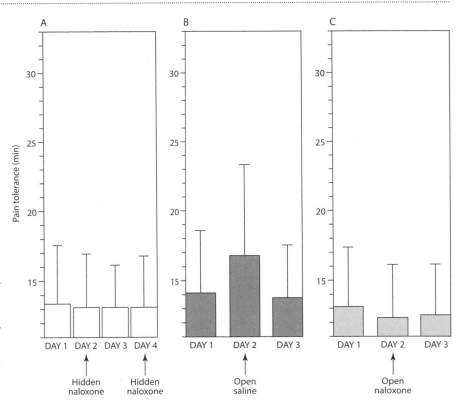

Figure 22.3. Expectation-induced placebo analgesia and its blockade by naloxone. A, A hidden injection of naloxone on days 2 and 4 (group 2) does not produce any change in pain tolerance compared with days 1 and 3, indicating that naloxone per se does not affect this type of experimental pain. B, An open injection of saline (group 3) produces a placebo analgesic effect. Days 1 and 3 represent preinjection and postinjection controls. C, An open injection of naloxone on day 2 (group 4) blocks the placebo effect completely. In fact, pain tolerance on day 2 is equal to preinjection and postinjection controls.

injecting saline which the subjects believed to be a potent painkiller (group 3); a clear-cut placebo effect could be observed compared with days 1 and 3 ($F_{(1,15)} = 12.36$; $p < 0.003$) (Fig. 22.3B). If, however, the open injection contained naloxone (group 4), no effect could be observed (Fig. 22.3C); in fact, no difference was found between days 2 and 1 ($F_{(1,14)} = 4.41$; $p = 0.054$). It is worth noting that, albeit nonsignificant, there was a tendency for pain tolerance on day 2 to be smaller than on day 1. Therefore, we can conclude that this type of experimental pain (1) is not affected by naloxone, (2) can produce placebo responses, and (3) these placebo responses are blocked by naloxone.

Conditioning with Morphine Hydrochloride

When morphine was administered on days 2 and 3, a significant increase in pain tolerance was found ($F_{(1,12)} = 274.46$; $p < 0.0001$ and $F_{(1,12)} = 157.25$; $p < 0.0001$, respectively) (Fig. 22.4A). A saline injection on day 4, which the subjects believed to be morphine (group 5), mimicked the morphine responses of the previous days ($F_{(1,12)} = 69.12$; $p < 0.001$), whereas pain tolerance returned to baseline on day 5 ($F_{(1,12)} = 0.03$; $p = 0.862$) (Fig. 22.4A). If the same procedure was performed but naloxone, which was believed to be morphine, was injected on day 4 (group 6), no morphine-mimicking response could be observed ($F_{(1,13)} = 0.09$; $p = 0.765$) (Fig. 22.4B). The same procedure was also used in groups 7 (Fig. 22.4C) and 8 (Fig. 22.4D). However, the subjects were told that the injection of day 4 was an antibiotic, and, thus, they did not expect any pain relief. In group 7 (Fig. 22.4C), a

morphine-mimicking response was found after saline injection on day 4, even if no expectation of pain relief was present ($F_{(1,13)} = 78$; $p < 0.001$), indicating that the previous morphine conditioning per se was sufficient to evoke a placebo effect. There was a significant difference between the placebo effects of groups 5 (Fig. 22.4A) and 7 (Fig. 22.4C) ($F_{(1,25)} = 5.5$; $p < 0.03$), indicating that conditioning plus expectation produces a placebo response that is larger than conditioning alone. The conditioning-induced placebo effect was completely blocked by naloxone (group 8) because no effect was observed after an open injection of naloxone that the subjects believed to be an antibiotic ($F_{(1,15)} = 0.32$; $p = 0.580$) (Fig. 22.4D). It is important to note that pain tolerance returned to baseline on day 5 in all cases.

We also performed a linear regression analysis by considering the data from single subjects. We found a high correlation between the response to morphine on day 3 and the response to saline on day 4, according to the rule "the larger the morphine responses, the larger the placebo responses." The analgesic response to morphine was expressed as Δt, that is, the difference between pain tolerance on days 3 and 1. Similarly, the analgesic response to placebo was expressed as the difference of pain tolerance on days 4 and 1. This was true for both groups 5 and 7 ($r = 0.627$; $t_{(11)} = 2.669$; $p < 0.025$ and $r = 0.855$; $t_{(12)} = 5.704$; $p < 0.001$, respectively) (Fig. 22.5, *black circles*). Naloxone disrupted completely this correlation in both groups 6 and 8 ($r = 0.187$; $t_{(12)} = 0.661$; $p = 0.521$ and $r = 20.282$; $t_{(14)} = 21.1$; $p = 0.290$, respectively) (Fig. 22.5, *white circles*).

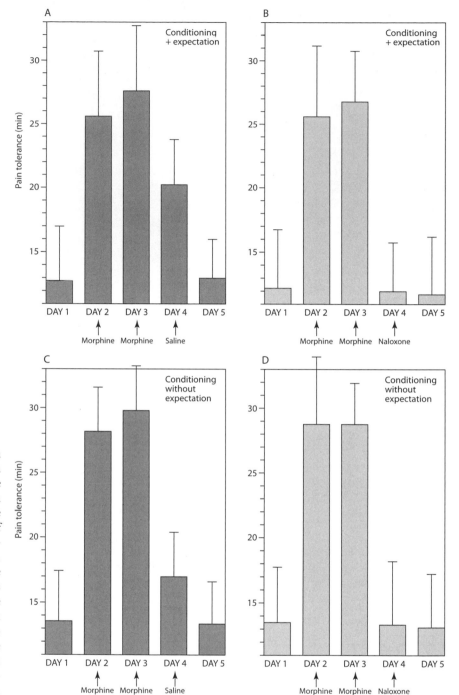

Figure 22.4. A, After morphine conditioning on days 2 and 3, an open injection of saline, which is believed to be morphine (group 5), mimics the morphine analgesic response. B, If an open injection of naloxone, which is believed to be morphine (group 6), is performed after 2 days of morphine conditioning, the morphine-mimicking effect is completely abolished. C, After morphine conditioning for 2 consecutive days, an open injection of saline, which is believed to be an antibiotic (group 7), mimics the morphine response (albeit less than in A). D, An open injection of naloxone, which is believed to be an antibiotic (group 8), completely blocks the morphine-mimicking effect. In all cases, days 1 and 5 represent preconditioning and postconditioning controls.

In conclusion, the placebo responses induced by morphine conditioning plus expectation and morphine conditioning alone could be blocked completely by naloxone.

Conditioning with Ketorolac Tromethamine

The same procedures used for morphine conditioning and described above were repeated with the nonopioid ketorolac. Administration of ketorolac on days 2 and 3 produced strong analgesic responses ($F_{(1,16)} = 193.88$; $p < 0.0001$ and $F_{(1,16)} = 83.22$; $p < 0.001$, respectively) (Fig. 22.6A). In both groups 9 (Fig. 22.6A) and 11 (Fig. 22.6C), the saline injection produced ketorolac-mimicking responses ($F_{(1,16)} = 68.36$;

$p < 0.001$ and $F_{(1,13)} = 28.04$; $p < 0.001$, respectively). If naloxone was administered on day 4 (group 10) and was believed to be ketorolac (Fig. 22.6B), the ketorolac-mimicking response was still present ($F_{(1,14)} = 56$; $p < 0.001$), but was significantly smaller than the mimicking response of group 9 ($F_{(1,30)} = 5.65$; $p < 0.025$). Therefore, in this case the placebo response was only partially abolished by naloxone. By contrast, if naloxone was administered on day 4 (group 12) and was believed to be an antibiotic (no-expectation, Fig. 22.6D), it was completely ineffective in blocking the conditioning-induced placebo response. In fact, the ketorolac-mimicking response was still present ($F_{(1,13)} = 59.47$; $p < 0.001$).

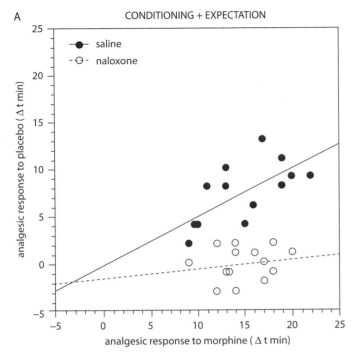

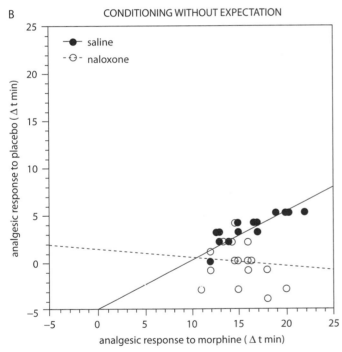

Figure 22.5. Relationship between the analgesic response to morphine on day 3 and the placebo analgesic response on day 4. Each circle represents the response of a single subject. The responses are expressed as Δt, that is, the difference of pain tolerance between days 3 and 4 and day 1. A, In group 5 (*black circles*), the larger the morphine response, the larger the placebo response after a saline injection that is believed to be morphine. This correlation is completely disrupted by naloxone in group 6 (*white circles*). B, Same as in A but the saline injection is believed to be an antibiotic (groups 7 and 8).

The linear regression analysis performed with the data from single subjects gave the same results (Fig. 22.7). A correlation between ketorolac responses on day 3 and placebo

responses on day 4 was present in groups 9 and 11, which received saline ($r = 0.815$; $t_{(15)} = 5.44$; $p < 0.001$ and $r = 0.645$; $t_{(12)} = 2.924$; $p < 0.015$, respectively) and in groups 10 and 12, which received naloxone ($r = 0.580$; $t_{(13)} = 2.566$; $p < 0.025$ and $r = 0.554$; $t_{(12)} = 2.308$; $p < 0.04$, respectively).

Therefore, the placebo responses induced by ketorolac conditioning plus expectation were only partially blocked by naloxone, whereas those induced by ketorolac conditioning alone were naloxone-insensitive.

The Naloxone-Reversible and Naloxone-Insensitive Components of Placebo

Because of the complex experimental design, a brief summary of the statistical analysis previously described is reported below. Expectation alone (group 3) produces a placebo response that can be blocked completely by naloxone (group 4) (Fig. 22.8A). Conditioning with morphine plus expectation cues (group 5) produce a placebo effect that is larger than morphine conditioning alone (group 7); both can be blocked completely by naloxone (groups 6 and 8) (Fig. 22.8B). Conditioning with ketorolac plus expectation cues (group 9) produce a placebo effect that has the tendency ($F_{(1,29)} = 2.92$; $p = 0.098$) to be larger than ketorolac conditioning alone (group 11). The former can be blocked by naloxone only partially (group 10), whereas the latter is completely insensitive to naloxone (group 12) (Fig. 22.8C).

Discussion

In the present study we have produced different types of placebo response that can be totally blocked, partially blocked, or totally unaffected by naloxone. This indicates that placebo analgesia can be dissected into opioid and nonopioid components, depending on the procedure used to induce the placebo response. These findings were obtained by using a model of experimental pain that has been shown to be sensitive to morphine (Smith et al., 1966, 1972) and to produce well measurable placebo responses (Grevert et al., 1983; Benedetti, 1996). Most important, this type of experimental ischemic arm pain was found to be unaffected by naloxone (Grevert and Goldstein, 1977, 1978; Benedetti, 1996), a necessary condition when naloxone is used to study placebo analgesia. Therefore, the present results are in accordance with previous investigations, confirming that naloxone per se does not influence ischemic arm pain (Fig. 22.3A). In addition, we also produced an increase of pain tolerance by means of ketorolac, an NSAID with powerful analgesic activity and no opioid action. It should be pointed out that NSAIDs are known to act at peripheral sites during inflammation by inhibiting the cyclo-oxygenase enzyme necessary for the conversion of arachidonic acid into prostaglandins (Levine and Taiwo, 1994). However, recently it was shown that NSAIDs have a central site of action at the spinal level (Malmberg and Yaksh, 1992). Thus, inflammation is not a necessary condition for the analgesic action of NSAIDs, and the findings of the present study show that

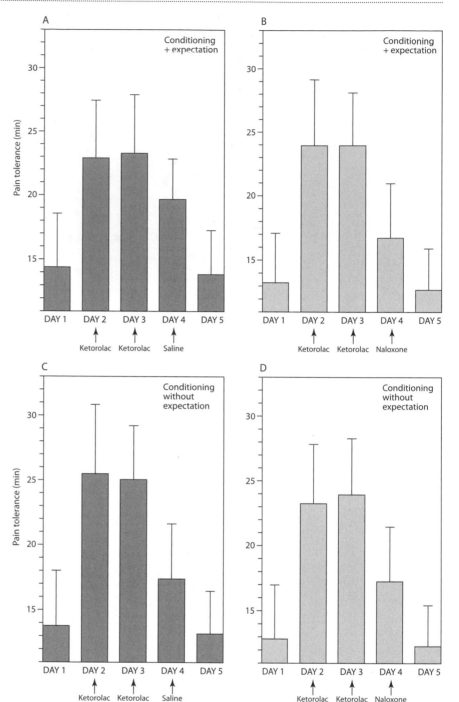

Figure 22.6. A, After ketorolac conditioning on days 2 and 3, an open injection of saline that is believed to be ketorolac (group 9) mimics the ketorolac analgesic response. B, An open injection of naloxone, which is believed to be ketorolac (group 10), blocks the ketorolac-mimicking effect only partially. C, After ketorolac conditioning for 2 consecutive days, an open injection of saline that is believed to be an antibiotic (group 11), mimics the ketorolac response. D, An open injection of naloxone, which is believed to be an antibiotic (group 12), is ineffective in abolishing the ketorolac-mimicking effect. Preconditioning and postconditioning control tests are shown on days 1 and 5 in all cases.

ketorolac is a powerful analgesic in experimental ischemic arm pain (Fig. 22.6).

In a previous study (Benedetti, 1996), we observed that the tourniquet technique induces an increase of pain over time that is variable among different subjects. To reduce this variability, we inflated the sphygmomanometer cuff up to 300 mmHg, maintained the Esmarch bandage around the forearm throughout the test, and used a hand exerciser with a force of 7.2 kg. These modifications, compared with the study by Benedetti (1996), produced a quick increase of pain, such that pain tolerances were reduced and variability decreased. In addition, drugs were administered 10 min before cuff inflation, so that a long time interval was allowed for the drug to produce its effects (~25 min; 11 min before the last squeeze plus ~14 min of pain tolerance). Therefore, by reducing both pain tolerance and variability, and by maintaining constant the time interval for drug peak effects, we could obtain homogeneous populations of subjects. In addition, the use of tolerance as a measure of pain needs some considerations. In fact, tolerance is a complex variable in which the motivational-affective dimension of pain appears to be more important than the sensory dimension (Price, 1988). We measured pain tolerance because it has been shown to be affected by analgesics like morphine (Smith et al., 1966), thus indicat-

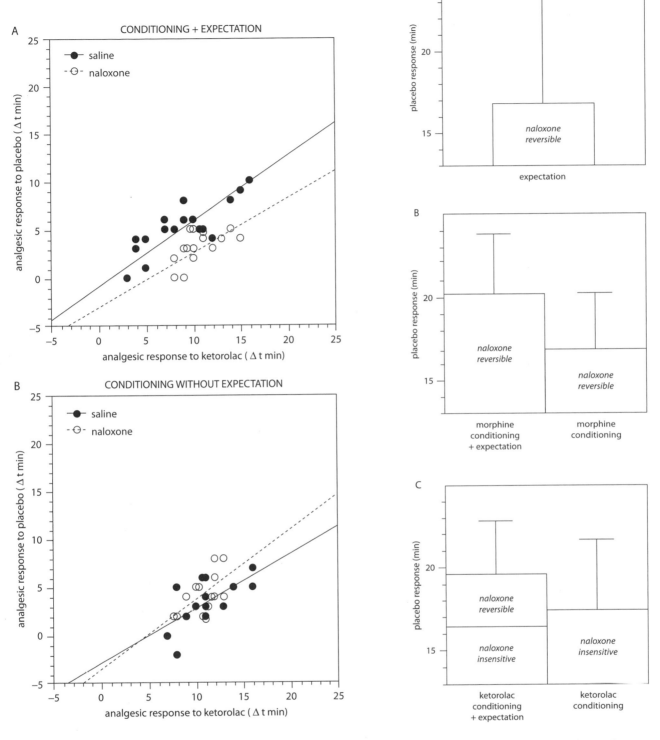

Figure 22.7. Relationship between the analgesic response to ketorolac on day 3 and the placebo analgesic response on day 4. Each *circle* represents the response of a single subject. As in Figure 22.5, the responses are expressed as Δt, that is, the difference of pain tolerance between days 3 and 4 and day 1. A, In group 9 (*black circles*), the larger the ketorolac response, the larger the placebo response after a saline injection that is believed to be ketorolac. This correlation is maintained after naloxone injection in group 10 (*white circles*). B, Same as in A but the saline injection is believed to be an antibiotic (groups 11 and 12). In this case, naloxone is completely ineffective in disrupting the correlation.

Figure 22.8. Dissection of placebo analgesia into naloxone-reversible and naloxone-insensitive components. A, Expectation-induced placebo analgesia is completely blocked by naloxone. B, Morphine conditioning plus expectation produces a placebo response that is totally blocked by naloxone. Morphine conditioning alone induces placebo responses that, similarly, are completely blocked by naloxone. C, Nonopioid ketorolac conditioning plus expectation produces a placebo response that is only partially antagonized by naloxone. By contrast, nonopioid ketorolac conditioning alone induces placebo responses that are completely insensitive to naloxone.

ing that such a measure of pain can be used to test analgesic drugs. Accordingly, we wanted to see whether placebos produced analgesic-like effects, that is, an increase in tolerance. Even if tolerance measures both the sensory and the motivational-affective component of pain, as carefully stated by Price (1988), this is not against our findings.

One of the main findings emerging from this study is that cognitive factors like expectation appear to trigger endogenous opioid systems in all cases. When we talk of expectation, we refer to verbal expectation. In fact, the subjects believed to receive an analgesic, such that they expected a relief of pain. Although we have not actually measured a change in expectation, the verbal cues (analgesic or antibiotic) are clearly directed in two opposite directions: the first increasing, the second reducing expectation. Unfortunately, we do not know whether in group 3 (expectation) a previous conditioning occurred (Fig. 22.8A). In fact, most of the subjects had a previous experience with either opioids or nonopioids (e.g., headache or surgery). Nonetheless, the conditioning experiments with morphine and ketorolac clearly indicate that expectation-induced placebo responses are mediated by endogenous opioids. For example, it is worth emphasizing that ketorolac conditioning alone was naloxone-insensitive, whereas ketorolac conditioning plus expectation was partially naloxone-reversible (Fig. 22.8C). This indicates that, by adding expectation cues, an opioid component comes out.

On the other hand, conditioning-induced placebo responses are not mediated by endogenous opioids per se but by specific subsystems, depending on the drug used for conditioning (Fig. 22.9). If an opioid like morphine is used, conditioning occurs via opioid receptors such that the resulting conditioned placebo response will be naloxone-reversible. Conversely, if conditioning is performed with a nonopioid drug like ketorolac, the resulting placebo response will be naloxone-insensitive. This is probably caused by the involvement of specific mechanisms during conditioning. For instance, the NSAIDs, like ketorolac, act at both peripheral and central sites in the spinal cord (Malmberg and Yaksh, 1992), inhibiting the cyclo-oxygenase enzyme necessary for the conversion of arachidonic acid into prostaglandins. Therefore, conditioning might occur via these nonopioid pathways. We further propose that, if other analgesics (e.g., the $\alpha 2$ adrenergic receptor agonist clonidine or the tricyclic-type antidepressant amitriptyline) are used for conditioning, other mechanisms may result to be involved (e.g., via adrenergic pathways), thus producing a naloxone-insensitive placebo analgesia (Fig. 22.9).

These findings clarify some previous contrasting studies showing that placebo analgesia is unaffected (Gracely et al., 1983) or reversed (Levine et al., 1978; Grevert et al., 1983; Benedetti, 1996) by naloxone. In fact, if we ignore the strength of the expectation cues and the previous experience (conditioning) with opioids or nonopioids, different subjects with different past experiences can be mistakenly considered to be homogeneous. This issue was first raised by Fields

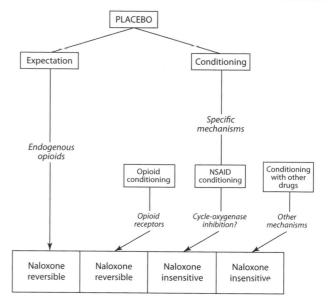

Figure 22.9. Schematic diagram of the mechanisms activating endogenous opioid systems and nonopioid systems in placebo analgesia. The administration of a placebo can trigger both cognitive (expectation) and conditioning mechanisms. Expectation activates endogenous opioid systems, whereas conditioning is mediated by specific mechanisms. If conditioning is performed with opioids, placebo analgesia is mediated via opioid receptors. However, if conditioning is performed with nonopioid drugs, other mechanisms result to be involved. Therefore, placebo analgesia can result to be either naloxone-reversible or partially naloxone-reversible or, otherwise, naloxone-insensitive, depending on the procedure used to evoke the placebo response.

and Levine (1984), who analyzed the different circumstances that might determine whether the placebo response has an opioid component. In particular, Fields and Levine stressed that complex psychological factors, such as instructions, consent form, remuneration, time of placebo administration, method of pain rating, site, and cause of pain may be relevant for the activation of endogenous opioid systems. Thus, it is not surprising that previous studies found placebo effects that respond totally, partially, or do not respond at all to naloxone. If, for example, expectation cues are not adequate, and the subject has been previously conditioned with nonopioid drugs, the placebo response is likely to be naloxone-insensitive. By contrast, if the subject had a previous experience with opioids, and the expectation cues are strong, the placebo response will result to be naloxone-reversible.

It is interesting that placebo responses occurred even without expectation of pain relief. In other words, if the subject was previously conditioned with either morphine or ketorolac, the lack of expectation cues only reduced but did not prevent the occurrence of a placebo effect. These findings are in agreement with those by Voudouris et al. (1990), who showed that conditioned placebo responses can be obtained without expectancy. Thus, previously conditioned subjects experience an analgesic effect even if they do not expect it. Nonetheless, it should be reminded that in a recent work,

Montgomery and Kirsch (1997) showed that placebo analgesia can result from conditioning but is mediated by expectation. This is consistent with our findings that, by reducing expectation in conditioned subjects (belief to receive an antibiotic), the placebo effect results to be smaller. However, this small residual effect is likely to represent a sequence effect caused by learning (conditioning), with little or no involvement of expectation. This notion is supported by a recent study (Benedetti et al., 1999), showing that a similar conditioning can be found in placebo respiratory depression, a phenomenon mediated by endogenous opioids and in which expectation cues are not present.

Several studies showed that conditioning plays an important role in the placebo response, and this is true for pain, the immune system and, in general, for pharmacotherapy (Gleidman et al., 1957; Herrnstein, 1962; Batterman, 1966; Batterman and Lower, 1968; Laska and Sunshine, 1973; Ader, 1985; Siegel, 1985; Wickramasekera, 1985; Voudouris et al., 1989, 1990; Ader, 1997; Benedetti et al., 1998). Similarly, cognitive and motivational factors, such as expectation and desire of pain relief, appear to play an essential role (Fields and Price, 1997; Price and Fields, 1997). The findings of the present study and the experimental approach by itself show that cognition and conditioning can be balanced in different ways during a placebo procedure. This balance is crucial for the activation of opioid systems or other specific subsystems and has at least three important implications. First, a complex cognitive function, like expectation of pain relief, is capable to interact with neurochemical systems and to produce a specific analgesic effect. Second, the placebo response depends on past experience, being mediated by specific subsystems that are likely to be activated during learning. Third, the understanding of the intricate mechanisms linking mental activity and pain will help in planning new therapeutic strategies.

REFERENCES

Ader R (1985) Conditioned immunopharmacological effects in animals: implications for a conditioning model of pharmacotherapy. In: Placebo: theory, research, and mechanisms (White L, Tursky B, Schwartz GE, eds.), pp. 306–323. New York: Guilford.

Ader R (1997) The role of conditioning in pharmacotherapy. In: The placebo effect: an interdisciplinary exploration (Harrington A, ed.), pp. 138–165. Cambridge, Mass.: Harvard UP.

Amanzio M, Pollo A, Benedetti F (1998) Endogenous opioids mediate both placebo analgesia and placebo respiratory depression. Soc Neurosci Abstr 495.11.

Batterman RC (1966) Persistence of responsiveness with placebo therapy following an effective drug trial. J New Drugs 6:137–141.

Batterman RC, Lower WR (1968) Placebo responsiveness: influence of previous therapy. Curr Ther Res 10:136–143.

Benedetti F (1996) The opposite effects of the opiate antagonist naloxone and the cholecystokinin antagonist proglumide on placebo analgesia. Pain 64:535–543.

Benedetti F, Amanzio M (1997) The neurobiology of placebo analgesia: from endogenous opioids to cholecystokinin. Prog Neurobiol 52:109–125.

Benedetti F, Amanzio M, Maggi G (1995) Potentiation of placebo analgesia by proglumide. Lancet 346:1231.

Benedetti F, Amanzio M, Baldi S, et al. (1998) The specific effects of prior opioid exposure on placebo analgesia and placebo respiratory depression. Pain 75:313–319.

Benedetti F, Amanzio M, Baldi S, Casadio C, Maggi G (1999) Inducing placebo respiratory depressant responses in humans via opioid receptors. Eur J Neurosci 11:625–631.

Evans FJ (1985) Expectancy, therapeutic instructions, and the placebo response. In: Placebo: theory, research, and mechanisms (White L, Tursky B, Schwartz GE, eds.), pp. 215–228. New York: Guilford.

Fields HL, Levine JD (1984) Placebo analgesia: a role for endorphins? Trends Neurosci 7:271–273.

Fields HL, Price DD (1997) Toward a neurobiology of placebo analgesia. In: The placebo effect: an interdisciplinary exploration (Harrington A, ed.), pp. 93–116. Cambridge, Mass.: Harvard UP.

Gleidman LH, Grantt WH, Teitelbaum HA (1957) Some implications of conditional reflex studies for placebo research. Am J Psychiatry 113:1103–1107.

Gracely RH, Dubner R, Wolskee PJ, Deeter WR (1983) Placebo and naloxone can alter postsurgical pain by separate mechanisms. Nature 306:264–265.

Grevert P, Goldstein A (1977) Effects of naloxone on experimentally induced ischemic pain and on mood in human subjects. Proc Natl Acad Sci USA 74:1291–1294.

Grevert P, Goldstein A (1978) Endorphins: naloxone fails to alter experimental pain or mood in humans. Science 199:1093–1095.

Grevert P, Albert LH, Goldstein A (1983) Partial antagonism of placebo analgesia by naloxone. Pain 16:129–143.

Herrnstein RJ (1962) Placebo effect in the rat. Science 138:677–678.

Laska E, Sunshine A (1973) Anticipation of analgesia: a placebo effect. Headache 13:1–11.

Levine JD, Gordon NC (1984) Influence of the method of drug administration on analgesic response. Nature 312:755–756.

Levine JD, Taiwo Y (1994) Inflammatory pain. In: Textbook of pain (Wall PD, Melzack R, eds.), pp. 45–56. Edinburgh: Churchill Livingstone.

Levine JD, Gordon NC, Fields HL (1978) The mechanism of placebo analgesia. Lancet 2:654–657.

Malmberg AB, Yaksh TL (1992) Hyperalgesia mediated by spinal glutamate or substance P receptor blocked by spinal cyclo-oxygenase inhibition. Science 257:1277–1280.

Montgomery GH, Kirsch I (1997) Classical conditioning and the placebo effect. Pain 72:107–113.

Price DD (1988) Psychological and neural mechanisms of pain. New York: Raven.

Price DD, Fields HL (1997) The contribution of desire and expectation to placebo analgesia: implications for new research strategies. In: The placebo effect: an interdisciplinary exploration (Harrington A, ed.), pp. 117–137. Cambridge, Mass.: Harvard UP.

Siegel S (1985) Drug anticipatory responses in animals. In: Placebo: theory, research, and mechanisms (White L, Tursky B, Schwartz GE, eds.), pp. 288–305. New York: Guilford.

Smith GM, Egbert LD, Markowitz RA, Mosteller F, Beecher HK (1966) An experimental pain method sensitive to morphine in man: the submaximum effort tourniquet technique. J Pharmacol Exp Ther 154:324–332.

Smith GM, Lowenstein E, Hubbard JH, Beecher HK (1972) Experimental pain produced by the submaximum effort tourniquet technique: further evidence of validity. J Pharmacol Exp Ther 163:468–474.

ter Riet G, de Craen AJM, de Boer A, Kessels AGH (1998) Is placebo analgesia mediated by endogenous opioids? A systematic review. Pain 76:273–275.

Voudouris NJ, Peck CL, Coleman G (1989) Conditioned response models of placebo phenomena: further support. Pain 38:109–116.

Voudouris NJ, Peck CL, Coleman G (1990) The role of conditioning and verbal expectancy in the placebo response. Pain 43:121–128.

Wall PD (1992) The placebo effect: an unpopular topic. Pain 51:1–3.

Wall PD (1993) Pain and the placebo response. In: Ciba foundation symposium 174— experimental and theoretical studies of consciousness (Bock GR, Marsh J, eds.), pp. 187–216. New York: Wiley.

Wickramasekera I (1985) A conditioned response model of the placebo effect: predictions from the model. In: Placebo: theory, research, and mechanisms (White L, Tursky B, Schwartz GE, eds.), pp. 255–287. New York: Guilford.

23

Placebo Analgesia Induced by Social Observational Learning

LUANA COLLOCA AND FABRIZIO BENEDETTI

Luana Colloca and Fabrizio Benedetti, "Placebo Analgesia Induced by Social Observational Learning," Pain 2009;144:28–34.

1. Introduction

Placebo effects are known to be mediated by a variety of mechanisms, such as expectation, reward, and conditioning [11,13,28,39,40]. However, a common factor that appears to be present across different conditions is represented by learning, as previous experience has been found to powerfully modulate the magnitude of placebo responses. For example, early clinical observations [1,7,27,31,32] as well as more recent experimental findings [2,9,14–16,29,33,37,38,41–43] indicate that prior experience can either lead to conditioned responses or reinforce expectations. Placebo effects might also occur without a history of actual firsthand experience, because other signaling systems such as language and/or observation may convey information that is necessary to build up learned responses. On the basis of these considerations, it is worth investigating the potential of other forms of learning in the modulation of placebo responses. So far, only conditioning and reinforced expectations have been tested, whereas no attempt has been made to understand whether social observation influences placebo analgesia. Social learning refers to instances of learning where the behavior of a demonstrator, or its by-products, modifies the subsequent behavior of an observer [21], and a substantial body of work highlights its critical function in a wide range of models, both human, and non-human for reviews see [24,25,34]. In addition, Bootzin and Caspi [12] postulated the possible involvement of social learning in placebo responsiveness.

In the present study, we investigated the role of observational social learning in placebo analgesia in a human experimental setting, whereby subjects learn by observing the analgesic experience of others. In order to compare these observation-induced effects with other kinds of learning, we replicated our earlier findings (e.g., [14]) demonstrating that learning, via a typical conditioning procedure, can elicit placebo responses that are substantially larger than those induced by verbal suggestions alone.

2. Materials and Methods

2.1. Subjects

A total of 48 healthy female volunteers (mean age 22.6 ± 4.7 years) were recruited from the University of Turin Medical School, Turin, Italy, to participate in a research on pain mechanisms. They were randomly assigned to one of three experimental groups: social learning, through the observation of another subject (Group 1), conditioning (Group 2), and verbal suggestions alone (Group 3) (Table 23.1). None of them had any kind of disease or were taking any type of medication. All the experimental procedures were conducted in conformance with the policies and principles contained in the Declaration of Helsinki. Subjects gave their written informed consent to receive repeated phasic painful and non-painful stimuli for a study on a procedure of pain inhibition. Those who were enrolled in Group 1 were informed that the experimental details would be shown by one of the experimenters. Conversely, subjects who were assigned to Groups 2 and 3 were deceptively informed that a red light would anticipate painful electrical stimuli, whereas a green light would anticipate a stimulus that would be made less painful through a sub-threshold stimulation of a different body part. All the subjects were debriefed at the end of the study.

2.2. Tactile and Painful Stimuli

The stimulus was an electric shock delivered to the back of the non-dominant hand through two silver chloride electrodes (size = 1×2.5 cm) connected to a constant current unit, thus avoiding the variability of skin-electrode impedance, according to the procedure previously used by Colloca and Benedetti [14] and Colloca et al. [15]. Stimuli were square pulses delivered by a somatosensory stimulator (Galileo Mizar NT, EBNeuro, Florence, Italy), with a duration of 100 μs. The stimuli were delivered at the end of either a red or a green light, repetitively (18 red + 18 green), and randomly administered.

Table 23.1.
Characteristics of subjects for each experimental group

Group	Experimental procedure	n	Sex	Age	PT	FS	EC	PD	Total IRI
							IRI		
1	Social observation	16	F	21.7±3.4	20.8±2.6	22.4±2.4	24.1±3	15.9±3.3	83.3±5.7
2	Conditioning	16	F	22.8±3.1	22.7±4.7	21.5±3.7	23.7±2.5	14.2±3.1	82.1±6.4
3	Verbal suggestion	16	F	23.5±6.9	21.8±4	22.7±2.4	23.6±3.8	15.1±3.3	83.2±6.8

Note: IRI = Interpersonal Reactivity Index; PT = Perspective Taking; FS = Fantasy Score; EC = Empathic Concern; PD = Personal Distress.

2.3. Design and Procedures

We first assessed tactile (t) and pain threshold (T) according to the following procedure: an ascending series of stimuli (steps of 1 mA) were delivered starting at sub-tactile threshold, until tactile sensation and pain sensation were induced. After determination of T, each subject was randomly assigned to one of the three experimental groups. Depending on the experimental group, the stimulus paired to the green light had either the same intensity as the stimulus following the red light (Groups 1 and 3) or a surreptitiously reduced intensity with respect to the stimulus intensity following the red light (Group 2, conditioning phase).

The placebo was administered according to the following procedure: a placebo electrode was applied to the middle finger of the non-dominant hand, but it was not connected to any pulse generator, and no electric shock was ever delivered. However, the subjects believed that the stimulation of the middle finger through this electrode, which was anticipated by the green light on the computer screen, was analgesic, thus they expected a green light–associated non-painful stimulus. By contrast, the red light indicated that the electrode was not activated, thus they expected a red light–associated painful stimulus. Each trial lasted about 20 s. Either the red or the green light was presented for 5 s and ended with the electric shock. The inter-stimulus interval (ISI) was about 15 s. Before each session started, the green and red stimuli were delivered once in order to make the subjects familiarize with the experimental protocol.

2.3.1. GROUP 1

To evaluate the effects of observational social learning, the subjects were asked to sit beside a demonstrator (actually a simulator) who underwent the whole experimental session (Fig. 23.1). The demonstrator was the same for all the experimental subjects: he was a 26-year-old male Ph.D. student visiting our laboratory from the University of Sydney, Australia, carefully trained to simulate the experimental session. To do this, two silver chloride electrodes were applied to the back of the non-dominant hand, and a sham electrode was pasted above his middle finger. The demonstrator received a total of 36 stimuli (18 red + 18 green) delivered according to a pseudorandom sequence. He always rated as painful the stimuli paired to red light and as non-painful the stimuli paired to green light. In this way, he simulated an analgesic benefit following the presentation of the green light. The experimental subjects had to pay attention to the lights displayed on a monitor, with particular regard to their meaning. To be sure that attention was kept constant throughout the experimental session, the subjects were asked to furnish some details about the experiment (total number of red and green lights as well as evaluation of demonstrator's reports). This observational phase lasted about 12 minutes (Phase I of Fig. 23.1 [left]). At the end of this phase, the subjects were asked to undergo a similar experimental session (Phase II of Fig. 23.1 [right]). After t and T assessment, stimulus intensity was set at 2T for both the green and the red stimuli.

2.3.2. GROUP 2

In order to assess the effect of direct experience of benefit, the placebo responses were tested after a conditioning phase according to the procedure used in our previous studies [14,15]. Subjects were informed that the green and red lights indicated the activation and deactivation, respectively, of the electrode on their middle finger, which, in turn, would induce an analgesic effect by delivering a sub-threshold electrical shock. However, this electrode never delivered electrical pulses (placebo electrode).

Phase I: simulation

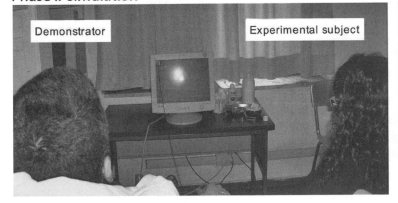

Phase II: testing

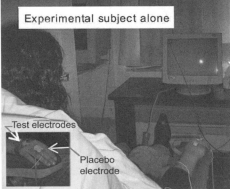

Fig. 23.1. Experimental setting of the social observational learning. An experimental subject sits beside a demonstrator who rates as painful red-associated stimuli and as non-painful green-associated stimuli (Phase I). Then a phase of testing is run, whereby the experimental subject receives a series of red- and green-associated stimuli in the same way as the demonstrator, but the intensity of all the stimuli is set at twice the pain threshold (Phase II). The insert (*bottom left* [of picture on right]) shows some details of the placebo electrode on the middle finger and the test electrodes on the dorsum of the same hand. The subjects believe that the stimulation of the middle finger induces analgesia on the dorsum of the hand.

A total of 36 stimuli (18 red + 18 green) were delivered according to the same pseudorandom sequence of Group 1. In this case, subjects received a pseudorandom series of 12 red-stimuli at 2T and 12 green stimuli at T–2 (T minus 2 mA), so that they had a firsthand experience of green light–associated non-painful stimulation. It is important to stress that the stimulus intensity was surreptitiously reduced, so that the subjects believed that the green light anticipated analgesic effects. This conditioning phase was followed by a testing period whereby the intensity of green light was increased up to 2T.

2.3.3. GROUP 3

As in Group 2, subjects were informed that green and red lights would indicate the activation and deactivation, respectively, of the electrode on their middle finger. In fact, the subjects were told that a green light would anticipate a stimulus that was made analgesic by delivering a sub-threshold electrical shock on their middle finger. Conversely, a red light would anticipate the deactivation of this electrode and thus a painful stimulation on the dorsum of the hand. Actually, all the stimuli were set at 2T. A total of 36 stimuli (18 red + 18 green) were delivered according to the same pseudorandom sequence of Groups 1 and 2.

2.4. Psychophysical Scale and Empathy Questionnaire

In all the experimental groups, the subjects rated pain intensity at the end of each stimulus by means of Numerical Rating Scale (NRS) ranging from 0 = no pain to 10 = maximum imaginable pain. Subjects were also required to complete the Interpersonal Reactivity Index (IRI; [18]), a commonly used trait empathy questionnaire which includes the following four subscales: Perspective Taking (PT), Fantasy Score (FS), Empathic Concern (EC), and Personal Distress (PD).

2.5. Cardiac Data Analysis

Heart rate (HR) was obtained by recording conventional electrocardiogram (ECG) from the arms. ECG signals were amplified, digitalized, and stored. Cardiac data analysis was performed on beat-to-beat series which did not present ectopic beats or artifacts. After the extrapolation of R–R intervals (Spectrum Cartoon Galileo, EBNeuro, Firenze, Italy), HR was calculated by transforming them into frequency (1/R–R). We evaluated 10 R–R intervals immediately preceding and following each stimulus. Because the testing phase in Group 2 consisted of 6 red + 6 green stimuli, we restricted the cardiac data analysis to the initial 6 red + 6 green testing series in all the experimental groups.

2.6. Statistical Analysis

The normal distribution of data was tested with the Kolmogorov-Smirnov test. As in no case we found a significant difference between our data set and a normal distribution, statistical comparisons were performed by means of ANOVA for repeated measures. Sphericity condition was assessed and when it was not verified, the Greenhouse-Geisser correction was applied. In Groups 1 and 3, ANOVA included the following within-subjects factors: treatment (red and green stimuli) and time (trials). In Group 2, ANOVA was performed with the factors: treatment (red and green stimuli), run (1, 2, and 3), and time (trials). In this case, the F-tests were followed by the Bonferroni post hoc tests for multiple comparisons. In addition, a series of single-sample paired t-tests were performed on red against green ratings to determine whether each green stimulus was rated as analgesic or not. In order to compare the effects of the different conditions, we expressed the placebo responses as the difference between green-associated and red-associated NRS scores and performed a supplementary ANOVA with Group as between factor. Linear regression analysis was done to correlate IRI scores with placebo responses. Linear regressions were also used to examine the relationship between the ratings by the demonstrator and the placebo responses in Group 1. Finally, HR changes were estimated by performing repeated measures ANOVA with treatment (red and green stimuli), phase (pre- and post-stimuli), and time (six trials), as within factors. All the analyses were carried out using SPSS software package (SPSS Inc., Chicago, Illinois, USA). The level of significance was set at $p < 0.05$.

3. Results

3.1. Psychophysical Data

3.1.1. GROUP 1

Repeated measures ANOVA of the NRS scores revealed a main effect for treatment ($F_{(1,15)} = 87.677$; $p < 0.0001$) but not for time ($F_{(17,255)} = 1.222$; $p = 0.247$), indicating that the subjects who had observed the analgesic effect in the demonstrator rated the green stimuli consistently less painful than the red stimuli. An additional series of single-sample paired t-tests were performed to determine whether each green-associated stimulus was rated as analgesic or not. We found that all the 18 green stimuli were deemed less painful compared to the red-associated stimuli, which indicates stable conditions of the responses over the entire experimental session, with neither habituation nor sensitization effects ($p < 0.01$ for all the 18 pairs; Fig. 23.2A). We also examined the relationship between demonstrator's and subjects' reports. The correlation between the differences in demonstrator's and participant's NRS scores (red–green values) did not show any significance ($r = 0.135$; $p = 0.617$), which suggests that the subjects rated their own perception rather than repeating what they heard from the demonstrator.

In order to test whether empathy itself modulated these socially learned placebo responses, we correlated the differences in NRS with IRI scores. We found a positive correlation for EC ($r = 0.555$, $p < 0.026$; see Fig. 23.3), but not for the other IRI subscales (PT [$r = 0.154$; $p = 0.569$], FS [$r = 0.172$; $p = 0.523$], PD [$r = -0.084$; $p = 0.756$]), and total IRI ($r = 0.42$; $p = 0.106$). Thus social observational learning induced pla-

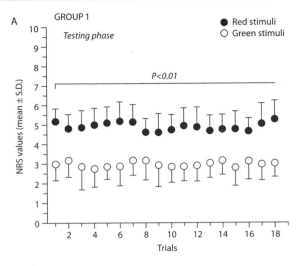

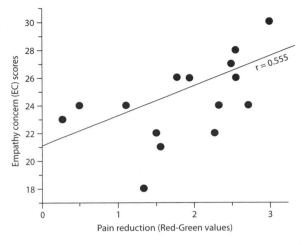

Fig. 23.3. Correlations between empathy concern (EC) scores and numerical rating scale (NRS) differences in Group 1. Note that the placebo analgesic responses were positively correlated with the subjects' empathy trait.

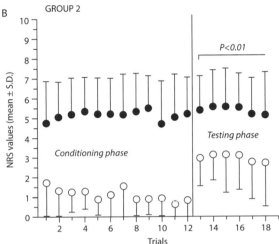

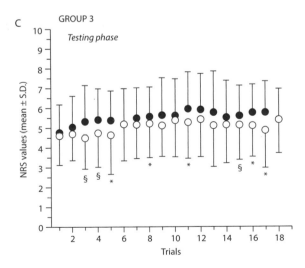

Fig. 23.2. The graphics show the placebo responses following prior observation (A), first-person experience of benefit (B, testing phase), and verbal suggestions of benefit (C). Stimuli that were paired to the green light were constantly rated as non-painful in Groups 1 and 2 (testing phase). Conversely, verbal suggestions alone produced smaller and more variable placebo responses (§ p < 0.01; * p < 0.05).

cebo responses that were independent of the demonstrator's NRS reports. Rather, they were linked to the individual empathy trait.

3.1.2. GROUP 2

After firsthand experience of analgesia by means of the conditioning procedure, the green-associated stimuli were rated significantly less painful compared with the red-associated stimuli. In this case, we performed a repeated measures ANOVA of the NRS scores, including both conditioning (runs 1 and 2) and testing (run 3) phases. We found a main effect for treatment ($F_{(1,15)} = 197.08$; $p < 0.0001$) and run ($F_{(2,30)} = 10.598$; $p < 0.0001$) with a significant interaction between the two factors ($F_{(2,30)} = 30.813$; $p < 0.0001$), indicating variability across the three experimental runs, as expected. The post hoc Bonferroni test for multiple comparisons showed that the NRS reports of run 3 were different with respect to run 1 ($p < 0.036$) and run 2 ($p < 0.0001$); no difference was present between runs 1 and 2 ($p = 1.000$). A separate analysis in the testing run demonstrated that subjects rated noxious stimuli consistently less painful when they expected an analgesic effect following the green light (treatment: $F_{(1,15)} = 94.433$, $p < 0.0001$; time: $F_{(5,75)} = 0.972$, $p = 0.440$). The single-sample t-tests confirmed that each green-associated stimulus of the testing series was rated less painful with respect to the red stimuli ($p < 0.01$ for all the six pairs; Fig. 23.2B).

Correlation analyses between the differences in NRS and IRI scores did not show any significance (EC [$r = -0.144$; $p = 0.608$], PT [$r = 0.08$; $p = 0.778$], FS [$r = 0.06$; $p = 0.828$], PD [$r = -0.01$; $p = 0.967$], and total IRI [$r = 0.04$; $p = 0.875$]).

3.1.3. GROUP 3

Repeated measures ANOVA of the NRS scores showed that subjects rated a green-associated painful stimulus less

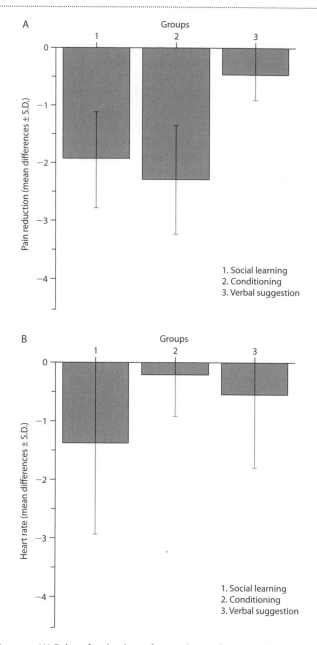

Fig. 23.4. (A) Pain reduction in each experimental group. The mean differences (red–green values) in Group 1 were not different from those found in Group 2. Both Group 1 and Group 2 showed a substantial difference in the magnitude of placebo responses with respect to Group 3 (Group 1 versus 3, $p < 0.01$; Group 2 versus 3, $p < 0.01$). (B) HR changes in each experimental group. The bars represent the HR mean difference (red–green values) during the anticipation of the red- and green-associated stimuli in the testing phase. The presentation of green-associated stimuli resulted in heart rate acceleration, whereas heart rate deceleration was found during presentation of red-associated stimuli in all three experimental groups. However, only HR changes of Group 1 reached significance ($p < 0.026$).

painful than a red-associated pain stimulus (main effect for treatment [$F_{(1,15)} = 16.977$; $p < 0.001$] and for time [$F_{(17,255)} = 1.883$; $p < 0.02$], with a non-significant interaction between the two factors [$F_{(17,255)} = 1.166$; $p = 0.293$]). However, this effect was smaller and less consistent over time (Fig.

23.2C). Indeed, paired *t*-tests revealed that only some of the 18 green-associated stimuli were rated less painful than the red-associated stimuli (Fig. 23.2C). No correlation was present between NRS and IRI subscale scores (EC [$r = 0.03$; $p = 0.919$], PT [$r = -0.393$; $p = 0.132$], FS [$r = -0.04$; $p = 0.876$], PD [$r = 0.284$; $p = 0.286$], and total IRI [$r = -0.1$; $p = 0.714$]).

In order to compare the effects of the three placebo conditions, after expressing the pain reports as the difference between red and green stimuli, we calculated the ANOVA with Group as between factor. We found a significant difference between Groups 1, 2, and 3 ($F_{(2,45)} = 26.543$; $p < 0.0001$). The post hoc Bonferroni test for multiple comparisons showed that Group 1 was not different from Group 2 ($p = 1.000$), whereas both Groups 1 and 2 differed from Group 3 (Group 1 versus 3, $p < 0.0001$; Group 2 versus 3, $p < 0.0001$). As shown in Fig. 23.4A, the mean difference between red and green pain reports was 1.92 ± 0.82 in Group 1, 2.29 ± 0.94 in Group 2, and 0.46 ± 0.45 in Group 3, which corresponds to a percentage reduction of 39.18% in Group 1, 43.35% in Group 2, and 8.42% in Group 3.

3.2. Heart Rate Responses

3.2.1. GROUP 1

Repeated measures ANOVA showed a trend for HR to be differently affected by treatment ($F_{(1,12)} = 4.475$; $p = 0.056$) and experimental phase ($F_{(1,12)} = 8.251$; $p < 0.014$). The interaction between the two factors was not significant ($F_{(1,12)} = 0.282$; $p = 0.605$). Thus we performed a separate analysis of HR responses to red- and green-associated stimuli in the anticipatory and in the post-stimulus phases. We found a main effect of treatment only during the anticipatory phase ($F_{(1,12)} = 6.425$; $p < 0.026$). Presentation of green-associated stimuli resulted in heart rate acceleration, whereas heart rate deceleration was found during presentation of red-associated stimuli. Fig. 23.4B shows the HR mean difference (red–green values) during the anticipation of the red- and green-associated stimuli. HR changes did not correlate with NRS differences (anticipation phase: $r = -0.06$, $p = 0.844$; post-stimulus phase: $r = -0.105$, $p = 0.720$).

3.2.2. GROUP 2

HR did not present differences related to either red- or green-associated stimuli ($F_{(1,13)} = 0.307$; $p = 0.589$). It should be noted that this group underwent repetitive stimulation during the conditioning phases, thus habituation may have occurred. Conversely, a significant HR increase was observed in the post-stimulus phase with respect to the anticipatory phase ($F_{(1,13)} = 25.756$; $p < 0.0001$).

3.2.3. GROUP 3

As in Group 2, HR showed a difference between pre- and post-stimulus ($F_{(1,13)} = 55.887$; $p < 0.0001$), but not with respect to either red- or green-associated stimulus ($F_{(1,13)} = 0.287$; $p = 0.601$).

4. Discussion

This is the first study which investigates the effects of observational social learning on placebo analgesia in the experimental setting. Bootzin and Caspi [12] postulated the involvement of social learning in placebo responsiveness as one of the underlying mechanisms. Indeed we found substantial placebo responses following observation of another subject undergoing a beneficial treatment. These responses were positively correlated with EC scores of the empathy questionnaire, suggesting that emphatic concern may modulate socially learned placebo analgesic responses. Interestingly, observational social learning produced placebo responses that were similar in magnitude to those induced by directly experiencing the benefit through the conditioning procedure. In addition, these two conditions induced placebo responses that were significantly larger than those induced by verbal suggestions alone. These findings extend and confirm our previous works [14,15], demonstrating the key role of different forms of learning in the placebo phenomenon.

Today several lines of research indicate that the placebo analgesic response is a learned phenomenon. In a previous study [14], we showed that a conditioning manipulation can produce substantial placebo responses that lasted several days and that depended on prior experience. In fact, after exposure to an effective treatment, we observed that conditioned placebo responses were present after both a few minutes and four to seven days. Conversely, when the same conditioning procedure was repeated after a totally ineffective verbal suggestion procedure, the placebo responses were remarkably reduced compared to the first group, pointing out that prior experience, both effective and ineffective, may have long-lasting effects on the outcome of a subsequent treatment.

The importance of previous experience in placebo responsiveness is also confirmed by recent findings illustrating the effects of conditioning and verbal suggestions at the level of central early nociceptive processing. Compared to natural history, conditioning produced more robust reductions in the amplitudes of N2–P2 components of laser-evoked potentials (LEPs) than verbal suggestions alone [16]. In the case of placebo analgesia conditioning elicits larger reductions in pain than verbal suggestions alone, whereas in nocebo hyperalgesia both negative verbal suggestions and conditioning induce significant nocebo responses [15], suggesting the presence of some distinctly different neural mechanisms in placebo and nocebo phenomenon [35]; for a review see [19].

In the present study, we extend these findings on learning by demonstrating for the first time that robust placebo analgesic responses can be evoked through social observation in the experimental setting. On the one hand, it has long been known that social and contextual cues and the whole atmosphere around the patient [5], such as words, attitudes, providers' behavior, drug's color and smell, medical devices, all contribute to evoke placebo responses [8]. On the other hand, an extensive literature investigating prosocial behaviors (e.g., ability to share the others' feelings, imitation, mimicry) suggests that social modeling is critical in developing learning processes across species [24,25,34], including social influences on psychophysical judgments of pain [17].

In our experimental condition, subjects constantly reported as less painful those stimuli that were paired to the analgesic procedure during the demonstrator's simulation (i.e., the green light), suggesting that the information drawn from observation of another person may establish a self-projection into the future outcome. These effects exhibited no extinction over the entire experimental session, indicating implicit acquisition and retention of behavioral output. It is also worth noting that the participants' NRS ratings did not correlate with those provided by the demonstrator, indicating that they evaluated their own perception rather than reporting merely what they heard during the simulation.

The larger HR changes for green-associated versus red-associated stimuli replicate earlier findings on heart rate responses to low- and high-painful stimuli [36].

At least in our experimental conditions, the magnitude of observation-induced placebo responses was similar to that found in Group 2, in which subjects underwent firsthand experience of the conditioning procedure. This suggests that observation of the demonstrator's benefit served as an unconditioned stimulus, underscoring some possible similarities between social learning and classical conditioning. Indeed, attempts to analyze social learning phenomena within an associative learning framework have been made in the field of fear. Some studies on observational aversive learning in rats fail to find blocking, latent inhibition, and overshadowing—three well-documented features of classical conditioning [22,44], whilst studies in humans reported classical conditioning features for social aversive learning, including overshadowing and blocking [30]. By contrast, other theories move beyond classical learning interpretation. Humans might alter their behavior without any practice and direct reinforcement, due to their ability to use symbols, thus setting them apart from the limited stimulus–response world of animals [6].

In our study, major gains in social learning occurred when the experimental subjects presented high EC scores of the empathy questionnaire. In fact, the analgesic placebo responses acquired through observation were highly correlated with EC scores, demonstrating a link between prosocial features and placebo effects. This is in line with several studies investigating inter-individual differences in trait measures of empathy in questionnaires such as IRI, as well as in pain modulation for reviews; see [23,26]. Usually, the higher the subjects scored on IRI, the higher the activation of part of the neural pain network was. Results of recent neuroimaging studies show that the neural system involved in the perception of pain in others partially overlap with some areas such as anterior cingulate, insular, and somatosensory cortices, which are activated by the firsthand perception of noxious stimuli [26]. Nevertheless, it is important to note that where these studies investigated the affective link between the empathizer and person in pain, our present work focused on instances of learning in which the behavior of a demonstrator modifies the subsequent behavior of an experimental subject. This type of cognitive processing likely requires the involvement of the medial prefrontal cortex which has a predominant role in making inferences and in social cognition [3].

Some limitations of our study need to be discussed. First, this work is based on phasic and acute experimental pain, whilst clinical pain is usually chronic and long-lasting. A second limitation is represented by the fact that we did not assess expectations and motivation, thus limiting our understanding about the weight of subject's expectations on potential outcomes. A third limitation is about the involvement of a male subject as a demonstrator and female subjects as experimental subjects, thus not allowing definitive conclusions about possible gender differences in empathy. In fact, there is some experimental evidence that gender (of both experimenter and experimental subject) is important in both placebo responsiveness and pain reports [4,18–20]. It is also worth discussing the relative magnitude of placebo responses induced by verbal suggestions alone. The duration of the experimental pain and the placebo instruction set may have been critical factors. For example, in previous studies we observed a substantial effect of suggestions on the submaximal effort tourniquet technique [2,10], but not on electrical shock [14,15]. Moreover, different types of placebos, such as an intra-muscular saline injection [10] versus the application of a sham electrode [14,15], can make a difference.

The main point that emerges from this work is that social learning, which humans share with many other species, is important in placebo analgesia. Thus many forms of learning appear to be involved in placebo responsiveness, making the placebo effect a highly complex phenomenon which is attributable to the intricate interplay of many factors. Further investigations of the neural mechanisms underlying socially-induced placebo responses are essential to integrate observational learning into the neurobiological placebo literature. From a clinical point of view, a better understanding of social learning in the placebo phenomenon may have important implications in the everyday clinical setting, whereby social interactions of patients with healthcare providers and other patients represent routine medical practice.

REFERENCES

[1] Ader R. The role of conditioning in pharmacotherapy. In: Harrington A, editor. The placebo effect: an interdisciplinary exploration. Cambridge, Mass.: Harvard UP; 1997. p. 138–165.

[2] Amanzio M, Benedetti F. Neuropharmacological dissection of placebo analgesia: expectation-activated opioid systems versus conditioning-activated specific subsystems. J Neurosci 1999;19:484–494.

[3] Amodio DM, Frith CD. Meeting of minds: the medial frontal cortex and social cognition. Nat Rev Neurosci 2006;7:268–277.

[4] Aslaksen PM, Myrbakk IN, Hoifodt RS, Flaten MA. The effect of experimenter gender on autonomic and subjective responses to pain stimuli. Pain 2007,129:260–268.

[5] Balint M. The doctor, his patient, and the illness. Lancet 1955;268:683–688.

[6] Bandura A. Social learning theory. New York: General Learning Press; 1977.

[7] Batterman RC, Lower WR. Placebo responsiveness—influence of previous therapy. Curr Ther Res Clin Exp 1968;10:136–143.

[8] Benedetti F. How the doctor's words affect the patient's brain. Eval Health Prof 2002;25:369–386.

[9] Benedetti F, Pollo A, Lopiano L, et al. Conscious expectation and unconscious conditioning in analgesic, motor, and hormonal placebo/nocebo responses. J Neurosci 2003;23:4315–4323.

[10] Benedetti F, Pollo A, Colloca L. Opioid-mediated placebo responses boost pain endurance and physical performance. Is it doping in sport competitions? J Neurosci 2007;27:11934–11939.

[11] Benedetti F. Mechanisms of placebo and placebo-related effects across diseases and treatments. Annu Rev Pharmacol Toxicol 2008;48:33–60.

[12] Bootzin RR, Caspi O. Explanatory mechanisms for placebo effects: cognition, personality and social learning. In: Guess HA, Kleinman A, Kusek JW, Engel LW, editors. The science of the placebo: toward an interdisciplinary research agenda. London: BMJ Books; 2002. p. 108–132.

[13] Colloca L, Benedetti F. Placebos and painkillers: is mind as real as matter? Nat Rev Neurosci 2005;6:545–552.

[14] Colloca L, Benedetti F. How prior experience shapes placebo analgesia. Pain 2006;124:126–133.

[15] Colloca L, Sigaudo M, Benedetti F. The role of learning in nocebo and placebo effects. Pain 2008;136:211–218.

[16] Colloca L, Tinazzi M, Recchia S, et al. Learning potentiates neuro-physiological and behavioral placebo analgesic responses. Pain 2008;139:306–314.

[17] Craig KD. Social modelling determinants of pain processes. Pain 1975;1:375–378.

[18] Davis MA. A multidimensional approach to individual differences in empathy. JSAS Cat Selected Docs Psychol 1980;10:85.

[19] Enck P, Benedetti F, Schedlowski M. New insights into the placebo and nocebo responses. Neuron 2008;59:195–206.

[20] Flaten MA, Aslaksen PM, Finset A, Simonsen T, Johansen O. Cognitive and emotional factors in placebo analgesia. J Psychosom Res 2006; 61:81–89.

[21] Galef BG Jr. Imitation in animals: history, definition, and interpretation of data from the psychological laboratory. In: Zentall TR, Galef BG Jr, editors. Social learning: psychological and biological perspectives. Hillsdale, N.J.: Lawrence Erlbaum Associates; 1988. p. 3–28.

[22] Galef BG Jr, Durlach PJ. Absence of blocking, overshadowing, and latent inhibition in social enhancement of food preferences. Anim Learn Behav 1993;21:214–220.

[23] Hein G, Singer T. I feel how you feel but not always: the empathic brain and its modulation. Curr Opin Neurobiol 2008;18:153–158.

[24] Heyes CM. Social learning in animals: categories and mechanisms. Biol Rev 1994;69:207–231.

[25] Iacoboni M. Imitation, empathy, and mirror neurons. Annu Rev Psychol 2009;60:653–670.

[26] Jackson PL, Rainville P, Decety J. To what extent do we share the pain of others? Insight from the neural bases of pain empathy. Pain 2006;125:5–9.

[27] Kantor TG, Sunshine A, Laska E, Meisner M, Hopper M. Oral analgesic studies: pentazocine hydrochloride, codeine, aspirin, and placebo and their influence on response to placebo. Clin Pharmacol Ther 1966;7:447–454.

[28] Kirsch I. Conditioning, expectancy, and the placebo effect: comment on Stewart-Williams and Podd (2004). Psychol Bull 2004;130:341–343.

[29] Klinger R, Soost S, Flor H, Worm M. Classical conditioning and expectancy in placebo hypoalgesia: a randomized controlled study in patients with atopic dermatitis and persons with healthy skin. Pain 2007;128:31–39.

[30] Lanzetta JT, Orr SP. Influence of facial expressions on the classical conditioning of fear. J Pers Soc Psychol 1980;39:1081–1087.

[31] Lasagna L, Mosteller F, von Felsinger JM, Beecher HK. A study of the placebo response. Am J Med 1954;16:770–779.

[32] Laska E, Sunshine A. Anticipation of analgesia, a placebo effect. Headache 1973;13:1–11.

[33] Montgomery GH, Kirsch I. Classical conditioning and the placebo effect. Pain 1997;72:107–113.

[34] Olsson A, Phelps EA. Social learning of fear. Nat Neurosci 2007;10:1095–1102.

[35] Petrovic P. Placebo analgesia and nocebo hyperalgesia—two sides of the same coin? Pain 2008;136:5–6.

[36] Ploghaus A, Narain C, Beckmann CF, et al. Exacerbation of pain by anxiety is associated with activity in a hippocampal network. J Neurosci 2001;21:9896–9903.

[37] Pollo A, Carlino E, Benedetti F. The top-down influence of ergogenic placebos on muscle work and fatigue. Eur J Neurosci 2008;28:379–388.

[38] Price DD, Milling LS, Kirsch I, et al. An analysis of factors that contribute to the magnitude of placebo analgesia in an experimental paradigm. Pain 1999;83:147–156.

[39] Price DD, Finniss DG, Benedetti F. A comprehensive review of the placebo effect: recent advances and current thought. Annu Rev Psychol 2008;59:565–590.

[40] Stewart-Williams S, Podd J. The placebo effect: dissolving the expectancy versus conditioning debate. Psychol Bull 2004;130:324–340.

[41] Voudouris NJ, Peck CL, Coleman G. Conditioned placebo responses. J Pers Soc Psychol 1985;48:47–53.

[42] Voudouris NJ, Peck CL, Coleman G. Conditioned response models of placebo phenomena: further support. Pain 1989;38:109–116.

[43] Voudouris NJ, Peck CL, Coleman G. The role of conditioning and verbal expectancy in the placebo response. Pain 1990;43:121–128.

[44] White DJ, Galef BG Jr. Social influence on avoidance of dangerous stimuli by rats. Anim Learn Behav 1998;26:433–438.

SECTION C. NEUROBIOLOGICAL MECHANISMS

24
Placebo and Opioid Analgesia
Imaging a Shared Neuronal Network

Predrag Petrovic, Eija Kalso, Karl Magnus Petersson, and Martin Ingvar

Predrag Petrovic, Eija Kalso, Karl Magnus Petersson, and Martin Ingvar, "Placebo and Opioid Analgesia—Imaging a Shared Neuronal Network," Science 2002;295:1737–1740.

Placebo analgesia is an important component in pain management (1), although the basic mechanisms are still poorly understood. At least some aspects of placebo analgesia are dependent upon endogenous opioid systems (1–3) because the effect may be partly abolished by the opioid antagonist naloxone (2). Therefore, the underlying neurophysiology of opioid-dependent placebo analgesia can be elucidated by studying similarities and differences in the function of the opioid and placebo systems in the brain. The opioid system consists of a well-studied subsystem in the brainstem and a less well elaborated cortical opioid-dependent network (4, 5). This system appears to be a likely candidate for the mediation of opioid-dependent placebo analgesia. The importance of the ACC in opioid effects has been suggested in several receptor-imaging studies of the brain (6–10), activation studies of opioid compounds (11–14), and theoretical frameworks of opioid analgesia (15). The rostral ACC (rACC)/ventromedial prefrontal cortex has been suggested as an important region in opioid analgesia and in other forms of pain modulation (16–26), which may suggest a similar involvement of higher-order control of opioid-dependent placebo analgesia.

We compared the analgesic effects of a placebo treatment and a rapidly acting opioid (remifentanil) [supplement A (27)] in a standard pain-stimulus paradigm (28). We used six different conditions in the study: heat pain and opioid treatment (POP), nonpainful warm stimulation and opioid treatment (WOP), heat pain and placebo treatment (PPL), nonpainful warm stimulation and placebo treatment (WPL), heat pain only (P), and nonpainful warm stimulation only (W). We studied concomitant behavioral responses and regional cerebral blood flow (rCBF) using positron emission tomography (PET) (29, 30) and compared the functional anatomy of the placebo analgesic response with that of the opioid response. We were especially interested in whether placebo analgesia and opioid effects induce a similar rCBF response in the rACC and the brainstem.

Comparison of scans in the pain conditions and in the warm conditions showed increased activity in the contralateral thalamus, in the insula bilaterally, and in the caudal ACC [Web table 1 (27) and Fig. 24.1A], all regions that have shown increased activity in previous imaging studies of pain (31). The opioid agonist remifentanil activated the cerebral network [Web table 2 (27) and Figs. 24.1B and 24.2A], which has been described previously in opioid receptor binding (6–9) and in rCBF studies (11–14). One of the major increases in rCBF was observed in the ACC and especially in the rACC. We also observed an increased activity in the lower brainstem. The subjects rated the pain intensity lower during POP compared with P in every experimental block [Web fig. 1 (27)]. The rCBF analysis showed that the insula, one of the major regions involved in pain processing, had an attenuated rCBF response bilaterally during POP–WOP as compared with P–W [Web table 2 (27)].

Although there was high interindividual variability in placebo ratings, most subjects decreased their pain intensity rating during PPL as compared with the P condition [Web fig. 1 (27)]. Recent experiments have revealed different types of placebo analgesia and indicate that some are dependent upon opioid systems (32, 33). Placebo responses were induced in subjects as a result of suggestions that each of the

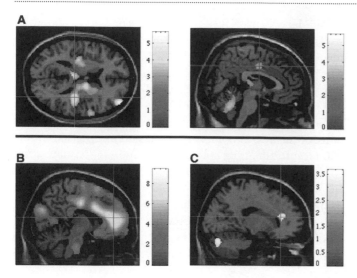

Fig. 24.1. (**A**) Increased activity was observed in the right (*cross*) and left insula (*left panel*, horizontal section), in the thalamus (*left panel*), and in the caudal ACC (*right panel*, sagittal section) during the main effect of pain [(POP + PPL + P)−(WOP + WPL + W)]. (**B**) The activation was most pronounced in the rACC during the main effect of opioids [(POP + WOP)−(P + W)]. Increased activity is apparent in the lower pons. (**C**) Increased activity in the same area of the rACC was also seen in the placebo effect during pain (PPL−P). The activations are presented on an SPM99-template. The activation threshold is at P = 0.005.

drugs used in the experiment was a potent analgesic (28) (i.e., expectation of pain relief) and by preceding the placebo treatment by active opioid during noxious stimulation in the first (five subjects) or second experimental block (four subjects) (i.e., opioid conditioning). Both of these placebo mechanisms can be abolished by the opioid antagonist naloxone and thus appear to be opioid dependent (32). Therefore, we expected similarities between activity observed in the opioid network and in the placebo analgesia network. The placebo analgesia was accompanied by increased activity in the orbitofrontal and ACC areas during PPL when compared with P [Web table 3 (27); Figs. 24.1C and 24.2B]. When we controlled for unspecific placebo effects (WPL−W), we observed an activation in the ACC [Web table 3 (27)], somewhat caudal to the rACC effect in PPL−P but rostral to the ACC activation during pain.

Previous imaging studies have shown that the rACC is more reliably activated by opioids, whereas the caudal ACC is more reliably activated by pain (11, 12). This distinction was also observed here, pointing to the importance of the rACC in opioid analgesia. This area of the human ACC contains a high concentration of opioid receptors (9). Moreover, studies examining stimulus-induced analgesia (16, 18, 19, 21, 23), nitrous oxide–induced analgesia (22), and hypnosis-induced change in pain perception (24, 25) have shown an increased activation in the rACC associated with the modulation mechanism. Rainville *et al.* (25) noted a similar functional division of the ACC: Pain (and unpleasantness) activated a more caudal region in the ACC, whereas the conditions involving suggestion, resulting in modulation of the pain experience, activated a more rostral part in the ACC. Hence, the increased activity in the rACC during PPL–P may support its involvement in the analgesic response mechanism during placebo. In addition, a post hoc analysis indicated that during opioid analgesia, the high placebo responders activated this area, whereas the low responders did not (Fig. 24.3). This suggests a relation between how effectively opioids may activate the rACC and adjacent areas and how well subjects respond to placebo during pain. Earlier studies have shown a behavioral correlation between opioid analgesia and placebo analgesia (32). The suggestion that the opioid system may vary among subjects is supported by the finding that the opioid receptor binding potential during rest and pain is highly specific to an individual (10), leading to the hypothesis that high placebo responders have a more efficient opioid system.

The placebo analgesic effect is dependent on complex cognitive information processing, including analysis of threat in a given context, expectations of treatment outcome, and desire for relief (1, 3, 4). The brainstem opioid system may thus be under cognitive control from higher order cortical regions. The ACC might play a key role in the cortical control of the brainstem during opioid analgesia (15, 34) by way of fiber tracts projecting directly to the periaqueductal gray (PAG) (35) or by way of the medial thalamic nucleus (36). A similar mechanism may be necessary in placebo analgesia, which implies that a functional connection should exist between these regions, both in opioid and placebo analgesia. Regression analysis supported this hypothesis (30) [Web table 4 (27) and Fig. 24.4]. The activity in the rACC covaried with activity in areas close to the PAG and the pons in the POP condition. We also observed a significant covariation in activity between the rACC and the pons, and a subsignificant covariation in activity between the rACC and the PAG, during PPL. No effect was observed in the pain-only condition (P), and the differences between these regressions (POP versus P and PPL versus P) were significant. The area in the pons is in the same region as the area activated in the main effect of opioids (Fig. 24.1). The brainstem opioid system consists of the PAG, which alters the neuronal activity in the rostral ventromedial medulla (4, 5). Additional nuclei in the pons, such as the parabrachial nuclei, also contain opioid-dependent neurons (4, 5). The positive covariation between rACC and these regions during POP and PPL, but not during P, may thus indicate that the higher cortical systems may, in specific circumstances, exert direct control over the analgesic systems of the brainstem not only during opioid analgesia but also during placebo analgesia.

The increased activity in the lateral orbitofrontal cortex during placebo analgesia is of interest because previous PET studies have implicated this region in cognitively driven pain modulation (25, 37). Stimulation of this region in rats (38) and primates (39) also induces analgesia. A right predominance of the orbitofrontal activation was observed during placebo analgesia, but interpretation of this finding is uncertain

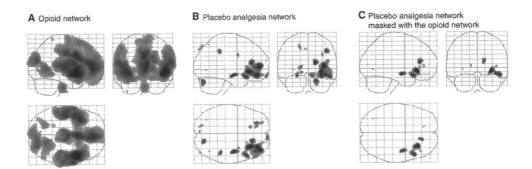

A Opioid network **B** Placebo analgesia network **C** Placebo analgesia network masked with the opioid network

Fig. 24.2. (**A**) The main effect of remifentanil [(POP + WOP)−(P + W)] showed increased activity bilaterally in the rostral and caudal ACC (extending into the ventromedial prefrontal cortex), insula, orbitofrontal cortex (extending into the temporopolar areas), and lower pons. The effect was widespread in the rACC and bilaterally in the anterior insula. (**B**) The placebo effect during pain (PPL−P) showed increased activity in the orbitofrontal regions bilaterally (most extensively in the right hemisphere) and in the contralateral rACC. (**C**) To observe the overlapping activation in the two different conditions, we used the placebo analgesia effect (activation threshold at P = 0.001) and masked the main effect of remifentanil (same activation threshold). Several of the orbitofrontal regions in the right hemisphere and in the rACC remained after the high-threshold masking, indicating that these regions were activated both during opioid stimulation and during the pain and placebo conditions. Thus, these regions were activated both by opioids in general and by placebo during pain. The activations are presented on an SPM99-template. The activation threshold is at P = 0.005.

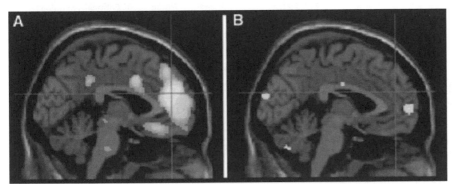

Fig. 24.3. Post hoc analysis comparing the activation of the rACC in high placebo responders with that in low responders revealed no significant differences in PPL−P between groups. However, activation of the rACC and adjacent areas by the high placebo responders was significant during POP−P [(x, y, z) = (−2, 46, 22); Z = 4.77] (**A**), whereas activation by the low responders was not significant (**B**). The difference between groups was significant in the rACC/ventromedial prefrontal cortex [(x, y, z) = (−2, 46, 26); Z = 3.24]. The activation threshold is at P = 0.005.

Covariation between rACC and the brainstem

A POP **B** PPL **C** P

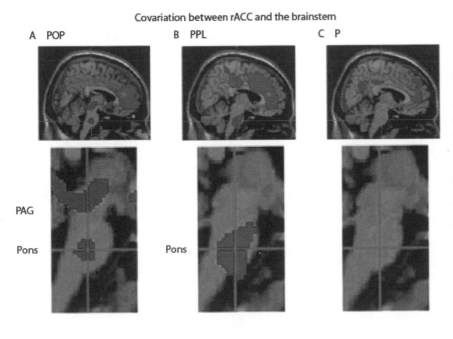

PAG

Pons   Pons

Fig. 24.4. (**A** to **C**) Covariation of activity in brainstem regions with activity in the rACC in different pain conditions. (**A**) Activity in the rACC covaried with activity in the PAG and in the lower pons/medulla during the POP condition. These covariations were significantly greater during POP as compared with P [Web table 4 (27)]. (**B**) A similar covariation between the rACC and the lower pons/medulla was observed during the PPL condition. This covariation was significantly greater during PPL as compared with P [Web table 4 (27)]. (**C**) No such regressions were observed during the P condition. The activations are presented on an SPM99-template and a more detailed image of the brainstem indicating the approximate position of the PAG and the pons. The threshold of activation is at P = 0.005.

because it may reflect a threshold effect. Placebo analgesia seems to activate a more rostral part of the orbitofrontal cortex as compared with the general opioid effect. Because the orbitofrontal cortex has dense connections with both the ACC and the brainstem (40), which have also been implicated in placebo analgesia, we suggest that these regions belong to a network that uses cognitive cues to activate the endogenous opioid system.

REFERENCES AND NOTES

1. P. Wall, in *Textbook of Pain*, P. Wall, R. Melzack, Eds. (Churchill Livingstone, Edinburgh, 1999), pp. 1419–1430.
2. J. D. Levine, N. C. Gordon, H. L. Fields, *Lancet* **312**, 654 (1978).
3. D. Price, in *Psychological Mechanisms of Pain and Analgesia* (International Association for the Study of Pain, Seattle, Wash., 1999), pp. 155–181.
4. D. Price, in *Psychological Mechanisms of Pain and Analgesia* (International Association for the Study of Pain, Seattle, Wash., 1999), pp. 137–153.
5. H. Fields, A. Basbaum, in *Textbook of Pain*, P. Wall, R. Melzack, Eds. (Churchill Livingstone, Edinburgh, 1999), pp. 309–329.
6. A. K. Jones et al., *J. Cereb. Blood Flow Metab.* **19**, 803 (1999).
7. A. K. Jones et al., *Br. J. Rheumatol.* **33**, 909 (1994).
8. A. K. Jones et al., *Neurosci. Lett.* **126**, 25 (1991).
9. F. Willoch et al., *Am. J. Neuroradiol.* **20**, 686 (1999).
10. J.-K. Zubieta et al., *Science* **293**, 311 (2001).
11. K. L. Casey et al., *J. Neurophysiol.* **84**, 525 (2000).
12. L. J. Adler et al., *Anesth. Analg.* **84**, 120 (1997).
13. L. L. Firestone et al., *Anesth. Analg.* **82**, 1247 (1996).
14. K. J. Wagner, F. Willoch, E. F. Kochs, T. Siessmeier, T. R. Tölle, *Anesthesiology* **94**, 732 (2001).
15. B. A. Vogt, R. W. Sikes, L. J. Vogt, in *Neurobiology of Cingulate Cortex and Limbic Thalamus: A Comprehensive Handbook*, B. A. Vogt, M. Gabriel, Eds. (Birkhäuser, Boston, Mass., 1993), pp. 313–344.
16. K. D. Davis et al., *J. Neurosurg.* **92**, 64 (2000).
17. G. H. Duncan et al., *J. Neurophysiol.* **80**, 3326 (1998).
18. L. Garcia-Larrea et al., *Stereotact. Funct. Neurosurg.* **68**, 141 (1997).
19. L. Garcia-Larrea et al., *Pain* **83**, 259 (1999).
20. R. C. Kupers, J. M. Gybels, A. Gjedde, *Pain* **87**, 295 (2000).
21. R. Peyron et al., *Pain* **62**, 275 (1995).
22. F. E. Gyulai, L. L. Firestone, M. A. Mintun, P. M. Winter, *Anesthesiology* **86**, 538 (1997).
23. F. Willoch, thesis, University of Oslo (2001).
24. M. E. Faymonville et al., *Anesthesiology* **92**, 1257 (2000).
25. P. Rainville et al., *J. Cogn. Neurosci.* **11**, 110 (1999).
26. S. G. P. Hardy, *Brain Res.* **339**, 281 (1985).
27. Supplementary Web material is available on *Science* Online at www.sciencemag.org/cgi/content/full/1067176/DC1.
28. Nine subjects participated in the study, which was approved by the local ethics and radiation safety committees [supplement B (27)]. Tonic pain was induced by heat stimulation (48°C, 70-s duration) on the dorsum of the left hand. The control stimulation consisted of a tonic stimulation of 38°C. The stimulation onset time was 10 s before the scan. The subjects were informed that two potent analgesics would be used in the experiment and that one of these drugs was an opioid. The drugs—either remifentanil (0.5 μg/kg) [(41, 42); supplement A (27)] or saline (placebo)—were injected intravenously (i.v.) 40 s before each stimulation. In one-third of the scans (both pain and warm stimulation), no drug was injected, and the subjects were told that these stimuli would be given without prior analgesics. Each subject underwent twelve scans in two blocks with the order of the conditions randomized within the block. Each subject tested the painful stimulation in a training session during the week preceding the PET study. The subjects rated the pain intensity after each scan using a visual analog scale (VAS) [supplement B (27)].
29. Standard rCBF PET procedures were used (www.fil.ion.ucl.ac.uk/spm) (31, 43, 44). Limiting the search area to a predefined network allowed us to consider any activation with P < 0.001 as significant [supplement C (27)].
30. A regression analysis was performed between rACC and the brainstem. Limiting the search area allowed for a threshold of P < 0.005 [(45, 46); supplement D (27)].
31. M. Ingvar, *Philos. Trans. R. Soc. London Ser. B* **54**, 1347 (1999).
32. M. Amanzio, F. Benedetti, *J. Neurosci.* **19**, 484 (1999).
33. F. Benedetti, C. Arduino, M. Amanzio, *J. Neurosci.* **19**, 3639 (1999).
34. O. Devinsky, M. J. Morrell, B. A. Vogt, *Brain* **118**, 279 (1995).
35. S. G. Hardy, G. R. Leichnetz, *Neurosci. Lett.* **22**, 97 (1981).
36. G. J. Royce, *Exp. Brain Res.* **50**, 157 (1983).
37. P. Petrovic, K. M. Petersson, P. H. Ghatan, S. Stone-Elander, M. Ingvar, *Pain* **85**, 19 (2000).
38. Y.-Q. Zhang, J.-S. Tang, B. Yuan, H. Jia, *Pain* **72**, 127 (1997).
39. T. D. Oleson, D. B. Kirkpatrick, S. J. Goodman, *Brain Res.* **194**, 79 (1980).
40. C. Cavada, T. Company, J. Tejedor, R. J. Cruz-Rizzolo, F. Reinoso-Suarez, *Cereb. Cortex* **10**, 220 (2000).
41. P. Feldman et al., *J. Med. Chem.* **34**, 2202 (1991).
42. C. L. Westmoreland, J. F. Hoke, P. S. Sebel, C. C. Hug, Jr., K. T. Muir, *Anesthesiology* **79**, 893 (1993).
43. J. Talairach, P. Tournoux, *Co-Planar Stereotaxic Atlas of the Human Brain* (George Thieme Verlag, Stuttgart, Germany, 1988).
44. K. J. Friston, A. P. Holmes, K. J. Worsley, J.-P. Poline, R. S. J. Frackowiak, *Hum. Brain Mapp.* **2**, 189 (1995).
45. K. Friston, *Hum. Brain Mapp.* **2**, 56 (1994).
46. K. J. Friston et al., *NeuroImage* **6**, 218 (1997).

25

Placebo-Induced Changes in fMRI in the Anticipation and Experience of Pain

TOR D. WAGER, JAMES K. RILLING, EDWARD E. SMITH, ALEX SOKOLIK, KENNETH L. CASEY, RICHARD J. DAVIDSON, STEPHEN M. KOSSLYN, ROBERT M. ROSE, AND JONATHAN D. COHEN

Tor D. Wager, James K. Rilling, Edward E. Smith, Alex Sokolik, Kenneth L. Casey, Richard J. Davidson, Stephen M. Kosslyn, Robert M. Rose, and Jonathan D. Cohen, "Placebo-Induced Changes in fMRI in the Anticipation and Experience of Pain," *Science* 2004;303:1162–1167.

The idea that sensory experience is shaped by one's attitudes and beliefs has gained currency among psychologists, physicians, and the general public. Perhaps nowhere is this more apparent than in our ability to modulate pain perception. A special case of this phenomenon is placebo analgesia, in which the mere belief that one is receiving an effective analgesic treatment can reduce pain (1–5). Recently, some researchers have attributed placebo effects to response bias and/or to publication biases (6), which raises the issue of whether placebo treatments actually influence the sensory, affective, and cognitive processes that mediate the experience of pain.

One important piece of evidence that placebo effects are not simply due to response or publication bias is that such effects can be reversed by the mu-opioid antagonist naloxone (2, 3, 7), suggesting that some kinds of placebo effects may be mediated by the opioid system. However, naloxone has also been shown to produce hyperalgesia independent of placebo, in some cases offsetting rather than blocking the effects of placebo analgesia (8). Although pharmacological blockade provides suggestive evidence regarding the neurochemical mechanisms mediating placebo effects, such data do not illuminate the nature of the information-processing system that gives rise to such effects. Neuroimaging data can provide complementary evidence of how pain processing in the brain is affected by placebos and about the time course of pain processing. Identifying placebo-induced changes in brain activity in regions associated with sensory, affective, and cognitive pain processing (9) may provide insight into which components of pain processing are affected by placebo. In addition, identifying changes that occur at particular times—in anticipation of pain, early or late during pain processing—may shed light on how cognitive systems mediating expectancy interact with pain and opioid systems.

In two functional magnetic resonance imaging (fMRI) experiments (n = 24 and n = 23), we examined two hypotheses regarding the psychological and neural mechanisms that underlie placebo analgesia. Our first hypothesis was that if placebo manipulations reduce the experience of pain, pain-responsive regions of the brain should show a reduced fMRI blood oxygen level–dependent (BOLD) signal (a measure related to neural activity) during pain. (Pain-responsive regions, or the "pain matrix," include thalamus, somatosensory cortex, insula, and anterior cingulate cortex (10–14).) Our second hypothesis was that placebo modulates activity of the pain matrix by creating expectations for pain relief, which in turn inhibit activity in pain-processing regions. Converging evidence suggests that the prefrontal cortex (PFC), the dorsolateral aspect (DLPFC) in particular, acts to maintain and appropriately update internal representations of goals and expectations, which modulate processing in other brain areas (15, 16). Thus, stronger PFC activation during the anticipation of pain should correlate with greater placebo-induced pain relief as reported by participants and greater placebo-induced reductions in neural activity within pain regions (17).

Placebo Reduces Reported Pain and Brain Activity in Study 1 (Shock Pain)

The design of Study 1 is illustrated in Fig. 25.1A (see the figure legend for a description) (18). First, to confirm that application of shock elicited a neural response in pain-related areas, we compared brain activity in the intense shock versus no shock conditions. This revealed activation of the classic pain matrix (11, 14, 19, 20), including thalamus, primary somatosensory cortex/ primary motor cortex (SI/MI), secondary somatosensory cortex (SII), midbrain, anterior insula, anterior cingulate cortex (ACC), ventrolateral prefrontal cortex, and cerebellum (fig. S1). As expected, activations in thalamus, SI, SII, and MI were larger in the left hemisphere, con-

tralateral to the wrist where shocks were applied, whereas cerebellar activation was ipsilateral, although some bilateral activation was observed in each of these areas. We also compared intense shock with mild shock to determine which pain regions responded more specifically to the painful aspects of the stimulus, which produced a similar network of activated regions (Fig. 25.1C and table S1). These regions, which we refer to as "pain-responsive" regions because they track the magnitude of painful stimulation (10), constituted the pain-sensitive regions of interest (ROIs) in which we expected to find placebo effects (21). Anticipation of shock activated contralateral SI, SII, MI, and dorsal amygdala (fig. S2).

Turning to placebo effects, we first assessed the placebo effect based on participants' reports, calculated as the difference between the average rating of intense shocks in the placebo and control conditions. Reported pain was greater for control than for placebo conditions across participants ($\bar{x} = 0.21$, $\sigma = 0.47$, $t(23) = 2.20$, $P < 0.05$), indicating a significant analgesic effect of the placebo. However, the relatively high variability in the placebo response across participants (only 8 of the 24 participants both showed a placebo effect in our measure and reported some pain relief in a post-session debriefing) allowed us to examine correlations between measures of reported pain relief and corresponding neural responses, as discussed below. In contrast to intense shocks, we found no placebo effect for the ratings of mild shocks for the group as a whole ($\bar{x} = 0.04$, $\sigma = 0.54$, $t(23) = 0.36$), and thus will not further discuss findings from this condition.

Our first prediction was that the placebo treatment would attenuate activation within pain ROIs. We found that the magnitude of the reduction between control and placebo trials in reported pain (hereafter referred to as control > placebo, a measure of experienced placebo analgesia) correlated with the magnitude of reduction in neural activity during the shock period (control > placebo, a measure of placebo analgesia in the brain) in pain-responsive portions of several brain structures. These structures included the rostral anterior cingulate cortex (rACC) at the junction between rostral and caudal ACC ($r = 0.66$), contralateral insula ($r = 0.59$), and the contralateral thalamus ($r = 0.53$) (22). These findings were all significant at $P < 0.005$, and are shown in Fig. 25.2A, C, and E, respectively. (All brain-behavior correlations we report compare the magnitudes of placebo effects (control–placebo) on reported pain with magnitudes of placebo effects in neural activity (control–placebo).) Because the thalamus is the major cortical relay for afferent pain fibers, this correlation is predicted by theories of placebo that hypothesize inhibition of afferent sensory pain transmission (23). The insula has been associated with both the sensory-discriminative and affective components of pain (10, 24), and the rACC has been shown to track changes in reported pain induced by hypnosis (25), at coordinates [7 20 29], 5 mm from the center of our activation.

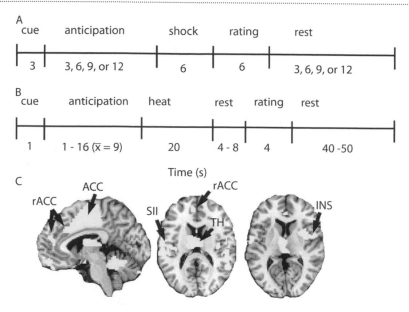

Figure 25.1. (A) Time course of a single trial in Study 1. Twenty-four participants were scanned by fMRI as they received painful and nonpainful electric shocks to their right wrist. We modeled our design after a study by Ploghaus et al. (58), which allowed us to distinguish the brain's response to pain from its anticipation of pain. The experiment consisted of five blocks of fifteen trials. Each trial lasted 30 s and began with a 3-s warning cue–a red or blue spiral icon–that indicated whether the upcoming shock would be intense or mild, respectively (18). An ensuing anticipation epoch varied between 3 and 12 s, and was followed by a 6-s epoch of either intense or mild shock. After the shock, participants rated the intensity of the shock on a 10-point scale, followed by a variable rest period until the end of the trial. Shocks were randomly omitted on one-third of all trials, in order to increase the number of total test trials without compromising expectations regarding pain. Participants were told that they were taking part in a study of brain responses to a new analgesic cream. In the first block of trials, participants received shocks without any treatment. After Block 1, an investigator applied a skin cream to the participant's right wrist with the participant still in the scanner. Half the participants were told that this was an analgesic cream that would reduce but not eliminate the pain of the shocks. After Blocks 2 and 3 were completed in this placebo condition, the cream was removed and the same cream was reapplied. Then participants were told that the cream was actually a different, ineffective cream needed as a control. Participants then completed Blocks 4 and 5. For the other half of the participants, we reversed the order of placebo and control conditions. Our measures of the placebo effect were the differences in reported ratings of pain and regional brain activity in the control versus placebo conditions (control–placebo in both behavior and brain). During pain and rest periods, participants saw a fixation cross.

   (B) Time course of a trial in Study 2. The design was similar to that of Study 1, with the following differences. The cue was the words "Get ready!" in red letters (1-s duration). A painful thermal stimulus was applied for 20 s (17 s peak, 1.5 s ramp up/down), allowing us to analyze pain responses in three separate segments (early, peak, and late). Different patches of skin on the left forearm (38) were treated with placebo and control topical creams (which were identical). Thermal stimuli were applied to these patches of skin in three phases. During the calibration phase, the stimulus was varied to identify temperatures corresponding to reported pain levels of 2, 5, and 8 on a 10-point scale (1 = just painful; 10 = unbearable pain) for each participant (59). This was followed by the manipulation phase, included to enhance participants' expectations of pain relief and thereby increase placebo responding. In this phase, pain was surreptitiously reduced in the placebo condition (5, 60). During one block of trials the stimuli were applied to the placebo-treated patch of skin, and during another block the stimuli were applied to the control-treated patch (order counterbalanced across participants). Participants were told that all stimuli were at level 8. However, they were administered at level 2 in the placebo-treated patch and at level 8 in the control-treated patch. Finally, during the test phase, two additional blocks of stimuli were administered to placebo- and control-treated patches of skin. Again, participants were told these were at level 8, but both were delivered at level 5, in keeping with the paradigm used in (5). Because the stimuli were identical, any differences in reported pain (control–placebo) during this phase are attributable to placebo effects.

   (C) Pain-responsive regions identified by their significance in (intense–mild stimulation) contrasts in Study 1 or Study 2. These regions were regions of interest (ROIs) in which we looked for placebo effects. ACC: anterior cingulate; rACC: rostral anterior cingulate; SII: secondary somatosensory cortex; INS: insula; TH: thalamus.

Placebo Increases Prefrontal Activity in Anticipation of Painful Shock

To evaluate our second hypothesis—that expectation of pain relief is represented in PFC and mediates placebo analgesia—we examined correlations between reported placebo effects in ratings (control > placebo) and fMRI activity in the anticipation period (placebo > control). We restricted our analysis to DLPFC and orbitofrontal cortex (OFC), based on our hypothesis. OFC is thought to play an important role in configuring control mechanisms and learning based on reward information (26–31). Regions within bilateral DLPFC showed significant correlations (r = 0.62 within both left (L) and right (R) hemispheres) (32). Regions within bilateral OFC showed similar correlations (OFC; r = 0.65/0.76 in L/R hemispheres, respectively) (Fig. 25.3B) (32). Previous research (33) suggests that rACC may also serve as a control region, because it was activated in placebo relative to control condi-

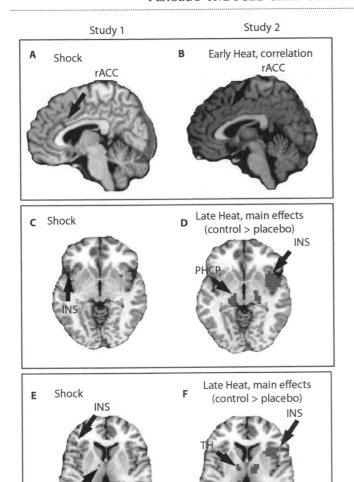

Figure 25.2. Pain regions showing correlations between placebo effects in reported pain (control–placebo) and placebo effects in neural pain (control–placebo). (**A**) Rostral anterior cingulate (rACC) effects in Study 1. (**B**) rACC effects in early heat in Study 2. (**C**) Contralateral (*left*) insula (INS) in Study 1, z = −4 mm. (**D**) Contralateral (*right*) INS effects in Study 2, z = −4 mm. The parahippocampal cortex (PHCP) activations extended into the basal forebrain and are contiguous with thalamic activations; however, only thalamic activations are in pain-sensitive regions. (**E**) Contralateral INS and thalamus (TH) in Study 1, z = 6 mm. (**F**) Contralateral INS and TH in Study 2, z = 6 mm.

tions. Our data support this notion, as we also found correlations of the form described above for rACC (32). Correlations between reported placebo effects and prefrontal activation are consistent with the hypothesis that regions involved in generating and maintaining expectations contribute to placebo-related analgesia.

We also tested for correlations between anticipation activity in expectancy areas and pain activity in pain regions. Negative correlations would support the view that prefrontal activity is an antecedent to reduction in pain. Placebo-induced increases in DLPFC were correlated with placebo-induced reductions during pain in several regions: (i) contralateral thalamus, r = −0.56/−0.38 for L and R DLPFC; correlations

whose absolute value is greater than 0.4 are significant at P < 0.05; (ii) insula, r = −0.59/−0.26 for L and R DLPFC; and (iii) rACC, r = −0.44/−0.45 for L and R DLPFC. Similar correlations were observed between placebo increases in OFC and placebo reductions in pain activity: (i) thalamus, r = −0.52/−0.63 for L and R OFC; (ii) insula, r = −0.61/−0.56 for L and R OFC; (iii) rACC: r = −0.65/−0.70 for L and R OFC.

We also found increased activity (placebo > control) during the anticipation period in the midbrain, in the vicinity of the periaqueductal grey (PAG), which contains a high concentration of opiate neurons with descending spinal efferents (23, 34). Midbrain placebo increases (placebo > control, at coordinates [10 −26 −14]) (35), were positively correlated with both reported placebo effects (control > placebo) and brain placebo effects (control > placebo) in some pain areas (r = 0.47 for thalamus and r = 0.48 for rACC) (36). Furthermore, midbrain placebo > control activity was correlated with anticipation-period activation (placebo > control) of the right PFC (r = 0.51) and OFC (r = 0.48/0.39 for L and R hemispheres) (37).

Placebo Reduces Reported Pain and Brain Activity in Study 2 (Thermal Pain)

In Study 2 we used a stronger placebo induction, a different pain modality, and an experimental design that allowed us to analyze the time course of placebo-related effects during the pain epoch. These manipulations provided greater power to test the influence of the placebo manipulation on activation of the pain matrix, and to test further hypotheses regarding the mechanisms of placebo action. For example, if placebo can affect the pain matrix through expectation alone, we expect such effects to occur early during pain, whereas if placebo effects also involve direct (e.g., opioid release) or indirect (cognitive reappraisal) processes that evolve over time (e.g., in response to the sensory stimulus), we expect them to occur later during pain stimulation. The sequence of events on each trial is shown in Fig. 25.1B, and other aspects of the design are discussed in the figure legend (18, 38, 39).

Fifty participants were studied using the procedures described above before fMRI scanning, including a manipulation phase designed to enhance placebo-related expectations. On average, placebo resulted in a 22% decrease in reported pain during the test phase, with 72% of participants showing effects in the expected direction (t(49) = 5.87, P < 0.0001) (fig. S3A). This high rate of response confirmed that we had effectively enhanced participants' belief in the placebo. Placebo responders were invited to return for fMRI scanning (40, 41).

As in Study 1, we found significant pain activation in expected regions (averaging over control and placebo), shown in red in fig. S1. These included bilateral insula, SI/MI, SII, thalamus, and anterior and dorsolateral PFC, as well as ACC, medial PFC, and cerebellar vermis. Comparing intense (level 8) pain with mild (level 2) pain during the manipulation phase produced activations within all of these regions (table S1). We used these regions to test for placebo effects.

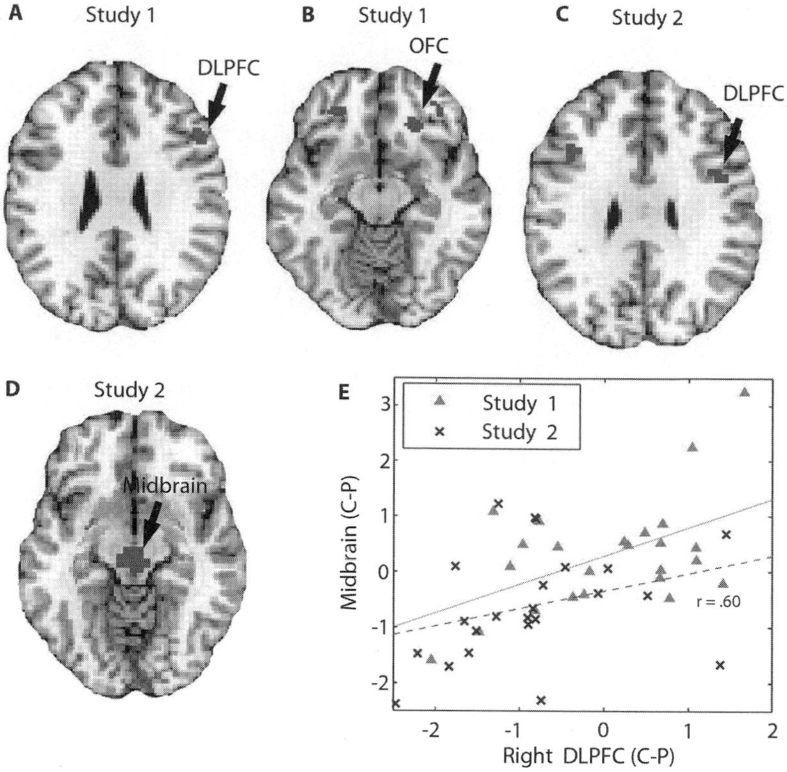

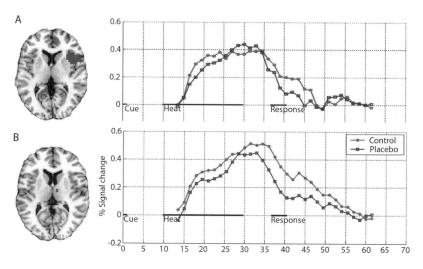

Figure 25.3. Prefrontal regions activated with placebo during anticipation. Regions in Study 1 showed positive correlations between reported placebo effects (placebo > control) and brain placebo effects (placebo > control). Regions in Study 2, in which placebo responders were preselected for fMRI, showed main effects of placebo (placebo > control). **(A)** Right dorsolateral prefrontal cortex (DLPFC) in Study 1, z = 28 mm. Left DLPFC activation (found superior to this slice) is not shown. **(B)** Regions of orbitofrontal cortex (OFC) showing correlations in Study 1, z = −12 mm. **(C)** Right and left DLPFC showing main effects (placebo > control) in Study 2, z = 30 mm. **(D)** Midbrain placebo-induced activations (placebo > control) in anticipation, z = −10 mm, Study 2. **(E)** Scatterplot showing the correlation between midbrain placebo effects and right DLPFC placebo effects in Study 1 (triangles, solid line) and Study 2 (x's, dashed line).

Figure 25.4. Time courses of pain responses for regions showing main effects of placebo (control > placebo) in late heat in Study 2. For display, time courses were extracted from regions showing a main effect of pain at Z > 4.1. **(A)** Group-averaged, finite impulse-response deconvolved responses to pain for placebo (squares on graph) and control (circles on graph) in the contralateral insula (the exact region is shown in the slice at left), partialing out signal contributions from the anticipation and response periods. Black bars show average timing of trial events, although timing varied from trial to trial. **(B)** Time courses in contralateral thalamus, as in **(A)**.

The results provided further support for our first hypothesis, that placebo would reduce activity in pain-responsive areas. We expected main effects of placebo (control > placebo) in Study 2, because only placebo responders were selected as participants; thus, the range of the placebo response was restricted in Study 2, although this selection procedure does not preclude finding correlations as well. As in Study 1, contralateral thalamus, anterior insula, and rACC all showed significant placebo effects. In the rACC pain region (Fig. 25.2B), reported placebo effects (control > placebo) were correlated with neural placebo effects (control > placebo) in the early heat period (r = 0.58) (42). In contralateral insula and thalamus

(Fig. 25.2, D and F), main effects of placebo (control > placebo) were found in the late heat period (43). Thalamic activations extended into the basal forebrain and medial temporal cortex (Fig. 25.2E), which has been implicated in enhanced pain due to anxiety (44). All these placebo activations fell within pain-sensitive regions, consistent with the hypothesis that they reflect modulation of the pain experience.

Time courses of neural placebo effects (Fig. 25.4) show the predominant decrease late in the pain response, after stimulus offset (although there is a trend toward control > placebo effects earlier in stimulation as well) (45). The late decreases suggest that placebo effects may require a period of pain to develop, and may modulate pain signals most strongly after stimulation is removed. This may be especially true of protracted painful stimuli, such as the thermal stimulus used in Study 2. The late decreases may reflect cognitive reappraisal of the significance of pain, resulting in decreases in pain affect and pain experience (5, 8). Alternatively, the late decreases may reflect engagement of opioid mechanisms triggered by prolonged pain.

Placebo Increases Prefrontal Cortex and Midbrain Activity in Anticipation of Thermal Pain

Study 2 also provided further support for our second hypothesis, that the expectation of pain relief is mediated by PFC. Regions within both right and left DLPFC, similar to those observed in Study 1 and shown in Fig. 25.3C, were significantly more active during anticipation in the placebo versus control conditions (placebo > control) (46). Study 2 also confirmed placebo- increased activation during the anticipation period of a midbrain region containing the PAG (46) (Fig. 25.3D), which again correlated significantly with DLPFC activity ($r = 0.60$ for both L and R DLPFC) (Fig. 25.3E). Finally, Study 2 showed the expected placebo-induced activation of rACC (47). Interestingly, this is the same area in which we found placebo-induced decreases during early heat, suggesting that this pain-responsive region may also serve as part of the network for cognitive control.

Overall Impact of the Studies

These two studies provide important insights into the neural mechanisms underlying placebo analgesia. First, they support the hypothesis that placebo manipulations decrease neural responses in brain regions that are pain sensitive. In addition, the magnitude of these neural decreases correlates with reduction in reported pain. These findings provide strong refutation of the conjecture that placebo responses reflect nothing more than report bias (6).

Our findings also provide support for a specific hypothesis regarding one potential mechanism of placebo action, the representation of expectations within regions of PFC that modulate activity in pain-responsive areas. We found significant correlations of DLPFC and OFC activity with placebo response, measured both behaviorally (as the reported experience of pain) and neurally (as activity in pain-responsive areas). The DLPFC is an area that has consistently been associated with the representation and maintenance of information needed for cognitive control (16, 48), whereas the OFC is more frequently associated with representing evaluative and reward information relevant to the allocation of control (26, 27, 29).

Previously, Petrovic et al. (33) found increases in OFC in placebo during pain, whereas the current studies found it during anticipation (49). However, the Petrovic study used positron emission tomography and did not include an anticipation period, and so could not discriminate neural responses during anticipation from those associated with the painful stimulus itself. Nevertheless, it may be that the OFC is involved in processes that occur in advance of pain only if warning stimuli signal that pain is imminent, and otherwise occur during pain itself. Affective and motivational responses to pain are examples of such processes.

Both DLPFC and OFC activation correlated with midbrain activation during anticipation, consistent with the idea that prefrontal mechanisms trigger opioid release in the midbrain. An alternative interpretation is that DLPFC redirects attention away from pain, as it has also been implicated in general attentional processes (10, 50). However, OFC and midbrain regions are not typically associated with directed attention; rather, activation of these regions seems more consistent with the view that anticipation during placebo involves a specific expectancy process that may be related to opioid system activation. Although the results do not provide definitive evidence for a causal role of PFC in placebo, they were predicted by and are consistent with the hypothesis that PFC activation reflects a form of externally elicited top-down control that modulates the experience of pain.

The studies also provide additional information about which aspects of pain—sensory, affective, or cognitive evaluation—are affected by placebo. Previous studies showing reversal of placebo effects by opioid antagonists (2, 3), coupled with theories implicating opioids in the inhibition of spinal pain afferents (23), suggest that placebo affects sensory pain transmission at the earliest stages. Inhibition of spinal afferents might be expected to produce placebo decreases throughout the pain matrix; however, we found such reductions only in a few regions (table S1). Our findings provide evidence for multiple components of expectation-induced placebo effects, with (potentially) opioid-containing regions in the midbrain active during anticipation, anterior cingulate showing decreased responses early in pain, and contralateral thalamus and insula showing decreases only after more prolonged pain (Study 2). Although our results are consistent with the hypotheses that at least a part of the placebo effect is mediated by afferent pain fiber inhibition, a major portion of the placebo effect may be mediated centrally by changes in specific pain regions. This account acknowledges that pain is a psychologically constructed experience that includes cognitive evaluation of the potential for harm and affect as well as sensory components (24, 51).

REFERENCES AND NOTES

1. P. Wall, in *Textbook of Pain*, P. Wall, R. Melzack, Eds. (Churchill Livingstone, Edinburgh, 1999), pp. 1419–1430.
2. M. Amanzio, F. Benedetti, *J. Neurosci.* **19**, 484 (1999).
3. F. Benedetti, C. Arduino, M. Amanzio, *J. Neurosci.* **19**, 3639 (1999).
4. D. D. Price, J. J. Barrell, *Prog. Brain Res.* **122**, 255 (2000).
5. D. D. Price et al., *Pain* **83**, 147 (1999).
6. A. Hróbjartsson, P. C. Gøtzsche, *N. Engl. J. Med.* **344**, 1594 (2001).
7. J. D. Levine, N. C. Gordon, H. L. Fields, *Lancet* **2**, 654 (1978).
8. R. H. Gracely, R. Dubner, P. J. Wolskee, W. R. Deeter, *Nature* **306**, 264 (1983).
9. R. Melzack, K. L. Casey, in *The Skin Senses*, D. R. Kenshalo, Ed. (Thomas, Springfield, Ill., 1968), pp. 423–439.

10. R. Peyron *et al.*, *Brain* **122**, 1765 (1999).

11. R. Peyron, B. Laurent, L. Garcia-Larrea, *Neurophysiol. Clin.* **30**, 263 (2000).

12. F. Schneider *et al.*, *Neuropsychobiology* **43**, 175 (2001).

13. K. D. Davis, S. J. Taylor, A. P. Crawley, M. L. Wood, D. J. Mikulis, *J. Neurophysiol.* **77**, 3370 (1997).

14. K. L. Casey, *Proc. Natl. Acad. Sci. U.S.A.* **96**, 7668 (1999).

15. J. D. Cohen, D. Servan-Schreiber, *Psychol. Rev.* **99**, 45 (1992).

16. E. K. Miller, J. D. Cohen, *Annu. Rev. Neurosci.* **24**, 167 (2001).

17. Expectation generation is conceptually distinct from simple direction of attention away from painful stimuli, which has also been shown to modulate pain (52–55). The critical distinction is that expectation-induced analgesia should (i) engage prefrontal regions primarily during anticipation of pain; (ii) potentially activate opioid systems in the midbrain PAG; and (iii) activate affective regulation mechanisms in OFC and anterior medial PFC (56, 57). General attention effects, on the other hand, should be mediated by a distributed attentional network that remains active throughout pain and is not linked to affective regulation and/or opioid activity.

18. Materials and methods are available as supporting material on *Science* Online.

19. M. Ingvar, *Philos. Trans. R. Soc. London B Biol. Sci.* **354**, 1347 (1999).

20. K. D. Davis, *Neurol. Res.* **22**, 313 (2000).

21. To avoid missing pain regions due to power issues, we defined stimulation-responsive (intense–none) and pain-responsive regions (intense–mild) as those that responded in these comparisons in either Study 1 or Study 2. This procedure also makes the pain masks comparable across the two studies.

22. Placebo effects in brain (control > placebo) that were positively correlated with experienced pain (control > placebo) in stimulation-responsive ROIs (defined by pain–baseline) included rACC ([4 23 27], 27 contiguous voxels, $Z = 3.56$; and [−2 32 19], 16 voxels, $Z = 3.12$) and left (contralateral) insula ([−44 14 −3], 19 voxels, $Z = 3.04$). These activations overlapped with pain-responsive ROIs (defined by intense–mild pain) in 3, 5, and 8 voxels, respectively. Thalamic placebo effects were just below the 10-voxel extent threshold ([11 −5 14], 8 voxels, $Z = 2.65$, 3 voxels in pain-sensitive regions), but stronger support for thalamic involvement was found in Study 2.

23. R. Melzack, P. D. Wall, *Science* **150**, 971 (1965).

24. A. D. Craig, K. Chen, D. Bandy, E. M. Reiman, *Nature Neurosci.* **3**, 184 (2000).

25. P. Rainville, G. H. Duncan, D. D. Price, B. Carrier, M. C. Bushnell, *Science* **277**, 968 (1997).

26. W. C. Drevets, *Biol. Psychiatry* **48**, 813 (2000).

27. E. T. Rolls, in *The Cognitive Neurosciences*, M. S. Gazzaniga, Ed. (MIT Press, Cambridge, Mass., 1995), pp. 1091–1106.

28. R. C. O'Reilly, D. C. Noelle, T. S. Braver, J. D. Cohen, *Cereb. Cortex* **12**, 246 (2002).

29. R. Dias, T. W. Robbins, A. C. Roberts, *J. Neurosci.* **17**, 9285 (1997).

30. J. O'Doherty, M. L. Kringelbach, E. T. Rolls, J. Hornak, C. Andrews, *Nature Neurosci.* **4**, 95 (2001).

31. G. Schoenbaum, B. Setlow, *Learn. Mem.* **8**, 134 (2001).

32. DLPFC correlations were [52 18 28], 42 voxels, $Z = 3.3$; [42 6 30], 14 voxels, $Z = 3.3$; [36 20 38], 13 voxels, $Z = 3.00$; [−30 4 42], 22 voxels, $Z = 3.30$. OFC correlations were [−26 38 −12], 32 voxels, $r = 0.64$; [24 30 −12], 62 voxels; $r = 0.79$. Correlations were also found in other areas, including rostral (rACC) and caudal (cACC) anterior cingulate, which may be part of an "executive" circuit mediating cognitive control functions. rACC correlation loci were [6 14 26], 40 voxels, $Z = 4.23$; [−4 26 26], 21 voxels, $Z = 3.68$; [10 32 32], 20 voxels, $Z = 3.36$. The cACC correlation locus was [−2 −8 24], 68 voxels, $Z = 3.5$.

33. P. Petrovic, E. Kalso, K. M. Petersson, M. Ingvar, *Science* **295**, 1737 (2002).

34. I. Tracey *et al.*, *J. Neurosci.* **22**, 2748 (2002).

35. Only one voxel was significant at $P < 0.005$ in Study 1. However, Study 2 replicated this finding with a substantially larger activation.

36. Pearson's $r > 0.4$ are significant at $P < 0.05$.

37. If midbrain activation were related to opioid system activity, we might expect placebo increases in activation throughout the period when participants experienced pain, rather than during the period when they anticipated it. However, pain-induced opioid release—an endogenous response to pain expected to be greater in the more painful control condition—may have offset placebo increases during pain, resulting in no overall placebo–control differences.

38. Stimulation of the left arm in Study 2 (as opposed to the right arm in Study 1) allowed us to test whether placebo effects occurred contralateral to stimulation, or always occurred in the same hemisphere.

39. At the conclusion of the manipulation phase, participants were asked to rate how effective they expected the analgesic to be during subsequent testing. We administered stimulation on separate, nonoverlapping patches of skin in the calibration, manipulation, and test phases to avoid physiological sensitization and habituation effects due to repeated stimulation.

40. Of the 24 participants who returned, 22 reported a reduction of pain in the placebo condition during the fMRI scanning session, revealing a highly significant test-retest reliability of the placebo effect ($r = 0.62$, $P < 0.05$).

41. Data were analyzed in the general linear model framework, with five regressors to model BOLD responses during the trials. Regressors were unconvolved epochs (to avoid assuming a particular response shape) shifted by 4 s to allow for the hemodynamic lag. The five time periods modeled were (i) early anticipation, 4 to 8 s after the cue; (ii) late anticipation, 8 to 13 s after cue offset; (iii) early pain, 4 to 14 s after stimulation onset; (iv) peak pain, 14 to 24 s after stimulation onset; and (v) late pain, 24 to 34 s after heat onset (stimulation offset was at 20 s). During fMRI scanning, each block of six C or P test trials constituted a separate scanner run, and BOLD responses to anticipation and pain were compared to the baseline interval immediately after each trial. An additional regressor for the behavioral response (4 to 8 s after cue to respond) was included but not analyzed further.

42. rACC: [3 18 34], 37 contiguous voxels within pain-responsive regions, $Z = 2.92$.

43. The following pain-responsive regions showing placebo effects in late heat: Right (contralateral) insula ([41 7 1], 207 voxels, $Z = 3.24$); right medial thalamus ([2 −15 9], 10 voxels, $Z = 2.63$). Additional effects in left SII ([−58 −6 10], 145 voxels, $Z = 3.37$) were found in Study 2 but not in Study 1. See table S2 for additional regions.

44. A. Ploghaus *et al.*, *J. Neurosci.* **21**, 9896 (2001).

45. Placebo-induced decreases in right insula and medial thalamus pain-responsive regions were significantly greater during the late heat period than during the early heat period. Results from ROIs, averaging over voxels, for the insula: 41% larger placebo decreases in late heat; $t(22) = 1.75$, $P = 0.09$; for early heat, $t(22) = 3.73$, $P < 0.001$ for late heat, and $t(22) = 2.33$, $P < 0.05$ in a paired t test for the difference. For the thalamus: 20-fold larger placebo decreases in late heat; $t(22) = 0.18$. $P = 0.86$ for early heat, $t(22) = 2.95$, $P = 0.008$ for late heat, and $t(22) = 2.94$, $P = 0.008$ in a paired t test for the difference.

46. Right DLPFC: [42 4 30], 55 voxels, $Z − 2.79$; left DLPFC: [−42 14 30], 100 voxels, $Z = 3.34$. Midbrain: [−2 −26 −12], 251 voxels, $Z = 3.56$. Midbrain and DLPFC activations did not correlate with the magnitude of the behavioral placebo effect in Study 2. However, Study 2 was conducted only on placebo responders, and so was expected to produce main effects rather than correlations. Study 2 also failed to replicate the correlation of OFC activity with reported placebo effects. However, this may be due to the use of spiral gradient-echo imaging at 3 T in Study 2, which was subject to substantially more signal dropout in the relevant regions of OFC than was the echo-planar magnetic resonance imaging sequence used in Study 1 (fig. S4).

47. rACC placebo–control: [10 16 20], 79 voxels, $Z = 2.91$, 3 mm from similar findings in Study 1.

48. A. W. MacDonald III, J. D. Cohen, V. A. Stenger, C. S. Carter, *Science* **288**, 1835 (2000).

49. The correlation between placebo-induced increases in OFC and reported placebo effects was significantly greater during the anticipation period than during the shock period (right OFC: Z=−4.50 for anticipation, Z=0.49 for shock, difference Z=5.01, P<0.0001; left OFC: Z=−3.55 for anticipation, Z=2.02 for shock, difference Z=5.57, P<0.0001).

50. We also observed placebo activations (placebo > control) during pain in frontal and parietal cortical areas, consistent with activation of a general attentional network. However, these regions did not correlate with placebo reductions in experienced pain in either study, and they lie outside the scope of the current hypotheses.

51. D. D. Price, Science 288, 1769 (2000).

52. R. Peyron et al., Brain 122, 1765 (1999).

53. P. Petrovic, K. M. Petersson, P. H. Ghatan, S. Stone-Elander, M. Ingvar, Pain 85, 19 (2000).

54. J. C. Brooks, T. J. Nurmikko, W. E. Bimson, K. D. Singh, N. Roberts, NeuroImage 15, 293 (2002).

55. S. J. Bantick et al., Brain 125, 310 (2002).

56. E. T. Rolls, in The Cognitive Neurosciences, M. S. Gazzanaga, Ed. (MIT Press, Cambridge, Mass., 1995), pp. 1091–1106.

57. W. C. Drevets, Biol. Psychiatry 48, 813 (2000).

58. A. Ploghaus et al., Science 284, 1979 (1999).

59. Temperatures were 45.4°C ± 1.1 (mean ± SD) for level 2, 47.0°C ± 0.9 for level 5, and 48.1°C ± 1.0 for level 8.

60. N. J. Voudouris, C. L. Peck, G. Coleman, Pain 38, 109 (1989).

Supporting Online Material

www.sciencemag.org/cgi/content/full/303/5661/1162/DC1
Materials and Methods
Tables S1 to S3
Figs. S1 to S5
References

26

Placebo Effects Mediated by Endogenous Opioid Activity on μ-Opioid Receptors

Jon-Kar Zubieta, Joshua A. Bueller, Lisa R. Jackson, David J. Scott, Yanjun Xu, Robert A. Koeppe, Thomas E. Nichols, and Christian S. Stohler

Jon-Kar Zubieta, Joshua A. Bueller, Lisa R. Jackson, David J. Scott, Yanjun Xu, Robert A. Koeppe, Thomas E. Nichols, and Christian S. Stohler, "Placebo Effects Mediated by Endogenous Opioid Activity on μ-Opioid Receptors," Journal of Neuroscience 2005;25:7754–7762.

Introduction

Placebo effects, the positive physiological or psychological changes associated with the administration of inert substances or procedures, can both enhance and obscure the effects of therapeutic interventions. However, they also represent an instance in which neural processes, through positive cognitive expectations, influence physical and neuropsychiatric states, a veritable example of "mind-body" interactions. It is therefore not surprising that interest is emerging in understanding their underlying mechanisms.

Substantial evidence implicates the endogenous opioid system in the mediation of placebo effects under conditions of expectation of analgesia. During both clinical and experimentally induced pain, placebo administration with expectation of analgesia has been associated with reductions in pain ratings that were reversed by either the open or hidden administration of naloxone (i.e., they were mediated by the activation of pain-suppressive endogenous opioid neurotransmission) (Gracely et al., 1983; Grevert et al., 1983; Levine and Gordon, 1984; Benedetti, 1996; Amanzio and Benedetti, 1999).

The endogenous opioid system, and specifically its activation of μ-opioid receptors, thought to primarily mediate the observed effects of placebo and naloxone, is implicated in a number of functions, from the regulation of stress responses and pain, particularly if sustained or threatening to the organism (Watkins and Mayer, 1982; Akil et al., 1984; Rubinstein et al., 1996; Sora et al., 1997; Zubieta et al., 2001), to reproductive and stress-related neuroendocrine functions (Smith et al., 1998; Drolet et al., 2001). Substantial evidence has also accumulated as to the involvement of this neurotransmitter system in the adaptation and response to novel and emotionally salient stimuli in both animal models and humans (Kalin et al., 1988; Nelson and Panksepp, 1998; Filliol et al., 2000; Zubieta et al., 2003b; Moles et al., 2004).

High placebo responders have shown more pronounced rostral anterior cingulate blood-flow responses to the systemic administration of a μ-opioid receptor agonist, remifentanil, suggesting the presence of variations in the responses of this receptor system as a function of placebo response (Petrovic et al., 2002). More recently, using functional magnetic resonance imaging (fMRI), the administration of a placebo with expectation of analgesia has also been associated with reductions in the activity of pain-responsive regions, namely, the rostral anterior cingulate, the insular cortex, and the thalamus (Wager et al., 2004).

The present study directly examines whether the introduction of a placebo with expectation of analgesia indeed activates endogenous opioid neurotransmission, using positron emission tomography (PET) and molecular imaging with a μ-opioid receptor selective radiotracer. Under these conditions, activation of this neurotransmitter system is evidenced by reductions in the in vivo availability of synaptic μ-opioid receptors to bind the radiolabeled tracer (Zubieta et al., 2001, 2002, 2003a; Bencherif et al., 2002).

From a methodological perspective, one of the difficulties inherent to the use of molecular imaging is the length of time required for the acquisition of quantitative measures of receptor availability (Zubieta et al., 2001, 2002), requiring that pain be maintained for a period of time. However, sustained pain also induces the activation of antinociceptive responses (Levine et al., 1978; Watkins and Mayer, 1982; Zubieta et al., 2001), which by substantially reducing pain ratings over time (Bencherif et al., 2002) may interfere with the subsequent formation of the placebo effect (Price et al., 1999). These issues were addressed by using an adaptive system that maintained pain over time by increasing the magnitude of the algesic stimulus as the rating of pain intensity reported by the volunteers declined over time (Zhang et al., 1993). The increases in algesic requirement then provided an objective psychophysical measure of antinociceptive activity, whereas the relationship between stimulus magnitude and pain ratings relate it to the subjective individual experiences of pain.

Materials and Methods

Subjects

Volunteers were 20- to 30-year-old, right-handed males, who were nonsmokers and had no personal history of medical, psychiatric illness, substance abuse or dependence, and no family history of inheritable illnesses. This study was restricted to males within a narrow age range, because both age and sex effects have been described for μ-opioid receptor concentrations and the capacity to activate this neurotransmitter system (Gabilondo et al., 1995; Zubieta et al., 1999, 2002). Volunteers were not taking psychotropic medications or hormone treatments and did not exercise in excess of 1 h three times a week. Subjects were instructed not to drink alcohol for at least 24 h nor to exercise or eat for at least 3 h before the study. Written informed consent was obtained in all cases. All the procedures used were approved by the University of Michigan Institutional Review Board and the Subcommittee for Human Use of Radioisotopes.

Experimental Design

Each volunteer was scanned three times with PET and [^{11}C] carfentanil. An initial study was performed without any intervention (baseline), and the second and third studies included either a sustained pain challenge or sustained pain with placebo with implied analgesic properties. Radiotracer administrations were separated by at least 2 h to allow for radiotracer decay and to eliminate any possible residual effects of the preceding challenge.

Pain and pain plus placebo conditions were introduced 40 min after radiotracer administration in a blind, randomized, and counterbalanced design (one-half of the volunteers receiving pain first and one-half receiving pain plus placebo). Deep sustained muscle pain was maintained from 40 to 60 min after radiotracer administration by the infusion of medication-grade 5% hypertonic saline into the relaxed masseter (jaw) muscle via a computer-controlled pump (total volume, 2.91 ± 0.96 ml), as described previously (Zhang et al., 1993; Stohler and Kowalski, 1999). Briefly, after the standardized bolus injection of 0.15 ml of hypertonic saline, infused over 15 s, subjects were required to report the present pain intensity every 15 s on an electronic version of 100 mm visual analog scale (VAS), with the lower and upper bound of the scale marked with numbers 0 and 100, respectively representing the range from "no pain" to "the most pain intensity imaginable." Based on pain intensity scores provided by the subject every 15 s for the reminder of the experiment, individual infusion requirements were continuously modeled

and updated to keep the present pain intensity scores in the preset range for the full duration of the experiment. Infusion volumes, required to maintain the preset pain intensity, were recorded every 15 s, and the cumulative infusion volume required over time was used as an indicator of subjects' pain sensitivity. Using this model, pain disappears 5–10 min after completion of the algesic infusion. To avoid swelling and possible tissue damage, the maximum infusion rate was limited to 250 μl/min.

Immediately after completion of the trials, the subjective pain experience was evaluated using the comprehensive version of the McGill Pain Questionnaire (MPQ) (Melzack and Torgerson, 1971) and overall VAS scores (rated from 0 to 100) of pain intensity and pain unpleasantness. The internal affective state of the volunteers was rated with the Positive and Negative Affectivity Scale (PANAS) (Watson et al., 1988) and the Profile of Mood States (POMS). The composite Total Mood Disturbance score (TMD) was used to evaluate the transient negative mood elicited by the pain stimulus (POMS-TMD) (McNair et al., 1992). These scores were related to the algesic input (subjective scores per volume of hypertonic saline, in milliliters) to provide with assessments of the pain experience as a function of the pain stimulus administered to the subject in each of the experimental conditions.

Subjects were given the following clinical trial–type instructions before administration of the placebo, so that the conditions of the study would be similar to those encountered in typical placebo-controlled drug trials: "We are studying the effect of a medication that may or may not relieve pain. This medication is thought to have analgesic effects through the activation of brain systems that suppress pain." In the written consent form, it was further explained that they could receive an active drug or a substance with no intrinsic pain relief properties. Subjects were also informed that they may not be able to ascertain whether the drug was actually working to relieve the pain but that the investigators would be able to ascertain its analgesic properties through their monitoring equipment.

The placebo condition consisted of the introduction of 1 ml of 0.9% physiological saline into one of the intravenous ports, every 4 min, starting 4 min after the initiation of the pain challenge and lasting for 15 s each time. Subjects were informed that the study drug was to be administered by means of a warning that was followed by a second-by-second count of the infusion timing (15 s), using a computer-generated human voice recording. Subjects were also asked to estimate the expected analgesia before the introduction of the placebo and afterward, estimating the analgesic properties using a VAS scale from 0 (no analgesic effect) to 100 (maximum analgesia).

Neuroimaging Methods

MRI scans were acquired in all subjects on a 1.5 tesla scanner (Signa; General Electric, Milwaukee, WI). Acquisition sequences were axial spoiled gradient-recalled echo (SPGR) inverse recovery-Prep MR (echo time [TE], 5.5; repetition time [TR], 14; inversion time, 300; flip angle, 20°; number of excitations [NEX], 1; 124 contiguous images; 1.5 mm thickness), followed by axial T2 and proton density images (TR, 4000; TE, 20 and 100, respectively; NEX, 1; 62 contiguous images; 3 mm thick).

PET scans were acquired with a Siemens AG (Erlangen, Germany) HR+ scanner in three-dimensional mode (reconstructed full width at half maximum [FWHM] resolution, ~5.5 mm in-plane and 5.0 mm axially), with septa retracted and scatter correction. Participants were positioned in the PET scanner gantry, and two intravenous (antecubital) lines were placed. A light forehead restraint was used to eliminate intrascan head movement. [^{11}C]carfentanil was synthesized at high specific activity (>2000 Ci/mmol) by the reaction of ^{11}C-methyliodide and a nonmethyl precursor as described previously (Dannals et al., 1985), with minor modifications to improve its synthetic yield (Jewett, 2001); 10–15 mCi (370–555 MBq) were administered to each subject for each of the three PET scans. The baseline study was always performed first, typically 24–48 h before the challenge studies. Pain and pain plus placebo studies were separated by at least 2 h to allow for tracer decay. The maximum mass of carfentanil injected was 0.03 μg/kg per scan, ensuring that the compound was administered in tracer quantities (i.e., subpharmacological doses). Receptor occupancy by carfentanil was calculated to be between 0.2 and 0.6% for brain regions with low, intermediate, and high μ-opioid receptor concentrations, based on the mass of carfentanil administered and the known concentration of μ-opioid receptors in the postmortem human brain (Gross-Isseroff et al., 1990; Gabilondo et al., 1995). Fifty percent of the [^{11}C]carfentanil dose was administered as a bolus, and the remainder as a continuous infusion using a computer-controlled pump to achieve steady-state tracer levels at ~35–40 min after tracer administration. Twenty-eight frames were acquired over 90 min with an increasing duration (30 s to 5 min).

Images were reconstructed using iterative algorithms (brain mode; FORE/OSEM, 4 iterations; 16 subsets; no smoothing) into a 128 × 128 pixel matrix in a 28.8-cm-diameter field of view. Attenuation correction was performed through a 6 min transmission scan (^{68}Ge source) obtained before the PET study, also with iterative reconstruction of the blank/transmission data followed by segmentation of the attenuation image. Small head motions during emission scans were corrected by an automated computer algorithm for each subject before analysis, and the images coregistered to each other with the same software (Minoshima et al., 1993). Time points were then decay-corrected during reconstruction of the PET data. Image data were then transformed on a voxel-by-voxel basis into two sets of parametric maps: (1) a tracer transport measure (K_1 ratio) and (2) a receptor-related measure at equilibrium (DVReq), the latter using data obtained from 40–90 min after tracer administration. The tracer transport and binding measures were calculated using a modified Logan graphical analysis (Logan et al., 1996), using the occipital cortex (an area devoid of μ-opioid receptors) as the reference region. With the bolus-continuous infusion tracer administration protocol used, all regions achieved steady state by between 35 and 40 min after tracer administration (e.g., they are not susceptible to biases introduced by blood flow and therefore tracer transport changes). The slope of the Logan plot was used for the estimation of the distribution volume ratio (DVReq), a measure equal to the $(B_{max}/K_d) + 1$ for this receptor site and radiotracer. B_{max}/K_d (or DVReq − 1) was the receptor-related measure (μ-opioid receptor availability or binding potential). K_1 and DVReq images for each experimental period and MR images were coregistered to each other and to the International Consortium for Brain Mapping (ICBM) stereotactic atlas orientation (Meyer et al., 1997).

Statistical parametric maps of differences between conditions (control–pain, pain plus placebo–pain) were generated by anatomically standardizing the T1-SPGR MRI of each subject to the ICBM stereotactic atlas coordinates, with subsequent application of this transformation to the μ-opioid receptor binding maps (Meyer et al., 1997). The accuracy of coregistration and nonlinear warping algorithms was confirmed for each subject individually by comparing the transformed MRI and PET images to each other and the ICBM atlas template.

Differences between conditions and groups were then mapped into stereotactic space using z-maps of statistical significance with statistical parametric mapping (SPM) (SPM 99; Wellcome Department of Cognitive Neurology, London, UK) and Matlab (WaveMetrics, Lake Oswego, Ore.) software, with a general linear model and correction for multiple comparisons (Friston et al., 1995). No global normalization was applied to the data, and therefore the calculations presented are based on absolute B_{max}/K_d estimates. Only regions with specific μ-opioid receptor binding were included in the analyses (voxels with DVR values > 1.2 times the mean global image value for μ-opioid receptor images as calculated with SMP 99). To compensate for small residual anatomic variations across subjects and to improve signal-to-noise ratios, a three-dimensional Gaussian filter (FWHM, 6 mm) was applied to each scan.

Comparisons between conditions, within subjects were then performed using paired, two-tailed t tests, on a voxel-by-voxel basis. Areas of significant differences were detected using a statistical threshold that controls a type-I error rate at $p < 0.05$ for multiple comparisons. These statistical thresholds were estimated using the Euler characteristic (Worsley, 1994) based on the number of voxels in the gray matter, image smoothness, and the extent of local changes (correction for cluster volume) (Friston et al., 1991). The only region for which a lower statistical threshold was allowed ($p < 0.0001$ uncorrected) was the periaqueductal gray, because of its small size, making the finding of significant effects difficult, and because of its central involvement in endogenous opioid modulation of pain. Numerical values for the graphs presented in Figures 26.2 and 26.3 and for the correlations described in the text were extracted from the image data by averaging the values of voxels contained in an area where significant differences were obtained in the voxel-by-voxel analysis, down to a threshold of $p = 0.01$. Correlations between activation of neurotransmission and the changes in psychophysical measures were calculated with one-tailed Pearson correlations at $p < 0.05$, given the known directionality of these relationships (Zubieta et al., 2001).

The within-subject, interexperimental variability in the binding measures was calculated previously from a separate sample of five healthy individuals, 20–30 years of age, studied twice without interventions. For the regions in which placebo effects were detected in this study (anterior cingulate, prefrontal cortex, insular cortex, nucleus accumbens), interexperimental differences ranged from 7.7 to −8.4% (mean, −3.2 ± 6.4%). A conservative cutoff of 10% was then used to assess the formation of a substantial neurochemical placebo effect for the analyses of its psychophysical correlates.

Results

Effects of Sustained Pain on μ-Opioid Receptor-Mediated Neurotransmission

Consistent with previous work (Zubieta et al., 2001), the sustained pain stimulus, which was always applied on the left side, was associated with a significant activation of endogenous opioid transmission and μ-opioid receptors (n = 14). The areas involved included the dorsal anterior cingulate; medial prefrontal cortex; right insular cortex; ventral basal ganglia, bilaterally (nucleus accumbens extending to the ventral pallidum); medial thalamus; right amygdala; left subamygdalar temporal cortex; and periaqueductal gray (Fig. 26.1).

Psychophysical Responses to Placebo Administration

Expectation of analgesia before the introduction of the placebo was rated at 50 ± 18% VAS units (range, 10–75%), with endpoints denoted as "no effect at all" and "complete pain relief," respectively. The analgesic effectiveness of the placebo was subjectively rated at 54 ± 24% VAS units (range, 10–90%) after completion of the study. This information confirmed that there was expectation of analgesia induced by our clinical trial–type of instructions.

Introduction of the placebo (1 ml of isotonic saline, i.v.; every 4 min) was associated with an increase in the average rate of algesic stimulus required to maintain pain, an objective assessment of the activation of antinociceptive mechanisms (Table 26.1, top). Pain intensity, as rated every 15 s by the volunteers, was maintained for the duration of the study, as expected given the adaptive nature of the algesic infusion system used. However, a small mean reduction of 4 points in the 0–100 scale used to rate momentary pain was noted after the introduction of the placebo, which reached statistical significance (Table 26.1, top). This was attributed to five subjects reaching the maximum allowable infusion rate to maintain pain (250 μl/min) when the placebo was administered, an unexpected occurrence. This maximum, safety-bound rate had been originally established to avoid tissue swelling and damage. However, because the subjective ratings of the pain experience were related to the volume of algesic substance introduced, the ceiling effect reached in some subjects was not felt to compromise these assessments. Just the opposite, reductions in the pain signal would tend to bias the experiments toward finding lower placebo effects as well.

The additional psychophysical variables used to assess the subjective experience of sustained pain with and without placebo administration are shown in Table 26.1 (bottom). With the exception of the momentary VAS ratings of pain intensity, which was acquired every 15 s for the duration of the studies, other rating scales (overall VAS ratings of pain intensity and unpleasantness, MPQ, PANAS, POMS-TMD) were administered immediately after completion of each of the challenges. For the entire sample, significant effects of placebo on the pain experience in terms of stimulus magnitude to stimulus response were observed for the ratings of pain intensity and unpleasantness, as well as for the affective information content of the pain, as measured with the MPQ (Table 26.1).

We then contrasted the response properties of high and low placebo responders using a 20% difference in the response-to-stimulus ratios (average of every 15 s VAS intensity ratings/volume infused) as the cutoff to classify placebo responders. In this manner, nine subjects were classified as high placebo responders, whereas five were classified as low placebo responders. High placebo responders demonstrated significant reductions in rating to stimulus ratios for VAS ratings of overall pain intensity (t = 2.12) and pain unpleasantness (t = 2.21), MPQ sensory subscale scores (t = 3.13), MPQ affective subscale scores (t = 2.66), and MPQ total scores (t = 3.16) and presented lower PANAS negative affect (t = 2.02) and higher PANAS positive affect scores during placebo administration (t = 2.25) (df = 12; unpaired, one-tailed t tests; p < 0.05). Trend effects were observed for POMS-TMD scores, which were also lower in the placebo responders, albeit below statistically significant thresholds (t = 1.62; p < 0.06).

Effect of Placebo on μ-Opioid Receptor-Mediated Neurotransmission

The activation of the endogenous opioid system and μ-opioid receptors was then compared between sustained pain and sustained pain plus placebo conditions for all subjects (n = 14). Significantly higher levels of activation were obtained for the condition in which placebo was administered. After correction for multiple comparisons, statistically significant effects of placebo on μ-opioid system activation were obtained in the left (ipsilateral to pain) dorsolateral prefrontal cortex (Brodmann areas 8 and 9), pregenual rostral right (contralateral) anterior cingulate (Brodmann areas 24 and 25), right (contralateral) anterior insular cortex, and

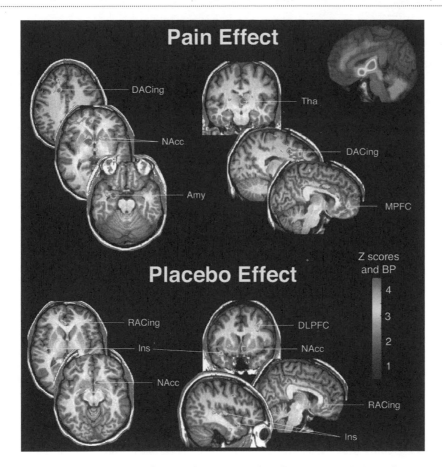

Figure 26.1. Effects of pain and placebo on the activation of μ-opioid receptor-mediated neurotransmission. After correction for multiple comparisons, significant μ-opioid system activations during the sustained pain challenge ($n = 14$) were obtained in the dorsal anterior cingulate (DACing; x,y,z coordinates [in millimeters]: 17,10,40; cluster size: 715mm^3; z score = 5.54; $p < 0.005$ after correction for multiple comparisons); medial prefrontal cortex (MPFC; x,y,z: 8,45,−5; cluster size: 1064 mm^3; z score = 3.90; $p < 0.001$); right (contralateral to pain) insular cortex (Ins; x,y,z: 49,16,6; cluster size: 257 mm^3; z score = 4.32; $p < 0.005$); ventral basal ganglia, bilaterally (nucleus accumbens [NAcc] extending to the ventral pallidum; right, x,y,z: 12,4,−2; cluster size: 1700 mm^3; z score = 9.26; $p < 0.0001$; left, x,y,z: −19,9,4; cluster size: 2177 mm^3; z score = 4.32; $p < 0.005$); medial thalamus (Tha; x,y,z: −3,−15,7; cluster size: 2283 mm^3; z score = 6.49; $p < 0.0001$); right amygdala (Amy; x,y,z: 25,−2,−21; cluster size: 464 mm^3; z score = 6.34; $p < 0.0001$); left subamygdalar temporal cortex (x,y,z: −28,10,−38; cluster size: 560 mm^3; z score = 5.36; $p < 0.005$); and periaqueductal gray (x,y,z: −5,−28,−3; cluster size: 122 mm^3; z score = 3.56; $p < 0.05$). Significant effects of placebo on the activation of the μ-opioid system ($n = 14$) were detected in the left dorsolateral prefrontal cortex (DLPFC; x,y,z peak coordinates: −36,13,39; cluster size: 1403 mm^3; z score = 4.27; $p < 0.0001$); rostral anterior cingulate (RACing; x,y,z: 14,49,13; cluster size: 3193 mm^3; z score = 4.18; $p < 0.0001$); left NAcc (x,y,z: −7,11,−11; cluster size: 1332 mm^3; z score = 4.83; $p < 0.0001$); and right anterior insula (Ins; x,y,z: 41,10,−17; cluster size: 844 mm^3; z score = 4.15; $p < 0.05$). The posterior right insula achieved subthreshold levels of significance (x,y,z: 44,−15,4; cluster size: 732 mm^3; z score = 3.81; $p < 0.0001$ uncorrected for multiple comparisons). Z scores of statistical significance are represented by the pseudocolor scale on the right side of the image (under the heading "Z scores and BP" and numbered 1 through 4) and are superimposed over an anatomically standardized MRI image in coronal views. The left side of the axial and coronal images corresponds to the right side of the body (contralateral to pain; radiological convention). A map of μ-opioid receptor distribution is shown in the top right corner of the figure in a sagittal view, with binding potential (BP) values (receptor availability in vivo; B_{max}/K_d) depicted by the same pseudocolor scale.

left (ipsilateral) nucleus accumbens (Fig. 26.1). A second area within the contralateral insular cortex, in its posterior region, also showed changes in neurotransmission; however, it did no longer reach statistical significance after correction for multiple comparisons (Fig. 26.1). Data points for significant regions are presented in Figure 26.2, confirming robust effects of the placebo on this neurotransmitter system. However, examination of the individual datasets showed that the degree of placebo-induced μ-opioid system activation was not of the same magnitude across all the brain sites in which these effects were detected. Overall, these data pointed to

the fact that an unselected sample of young healthy volunteers, when subjected to clinical trials instructions, showed robust placebo-induced activations of μ-opioid receptor-mediated neurotransmission that was relatively regionally specific for individual subjects.

Psychophysical Correlates of Placebo-Induced Activation of μ-Opioid Neurotransmission

In view of the differences in individual placebo-induced neurotransmitter activation patterns, regional psychophysical correlates were examined using a threshold of 10% change in

Table 26.1.

Psychophysiological responses during pain and pain plus placebo conditions, all subjects

	Pain	Pain + Plbo	t	p
Measure				
Mean q 15 s momentary VAS intensity	28.3±13.1	24.0±13.5	2.01	0.03
Volume 5% intramuscular saline (μl)	2796±956	3025±100	1.10	0.14
VAS overall intensity	37.5±19.9	27.4±15.7	3.40	0.002
VAS overall unpleasantness	40.4±25.5	32.9±21.6	2.05	0.03
MPQ sensory subscale	14.3±4.5	13.7±5.4	0.44	0.33
MPQ affective subscale	0.9±1.0	0.4±0.6	2.83	0.007
MPQ total	19.4±5.5	18.5±7.4	0.40	0.35
PANAS negative affect	2.1±2.1	2.6±3.5	0.97	0.44
PANAS positive affect	13.4±7.4	14.1±6.1	0.87	0.20
POMS-TMD score	9.7±7.9	10.7±9.5	0.99	0.17
Rating to stimulus (milliliters of algesic substance required) ratio				
Mean q 15 s momentary VAS intensity	14.7±16.1	10.8±1.0	1.40	0.09
VAS overall intensity	19.5±21.5	12.3±11.4	1.98	0.03
VAS overall unpleasantness	18.5±18.6	13.2±10.6	1.76	0.05
MPQ sensory subscale	6.0±3.3	5.5±4.4	0.43	0.38
MPQ affective subscale	0.5±0.6	0.2±0.4	2.32	0.02
MPQ total	8.4±5.1	7.6±6.6	0.41	0.34
PANAS negative affect	0.8±1.0	1.5±2.9	0.97	0.17
PANAS positive affect	5.8±4.6	5.7±4.4	0.15	0.44
POMS-TMD score	4.7±4.6	5.3±6.2	0.36	0.37

Note: Mean ±1 SD of psychophysical measures of pain during the sustained pain challenge in the absence (Pain) and presence (Pain + Plbo) of placebo in 14 males 20–30 years of age. Mean q 15 s momentary VAS intensity refers to the average ratings of momentary pain acquired every 15 s for the duration of the pain challenge (20 min). Volume 5% intramuscular saline (in microliters, μl) is the total volume of algesic substance introduced by the adaptive pain control system to maintain pain. The remainder of the scales (VAS, 0–100 of overall pain intensity and unpleasantness; MPQ; PANAS; and POMS-TMD) were obtained immediately after completion of the pain challenge. Data are also expressed as the relationship between the subject's ratings and the stimulus needed to maintain pain during the experimental period (rating to stimulus [in milliliters] ratio). These ratios are used as the subjective assessment of placebo effects. Paired, one-tailed t test, $p < 0.05$. [MPQ = McGill Pain Questionnaire; PANAS = Positive and Negative Affectivity Scale; POMS = Profile of Mood States; TMD = Total Mood Disturbance; VAS = visual analog scale—eds.].

the receptor binding measure to capture data points for which the formation of a substantial regional placebo effect could be ascertained (Fig. 26.2). This threshold clearly exceeded the typical variability of receptor binding measures obtained in separate experiments (see Materials and Methods). Correlations were conducted between these regional changes in receptor availability, the algesic infusion volume changes after placebo, and the placebo-induced changes in subjective reports of pain (overall VAS intensity and unpleasantness scores, MPQ sensory and affective subscales, PANAS negative and positive affect scales, and POMSTMD scores). No correction for multiple comparisons was applied to these correlations and should be considered exploratory in nature.

In the pregenual anterior cingulate, placebo-induced μ-opioid system activation above those levels (n = 7) was correlated with the changes in stimulus-to-response ratios for overall ratings of VAS pain intensity ($r = -0.87$; $p < 0.01$) and pain unpleasantness ($r = -0.74$; $p < 0.05$), MPQ sensory subscale ($r = -0.84$; $p < 0.01$), and total MPQ scores ($r = -0.89$; $p < 0.01$). Placebo-induced activation of endogenous opioid neurotransmission in this region was also highly and posi-

tively correlated with the increases in the volume of algesic substance required to maintain pain during the placebo condition ($r = 0.96$; $p < 0.0001$).

In the right anterior insular cortex (n = 9), significant correlations were obtained with the changes in VAS ratings of pain intensity ($r = -0.58$; $p < 0.05$), MPQ sensory ($r = -0.60$; $p < 0.05$), and total MPQ scores ($r = -0.58$; $p < 0.05$). At the level of the left nucleus accumbens (n = 8), significant correlations were obtained, in the same direction, with the change in VAS pain intensity ratings ($r = -0.80$; $p < 0.01$), MPQ affective subscale ($r = -0.81$; $p < 0.01$), and reductions in the POMS-TMD scores ($r = -0.71$; $p < 0.05$). No significant correlations were obtained between placebo-induced changes in these psychophysical measures and left dorsolateral prefrontal cortex (n = 10) μ-opioid neurotransmission. However, and uniquely for this region, μ-opioid system activation was negatively correlated with the expected analgesic effect as rated by the subjects before placebo administration, whether only placebo responders or all study participants were included in the analysis ($r = -0.55$ and -0.65, respectively; $p < 0.05$) (Fig. 26.3).

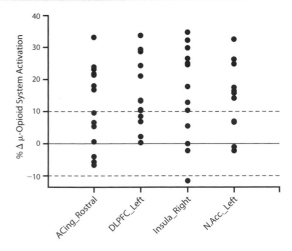

Figure 26.2. Individual data points for the magnitude of regional μ-opioid system activation in response to the placebo intervention. Individual data points for the change in the binding potential measure (BP; μ-opioid receptor availability *in vivo*; B_{max}/K_d) from the pain condition to the pain plus placebo condition are shown. A threshold of 10% increase in the activation of this neurotransmitter system, evidenced as a reduction in the BP measure during the placebo condition, was used to identify individuals that responded with a robust placebo effect on the activation of this system in each of the regions (dashed line). ACing_Rostral = Rostral (pregenual) region of the anterior cingulate; DLPFC_Left = left dorsolateral prefrontal cortex; Insula_Right = right insular cortex; N.Acc._Left = left nucleus accumbens.

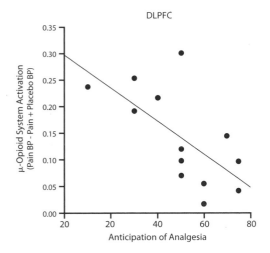

Figure 26.3. Relationship between placebo-induced regional μ-opioid system activation and expectation of analgesia. Negative correlation between the expected analgesic effects as rated by the volunteers before the study and the placebo-induced activation of dorsolateral prefrontal cortex (DLPFC) μ-opioid neurotransmission in placebo responders (black circles) and nonresponders (gray circles) are shown. BP = Binding potential.

Discussion

This report provides the first direct evidence that the administration of a placebo with implied analgesic properties regionally activates a pain and stress inhibitory neurotransmitter system, the endogenous opioid system, through direct effects on the μ-opioid receptors. Furthermore, this activation is associated with quantifiable reductions in the physical and emotional attributes of a sustained pain challenge. We also observe that the respective neurotransmitter activity took place directly in associative, higher-order brain regions, namely, the pregenual and subgenual area of the rostral anterior cingulate, the dorsolateral prefrontal and insular cortex, and in the nucleus accumbens, correlating with various aspects of the experience of pain. In the case of the rostral anterior cingulate, activation of this neurotransmitter system was highly associated with the algesic infusion requirements to maintain pain for the duration of the study, an objective measure of the activation of antinociceptive mechanisms. Dorsolateral prefrontal cortex endogenous opioid activity, on the other hand, was associated with the magnitude of analgesia expected by the volunteers before placebo administration.

For the regions in which placebo administration increased the endogenous opioid neurotransmission, with exception of the nucleus accumbens, their localization primarily coincided with that observed by Wager et al. (2004) as reductions in pain-induced metabolic demands as measured by blood oxygenation level–dependent fMRI (BOLD-fMRI) during placebo administration (i.e., prefrontal cortex, pregenual anterior cingulate, and insular cortex). Basal ganglia signals are often difficult to obtain with BOLD-fMRI techniques, which may explain the difference with respect to this region between their data and ours. The regions implicated in the placebo effect are, as would be expected, part of those where prominent endogenous opioid neurotransmission and μ-opioid receptor populations are present in rodent and human brains (e.g., cingulate, prefrontal, temporal and insular cortices, thalamus, basal ganglia, amygdala, hypothalamus, brainstem) (Gross-Isseroff et al., 1990; Gabilondo et al., 1995; Mansour et al., 1995). These are the areas in which increases in regional blood flow are registered after the exogenous administration of μ-opioid receptor agonists (Firestone et al., 1996; Adler et al., 1997; Schlaepfer et al., 1998; Casey et al., 2000; Wagner et al., 2001); some of them (i.e., rostral anterior cingulate) had also been noted to be more prominently activated in high placebo responders after μ-opioid agonist administration (Petrovic et al., 2002).

Our work takes the investigation of placebo effects directly into the realm of human brain neurotransmission, addressing the function of a single neurotransmitter system. In this regard, μ-opioid receptor-mediated neurotransmission is one of the principal systems involved in the modulation of pain (Matthes et al., 1996), stress responses (Akil et al., 1984), and stress-induced analgesia in animal models (Mogil et al., 1994; Rubinstein et al., 1996) as well as in humans (Zubieta et al., 2001, 2002, 2003a). The μ-opioid system has also been implicated in the regulation of behavioral responses to novel environments and stimulus-reward associations in studies using animal models devoid of these receptors (Filliol et al., 2000; Moles et al., 2004), as well as in the regulation of affective responses in humans (Zubieta et al., 2003b). As such, this neurotransmitter system appears to support the neurobiologies of pain, stress, and their modulation by cognitive-emotional influences.

Prominent effects of the placebo intervention on μ-opioid receptor-mediated neurotransmission were observed in Brodmann areas 24 and 25 of the pregenual and subgenual anterior cingulate, part of the so-called affective subdivision of the anterior cingulate (Bush et al., 2000). Notably, the metabolic activation of the anterior cingulate by pain (Talbot et al., 1991; Davis et al., 1995; Vogt et al., 1996; Aziz et al., 1997; Casey, 1999; Gelnar et al., 1999; Willoch et al., 2000) and by more specific aspects of the pain experience, such as the pain intensity (Coghill et al., 1999; Hofbauer et al., 2001), its affective qualities (Rainville et al., 1997; Tolle et al., 1999), pain anticipation (Hsieh et al., 1999; Ploghaus et al., 1999), the illusion of pain (Craig et al., 1996), or even empathy to pain experienced by others (Singer et al., 2004) have typically involved more dorsal subregions of the anterior cingulate. Conversely, the metabolic activity of the pregenual and subgenual anterior cingulate has been traditionally implicated in responses to stressful challenges of emotional significance (Phan et al., 2002) and, more recently, in the placebo effect (Petrovic et al., 2002; Wager et al., 2004). Of interest, reductions in its baseline metabolism and volume have been associated with familial and treatment-refractory major depression (Drevets et al., 1997; Mayberg et al., 1997), an illness thought to be mediated by alterations in homeostatic responses to salient or stressful environmental events. This illness otherwise presents with high responses to placebo administration in controlled trials (Schatzberg and Kraemer, 2000).

In the present report, placebo-induced activation of μ-opioid neurotransmission in the pregenual and subgenual anterior cingulate was not only significantly correlated with the suppression of volunteer's reports of perceived pain intensity and sensory pain qualities, but also with the increases in algesic infusion requirements for maintaining pain intensity during placebo administration. The connectivity of this region (Brodmann areas 24 and 25) with brain nuclei involved in pain, saliency-reward, affect, and autonomic and neuroendocrine regulatory (Carmichael and Price, 1995; Haber et al., 1995; An et al., 1998; Ongur et al., 1998), together with recent data on the effects of placebo on the metabolic activity (Petrovic et al., 2002; Wager et al., 2004), makes it a particularly likely site for the mediation of various placebo effects.

Placebo-induced activation of μ-opioid neurotransmission was also observed in the insular cortex, an area that becomes metabolically activated in response to painful stimuli in imaging studies in humans (Casey, 1999; Davis, 2000; Peyron et al., 2000). This region is thought to have a more general involvement in the representation and modulation of interoceptive, internal bodily responses to both physical and emotional stimuli (Casey, 1999; Cameron, 2001; Craig, 2002; Phan et al., 2002). Its posterior portions aid in the processing of somatosensory information, including muscular pain, such as is the case of the present study (Craig et al., 2000;

Kupers et al., 2004). The anterior insula, however, appears implicated in the more complex, subjective processing of the affective qualities of various physical and emotional stimuli (Craig, 2003; Singer et al., 2004). We also observed placebo-induced μ-opioid system activation in both posterior and anterior areas of the right insular cortex (contralateral to pain in the present study); however, only the anterior region reached statistical thresholds of significance, correlating with pain intensity and sensory qualities of the pain.

In the nucleus accumbens, placebo-induced activation of μ-opioid neurotransmission was significantly correlated with the suppression of pain intensity and pain affect, as well as with the negative mood state induced by the pain challenge. This is a dopamine-rich region in which both dopamine and opioid peptides have been shown to regulate responses to painful and stressful stimuli (Gear et al., 1999; Horvitz, 2000; Zubieta et al., 2003a) but also natural rewards (Berridge and Robinson, 1998; Will et al., 2003) and drugs of abuse (Unterwald, 2001; Volkow et al., 2004), in both animals and humans. As a result, it is thought to have broader role in responding to and modulating salient stimuli with both rewarding and nonrewarding valences (Berridge and Robinson, 1998; Horvitz, 2000; Lorenz et al., 2003; Pruessner et al., 2004; Zald et al., 2004; Zink et al., 2004). Activation of dopaminergic neurotransmission in this region, and reductions in the neuronal activity of some of its efferent targets (subthalamic nucleus), have also been shown under conditions of placebo administration and expectation of improvement in Parkinson's disease (de la Fuente-Fernández et al., 2001; Benedetti et al., 2004). Of relevance to the present results, Parkinson's disease is characterized by reductions in dopaminergic neurotransmission, which in turn has been associated with both a higher content of opioid peptides in this region (George and Kertesz, 1987; Steiner and Gerfen, 1998) and a more prominent activation of the μ-opioid system in response to pain (Zubieta et al., 2003a). These mechanisms may then underlie the particular responsiveness of this neurodegenerative illness to placebo-associated expectancies, previously observed by various authors (Shetty et al., 1999; Goetz et al., 2000).

Finally, although the activation of endogenous opioid neurotransmission in the left dorsolateral prefrontal cortex was not correlated with placebo-induced changes in the pain psychophysical measures obtained from our subjects, we did observe a negative relationship between μ-opioid system activation in this region and the magnitude of the analgesic effect expected by our subjects before the administration of the placebo. Consistent with this observation, this brain region was found bilaterally activated during placebo-induced anticipation of analgesia in an fMRI study (Wager et al., 2004). Lorenz et al. (2003) also found that the metabolic activity of this region was negatively correlated with that of other elements of the "pain matrix" (e.g., medial thalamus, midbrain, and insular cortex) during pain; it was also negatively correlated with the perceived intensity and unpleasantness of the painful stimulus. These authors then suggested a role for this region in the indirect modulation of responses to pain through other cortical (e.g., insular cortex) and subcortical (thalamus, midbrain) regions. If this were the case, a reduction in opioid inhibitory control in the dorsolateral prefrontal cortex would be associated with a permissive effect on the engagement of other pain control regions, a testable hypothesis for future studies. The hypothesized involvement of the dorsolateral prefrontal cortex in the temporal organization and adjustments in the control of behavior (Fuster, 2000; Kerns et al., 2004) may then extend into the metabolic (Wager et al., 2004) and neurotransmitter responses (as is the case in the present report) to placebo-induced expectations of analgesia. Conversely, Apkarian et al. (2004) reported progressive gray-matter atrophy in this brain region in chronic back pain patients as a function of pain duration. As more persistent forms of illness tend to present with lower placebo response rates, the contribution of variations in dorsolateral prefrontal function to the formation of a placebo effect warrants additional study.

The results presented are consistent with reports implicating the endogenous opioid system in the mediation of placebo analgesic effects, examined previously by their blockade after the systemic administration of naloxone (Gracely et al., 1983; Grevert et al., 1983; Levine and Gordon, 1984; Benedetti, 1996; Amanzio and Benedetti, 1999). Naloxone, however, is not a selective μ-opioid receptor antagonist, and it may influence other opioid receptor types. The present work, conversely, exclusively addresses the μ-opioid receptor and the psychophysical correlates of its activation, leaving open the question of whether other opioid receptor types or neurotransmitter mechanisms may also be involved in these effects. The data presented here also highlight that changes in neurochemical signaling induced by the introduction of a placebo do not represent an on–off phenomenon, but rather a graded effect that is influenced, with relative independence, by a number of brain regions with complex, "integrative-motivational" functions.

The results presented and recent data from animal models (Moles et al., 2004) are consistent with the notion that placebo-responding regions and neurochemical systems (e.g., the endogenous opioid system and μ-opioid receptors) are an intrinsic part of neuronal processes that mediate the interaction between positive environmental conditions (in the present case the suggestion of analgesia) and the corresponding physical and emotional responses of the individual. From a different perspective, disruptions in these normal regulatory processes, exemplified by the typically lower rates of placebo responding in the more persistent or severe forms of various illnesses, may then represent points of vulnerability for the expression or maintenance of various pathological states.

REFERENCES

Adler LJ, Gyulai FE, Diehl DJ, et al. (1997) Regional brain activity changes associated with fentanyl analgesia elucidated by positron emission tomography. Anesth Analg 84:120–126.

Akil H, Watson S, Young E, et al. (1984) Endogenous opioids: biology and function. Annu Rev Neurosci 7:223–255.

Amanzio M, Benedetti F (1999) Neuropharmacological dissection of placebo analgesia: expectation-activated opioid systems versus conditioning-activated specific subsystems. J Neurosci 19:484–494.

An X, Bandler R, Ongur D, Price JL (1998) Prefrontal cortical projections to longitudinal columns in the midbrain periaqueductal gray in macaque monkeys. J Comp Neurol 401:455–479.

Apkarian AV, Sosa Y, Sonty S, et al. (2004) Chronic back pain is associated with decreased prefrontal and thalamic gray matter density. J Neurosci 24:10410–10415.

Aziz Q, Andersson JL, Valind S, et al. (1997) Identification of human brain loci processing esophageal sensation using positron emission tomography. Gastroenterology 113:50–59.

Bencherif B, Fuchs PN, Sheth R, et al. (2002) Pain activation of human supraspinal opioid pathways as demonstrated by [^{11}C]carfentanil and positron emission tomography (PET). Pain 99:589–598.

Benedetti F (1996) The opposite effects of the opiate antagonist naloxone and the cholecystokinin antagonist proglumide on placebo analgesia. Pain 64:535–543.

Benedetti F, Colloca L, Torre E, et al. (2004) Placebo-responsive Parkinson patients show decreased activity in single neurons of subthalamic nucleus. Nat Neurosci 7:587–588.

Berridge KC, Robinson TE (1998) What is the role of dopamine in reward: hedonic impact, reward learning, or incentive salience? Brain Res Brain Res Rev 28:309–369.

Bush G, Luu P, Posner M (2000) Cognitive and emotional influences in anterior cingulate cortex. Trends Cogn Sci 4:215–222.

Cameron OG (2001) Interoception: the inside story—a model for psychosomatic processes. Psychosom Med 63:697–710.

Carmichael ST, Price JL (1995) Limbic connections of the orbital and medial prefrontal cortex in macaque monkeys. J Comp Neurol 363:615–641.

Casey K (1999) Forebrain mechanisms of nociception and pain: analysis through imaging. Proc Natl Acad Sci USA 96:7668–7674.

Casey K, Svensson P, Morrow T, et al. (2000) Selective opiate modulation of nociceptive processing in the human brain. J Neurophysiol 84:525–533.

Coghill R, Sang C, Maisog J, Iadarola M (1999) Pain intensity processing within the human brain: a bilateral, distributed mechanism. J Neurophysiol 82:1934–1943.

Craig A (2002) How do you feel? Interoception: the sense of the physiological condition of the body. Nat Rev Neurosci 3:655–666.

Craig A, Reiman E, Evans A, Bushnell M (1996) Functional imaging of an illusion of pain. Nature 384:258–260.

Craig AD (2003) Pain mechanisms: labeled lines versus convergence in central processing. Annu Rev Neurosci 26:1–30.

Craig AD, Chen K, Bandy D, Reiman EM (2000) Thermosensory activation of insular cortex. Nat Neurosci 3:184–190.

Dannals R, Ravert H, Frost J, et al. (1985) Radiosynthesis of an opiate receptor binding radiotracer: [^{11}C]carfentanil. Int J Appl Radiat Isot 36:303–306.

Davis K, Wood M, Crawley A, Mikulis D (1995) fMRI of human somatosensory and cingulate cortex during painful electrical nerve stimulation. NeuroReport 7:321–325.

Davis KD (2000) The neural circuitry of pain as explored with functional MRI. Neurol Res 22:313–317.

de la Fuente-Fernández R, Ruth TJ, Sossi V, et al. (2001) Expectation and dopamine release: mechanism of the placebo effect in Parkinson's disease. Science 293:1164–1166.

Drevets WC, Price JL, Simpson JR Jr., et al. (1997) Subgenual prefrontal cortex abnormalities in mood disorders. Nature 386:824–827.

Drolet G, Dumont EC, Gosselin I, et al. (2001) Role of endogenous opioid system in the regulation of the stress response. Prog Neuropsychopharmacol Biol Psychiatry 25:729–741.

Filliol D, Ghozland S, Chluba J, et al. (2000) Mice deficient for delta- and mu-opioid receptors exhibit opposing alterations of emotional responses. Nat Genet 25:195–200.

Firestone L, Gyulai F, Mintun M, et al. (1996) Human brain activity response to fentanyl imaged by positron emission tomography. Anesth Analg 82:1247–1251.

Friston KJ, Frith CD, Liddle PF, Frackowiak RSJ (1991) Comparing functional (PET) images: the assessment of significant change. J Cereb Blood Flow Metab 11:690–699.

Friston KJ, Holmes AP, Worsley KJ, et al. (1995) Statistical parametric maps in functional imaging: a general linear approach. Hum Brain Mapp 2:189–210.

Fuster JM (2000) Executive frontal functions. Exp Brain Res 133:66–70.

Gabilondo A, Meana J, Garcia-Sevilla J (1995) Increased density of mu-opioid receptors in the postmortem brain of suicide victims. Brain Res 682:245–250.

Gear R, Aley K, Levine J (1999) Pain-induced analgesia mediated by mesolimbic reward circuits. J Neurosci 19:7175–7181.

Gelnar P, Krauss B, Sheehe P, Szeverenyi N, Apkarian A (1999) A comparative fMRI study of cortical representations for thermal painful, vibrotactile, and motor performance tasks. NeuroImage 10:460–482.

George SR, Kertesz M (1987) Met-enkephalin concentrations in striatum respond reciprocally to alterations in dopamine neurotransmission. Peptides 8:487–492.

Goetz CG, Leurgans S, Raman R, Stebbins GT (2000) Objective changes in motor function during placebo treatment in PD. Neurology 54:710–714.

Gracely RH, Dubner R, Wolskee PJ, Deeter WR (1983) Placebo and naloxone can alter post-surgical pain by separate mechanisms. Nature 306:264–265.

Grevert P, Albert L, Goldstein A (1983) Partial antagonism of placebo analgesia by naloxone. Pain 16:129–143.

Gross-Isseroff R, Dillon K, Israeli M, Biegon A (1990) Regionally selective increases in mu-opioid receptor density in the brains of suicide victims. Brain Res 530:312–316.

Haber SN, Kunishio K, Mizobuchi M, Lynd-Balta E (1995) The orbital and medial prefrontal circuit through the primate basal ganglia. J Neurosci 15:4851–4867.

Hofbauer RK, Rainville P, Duncan GH, Bushnell MC (2001) Cortical representation of the sensory dimension of pain. J Neurophysiol 86:402–411.

Horvitz J (2000) Mesolimbic and nigrostriatal dopamine responses to salient non-rewarding stimuli. Neuroscience 96:651–656.

Hsieh J, Stone-Elander S, Ingvar M (1999) Anticipatory coping of pain expressed in the human anterior cingulate cortex: a positron emission tomography study. Neurosci Lett 262:61–64.

Jewett D (2001) A simple synthesis of [^{11}C]carfentanil. Nucl Med Biol 28:733–734.

Kalin N, Shelton S, Barksdale C (1988) Opiate modulation of separation-induced distress in non-human primates. Brain Res 440:285–292.

Kerns JG, Cohen JD, MacDonald III AW, et al. (2004) Anterior cingulate conflict monitoring and adjustments in control. Science 303:1023–1026.

Kupers RC, Svensson P, Jensen TS (2004) Central representation of muscle pain and mechanical hyperesthesia in the orofacial region: a positron emission tomography study. Pain 108:284–293.

Levine JD, Gordon NC, Jones RT, Fields HL (1978) The narcotic antagonist naloxone enhances clinical pain. Nature 272:826–827.

Levine JD, Gordon NC (1984) Influence of the method of drug administration on analgesic response. Nature 312:755–756.

Logan J, Fowler JS, Volkow ND, et al. (1996) Distribution volume ratios without blood sampling from graphical analysis of PET data. J Cereb Blood Flow Metab 16:834–840.

Lorenz J, Minoshima S, Casey KL (2003) Keeping pain out of mind: the role of the dorsolateral prefrontal cortex in pain modulation. Brain 126:1079–1091.

Mansour A, Fox CA, Akil H, Watson SJ (1995) Opioid-receptor mRNA expression in the rats CNS: anatomical and functional implications. Trends Neurosci 18:22–29.

Matthes HWD, Maldonado R, Simonin F, et al. (1996) Loss of morphine-induced analgesia, reward effect and withdrawal symptoms in mice lacking the μ-opioid-receptor gene. Nature 383:819–823.

Mayberg H, Brannan S, Mahurin RK, et al. (1997) Cingulate function in depression: a potential predictor of treatment response. NeuroReport 8:1057–1061.

McNair D, Lorr M, Droppleman L (1992) EdITS manual for the profile of mood states. San Diego: Educational and Industrial Testing Service (EdITS).

Melzack R, Torgerson W (1971) On the language of pain. Anesthesiology 34:50–59.

Meyer CR, Boes JL, Kim B, et al. (1997) Demonstration of accuracy and clinical versatility of mutual information for automatic multimodality image fusion using affine and thin-plate spline warped geometric deformations. Med Image Anal 1:195–206.

Minoshima S, Koeppe RA, Mintun MA, et al. (1993) Automated detection of the intercommissural line for stereotactic localization of functional brain images. J Nucl Med 34:322–329.

Mogil J, Marek P, O'Toole L, et al. (1994) Mu-opiate receptor binding is up-regulated in mice selectively bred for high stress-induced analgesia. Brain Res 653:16–22.

Moles A, Kieffer BL, D'Amato FR (2004) Deficit in attachment behavior in mice lacking the mu-opioid receptor gene. Science 304:1983–1986.

Nelson EE, Panksepp J (1998) Brain substrates of infant-mother attachment: contributions of opioids, oxytocin, and norepinephrine. Neurosci Biobehav Rev 22:437–452.

Ongur D, An X, Price JL (1998) Prefrontal cortical projections to the hypothalamus in macaque monkeys. J Comp Neurol 401:480–505.

Petrovic P, Kalso E, Petersson KM, Ingvar M (2002) Placebo and opioid analgesia—imaging a shared neuronal network. Science 295:1737–1740.

Peyron R, Laurent B, Garcia-Larrea L (2000) Functional imaging of brain responses to pain. A review and meta-analysis. Neurophysiol Clin 30:263–288.

Phan K, Wager T, Taylor S, Liberzon I (2002) Functional neuroanatomy of emotion: a meta-analysis of emotion activation studies in PET and fMRI. NeuroImage 16:331–348.

Ploghaus A, Tracey I, Gati J, et al. (1999) Dissociating pain from its anticipation in the human brain. Science 284:1979–1981.

Price DD, Milling LS, Kirsch I, et al. (1999) An analysis of factors that contribute to the magnitude of placebo analgesia in an experimental paradigm. Pain 83:147–156.

Pruessner JC, Champagne F, Meaney MJ, Dagher A (2004) Dopamine release in response to a psychological stress in humans and its relationship to early life maternal care: a positron emission tomography study using [^{11}C]raclopride. J Neurosci 24:2825–2831.

Rainville P, Duncan G, Price D, Carrier B, Bushnell M (1997) Pain affect encoded in human anterior cingulate but not somatosensory cortex. Science 277:968–971.

Rubinstein M, Mogil JS, Japon M, et al. (1996) Absence of opioid stress-induced analgesia in mice lacking β-endorphin by site directed mutagenesis. Proc Natl Acad Sci USA 93:3995–4000.

Schatzberg AF, Kraemer HC (2000) Use of placebo control groups in evaluating efficacy of treatment of unipolar major depression. Biol Psychiatry 47:736–744.

Schlaepfer T, Strain E, Greenberg B, et al. (1998) Site of opioid action in the human brain: mu and kappa agonists' subjective and cerebral blood flow effects. Am J Psychiatry 155:470–473.

Shetty N, Friedman JH, Kieburtz K, Marshall FJ, Oakes D (1999) The placebo response in Parkinson's disease. Parkinson Study Group. Clin Neuropharmacol 22:207–212.

Singer T, Seymour B, O'Doherty J, et al. (2004) Empathy for pain involves the affective but not sensory components of pain. Science 303:1157–1162.

Smith Y, Zubieta J, Del Carmen M, et al. (1998) Brain mu-opioid receptor measurements by positron emission tomography in normal cycling women: relationship to LH pulsatility and gonadal steroid hormones. J Clin Endocrinol Metab 83:4498–4505.

Sora I, Takahashi N, Funada M, et al. (1997) Opiate receptor knockout mice define μ receptor roles in endogenous nociceptive responses and morphine-induced analgesia. Proc Natl Acad Sci USA 94:1544–1549.

Steiner H, Gerfen CR (1998) Role of dynorphin and enkephalin in the regulation of striatal output pathways and behavior. Exp Brain Res 123:60–76.

Stohler C, Kowalski C (1999) Spatial and temporal summation of sensory and affective dimensions of deep somatic pain. Pain 79:165–173.

Talbot J, Marrett S, Evans A, et al. (1991) Multiple representations of pain in human cerebral cortex. Science 251:1355–1358.

Tolle T, Kaufmann T, Siessmeier T, et al. (1999) Region-specific encoding of sensory and affective components of pain in the human brain: a positron emission tomography correlation analysis. Ann Neurol 45:40–47.

Unterwald EM (2001) Regulation of opioid receptors by cocaine. Ann NY Acad Sci 937:74–92.

Vogt B, Derbyshire S, Jones A (1996) Pain processing in four regions of human cingulate cortex localized with co-registered PET and MR imaging. Eur J Neurosci 8:1461–1473.

Volkow ND, Fowler JS, Wang GJ, Swanson JM (2004) Dopamine in drug abuse and addiction: results from imaging studies and treatment implications. Mol Psychiatry 9:557–569.

Wager TD, Rilling JK, Smith EE, et al. (2004) Placebo-induced changes in fMRI in the anticipation and experience of pain. Science 303:1162–1167.

Wagner KJ, Willoch F, Kochs EF, et al. (2001) Dose-dependent regional cerebral blood flow changes during remifentanil infusion in humans: a positron emission tomography study. Anesthesiology 94:732–739.

Watkins L, Mayer D (1982) Organization of endogenous opiate and non-opiate pain control systems. Science 216:1185–1192.

Watson D, Clark LA, Tellegen A (1988) Development and validation of brief measures of positive and negative affect: the PANAS scales. J Pers Soc Psychol 54:1063–1070.

Will MJ, Franzblau EB, Kelley AE (2003) Nucleus accumbens μ-opioids regulate intake of a high-fat diet via activation of a distributed brain network. J Neurosci 23:2882–2888.

Willoch F, Rosen G, Tolle T, et al. (2000) Phantom limb pain in the human brain: unraveling neural circuitries of phantom limb sensations using positron emission tomography. Ann Neurol 48:842–849.

Worsley KJ (1994) Local maxima and the expected Euler characteristic of excursion sets of χ^2, F and t fields. Adv Appl Prob 26:13–42.

Zald DH, Boileau I, El-Dearedy W, et al. (2004) Dopamine transmission in the human striatum during monetary reward tasks. J Neurosci 24:4105–4112.

Zhang X, Ashton-Miller JA, Stohler CS (1993) A closed-loop system for maintaining constant experimental muscle pain in man. IEEE Trans Biomed Eng 40:344–352.

Zink CF, Pagnoni G, Martin-Skurski ME, Chappelow JC, Berns GS (2004) Human striatal responses to monetary reward depend on saliency. Neuron 42:509–517.

Zubieta JK, Dannals R, Frost J (1999) Gender and age influences on human brain mu-opioid receptor binding measured by PET. Am J Psychiatry 156:842–848.

Zubieta JK, Smith Y, Bueller J, et al. (2001) Regional mu-opioid receptor regulation of sensory and affective dimensions of pain. Science 293:311–315.

Zubieta JK, Smith Y, Bueller J, et al. (2002) μ-Opioid receptor–mediated antinociception differs in men and women. J Neurosci 22:5100–5107.

Zubieta JK, Heitzeg MM, Smith YR, et al. (2003a) COMT val158met genotype affects mu-opioid neurotransmitter responses to a pain stressor. Science 299:1240–1243.

Zubieta JK, Ketter TA, Bueller JA, et al. (2003b) Regulation of human affective responses by anterior cingulate and limbic mu-opioid neurotransmission. Arch Gen Psychiatry 60:1145–1153.

27

Direct Evidence for Spinal Cord Involvement in Placebo Analgesia

FALK EIPPERT, JÜRGEN FINSTERBUSCH, ULRIKE BINGEL, AND CHRISTIAN BÜCHEL

Falk Eippert, Jürgen Finsterbusch, Ulrike Bingel, and Christian Büchel, "Direct Evidence for Spinal Cord Involvement in Placebo Analgesia," Science 2009;326:404.

Placebo analgesia is a prime example of how psychological factors can influence pain perception (1). It refers to a situation where the administration of an inactive treatment has a pain-relieving effect, presumably because of the participant's belief in the analgesic effectiveness of the treatment. Neurobiologically, placebo analgesia is in many cases opioid-dependent and relies on frontal cortical areas and their projections to downstream effectors in the brainstem (1, 2). One possible mechanism of placebo analgesia is thus that cortical areas recruit the opioidergic descending pain control system in the brainstem (3), which ultimately inhibits nociceptive processing in the dorsal horn of the spinal cord in a gate-control manner (4). Behavioral data support the idea that placebo analgesia can act at the level of the spinal cord (5), but there is no direct evidence that nociceptive responses in the spinal cord are reduced under placebo analgesia. We combined high-resolution functional magnetic resonance imaging (fMRI) of the human cervical spinal cord with a robust placebo analgesia paradigm (6) (fig. S1; see "Supporting Online Material," below—eds.) to test the hypothesis that spinal cord blood oxygen level–dependent (BOLD) responses related to painful heat stimulation are reduced under placebo analgesia.

We first tested for the main effect of painful stimulation and observed the strongest BOLD responses in the dorsal horn ipsilateral to the side of painful stimulation at the expected segmental level (C6, approximately at the junction with C5; $t_{(12)} = 3.51$, $P = 0.002$; Fig. 27.1A). Pain ratings, which were obtained after each stimulus during the fMRI experiment, were significantly lower under the placebo condition as compared with the control condition (placebo rating of 52.3 ± 5.9 [mean $\pm$ SEM], control 71.1 ± 3.1; 26% reduction; $t_{(12)} = 3.56$, $P = 0.002$), indicating that our placebo induction was successful. We next tested whether the observed BOLD response in the ipsilateral dorsal horn (at the peak voxel of the main effect) would be decreased under the placebo condition. A reduction of BOLD responses under placebo compared

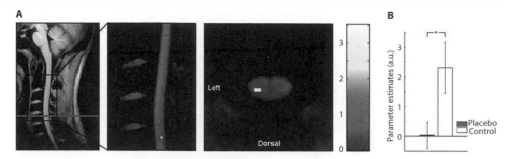

Fig. 27.1. Pain-related BOLD responses and their reduction by placebo. (A) (Left) The average structural image with the black box indicating the sagittal section (middle image) and the thick horizontal line near the bottom of the black box indicating the transverse section (right image). The sagittal and transverse sections show that BOLD responses (main effect of pain; visualization threshold $P < 0.01$ uncorrected) are present in the dorsal part of the spinal cord, ipsilateral to the side of painful stimulation (left). The location corresponds to segment C6. The shaded bar numbered 0 through 3 (at right) indicates t values. (B) Parameter estimates were extracted from the peak voxel for the main effect of pain in the ipsilateral spinal cord. The parameter estimates show that the BOLD response is significantly reduced under placebo (gray bar) in comparison with control (white bar). Error bars indicate standard error; $^*P \leq 0.05$.

with control was evident ($t_{(12)} = 1.81$, $P = 0.046$; Fig. 27.1B and fig. S2). To further demonstrate the spatial specificity of our approach, we also tested for motor responses in a reaction time task (middle finger button presses (6)) and found these to be localized more inferiorly and anteriorly (segments C7 and C8; fig. S3), consistent with the functional neuroanatomy of the sensory-motor system.

Our data provide direct evidence that psychological factors can influence nociceptive processing at the earliest stage of the central nervous system, namely, the dorsal horn of the spinal cord. They also reveal that one mechanism of placebo analgesia is inhibition of spinal cord nociceptive processing, possibly mediated by the descending pain control system (3) in a gate-control manner (4). It is likely that the decreased BOLD responses we observed are caused by endogenous opioids because opioid antagonists block placebo analgesia (1) and because recent fMRI data from rat spinal cord showed morphine depression of dorsal horn BOLD responses (7). However, our study cannot reveal the exact mechanism of spinal inhibition (i.e., effects on primary afferents [presynaptic], interneurons, or projection neurons [postsynaptic]) and whether the observed effect is specific for nociception, because we did not measure responses to innocuous stimuli. Nevertheless, the demonstration that modulatory influences on nociceptive spinal cord activity are measurable by fMRI in humans opens up new avenues for assessing the efficacy and possible site of action of new treatments for various forms of pain, including chronic pain.

REFERENCES AND NOTES

1. F. Benedetti, H. S. Mayberg, T. D. Wager, C. S. Stohler, J. K. Zubieta, J. Neurosci. **25**, 10390 (2005).
2. P. Petrovic, E. Kalso, K. M. Petersson, M. Ingvar, Science **295**, 1737 (2002).
3. H. L. Fields, A. I. Basbaum, M. M. Heinricher, in Wall and Melzack's Textbook of Pain, S. B. McMahon, M. Koltzenburg, Eds. (Elsevier, London, 2006), pp. 125–152.
4. R. Melzack, P. D. Wall, Science **150**, 971 (1965).
5. D. Matre, K. L. Casey, S. Knardahl, J. Neurosci. **26**, 559 (2006).
6. Materials and methods are available as supporting material on Science Online.
7. J. Lilja et al., J. Neurosci. **26**, 6330 (2006).

Supporting Online Material

www.sciencemag.org/cgi/content/full/326/5951/404/DC1
Materials and Methods
Figs. S1 to S3
References

28

The Biochemical and Neuroendocrine Bases of the Hyperalgesic Nocebo Effect

Fabrizio Benedetti, Martina Amanzio, Sergio Vighetti, and Giovanni Asteggiano

Fabrizio Benedetti, Martina Amanzio, Sergio Vighetti, and Giovanni Asteggiano, "The Biochemical and Neuroendocrine Bases of the Hyperalgesic Nocebo Effect," Journal of Neuroscience 2006;26:12014–12022.

Introduction

In recent times, the placebo effect has been analyzed with sophisticated neurobiological tools that have uncovered specific mechanisms at the biochemical, cellular, and anatomical level in different systems and conditions, such as pain, motor disorders, depression, and immune–endocrine responses (Benedetti et al., 2005; Colloca and Benedetti, 2005). It has been shown that this may occur through both expectation and conditioning mechanisms, although expectations and emotions seem to play a fundamental role (Benedetti et al., 2003; Price et al., 2005). Most of our knowledge about the placebo effect comes from the field of pain, in which both a neuropharmacological approach with opioid antagonists (Levine et al., 1978; Grevert et al., 1983; Levine and Gordon, 1984; Amanzio and Benedetti, 1999; Benedetti et al., 1999; Hoffman et al., 2005) and, more recently, brain imaging techniques (Petrovic et al., 2002, 2005; Wager et al.,

Table 28.1.
Characteristics (mean ± SD) of the subjects of each experimental group

	Sex (M/F)	Age (years)	Weight (kg)	Basal ACTH (pg/ml)	Basal cortisol (μg/L)	STAI-S	STAI-T
Group 1	6/6	37.4±12.4	63.1±11.5	22.7±3.4	106.4±8.7	40.6±4.3	41.1±5.9
Group 2	6/7	36.9±13.8	62.7±13.5	20.5±4.4	106.5±8.9	41.5±5.2	40.1±4.7
Group 3	6/6	39.1±13.3	64.0±13.1	19.4±3.4	103.8±7.8	41.6±6.2	39.2±4.7
Group 4	5/7	37.1±11.9	66.1±14.6	20.4±3.7	104.8±8.3	40.7±5.5	40.6±5.3

Note: M, male; F, female; [ACTH, adrenocorticotropic hormone; STAI-S, State–Trait Anxiety Inventory-State; STAI-T, State–Trait Anxiety Inventory-Trait—eds.].

2004, 2006; Zubieta et al., 2005; Keltner et al., 2006; Kong et al., 2006) have been used.

In contrast, the neurobiological mechanisms of the nocebo effect have been less investigated, despite them being interesting as those of the placebo effect. For example, hyperalgesia after expectation of painful stimulation is associated with changes in brain activation of different regions (Sawamoto et al., 2000; Koyama et al., 2005; Keltner et al., 2006). Expectation and/or conditioning mechanisms, which are similar and opposite to those of the placebo counterpart, are supposed to be involved (Benedetti et al., 2003). In a previous clinical study, we showed that nocebo hyperalgesia could be prevented by pretreatment with proglumide, a nonspecific cholecystokinin (CCK) antagonist for both CCK-A and CCK-B receptors, suggesting the possible involvement of CCKergic systems in the nocebo effect (Benedetti et al., 1997). However, because of ethical constraints in these patients, we did not have the possibility to investigate these effects further.

By using selective CCK-A and CCK-B receptor antagonists, several studies in animals and humans have shown the important role of CCKergic systems in the modulation of anxiety and in the link between anxiety and hyperalgesia (Hebb et al., 2005). For example, in a social-defeat model of anxiety in rats, it has been shown recently that CI-988 (4-[[2-[[3 -(1H-indol-3-yl) -2-methyl-1-oxo-2[[(tricyclo[3.3[12,17]dec-2-yloxy)-carbonyl] amino]-propyl]amino]-1-phenyethyl]amino]-4-oxo-[R-(R*, R*)]-butanoate N-methyl-D-glucamine), a selective CCK-B receptor antagonist, prevented anxiety-induced hyperalgesia, with an effect that was similar to that produced by the established anxiolytic chlordiazepoxide (Andre et al., 2005).

By taking all of these considerations into account and by considering the ethical limitations in the patients of our previous study (Benedetti et al., 1997), we performed a detailed neuropharmacological analysis of the hyperalgesic nocebo effect in healthy volunteers by using the nonselective CCK-A and CCK-B receptor antagonist proglumide. We decided to start this pharmacological investigation of nocebo hyperalgesia because the neuropharmacological approach in humans has represented a crucial step to unravel the opioid mechanisms of placebo analgesia (Levine et al., 1978; Grevert et al., 1983; Levine and Gordon, 1984; Amanzio and Benedetti, 1999; Benedetti et al., 1999), which have subsequently been confirmed by brain imaging and *in vivo* receptor binding techniques (Petrovic et al., 2002; Zubieta et al., 2005).

Materials and Methods

Subjects

A total of 49 healthy volunteers participated in the study after they signed a written informed consent form in which the experimental procedure and the use of the different drugs were described in detail. Each subject underwent a complete clinical examination to rule out main diseases. To avoid high variability in hormonal responses, we adopted the following criteria. The subjects were tested with the State–Trait Anxiety Inventory (STAI) to rule out both trait and state anxiety. In the Italian population, the normal STAI-S range is 45.2 ± 12.37 for adult women and 40.17 ± 10.01 for men, whereas the STAI-T normal range is 46.1 ± 11.53 for women and 39.53 ± 9.25 for men (Spielberg et al., 1980; Nattero et al., 1989). In our routine clinical experience, these values correspond to a range of ~32–52 for the STAI-S and ~30–55 for the STAI-T. Therefore, only subjects within these ranges were included in the study.

In addition, we decided to include only those subjects within a predetermined range of hormonal plasma concentrations. In the normal population, the range of adrenocorticotropic hormone (ACTH) plasma concentration in the morning is ~10–40 pg/ml, whereas the range of cortisol concentration is ~80–300 μg/L (Liddle, 1974). To make the subjects as similar as possible, we included only those subjects who showed ACTH plasma concentration between 14 and 30 pg/ml and cortisol concentration between 90 and 130 μg/L.

All of the experimental procedures were conducted in conformance with the policies and principles contained in the Declaration of Helsinki. The 49 subjects were randomly subdivided into four groups, whose characteristics are shown in Table 28.1.

Pain Induction

Pain was induced experimentally by means of the tourniquet technique, according to the procedures described by Amanzio and Benedetti (1999). Briefly, the subject reclined on a bed, his or her non-dominant forearm was extended vertically, and venous blood was drained by means of an Esmarch bandage. A sphygmomanometer was placed around the upper arm and inflated to a pressure of 300 mmHg. The Esmarch bandage was maintained around the forearm, which was lowered on the subject's side. After this, the subject started squeezing a hand spring exerciser twelve times while his or her arm rested on the bed. Each squeeze was timed to last 2 s, followed by a 2 s rest. The force necessary to bring the handles together was 7.2 kg. This type of ischemic pain increases over time very quickly, and the pain becomes unbearable after ~14 min (Amanzio and Benedetti, 1999). The tourniquet test lasted 10 min in all subjects, who had to rate their pain intensity every minute according to a numerical rating scale, ranging from 0 (no pain) to 10 (unbearable pain).

Drugs

Diazepam (Valium; Roche, Indianapolis, IN) was given intravenously 30 min before the beginning of the tourniquet at a dose of 0.28 mg/kg, with an infusion rate of 0.028 mg · kg^{-1} · min^{-1} and a total infusion time of 10 min. Likewise, proglumide (Milid; Rottapharm, Milan, Italy) was administered intravenously 30 min before the tourniquet at a dose of 1.5 mg/kg, with an infusion time of 0.15 mg · kg^{-1} · min^{-1} and a total infusion time of 10 min. As shown in Figure 28.1A, proglumide is a glutamic acid-based CCK antagonist and is a nonselective antagonist that binds to both CCK-A and CCK-B receptors, or CCK-1 and CCK-2 according to the new classification (Noble et al., 1999). Note that the binding affinity, expressed as the concentration required to inhibit by 50% the specific binding of ^{125}I-Bolton-Hunter CCK-8 (IC_{50}), is similar for CCK-A and CCK-B receptors, although it is a little bit higher for CCK-A receptors (Benedetti, 1997). The time interval from the sphygmomanometer cuff inflation (which lasted ~10 s) to the last squeeze was 50 s, for a total of 1 min of inflation plus squeezing. Thus, the time interval from the end of drug administration to the last squeeze during the tourniquet was the same in all subjects (31 min). By considering that the tourniquet lasted 10 min in all subjects, the time interval from the end of drug administration to the end of the tourniquet was 41 min.

Experimental Design

The experiments were always performed at 9:00 a.m. to avoid variability in the basal activity of the hypothalamic–pituitary–adrenal (HPA) axis, according to a randomized double-blind design in which neither the subject nor the experimenter knew what drug was being administered. To do this, either the active drug or saline solution was given. To avoid a large number of subjects, two or three additional subjects per group received an infusion of saline in place of the active drug 30 min before the tourniquet. These subjects were not included in the study because they were used only to allow the double-blind design, as described previously by Benedetti et al. (2003).

The complete experimental procedure is shown in Figure 28.1B. Group 1 (no-treatment or natural history group; n = 12) was tested twice (with an interval of 4 d) with the tourniquet without receiving any treatment. Likewise, group 2 (n = 13) was tested twice, with an intertest interval of 4 d. In the first test, these subjects did not receive any treatment, whereas in the second test, they underwent a nocebo procedure. This

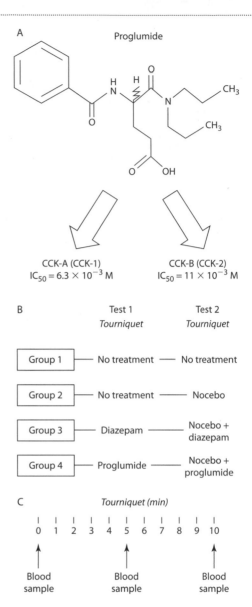

Figure 28.1. **A**, Proglumide is a nonselective CCK antagonist that binds to both CCK-A (or CCK-1) and CCK-B (or CCK-2) receptors. Note the similar binding affinity, expressed as the concentration required to inhibit by 50% the specific binding of ^{125}I-Bolton-Hunter CCK-8 (IC_{50}), for CCK-A and CCK-B receptors. **B**, Experimental design used in the present study. Each group was tested twice with tourniquet, and the interval between tests 1 and 2 was 4 d. **C**, Each tourniquet test lasted 10 min, and the subjects had to rate their pain every minute while a blood sample was taken just before and at 5 and 10 min during the tourniquet.

consisted in the oral administration of an inert talc pill 5 min before the tourniquet, along with the verbal suggestions that it was a powerful vasoconstrictor further increasing the tourniquet-induced ischemia. The subjects were further told that, because of the quick vasoconstriction, this would induce a faster and larger increase of pain intensity, so that a quite strong hyperalgesic effect should be expected. To further strengthen the nocebo verbal suggestions, the subjects were told that they could give up at any time. Therefore, this experimental paradigm represents a situation in which a stressor is anticipated. Group 3 ($n = 12$) was tested twice (intertest interval of 4 d), like group 2, but these subjects received a pretreatment with diazepam 30 min before the tourniquet. Similarly, group 4 ($n = 12$) was tested with the tourniquet, like groups 2 and 3, but 30 min after a pretreatment with proglumide.

ACTH and Cortisol Plasma Concentration

Plasma concentrations of ACTH and cortisol were assessed before the tourniquet and at 5 and 10 min during the tourniquet test (Fig. 28.1C), according to standard clinical practice and as described previously (Rainero et al., 2001; Benedetti et al., 2003). Briefly, blood samples were collected just before and at 5 and 10 min of the tourniquet in sterile tubes and immediately centrifuged at 4°C, and the plasma was stored at −80°C until assayed. Plasma ACTH and cortisol concentrations were measured using a commercially available kit [ACTH Allegro (Nichols Institute, San Juan Capistrano, CA); CORT-CTK-125 (Sorin, Saluggia, Italy)]. The sensitivity of ACTH was 1 pg/ml, and the intra-assay and interassay coefficient of variation were 3 and 7.8%. The sensitivity of cortisol was 5 μg/L, and the intra-assay and interassay coefficients of variation were 3.8 and 5.7%. All of the samples from each subject were analyzed in the same assay.

Statistical Analysis

Because the experimental design involves both a between- and a within-subjects design, statistical analysis was performed by means of one-way analysis of variance (ANOVA) and ANOVA for repeated measures, followed by the *post hoc* Newman-Keuls test for multiple comparisons and Dunnett's test for comparisons between a control group and different experimental groups. In addition, correlations were performed by using linear regression analysis. Data are presented as mean ± SD, and the level of significance is $p < 0.05$.

Results

As shown in Table 28.1, no difference was present in the four different groups for sex, age, weight, and basal plasma concentrations of ACTH and cortisol. In addition, STAI scores for both state and trait anxiety did not differ among the groups.

The induction of ischemic pain in the no-treatment group (group 1) produced a type of pain that increased over time (Fig. 28.2A), along with increases in plasma concentrations of both ACTH and cortisol (Fig. 28.2B,C, respectively). It is important to note that no difference was found between the first (black circles or squares) and second (white circles or squares) tests for all of these outcome measures (pain intensity, ACTH and cortisol). Therefore, our experimental conditions were stable in the two tests, because the repetition of the experimental pain and hormonal assessment after 4 d did not produce different results.

In group 2, the nocebo suggestions delivered on the second test (white circles or squares) induced both a significant

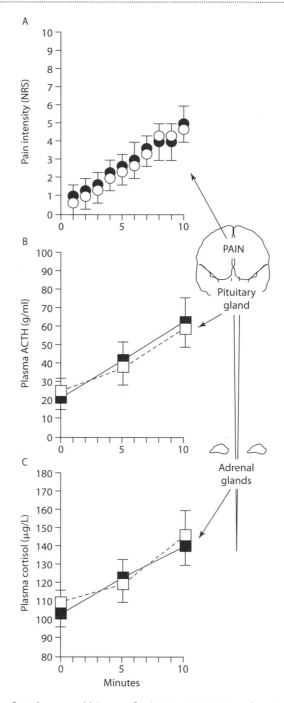

Figure 28.2. The natural history of pain (**A**), ACTH (**B**), and cortisol (**C**) in test 1 (black symbols) is compared with the natural history of test 2 (white symbols). Note that no difference was present between tests 1 and 2, indicating stable conditions of our experimental setup.

increase of subjective pain rating (Fig. 28.3A) and hyperactivity of the HPA axis, as shown by the increased plasma concentrations of ACTH and cortisol (Fig. 28.3B,C). Pain intensity increased in both the first (black circles) and second (white circles) tests ($F_{(19,228)} = 133.855$; $p < 0.001$), but the nocebo condition in the second test always induced higher pain scores compared with the first test, as assessed by the *post hoc* Newman-Keuls test for multiple comparisons (Fig. 28.3A).

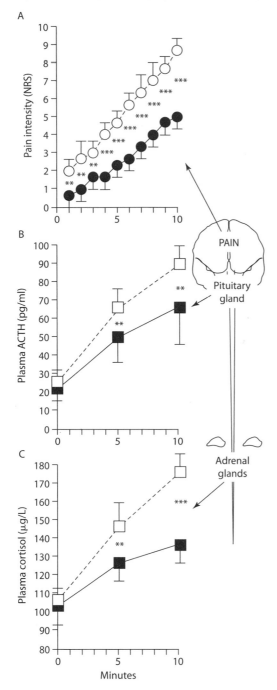

Figure 28.3. The natural history of pain (**A**), ACTH (**B**), and cortisol (**C**) in test 1 (black symbols) is compared with the nocebo condition of test 2 (white symbols), in which verbal suggestions of pain worsening were given. Note that, in the nocebo condition, there was a significant increase of both pain perception and ACTH and cortisol plasma concentrations. ** $p < 0.01$; *** $p < 0.001$.

In fact, at the end of the 10 min test, pain rating was 5.07 ± 0.95 in the non-nocebo condition and 8.61 ± 0.96 in the nocebo condition ($q_{(228)} = 18.304$; $p < 0.001$). Likewise, ACTH and cortisol increases occurred in both the first and second tests ($F_{(5,60)} = 135.113$, $p < 0.001$ for ACTH; $F_{(5,60)} = 141.248$, $p < 0.001$ for cortisol), but they were significantly larger in the no-

cebo condition (white squares) than in the first test (black squares), as assessed by means of the *post hoc* Newman-Keuls test (Fig. 28.3B,C). In fact, at the end of the 10 min test, ACTH plasma concentration was 66.46 ± 16.88 pg/ml in the non-nocebo condition and 86.69 ± 8.45 pg/ml in the nocebo condition ($q_{(60)} = 8.960$; $p < 0.01$), and cortisol was 138.2 ± 8.38 and 174.2 ± 12.46 μg/L, respectively ($q_{(60)} = 16.671$; $p < 0.001$).

The administration of diazepam blocked both the nocebo-induced hyperalgesia (Fig. 28.4A) and the nocebo-induced hyperactivity of the HPA axis (Fig. 28.4B,C). In fact, no difference was found between the first and the second tests, for both pain scores and hormone plasma concentrations. In contrast, proglumide only blocked the nocebo-induced hyperalgesia (Fig. 28.5A), but it was ineffective in reducing the nocebo-induced hyperactivity of the HPA axis (Fig. 28.5B,C). The plasma concentrations of both ACTH and cortisol increased in the two tests ($F_{(5,55)} = 204.083$, $p < 0.001$ for ACTH; $F_{(5,55)} = 147.952$, $p < 0.001$ for cortisol), and the *post hoc* Newman-Keuls test showed a significantly higher hormone increase in the nocebo condition. In fact, at the end of the 10 min test, ACTH plasma concentration was 68.33 ± 12.36 pg/ml in the non-nocebo condition and 87.5 ± 6.26 pg/ml in the nocebo condition ($q_{(55)} = 10.302$; $p < 0.001$), and cortisol was 140.9 ± 8.55 and 174.1 ± 14.48 μg/L, respectively ($q_{(55)} = 15.262$; $p < 0.001$).

An intergroup one-way ANOVA showed that neither diazepam nor proglumide had an analgesic effect in non-nocebo conditions. In fact, there was no significant difference in pain time course between diazepam in the non-nocebo condition (Fig. 28.4A, black circles) and the natural history of group 1 (Fig. 28.2A). Likewise, there was no difference in the time course of pain intensity between proglumide in the non-nocebo condition (Fig. 28.5A, black circles) and the natural history of group 1 (Fig. 28.2A). In contrast, a significant decrease of pain occurred in the nocebo condition with both diazepam and proglumide compared with the drug-free nocebo condition of Figure 28.3A (white circles). In fact, at the end of the 10 min test, pain rating was 5.16 ± 0.57 with diazepam and 5.58 ± 0.9 with proglumide compared with 8.61 ± 0.96 in the drug-free condition of group 2 ($F_{(1,23)} = 116.6$, $p < 0.001$; $F_{(1,23)} = 66.07$, $p < 0.001$, respectively). Therefore, whereas both diazepam and proglumide were ineffective as analgesics on basal pain, they proved to be effective in reducing the nocebo hyperalgesic component. In other words, both drugs affected only the nocebo component of pain.

The intergroup analysis of the hormonal responses produced similar results for diazepam but not for proglumide. In fact, there was no significant difference in ACTH–cortisol time course between diazepam in the non-nocebo condition (Fig. 28.4B,C, black squares) and the natural history of group 1 (Fig. 28.2B,C). In contrast, a significant decrease of both ACTH and cortisol plasma concentrations occurred in the nocebo condition with diazepam compared with the drug-free nocebo condition of Figure 28.3B,C (white squares). In fact, at the end of the 10 min test, ACTH plasma concentra-

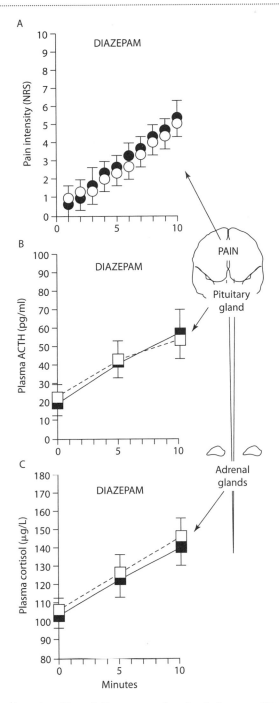

Figure 28.4. The effect of diazepam on basal pain increase (**A**), basal ACTH increase (**B**), and basal cortisol increase (**C**) in test 1 (black symbols) is compared with diazepam in the nocebo condition of test 2 (white symbols). Note that diazepam suppressed both nocebo hyperalgesia and nocebo increase of ACTH and cortisol plasma concentrations. In fact, no difference was present between tests 1 and 2.

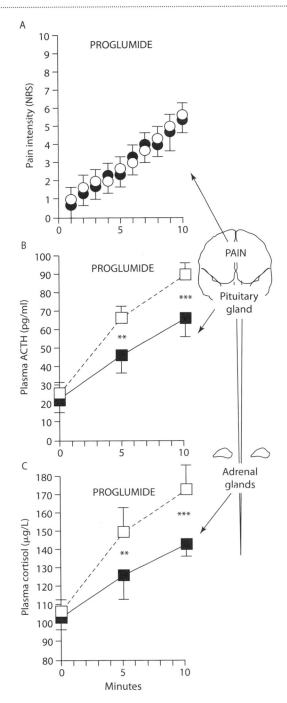

Figure 28.5. The effect of proglumide on basal pain increase (**A**), basal ACTH increase (**B**), and basal cortisol increase (**C**) in test 1 (black symbols) is compared with proglumide in the nocebo condition of test 2 (white symbols). Note that, whereas proglumide suppressed nocebo hyperalgesia, it was ineffective in suppressing the nocebo increase of ACTH and cortisol plasma concentrations. ** $p < 0.01$; *** $p < 0.001$.

tion was 54.75 ± 10.01 pg/ml with diazepam compared with 86.69 ± 8.45 pg/ml in the drug-free condition of group 2 ($F_{(1,23)} = 74.74$; $p < 0.001$), and cortisol concentration was $142 \pm 8.31\,\mu g/L$ compared with $174.2 \pm 12.46\,\mu g/L$ in group 2 ($F_{(1,23)} = 56.74$; $p < 0.001$). In contrast to the hormonal effects of diazepam, proglumide induced no effects on ACTH and

cortisol, in neither the non-nocebo nor nocebo condition, as shown by no significant differences in the intergroup analysis between groups 1, 2, and 4.

Finally, a correlation analysis between pain ratings and hormone plasma concentrations did not show any significant effect in the non-nocebo and the nocebo conditions.

Discussion

Most placebo research in recent times has focused on placebo effects in pain and Parkinson's disease. In the first case, there are now several converging lines of evidence indicating that placebo-induced expectations of analgesia activate the endogenous opioid systems in some circumstances (Benedetti et al., 2005; Colloca and Benedetti, 2005; Hoffman et al., 2005; Zubieta et al., 2005). In the second case, dopamine release in the striatum seems to play an important role (de la Fuente-Fernández et al., 2001), and the placebo response in Parkinson patients is associated with neuronal changes in the subthalamic nucleus (Benedetti et al., 2004).

In contrast, the study of the nocebo effect has not been carefully investigated, although some attempts to analyze its underlying neurobiological mechanisms have been performed (Benedetti et al., 1997, 2003; Johansen et al., 2003). For example, we tried to assess the role of CCK in nocebo hyperalgesia in postoperative patients by using a neuropharmacological approach with the CCK antagonist proglumide (Benedetti et al., 1997). Although in our previous study we showed a blockade of nocebo hyperalgesia by proglumide, the clinical experimental setting presented many ethical limitations. Therefore, in the present study, we addressed several unanswered questions of the study by Benedetti et al. (1997) by performing a careful analysis of the effects of proglumide on both pain and HPA axis in different nocebo and non-nocebo conditions and, moreover, by comparing the effects of proglumide with those of diazepam, a widely known anti-anxiety drug.

First of all, some methodological considerations and some limitations of the present study are worthy of discussion. We studied ACTH and cortisol because several studies have shown that the plasma concentrations of these hormones are sensitive to a number of stressors (Dickerson and Kemeny, 2004), including experimental ischemic arm pain (Gullner et al., 1982; Johansen et al., 2003). In particular, a short-latency response of cortisol has been shown in ischemic pain (Johansen et al., 2003), thus making our 10-min-long experimental pain a good model for HPA analysis. We used a neuropharmacological approach in humans with a nonspecific CCK antagonist for at least two reasons. First, the neuropharmacological approach to placebo analgesia with the opioid antagonist naloxone has been crucial to the understanding of the neurobiology of the placebo analgesic effect (Levine et al., 1978; Grevert et al., 1983; Levine and Gordon, 1984; Benedetti, 1996; Amanzio and Benedetti, 1999; Benedetti et al., 1999). In fact, these early pharmacological studies have been confirmed recently by several brain imaging studies, which basically show a similarity between narcotics and placebos in the activation of different brain regions (Petrovic et al., 2002) and the *in vivo* activation of the μ-opioid receptors following a placebo procedure (Zubieta et al., 2005). Therefore, the neuropharmacological study of placebo/nocebo phenomena with agonist and antagonist drugs in humans appears to be a reliable experimental approach that gives important information. The second reason why we decided to use the pharmacological approach with proglumide is that we were not so much interested in the involvement of specific CCK receptors but rather in studying CCK from a general point of view. In this sense, proglumide has proven to be useful in investigating placebo analgesia (Benedetti et al., 1995; Benedetti, 1996; Colloca and Benedetti, 2005).

Although proglumide is a weak CCK antagonist, its anti-CCK action in the brain has been demonstrated. There is behavioral and electrophysiological evidence that CCK is blocked by proglumide in the brain (Chiodo and Bunney, 1983; Suberg et al., 1985; Watkins et al., 1985a,b). The results obtained in humans on opioid potentiation by proglumide (Price et al., 1985; Lavigne et al., 1989; Benedetti et al., 1995; Benedetti, 1996) are in keeping with the potentiation of morphine analgesia by the CCK-A antagonist devazepide in the rat (Dourish et al., 1988) and with the results obtained in animal studies using CCK-B antagonists (Wiesenfeld-Hallin et al., 1990; Maldonado et al., 1993; Noble et al., 1993; Valverde et al., 1994; Xu et al., 1994; Andre et al., 2005). Proglumide has also been reported to block the anxiogenic effects of the tetrapeptide CCK-4 and caerulein, a CCK-8 agonist, indicating an anti-CCK action in the CNS at the level of affective mechanisms (Harro et al., 1990; Harro and Vasar, 1991; Van Megen et al., 1994).

By taking into consideration the limitations discussed above, the present study suggests that the nocebo hyperalgesic counterpart of the placebo/nocebo phenomenon is mediated by CCK. In particular, it suggests that the CCK antagonist proglumide does not act on the nocebo-induced anxiety but rather on anxiety-induced hyperalgesia. In fact, whereas diazepam reduced both HPA activation and pain perception, proglumide affected pain but not the HPA axis. The most plausible explanation of our findings is shown in Figure 28.6. The reduction of both pain and HPA hyperactivity by diazepam can be explained by its anxiolytic effect, thus affecting nocebo-induced anxiety. It should be noted, however, that nonspecific effects of diazepam, e.g., on arousal, cannot be ruled out completely. In this regard, it will be interesting to use measures of anxiety in future studies. In contrast, proglumide was likely to affect only the CCK-mediated link between anxiety and pain. Although we did not test naloxone in the present study, the involvement of endogenous opioids in the blockade of nocebo hyperalgesia seems to be unlikely, as shown by the ineffectiveness of naloxone in our previous study (Benedetti et al., 1997). This CCK link between anxiety and pain is in agreement with studies in rodents in which more selective CCK antagonists were used. For example, a recent study showed that CI-988, a specific CCK-B receptor antagonist, blocked anxiety-induced hyperalgesia, which indicates a biochemical link between anxiety and pain that is mediated by CCK-B receptors (Andre et al., 2005).

In recent years, there has been accumulating evidence that CCK acts as a neuromodulator of different functions,

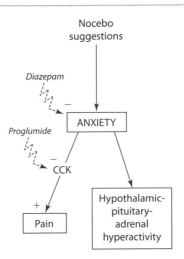

Figure 28.6. Model to explain the findings of the present study. Nocebo-induced anxiety affects both the HPA axis and pain mechanisms. The link between anxiety and pain is represented by CCK, which has a facilitating effect on pain. Benzodiazepines, like diazepam, can block anxiety, thus preventing both HPA hyperactivity and hyperalgesia. CCK antagonists, such as proglumide, only block the CCKergic anxiety–pain link. Therefore, CCK antagonists do not inhibit pain per se but rather the anxiety–pain link.

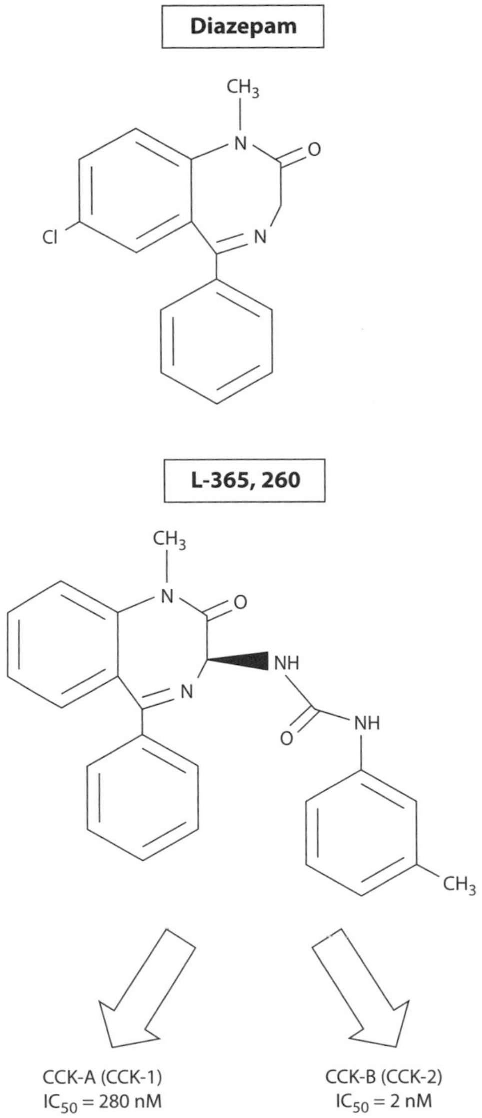

such as pain and anxiety, although the exact mechanisms are still unclear. CCK is found in the brain as an octapeptide (CCK-8) and has many functions, ranging from pain modulation to anxiety (Vanderhaegen et al., 1975; Beinfeld, 1983; Baber et al., 1989; Crawley and Corwin, 1994; Hebb et al., 2005). The distribution of CCK in the brain matches that of the opioid peptides at both the spinal and supraspinal level (Stengaard-Pedersen and Larsson, 1981; Gall et al., 1987; Gibbins et al., 1987), suggesting a close interaction between the two neuropeptides.

The involvement of CCK in both pain modulation and anxiety is particularly relevant to the present study. Interestingly, it is worth noting that some CCK-B receptor antagonists, such as L-365,260 [3S(—)[N'-2,3-dehydro-1-methyl-2-oxo-5-phenyl-1 H-1,4-benzodiazepin-3-yl]-1 H-indole-2-carboxamide], have a benzodiazepine-based chemical structure that is similar to the anxiolytic drug diazepam (Fig. 28.7), thus suggesting a similarity of action of CCK antagonists and benzodiazepines. In this regard, the recent work by Andre et al. (2005) in the rat shows that CCK-B receptor blockade antagonizes anxiety-induced hyperalgesia. This suggests a CCKergic link between anxiety and hyperalgesia, whereby anxiety-activated CCK has a facilitating action on pain. Our present study confirms these effects in humans and suggests that our nocebo procedure induced anticipatory anxiety about the impending pain.

It should also be stressed that the anti-CCK action of proglumide did not show any real analgesic effect, because the basal pain increase of the natural history group was unaffected. In other words, proglumide was effective only on the nocebo component of pain, that is, only on the anxiety-

Diazepam

L-365, 260

CCK-A (CCK-1)
$IC_{50} = 280$ nM

CCK-B (CCK-2)
$IC_{50} = 2$ nM

Figure 28.7. The structural formula of the anxiolytic drug diazepam, one of the most used benzodiazepines, is similar to L-365,260, a benzodiazepine-based CCK antagonist, thus suggesting similar mechanisms of action of benzodiazepines and CCK antagonists. Note the higher binding affinity of L-365,260 for CCK-B receptors compared with CCK-A receptors, expressed as the concentration required to inhibit by 50% the specific binding of ^{125}I-Bolton-Hunter CCK-8 (IC_{50}).

induced hyperalgesia. Therefore, CCK antagonists appear to be useful not so much as analgesics but rather as drugs suppressing the hyperalgesia induced by anxiety. Interestingly, the suppressing action of proglumide on nocebo (anxiety)-induced hyperalgesia was similar to that of diazepam, which further confirms the specific action of both benzodiazepines and CCK antagonists on anxiety-related pain.

The discrepancy between stress-induced hyperalgesia and stress-induced analgesia may be only apparent, because the nature of the stressor is likely to play a central role. In fact, whereas hyperalgesia may occur when the anticipatory anxiety is about the pain itself (Benedetti et al., 1997; Sawamoto et al., 2000; Koyama et al., 2005; Keltner et al., 2006), analgesia may occur when anxiety is about a stressor that shifts the attention from the pain (Willer and Albe-Fessard, 1980; Terman et al., 1986). The present study further suggests that there are two different pathways for anxiety-induced HPA hyperactivity and hyperalgesia (Fig. 28.6).

In conclusion, the hyperalgesic nocebo effect appears to be attributable to complex biochemical and neuroendocrine mechanisms that link anxiety to pain. On the one hand, nocebo suggestions induce anticipatory anxiety and thus the hyperactivity of the HPA axis. On the other hand, the nocebo-induced anxiety seems to activate CCKergic systems, which, in turn, facilitate pain transmission. Therefore, the placebo/nocebo phenomenon, with its opposite modulating effects on pain, is a very interesting model to understand the reciprocal and antagonist action of the opioidergic and CCKergic systems that are involved in the intricate mechanisms linking cognition and emotions to pain.

REFERENCES

Amanzio M, Benedetti F (1999) Neuropharmacological dissection of placebo analgesia: expectation-activated opioid systems versus conditioning-activated specific sub-systems. J Neurosci 19:484–494.

Andre J, Zeau B, Pohl M, et al. (2005) Involvement of cholecystokininergic systems in anxiety-induced hyperalgesia in male rats: behavioral and biochemical studies. J Neurosci 25:7896–7904.

Baber NS, Dourish CT, Hill DR (1989) The role of CCK, caerulein, and CCK antagonists in nociception. Pain 39:307–328.

Beinfeld MC (1983) Cholecystokinin in the central nervous system: a mini-review. Neuropeptides 3:411–427.

Benedetti F (1996) The opposite effects of the opiate antagonist naloxone and the cholecystokinin antagonist proglumide on placebo analgesia. Pain 64:535–543.

Benedetti F (1997) Cholecystokinin type A and type B receptors and their modulation of opioid analgesia. Physiol 12:263–268.

Benedetti F, Amanzio M, Maggi G (1995) Potentiation of placebo analgesia by proglumide. Lancet 346:1231.

Benedetti F, Amanzio M, Casadio C, Oliaro A, Maggi G (1997) Blockade of nocebo hyperalgesia by the cholecystokinin antagonist proglumide. Pain 71:135–140.

Benedetti F, Arduino C, Amanzio M (1999) Somatotopic activation of opioid systems by target-directed expectations of analgesia. J Neurosci 19:3639–3648.

Benedetti F, Pollo A, Lopiano L, et al. (2003) Conscious expectation and unconscious conditioning in analgesic; motor and hormonal placebo/nocebo responses. J Neurosci 23:4315–4323.

Benedetti F, Colloca L, Torre E, et al. (2004) Placebo-responsive Parkinson patients show decreased activity in single neurons of subthalamic nucleus. Nat Neurosci 7:587–588.

Benedetti F, Mayberg HS, Wager TD, Stohler CS, Zubieta JK (2005) Neurobiological mechanisms of the placebo effect. J Neurosci 25:10390–10402.

Chiodo LA, Bunney BS (1983) Proglumide: selective antagonism of excitatory effects of cholecystokinin in central nervous system. Science 219:1449–1451.

Colloca L, Benedetti F (2005) Placebos and painkillers: is mind as real as matter? Nat Rev Neurosci 6:545–552.

Crawley JN, Corwin RL (1994) Biological actions of cholecystokinin. Peptides 15:731–755.

de la Fuente-Fernández R, Ruth TJ, Sossi V, et al. (2001) Expectation and dopamine release: mechanism of the placebo effect in Parkinson's disease. Science 293:1164–1166.

Dickerson SS, Kemeny MME (2004) Acute stressors and cortisol responses: a theoretical integration and synthesis of laboratory research. Psychol Bull 130:355–391.

Dourish CT, Hawley D, Iversen SD (1988) Enhancement of morphine analgesia and prevention of morphine tolerance in the rat by the cholecystokinin antagonist L-364,718. Eur J Pharmacol 147:469–472.

Gall C, Lauterborn J, Burks D, Seroogy K (1987) Co-localization of enkephalin and cholecystokinin in discrete areas of the rat brain. Brain Res 403:403–408.

Gibbins IL, Furness JB, Costa M (1987) Pathway-specific patterns of coexistence of substance P, calcitonin gene-related peptide, cholecystokinin and dynorphin in neurons of the dorsal root ganglia of the guinea pig. Cell Tissue Res 248:417–437.

Grevert P, Albert LH, Goldstein A (1983) Partial antagonism of placebo analgesia by naloxone. Pain 16:129–143.

Gullner H-G, Nicholson WE, Wilson MG, Bartter FC, Orth DN (1982) The response of plasma immunoreactive adrenocorticotropin, beta-endorphin/beta-lipotropin, gamma-lipotropin and cortisol to experimentally induced pain in normal human subjects. Clin Sci 63:397–400.

Harro J, Vasar E (1991) Evidence that CCK-B receptors mediate the regulation of exploratory behaviour in the rat. Eur J Pharmacol 193:379–381.

Harro J, Pold M, Vasar E (1990) Anxiogenic-like action of caerulein, a CCK-8 receptor agonist in the mouse: influence of acute and subchronic diazepam treatment. Naunyn-Schmiedeberg's Arch Pharmacol 341:62–67.

Hebb ALO, Poulin J-F, Roach SP, Zacharko RM, Drolet G (2005) Cholecystokinin and endogenous opioid peptides: interactive influence on pain, cognition, and emotion. Prog Neuropsychopharmacol Biol Psychiatry 29:1225–1238.

Hoffman GA, Harrington A, Fields HL (2005) Pain and the placebo: what we have learned. Persp Biol Med 48:248–265.

Johansen O, Brox J, Flaten MA (2003) Placebo and nocebo responses, cortisol, and circulating beta-endorphin. Psychosom Med 65:786–790.

Keltner JR, Furst A, Fan C, et al. (2006) Isolating the modulatory effect of expectation on pain transmission: a functional magnetic resonance imaging study. J Neurosci 26:4437–4443.

Kong J, Gollub RL, Rosman IS, et al. (2006) Brain activity associated with expectancy-enhanced placebo analgesia as measured by functional magnetic resonance imaging. J Neurosci 26:381–388.

Koyama T, McHaffie JG, Laurienti PJ, Coghill RC (2005) The subjective experience of pain: where expectations become reality. Proc Natl Acad Sci USA 102:12950–12955.

Lavigne GJ, Hargreaves KM, Schmidt EA, Dionne RA (1989) Proglumide potentiates morphine analgesia for acute postsurgical pain. Clin Pharmacol Ther 45:666–673.

Levine JD, Gordon NC (1984) Influence of the method of drug administration on analgesic response. Nature 312:755–756.

Levine JD, Gordon NC, Fields HL (1978) The mechanisms of placebo analgesia. Lancet 312:654–657.

Liddle G (1974) The adrenal cortex. In: Textbook of endocrinology (Williams RH, ed.), Ed. 5. Philadelphia: Saunders.

Maldonado R, Derrien M, Noble F, Roques BP (1993) Association of a peptidase inhibitor and a CCK-B antagonist strongly potentiates antinociception mediated by endogenous enkephalins. NeuroReport 7:947–950.

Nattero G, De Lorenzo C, Biale L, et al. (1989) Psychological aspects of weekend headache sufferers in comparison with migraine patients. Headache 29:93–99.

Noble F, Derrien M, Roques BP (1993) Modulation of opioid antinociception by CCK at the supraspinal level: evidence of regulatory mechanisms between CCK and enkephalin systems in the control of pain. Br J Pharmacol 109:1064–1070.

Noble F, Wank SA, Crawley JN, et al. (1999) International Union of Pharmacology. XXI. Structure, distribution, and functions of cholecystokinin receptors. Pharmacol Rev 51:745–781.

Petrovic P, Kalso E, Petersson KM, Ingvar M (2002) Placebo and opioid analgesia: imaging a shared neuronal network. Science 295:1737–1740.

Petrovic P, Dietrich T, Fransson P, et al. (2005) Placebo in emotional processing: induced expectations of anxiety relief activate a generalized modulatory network. Neuron 46:957–969.

Price DD, von der Gruen A, Miller J, Rafii A, Price C (1985) Potentiation of systemic morphine analgesia in humans by proglumide, a cholecystokinin antagonist. Anesth Analg 64:801–806.

Price DD, Chung SK, Robinson ME (2005) Conditioning, expectation and desire for relief in placebo analgesia. Semin Pain Med 3:15–21.

Rainero I, Valfre W, Savi L, et al. (2001) Neuroendocrine effects of subcutaneous sumatriptan in patients with migraine. J Endocrinol Invest 24:310–315.

Sawamoto N, Honda M, Okada T, et al. (2000) Expectation of pain enhances responses to nonpainful somatosensory stimulation in the anterior cingulate cortex and parietal operculum/posterior insula: an event-related functional magnetic resonance imaging study. J Neurosci 20:7438–7445.

Spielberg CD, Gorsuch RL, Luschenne RE (1980) STAI. Questionario di autovalutazione per l'ansia di stato e di tratto. Florence, Italy: Organizzazioni Speciali.

Stengaard-Pedersen K, Larsson LI (1981) Localization and opiate receptor binding of enkephalin, CCK and ACTH/beta-endorphin in the rat central nervous system. Peptides 2 (Suppl. 1):3–19.

Suberg SN, Culhane ES, Carstens E, Watkins LR (1985) Behavioral and electrophysiological investigations of opiate/cholecystokinin interactions. In: Advances in pain research and therapy, Vol. 9 (Fields HL, Dubner R, Cervero F, eds.), pp. 541–553. New York: Raven.

Terman GW, Morgan MJ, Liebeskind JC (1986) Opioid and non-opioid stress analgesia from cold water swim: importance of stress severity. Brain Res 372:167–171.

Valverde O, Maldonado R, Fournie-Zaliski MC, Roques BP (1994) Cholecystokinin B antagonists strongly potentiate antinociception mediated by endogenous enkephalins. J Pharmacol Exp Ther 270:77–88.

Vanderhaegen JJ, Signeau JC, Gepts W (1975) New peptide in the vertebrate CNS reacting with antigastrin antibodies. Nature 257:604–605.

Van Megen HJGM, Den Boer JA, Westenberg HGM (1994) On the significance of cholecystokinin receptors in panic disorder. Prog Neuropsychopharmacol Biol Psychiatry 18:1235–1246.

Wager TD, Rilling JK, Smith EE, et al. (2004) Placebo-induced changes in fMRI in the anticipation and experience of pain. Science 303:1162–1166.

Wager TD, Matre D, Casey KL (2006) Placebo effects in laser-evoked pain potentials. Brain Behav Immunity 20:219–230.

Watkins LR, Kinscheck IB, Mayer DJ (1985a) Potentiation of morphine analgesia by the cholecystokinin antagonist proglumide. Brain Res 327:169–180.

Watkins LR, Kinscheck IB, Kaufmann EFS, et al. (1985b) Cholecystokinin antagonists selectively potentiate analgesia induced by endogenous opiates. Brain Res 327:181–190.

Wiesenfeld-Hallin Z, Xu X-J, Hyghes J, Horwell DC, Hokfelt T (1990) PD 134308, a selective antagonist of cholecystokinin type B receptor, enhances the analgesic effect of morphine and synergistically interacts with intrathecal galanin to depress spinal nociceptive reflexes. Proc Natl Acad Sci USA 87:7105–7109.

Willer JC, Albe-Fessard D (1980) Electrophysiological evidence for a release of endogenous opiates in stress-induced analgesia in man. Brain Res 198:419–426.

Xu X-J, Hokfelt T, Hughes J, Wiesenfeld-Hallin Z (1994) The CCK-B antagonist CI-988 enhances the reflex-depressive effect of morphine in axotomized rats. NeuroReport 5:718–720.

Zubieta JK, Bueller JA, Jackson LR, et al. (2005) Placebo effects mediated by endogenous opioid neurotransmission and μ-opioid receptors. J Neurosci 25:7754–7762.

29

Expectation and Dopamine Release

Mechanism of the Placebo Effect in Parkinson's Disease

RAÚL DE LA FUENTE-FERNÁNDEZ, THOMAS J. RUTH, VESNA SOSSI, MICHAEL SCHULZER, DONALD B. CALNE, A. JON STOESSL

Raúl de la Fuente-Fernández, Thomas J. Ruth, Vesna Sossi, Michael Schulzer, Donald B. Calne, A. Jon Stoessl, "Expectation and Dopamine Release: Mechanism of the Placebo Effect in Parkinson's Disease," *Science* 2001;293:1164–1166.

The simple act of receiving any treatment (active or not) may, in itself, be efficacious because of expectation of benefit (1). This is the placebo effect—a potential confounder in assessing the efficacy of any therapeutic intervention (2, 3). Placebo-controlled studies were designed precisely to control for such an effect (4). It has been assumed that the placebo response is not mediated directly through any physical or chemical effect of treatment (5). In Parkinson's disease (PD), the placebo effect can be prominent (6, 7).

We asked whether the placebo effect in PD is produced by activation of the pathway primarily damaged by degeneration (i.e., the nigrostriatal dopaminergic system (8, 9)). To answer this question, we took advantage of the ability of positron emission tomography (PET) to estimate pharmacologically or behaviorally induced dopamine release based on the competition between endogenous dopamine and [^{11}C]raclopride (RAC) for binding to dopamine D_2/D_3 receptors (10–14). We hypothesized that if the placebo effect is mediated through the activation of the pathway relevant to the disorder under study, we should be able to detect placebo-induced release of endogenous dopamine in PD.

We examined the striatal RAC binding potential of six patients with PD (group 1, placebo group) under two conditions (15): Condition 1, a placebo-controlled, blinded study in which the patients did not know when they were receiving placebo or active drug (apomorphine) (16)—all patients received both placebo and active drug; and condition 2, an open study in the same patients without placebo.

We found a significant decrease in striatal RAC binding potential (17% for the caudate nucleus [range, 8 to 25%]; 19% for the putamen [range, 8 to 28%]; $P < 0.005$ for both, two-tailed paired t test) when the patients received placebo compared with open baseline observations (Table 29.1). This

Table 29.1.
Striatal RAC binding potential (mean±SD) of PD patients (group 1) scanned at open baseline and after receiving placebo (n=6)

Site	Open baseline	Placebo	Mean percent change (range)
Head of caudate	1.964±0.221	1.638±0.230	16.6 (8.4–25.1)
Putamen			
Rostral	2.398±0.342	1.976±0.321	17.6 (5.3–26.3)
Intermediate	2.621±0.438	2.142±0.389	18.2 (7.4–27.0)
Caudal	2.095±0.269	1.646±0.261	21.2 (8.8–32.6)

[Note: PD=Parkinson's disease; RAC=[¹¹C]raclopride—eds.]

placebo-induced change in RAC binding potential was present in each patient and in each striatal subregion, although it was greatest in the posterolateral part of the putamen (Table 29.1). The magnitude of the placebo response was comparable to that of therapeutic doses of levodopa (17), or apomorphine (see below) (18). There were no differences in the striatal RAC binding potential between this group of patients when studied without placebo and a second group of patients matched by age and severity of parkinsonism studied exclusively in an open fashion (group 2, open group) (15) (Fig. 29.1).

These observations indicate that there is placebo-induced release of endogenous dopamine in the striatum (19). The estimated release of dopamine was greater in patients who perceived placebo benefit than in those who did not (20). This suggests a "dose-dependent" relation between the release of endogenous dopamine and the magnitude of the placebo effect.

We next asked whether there might be an interaction between the effects of the placebo and the active drug (21). The placebo response could synergistically enhance the benefit of an active drug, in which case double-blind, placebo-controlled studies would overestimate the active drug effect. Alternatively, the placebo effect could mask (or decrease) the specific effect of an active drug, which would lead to the opposite conclusion in the interpretation of a placebo-controlled study.

After adjusting for differences in "baseline" RAC binding potential, we found no significant differences in the response to apomorphine between the open group and the placebo group (combining patients who perceived a placebo effect and those who did not) (22). However, the degree of apomorphine-induced change in RAC binding potential tended to be lower in patients who perceived a placebo effect compared with those who did not and with patients studied in an open fashion (Fig. 29.2). We explored whether this observation could reflect a floor effect in the placebo group (i.e., whether the technique was insensitive for further reductions in RAC binding), but this did not appear to be the case (Fig. 29.3) (23). We conclude that the placebo response does not potentiate the effect of an active drug. Indeed, our results suggest that in some patients, most of the benefit obtained from an active drug might derive from a placebo effect.

The dopaminergic system is involved in the regulation of several cognitive, behavioral, and sensorimotor functions, and particularly in reward mechanisms (24–28). However, our experiments did not involve a direct reward. We conclude that dopamine release in the nigrostriatal system is linked to expectation of a reward—in this case, the anticipation of therapeutic benefit (29, 30). All patients were familiar with the effect of an active drug (levodopa), and such previous experience may have enhanced their expectation. We found that the level of expectation may determine experience (20)—patients who perceived a placebo effect had higher release of dopamine than those who did not.

Our observations indicate that the placebo effect in PD is mediated by an increase in the synaptic levels of dopamine in the striatum. Expectation-related dopamine release might be a common phenomenon in any medical condition susceptible to the placebo effect. PD patients receiving an active drug in the context of a placebo-controlled study benefit from the active drug being tested as well as from the placebo effect. By contrast, in the usual clinical practice setting, active drugs may be devoid of placebo effect. We found no evidence to suggest that the placebo effect synergistically augments the

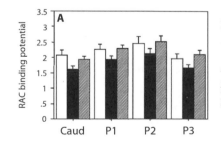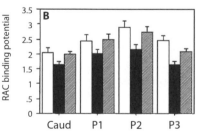

Figure. 29.1. Placebo-induced changes in [¹¹C]raclopride (RAC) binding potential in the striatum ipsilateral (**A**) and contralateral (**B**) to the more affected body side of patients with PD. The regions of interest (ROIs) are on the head of the caudate nucleus (Caud) and on the putamen, from rostral to caudal, P1, P2, P3 (15). Comparisons were made between the group of patients studied in an open fashion (group 2, open group; open bars) and the group of patients studied both with (solid bars) and without (hatched bars) placebo intervention (group 1, placebo group). Within-subject placebo-induced changes in RAC binding potential tended to be greater in the striatum contralateral to the more affected body side (20%) than in the ipsilateral striatum (17%). The placebo group and the open group did not differ in their baseline placebo-free RAC binding potential values (for the caudate nucleus, 1.96±0.22 (SD) versus 2.07±0.40, respectively; two-tailed t test, t=−0.55 (df=10), P=0.59; for the putamen, 2.37 ±0.34 versus 2.42±0.42, t=−0.20 (df=10), P=0.84). Error bars=SEM.

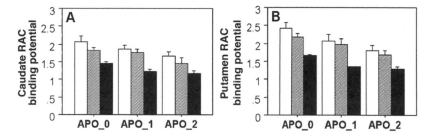

Figure. 29.2. Apomorphine-induced changes in RAC binding potential in the caudate nucleus (A) and putamen (B) before (APO_0) and after (APO_1 = 0.03 mg/kg, and APO_2 = 0.06 mg/kg) subcutaneous injection of apomorphine. Patients studied in an open fashion (open bars) had higher RAC binding potential values than those included in the placebo group (independently of whether they did not [hatched bars] or did [solid bars] perceive a placebo effect). The decline in RAC binding potential induced by an incremental dose of apomorphine tended to be less pronounced in patients who perceived a placebo effect as compared with those who did not, and with patients studied in an open fashion: interaction term (group × apomorphine dose) evaluated by repeated measures ANCOVA, $F = 4.66$ (df = 2,9), $P = 0.041$ for the caudate nucleus; $F = 3.40$ (df = 2,9), $P = 0.079$ for the putamen. Error bars = SEM.

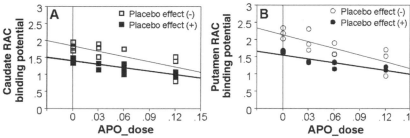

Figure. 29.3. Linear regression plots for patients without ($n = 3$; open symbols, thin lines) and with ($n = 3$; solid symbols, thick lines) perceived placebo effect: (A) caudate and (B) putamen RAC binding potential values against apomorphine dose (APO_dose). The four slopes were significantly different from zero ($P < 0.01$), but they did not differ significantly between patients with and without perceived placebo effect (for the caudate nucleus, −3.2 versus −5.1, respectively, $P = 0.28$; for the putamen, −3.8 versus −6.5, $P = 0.15$).

action of active drugs (in fact, a trend for the opposite was observed), so positive conclusions derived from placebo-controlled studies are not impugned by our findings.

REFERENCES AND NOTES

1. D.G. Altman, *Practical Statistics for Medical Research* (Chapman & Hall, London, 1991), pp. 450–451.
2. H.K. Beecher, J. Am. Med. Assoc. **159**, 1602 (1955).
3. E. Ernst, K.L. Resch, Br. Med. J. **311**, 551 (1995).
4. T.J. Kaptchuk, Lancet **351**, 1722 (1998).
5. L.D. Fisher, G. van Belle, *Biostatistics: A Methodology for the Health Sciences* (Wiley, New York, 1993), p. 22.
6. N. Shetty et al., Clin. Neuropharmacol. **22**, 207 (1999).
7. C.G. Goetz, S. Leurgans, R. Raman, G.T. Stebbins, Neurology **54**, 710 (2000).
8. J.M. Fearnley, A.J. Lees, Brain **114**, 2283 (1991).
9. S.J. Kish, K.S. Shannak, O. Hornykiewicz, N. Engl. J. Med. **318**, 876 (1988).
10. P. Seeman, H.C. Guan, H.B. Niznik, Synapse **3**, 96 (1989).
11. N.D. Volkow et al., Synapse **16**, 255 (1994).
12. M.J. Koepp et al., Nature **393**, 266 (1998).
13. A.J. Stoessl, T.J. Ruth, NeuroScience News **2**, 53 (1999).
14. M. Laruelle, J. Cereb. Blood Flow Metab. **20**, 423 (2000).
15. All PET scans were performed in three-dimensional (3D) mode using an ECAT 953B/31 tomograph. We obtained 16 sequential frames over 60 minutes, starting at the time of injection of 5 mCi of [^{11}C]raclopride (mean ± SEM specific activity = 4692 ± 349 Ci/mmol at ligand injection). A time-integrated image with 31 planes, each 3.37 mm thick, was made from the emission data (from 30 to 60 minutes) for each subject. The five axial planes in which the striatum was best visualized were summed. On this time- and spatially summed image, one circular region of interest (ROI) of 61.2 mm² was positioned on the

head of each caudate nucleus (Caud), and three circular ROIs of the same size were placed without overlap along the axis of each putamen (from rostral to caudal putamen: P1, P2, and P3); ROI position was adjusted to maximize the average radioactivity. The ROIs were replicated on the spatially summed image of each time frame. The background activity was averaged from a single elliptical ROI (2107 mm²) drawn over the cerebellum on the summed image of two contiguous axial planes. The binding potential ($BP = fNS \cdot B_{max}/K_d$, where fNS is the free fraction of tracer) was determined using a tissue input graphical approach (J. Logan et al., J. Cereb. Blood Flow Metab. **16**, 834 [1996]). Further details of the PET scan protocol are reported elsewhere (17). We studied two groups of PD patients, of six patients each, under two different protocols as described below. Both groups were matched by age and severity of parkinsonism as measured by the Modified Columbia Scale (MCS) (R.C. Duvoisin, in *Monoamines noyaux gris centraux et syndrome de Parkinson*, J. de Ajuriaguerra, G. Gauthier, Eds. [Georg and Cie SA, Geneva, 1971], pp. 313–325). Clinical details can be found on *Science* Online at www.sciencemag.org/cgi/content/full/sci;293/5532/1164/DC1. After being pretreated with domperidone for 48 hours to prevent side effects, all patients underwent three consecutive RAC PET scans on the same day according to the following protocol: (i) either baseline or placebo scan 12 to 18 hours after withdrawal of medications; (ii) after subcutaneous injection of 0.03 mg of apomorphine per kilogram of body weight; and (iii) after subcutaneous injection of 0.06 mg/kg of apomorphine. The treatment order was maintained constant for all patients. Group 1 (the placebo group) was studied in a blind fashion—patients did not know when they were receiving placebo (subcutaneous injection of saline) or apomorphine (all patients received all three treatments). This group also received a fourth injection, consisting of 0.12 mg/kg of apomorphine on the same day, to explore the possibility of a floor effect (see below). Group 2 (open group) was studied in an open fashion for comparison purposes (e.g., to investigate the effect of novelty on dopamine release). Here, recipients were scanned under all three conditions but knew explicitly if they were receiving no medication or which dose of apomorphine they were receiving at any given time. The advantages of this design are threefold: (i) It minimizes potential carry-over effects from the active drug (apomorphine) (17). (ii) It helps maintain the level of expectation throughout the study, which is crucial to this experiment. For example, the occurrence of apomorphine-induced side effects could "unblind" the study. (iii) It maximizes the tolerability of the procedure. In total, there was a 2.5-hour interval between scans (1-hour scan plus 1.5-hour break), sufficient to allow for decay of radioactivity, as well as for dopamine receptor recovery after apomorphine injection (16, 17). An additional open baseline scan was performed on group 1 patients on a different day to obtain placebo-free baseline values (interval between both sets of scans, 1 to 4 months). All patients had been contacted 1 month before the scans, and details of the protocol in which they were included were explained; they were reminded of these details 3 days before the scans. We avoided anticipation bias (e.g., patients' knowledge of the fact that the placebo effect can determine measurable changes in dopamine release might alter the results) by keeping the patients and the clinical staff unaware of the purpose of the study. In all cases, care was taken to optimize patient positioning in the scanner. Motion within and between scans was minimized by the use of a molded thermoplastic mask. All subjects gave written informed consent. The study was approved by the University of British Columbia (Vancouver, British Columbia, Canada) ethics committee.

16. S.T. Gancher, W.R. Woodward, B. Boucher, J.G. Nutt, *Ann. Neurol.* **26**, 232 (1989).

17. R. de la Fuente-Fernández *et al., Ann. Neurol.* **49**, 298 (2001).

18. The placebo-induced change in striatal RAC binding potential is much higher than the reported within-subject scan–rescan variation expected to occur within subject for scan and rescan (mean, 5%) (N.D. Volkow *et al., J. Nucl. Med.* **34**, 609 [1993]). The administration of 0.03 and 0.06 mg/kg of apomorphine led to a 14% and 26% decrease, respectively, in putamen RAC binding potential in the open group (see Fig. 29.2).

19. The increasing rostrocaudal gradient of the placebo effect (Table 29.1) eliminates the possibility that the results could be due to down-regulation of presynaptic D_2/D_3 receptors. Partial volume effects cannot explain the gradient in $BP_{open\ baseline} - BP_{placebo}$ reported here. Other considerations supporting our interpretation of the results can be found elsewhere (17).

20. Because the clinical benefit from apomorphine lasts typically about 1 hour (16), which is the duration of RAC PET scans, no objective measurements on changes in the clinical status after placebo or apomorphine injection were made (motor activity might confound the assessment of changes in striatal RAC binding potential). However, only half of the patients reported placebo-induced clinical improvement (comparable in magnitude to the clinical benefit obtained when they were on their regular treatment with levodopa). Although the number of subjects is small, those patients who perceived the placebo effect (n = 3) had higher changes in RAC binding potential than those who did not (n = 3) (for the caudate nucleus, 22% versus 12%; for the putamen, 24% versus 14%; P < 0.05 and P < 0.01, respectively, by analysis of covariance [ANCOVA]) (Fig. 29.2).

21. J. Kleijnen, A.J.M. de Craen, J. van Everdingen, L. Krol, *Lancet* **344**, 1347 (1994).

22. Repeated measures ANCOVA gave the following results: for the caudate nucleus, between-group differences, F = 0.03 (df = 1,9), P = 0.87; interaction term (group × apomorphine dose), F = 0.09 (df = 1,10), P = 0.77. For the putamen, between-group differences, F = 0.71 (df = 1,9), P = 0.42; interaction term, F = 1.81 (df = 1,10), P = 0.21. The power for the interaction terms may not have been sufficient.

23. An apomorphine dose of 0.12 mg/kg led to a further decrease in RAC binding potential in the placebo group (Fig. 29.3). The total reduction in RAC binding potential (compared with placebo-free baseline values) was 42% in the caudate nucleus (range, 19 to 59%) and 46% in the putamen (range, 24 to 60%).

24. R.A. Wise, *Trends Neurosci.* **3**, 91 (1980).

25. H.C. Fibiger, A.G. Phillips, in *Handbook of Physiology: The Nervous System*, vol. 4, *Intrinsic Systems of the Brain*, V.B. Mountcastle, F.E. Bloom, S.R. Geiger, Eds. (American Physiological Society, Bethesda, Md., 1986), pp. 647–675.

26. T.W. Robbins, B.J. Everitt, *Semin. Neurosci.* **4**, 119 (1992).

27. W. Schultz, *J. Neurophysiol.* **80**, 1 (1998).

28. S. Ikemoto, J. Panksepp, *Brain Res. Rev.* **31**, 6 (1999).

29. I. Kirsch, Ed., *How Expectancies Shape Experience* (American Psychological Association, Washington, D.C., 1999).

30. J.M. Fish, *Science* **284**, 914 (1999).

30

Placebo-Responsive Parkinson Patients Show Decreased Activity in Single Neurons of Subthalamic Nucleus

FABRIZIO BENEDETTI, LUANA COLLOCA, ELENA TORRE, MICHELE LANOTTE, ANTONIO MELCARNE, MARINA PESARE, BRUNO BERGAMASCO, AND LEONARDO LOPIANO

Fabrizio Benedetti, Luana Colloca, Elena Torre, Michele Lanotte, Antonio Melcarne, Marina Pesare, Bruno Bergamasco, and Leonardo Lopiano, "Placebo-Responsive Parkinson Patients Show Decreased Activity in Single Neurons of Subthalamic Nucleus," *Nature Neuroscience* 2004;7:587–588.

The placebo effect is a complex phenomenon whereby an inert treatment can induce a therapeutic benefit if the subject is made to believe that it is effective. This phenomenon has recently passed from nuisance in clinical research to target of scientific investigation.[1] Most of our understanding of its neurobiological mechanisms comes from the field of pain, where placebo analgesia has been found to be mediated by expectation-induced activation of opioid systems.[2-5] Recent research has shown that the placebo effect in Parkinson disease is also amenable to neurobiological investigation.[4,6-8] For example, a placebo-induced release of dopamine in the striatum has been described, which might affect different neuronal populations within the circuitry of the basal ganglia.[6,7]

The subthalamic nucleus (STN), which has a central role in basal ganglia functioning, is a major target in the surgical therapy of Parkinson disease,[9] and its identification requires the recording of intranuclear electrical activity.[10] Therefore, in our double-blind study, we recorded the activity from single neurons in the STN before and after placebo administration to see whether neuronal changes were linked to the clinical placebo response. As previous studies have shown, the placebo response is much stronger after repeated effective treatments.[2,4,5] Thus, we administered a placebo in the operating room after several pre-operative administrations of apomorphine, a powerful antiparkinsonian drug (see Supplementary Note online for details).

In 11 patients, before placebo administration, the activity of 100 neurons was recorded from one STN before implantation of the first electrode and used as a control. After the placebo, which consisted of a subcutaneous injection of saline solution along with the verbal suggestion of a motor improvement, neuronal activity was recorded from 110 neurons before implantation of the second electrode into the other STN (see Supplementary Note, below, for details).

A placebo response was defined as the decrease of arm rigidity of at least one point on the clinical evaluation scale (UPDRS; Supplementary Note). Those patients who showed a clear-cut clinical placebo response, assessed by means of arm rigidity and subjective report of well-being, also showed a significant decrease of neuronal discharge compared to the pre-placebo STN (Fig. 30.1, left; $F_{1,112} = 31.618$, $P < 0.001$). It is interesting to note the lack of neuronal activity decrease in the last placebo responder (left column) who, albeit responsive, showed a short-lasting placebo response (less than 15 min). In this individual, neuronal recording was done when the placebo response had already vanished. No significant difference between pre-placebo and post-placebo neuronal discharge was found in those patients who did not show any clinical placebo improvement (Fig. 30.1, right; $F_{1,94} = 0.564$, $P = 0.454$). Note that the arm rigidity decrease was paralleled by the person's subjective report of well-being (Fig. 30.1).

We also studied a no-treatment group (natural history) to address the possibility that the difference in neuronal frequency discharge between the pre- and post-placebo STN was independent of the placebo treatment itself. A total of 227 neurons were recorded from 12 patients in the left and right STN in the same conditions as those of the placebo group. The only difference was that these individuals did not undergo any placebo treatment between the implantation of the first and second electrode. They all showed no significant differences between the neuronal firing rates of the two STNs ($F_{1,225} = 0.023$, $P = 0.880$; Supplementary Note), indicating that the difference between the first and the second side of implantation in the placebo group was due to the placebo intervention *per se*.

Overall, the no-treatment group, the placebo responders and the placebo non-responders were significantly different from each other with regard to the pre–post placebo difference in neuronal firing rate ($F_{3,431} = 10.579$, $P < 0.001$). A post-hoc analysis by means of the Tukey test for multiple comparisons (see Supplementary Note) showed that the pre–post placebo difference in neuronal discharge in the responders was significantly different from that in the no-treatment group ($P < 0.001$). Likewise, the pre–post neuronal discharge difference in the placebo responders differed from that of the non-responders ($P < 0.001$). Conversely, no difference was present between the no-treatment group and the non-responders ($P = 0.398$).

Although the mean frequency of discharge of the STN neurons is a good parameter to assess STN activity, bursting and oscillatory patterns have also been described in Parkinson disease and related to motor symptoms and apomor-

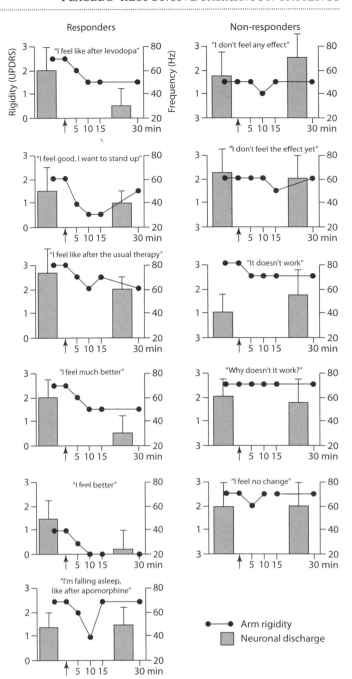

Figure 30.1. Correlation among arm rigidity (black circles), STN neuronal frequency discharge (bars), and subjective report in placebo responders (left) and non-responders (right). The black arrow on the abscissa indicates placebo administration. There was a decrease in neuronal activity after placebo administration in the placebo responders, but not in the non-responders. The sixth placebo responder (left column, bottom) showed no decrease in neuronal activity, as the single-neuron recording was performed when the placebo response had already vanished. Bars on the shaded columns represent standard deviations.

phine effects.[11,12] Therefore, we also analyzed the bursting activity of the STN neurons before and after placebo administration, to verify whether there was also a change in the pattern of discharge (other than frequency decrease; see Supplementary Note for burst and statistical analysis). Using

Table 30.1.
Bursting and non-bursting neurons before and after placebo administration in responders and non-responders

	Before placebo (burst/no burst)	After placebo (burst/no burst)	Odds ratio	Log odds ratio	95% confidence interval of odds ratio
Responders					
R1	8/2	2/7	14	2.64	1.6 to 121 (**$P<0.04$**)
R2	7/2	2/9	15.8	2.76	1.8 to 142 (**$P<0.027$**)
R3	5/1	2/8	20	2.99	1.4 to 280 (**$P<0.05$**)
R4	9/3	1/6	18	2.89	1.5 to 217 (**$P<0.037$**)
R5	8/1	3/9	24	3.18	2 to 279 (**$P<0.014$**)
R6	7/3	4/5	2.92	1.07	0.44 to 19 (P=0.508)
Total	44/12	14/44	11.5	2.44	4.8 to 27.8 (**$P<0.001$**)
Non-responders					
NR1	9/2	8/4	2.25	0.81	0.32 to 15.6 (P=0.725)
NR2	5/1	6/2	1.67	0.51	0.11 to 24 (P=0.778)
NR3	4/3	6/3	0.67	−0.41	0.09 to 5.09 (P=0.896)
NR4	8/3	5/5	2.67	0.98	0.43 to 16.5 (P=0.534)
NR5	7/2	9/4	1.56	0.44	0.22 to 11 (P=0.965)
Total	33/11	34/18	1.6	0.47	0.6 to 3.9 (P=0.424)

Note: Boldface indicates statistically significant difference (before versus after placebo).

a random-effects meta-analytic approach, we found that the STN neurons of all the placebo responders shifted significantly from a pattern of bursting activity to a pattern of non-bursting discharge (Table 30.1). The only exception was the last placebo responder, whose recordings were made when the placebo response had already vanished. All placebo non-responders did not show any difference in the number of bursting neurons before and after placebo administration (Table 30.1). Likewise, the no-treatment group did not show any significant difference in bursting activity between the first-side and second-side STN (see Supplementary Note), and no differences were present between the log odds ratios of the non-responders and of the no-treatment group ($t_{15}=0.767$, $P=0.455$). By contrast, a highly significant difference was present between the log odds ratios of the placebo responders and of the non-responders ($t_9=5.198$, $P<0.001$), and between the log odds ratios of the placebo responders and of the no-treatment group ($t_{16}=6.67$, $P<0.001$).

This is the first study of a placebo effect at the single-neuron level, showing that a placebo procedure affects specific neuronal populations. In particular, placebo clinical responses are accompanied by two types of neuronal changes in the STN of Parkinsonian patients: (i) a decrease of frequency discharge and (ii) a shift from bursting to non-bursting activity. In previous studies, some contrasting results were found, with either no change in STN mean frequency discharge[12] or a pronounced decrease[13] after apomorphine administration. Our present findings support the idea that the relief of Parkinsonian rigidity is associated with a decrease in neuronal firing rate. According to the classic pathophysiological view of Parkinson disease, the dopamine depletion in the striatum induces STN hyperactivity[14] and bursting activity.[11,12] The

high-frequency therapeutic stimulation of the STN would modify this abnormal activity.[9,15] The results of the present study, obtained by means of a placebo treatment, confirm this model by showing the tight correlation between reduction of rigidity on the one hand and reduction of STN frequency discharge and bursting activity on the other. As previous studies show a release of dopamine in the striatum after placebo intervention,[6,7] these STN neuronal changes are likely to be induced by the placebo-activated dopamine.

Supplementary Note: Supplementary information is available on the *Nature Neuroscience* website: http://www.nature.com /neuro/journal/v7/n6/suppinfo/nn1250_S1.html.

REFERENCES

1. Benedetti, F., Rainero, I., and Pollo, A. *Curr. Opin. Anaesthesiol.* 16, 515–519 (2003).
2. Amanzio, M., and Benedetti, F. *J. Neurosci.* 19, 484–494 (1999).
3. Benedetti, F., Arduino, C., and Amanzio, M. *J. Neurosci.* 19, 3639–3648 (1999).
4. Benedetti, F. et al. *J. Neurosci.* 23, 4315–4323 (2003).
5. Petrovic, P., Kalso, E., Petersson, K.M., and Ingvar, M. *Science* 295, 1737–1740 (2002).
6. de la Fuente-Fernández, R. et al. *Science* 293, 1164–1166 (2001).
7. de la Fuente-Fernández, R. et al. *Behav. Brain Res.* 136, 359–363 (2002).
8. Pollo, A. et al. *NeuroReport* 13, 1383–1386 (2002).
9. Limousin, P. et al. *N. Engl. J. Med.* 339, 1105–1111 (1998).
10. Hutchinson, W.D. et al. *Ann. Neurol.* 44, 622–628 (1998).
11. Bergman, H., Wichmann, T., Karmon, B., and DeLong, M.R. *J. Neurophysiol.* 72, 507–520 (1994).
12. Levy, R. et al. *J. Neurophysiol.* 86, 249–260 (2001).
13. Stefani, A. et al. *Clin. Neurophysiol.* 113, 91–100 (2002).
14. Blandini, F., Nappi, G., Tassorelli, C., and Martignoni, E. *Prog. Neurobiol.* 62, 63–88 (2000).
15. Benazzouz, A., and Hallett, M. *Neurology* 55(S6), S13–S17 (2000).

31

Expectation Enhances the Regional Brain Metabolic and the Reinforcing Effects of Stimulants in Cocaine Abusers

Nora D. Volkow, Gene-Jack Wang, Yemin Ma, Joanna S. Fowler, Wei Zhu, Laurence Maynard, Frank Telang, Paul Vaska, Yu-Shin Ding, Christopher Wong, and James M. Swanson

Nora D. Volkow, Gene-Jack Wang, Yemin Ma, Joanna S. Fowler, Wei Zhu, Laurence Maynard, Frank Telang, Paul Vaska, Yu-Shin Ding, Christopher Wong, and James M. Swanson, "Expectation Enhances the Regional Brain Metabolic and the Reinforcing Effects of Stimulants in Cocaine Abusers," *Journal of Neuroscience* 2003;23:11461–11468.

Introduction

The reinforcing effects of drugs of abuse are a result of complex interactions between pharmacological effects and conditioned responses (Robinson and Berridge, 1993). These nonpharmacological variables shape the expectation of the drug effects, which in turn modulates the responses to the drug (Mitchell et al., 1996). For example, in drug abusers, the subjective responses to the drug are more pleasurable when subjects expect to receive the drug than when they do not (Kirk et al., 1998).

The effects of expectation on brain responses to drugs of abuse have been studied in laboratory animals. For example, cocaine-induced increases in dopamine (DA) in nucleus accumbens (NAc), an effect associated with its reinforcing value (Di Chiara and Imperato, 1988), is larger when animals are given cocaine in an environment in which they had previously received it than in a novel environment (Duvauchelle et al., 2000) or when animals self-administer cocaine than when cocaine administration is involuntary (Hemby et al., 1997). Also, cocaine-induced changes in regional brain metabolism, which are an indicator of brain function (Sokoloff et al., 1977), are different when animals self-administer cocaine from when administration is involuntary (Graham and Porrino, 1995) and when cocaine is given in a conditioned environment versus their home cage (Knapp et al., 2002).

Not all studies, however, have shown that expectation enhances responses to a reinforcer. Indeed, there is evidence that for natural reinforcers, expected rewards do not induce activation of DA cells or of cells in orbitofrontal cortex (OFC), whereas unexpected rewards do (Schultz et al., 1998, 2000). Similarly, imaging studies in humans have documented that for natural reinforcers unpredictable reward induced larger activation than predictable reward in NAc and OFC (Berns et al., 2001).

The effects of expectation on the response of the human brain to drugs of abuse have not been reported. Here we assessed the effects of expectation on the regional brain metabolic responses induced by intravenous methylphenidate (MP) in cocaine abusers. We measured brain metabolism rather than changes in DA because it allows one to evaluate the brain response to the drug, which includes primary sites of action as well as downstream effects. Brain metabolism was measured with positron emission tomography (PET) and [^{18}F]deoxyglucose (FDG). For studies using FDG, we decided to use MP because it is pharmacologically similar to cocaine but has more favorable brain pharmacokinetic properties. Both drugs block DA transporters (DATs) with similar potencies (Volkow et al., 1995), and cocaine abusers report that the effects of intravenous MP are similar to those of cocaine (Wang et al., 1997). DAT blockade, however, is much longer for MP (half-life 90 min) than for cocaine (20 min), which is shorter than the interval evaluated by FDG (30 min). The effects of MP were measured when cocaine abusers were expecting as well as when they were not expecting to receive the drug. We hypothesized that the reinforcing effects of MP would be enhanced by expectation and that this would be paralleled by an enhanced activation of brain regions involved in its reinforcing effects.

Materials and Methods

Subjects

Twenty-five active cocaine abusers (21 male and 4 female; 41 ± 3 years of age) who responded to an advertisement were studied. Subjects fulfilled Diagnostic and Statistical Manual, Version IV of the American Psychiatric Association criteria for cocaine dependence and were active users for at least the previous six months (free-base or crack at least "4 gm" per week). Exclusion criteria included current or past psychiatric disease other than cocaine dependence; past or present history of neurological, cardiovascular, or endocrinological disease; history of head trauma with loss of consciousness >30 min; and current medical illness and drug dependence other than for cocaine or nicotine. Subjects had an average history of 13 ± 5 years of cocaine use. Written informed consent was obtained from all subjects after complete description of the study and following the guidelines set by the Institutional Review Board at Brookhaven National Laboratory.

Scans

PET scans were acquired on a whole-body, high-resolution positron emission tomograph (Siemens High Resolution +, with $4.6 \times 4.6 \times 4.2$ mm resolution at center of field of view and 63 slices) in three-dimensional dynamic acquisition mode using FDG. Methods for positioning of subjects, catheterizations, transmission scans, and blood sampling and analysis have been published (Wang et al., 1992). Briefly, a 20 min emission scan was started 35 min after injection of 4–6 mCi of FDG. Arterialized blood sampling was used to measure FDG in plasma. During the study, subjects were positioned supine in the PET camera with their eyes open; the room was dimly lit, and noise was kept to a minimum except for the periodic evaluation of drug effects.

Subjects were scanned on four different days with FDG under the four conditions defined by the expectation-by-drug combinations: (1) expecting placebo and receiving placebo (PL/PL; baseline); (2) expecting placebo and receiving MP (PL/MP; drug effects without expectation); (3) expecting MP and receiving MP (MP/MP; drug effects with expectation); (4) expecting MP and receiving placebo (MP/PL; expectation effects alone). The order of the conditions was randomized across subjects. Placebo (3 cc of saline) or MP (0.5 mg/kg, i.v.) was injected over 60 sec and 1 min before FDG injection. The plasma concentrations of MP were measured before and at 10, 25, 40, and 54 min after MP using capillary gas chromatography/mass spectrometry (Srinivas et al., 1991).

Behavioral Measures

Behavioral effects were evaluated using analog scales that assessed self-reports of "high," "drug liking," "feel drug," and "restlessness" from 0 (felt nothing) to 10 (felt intensely) (Wang et al., 1997). These self-reports of drug effects have been shown to be reliable and consistent across studies and to predict administration of drugs in human subjects (Fischman and Foltin, 1991). Subjective ratings were recorded 5 min before placebo or MP and then every minute for the first 20 min and at 25, 30, 45, and 67 min after administration. At the end of the study, subjects were asked to rate "drug liking" (1–10).

Analysis

The data were analyzed using statistical parametric mapping (SPM) (Friston et al., 1995), and the results were corroborated with manually drawn regions of interest (ROI). For the SPM analyses, the images were spatially normalized using the template provided in the SPM99 package and then normalized to the mean metabolic activity for the whole brain (mean of all voxels within the brain) and subsequently smoothed with a 16 mm isotropic Gaussian kernel. Paired samples t tests were performed for the following four planned but nonorthogonal comparisons: drug effects when unexpected (PL/PL vs. PL/MP) and drug effects when expected (PL/PL vs. MP/MP); effects of expectation on MP (PL/MP vs. MP/MP); and effects of expectation alone (PL/PL vs. MP/PL). Significance was set at $p < 0.005$, and the statistical maps were overlaid on a structural image derived from magnetic resonance imaging (MRI). Because of incomplete sampling in the upper brain levels, we were unable to do the spatial normalization in 2 of the subjects, and thus the SPM results reflect the analysis done in 23 subjects.

In addition to assessing the differences in the magnitude of metabolic activation, we also assessed the differences in the volumes that were activated by MP when it was unexpected (PL/MP) versus when it was expected (MP/MP). Although SPM provides activation volumes, it does not provide statistical tests to compare the differences in activation volumes between two conditions. For this purpose we applied the statistical resampling strategy using the jackknife method (Quenouille, 1956; Miller, 1974; Efron, 1982). The following procedures were performed. (1) The SPM maps for activation for unexpected MP (PL/PL vs. PL/MP) and expected MP (PL/PL vs. MP/MP) comparisons were obtained with all of the subjects ($n = 23$). (2) One at a time, each subject was taken out and the same SPM analyses were repeated using the remaining 22 subjects. (3) Pseudo values were generated using all of the SPM activation volumes generated in the previous jackknife procedures. These pseudo values are independent estimates of the activation volumes at the significance level of $p < 0.005$ (Miller, 1974). (4) Paired sample t tests were performed on the pseudo values to compare the activation volumes with unexpected versus expected MP within those brain regions identified by significant differences in magnitude of activation. The volumes of activations were expressed as a percentage of the activation of a given anatomical region as defined from the Talairach Daemon (Lancaster et al., 2000). We chose $p < 0.005$ rather than $p < 0.001$ because we wanted to avoid false negatives, and our design retested the SPM findings with the ROI method.

For the ROI analysis a template was used (Wang et al., 1992) that locates 114 ROIs. We averaged the values from the ROI from the different slices corresponding to the same anatomical region into ten "composite" brain regions including that for whole brain (average of metabolism in all slices). We compressed the original template into ten regions to increase the precision of our measures and decrease the multiplicity of comparisons. The errors on measurements of small regions from PET images are large because of the limited spatial resolution of PET (Bendriem et al., 1991) and the imprecision in locating a "functionally distinct" area in the brain, the location of which is likely to vary among individuals (Rademacher et al., 2001). A repeated measures ANOVA was used to identify the ROI that differed between conditions, and then post hoc t tests were used to determine for which of the conditions the differences were significant.

Pearson product moment correlations were used to assess the association between the regional metabolic changes that differed between the unexpected and expected MP conditions (expressed as a percentage of change from the PL/PL condition) and MP-induced behavioral effects both for the expected and the unexpected conditions.

Results

Effects of MP on Regional Brain Metabolism

Plasma MP concentrations did not differ for the unexpected (PL/MP) or the expected MP (MP/MP) conditions and at 10 min reached an average concentration of 158 ng/ml and at 25 min of 97 ng/ml for both conditions. MP significantly increased whole-brain glucose metabolism compared with the baseline condition (PL/PL) when it was both unexpected (2.9 ± 2.5 μmol/100 gm per minute; $t = 5.9$; $df = 24$; $p < 0.0001$) and expected (4.2 ± 5.4 μmol/100 gm per minute; $t = 3.8$; $df = 24$; $p < 0.001$). The increase was ~50% higher when MP was expected than when unexpected ($13.6 \pm 17\%$ vs. $9.3 \pm 8\%$ change). In contrast, the expectation effects when placebo

(MP/PL) was received in the global (0.2 ± 3 μmol/100 gm per minute; 1 ± 1% change; NS) and regional metabolic measures were negligible (Fig. 31.1).

The results from SPM revealed that the largest increases from MP (expected and unexpected) occurred in cerebellum, occipital cortex, and thalamus (Fig. 31.2, Table 31.1).

In the SPM analysis, normalization for the global increases induced by MP results in the identification of "relative decreases" in those regions in which the increases are smaller than in the rest of the brain. Relative decreases after MP (expected and unexpected) occurred in limbic brain regions (ventral striatum [including nucleus accumbens], parahippocampal gyri [including amygdala], and insular cortex) and frontal regions (including medial orbitofrontal cortex) (Fig. 31.3, Table 31.2).

The SPM comparison between unexpected (PL/MP) versus expected MP (MP/MP) showed significantly greater increases in the magnitude of the response in cerebellum (vermis) and thalamus for expected than unexpected MP (Fig. 31.4) and the opposite pattern (significantly greater increases for unexpected than expected MP) in left lateral OFC (Brodmann area 47) (Fig. 31.4).

The comparison of the volume of activation for these brain regions showed significantly larger areas of activation for expected MP (MP/MP) when compared with unexpected MP (PL/MP) in vermis (26% vs. 13%; $t = 2.5$; $df = 22$; $p < 0.05$) and in thalamus (44% vs. 5%; $t = 3.9$; $p < 0.001$)

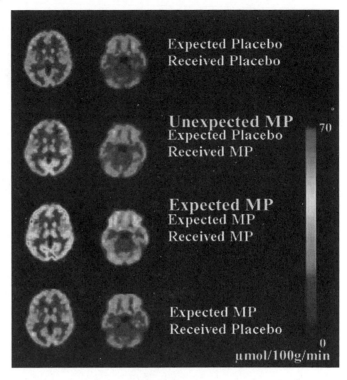

Figure 31.1. Brain metabolic images at the thalamic and cerebellar levels for the four conditions: (1) expected placebo received placebo, (2) expected placebo received MP, (3) expected MP received MP, and (4) expected MP received placebo. Scale is to the right and reflects micromoles/100 gm per minute. Note the larger increases in metabolism when MP was expected than when it was not expected.

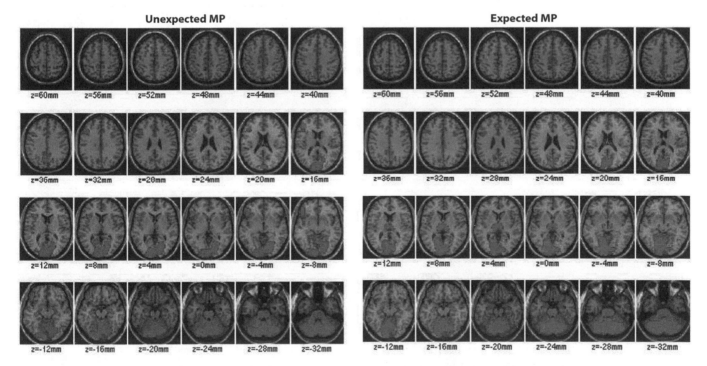

Figure 31.2. Brain maps obtained with SPM after normalization for the global metabolic increases to reveal the areas where MP induced the largest increases in metabolism both for unexpected and expected MP. Comparisons are with the "expected placebo received placebo" condition, and significance was set at $p < 0.005$. Note that the largest increases with MP occurred in cerebellum, occipital cortex, and thalamus. Note also the much larger areas of activation in thalamus for expected MP and in lateral orbitofrontal cortex for unexpected MP.

Table 31.1.
Location of the center of the areas in which MP induced significant increases (p<0.005; cluster size>100 pixels) in relative metabolic activity with respect to the x, y, z coordinates of the Talairach space and magnitude of the effects as assessed by the T values when MP was unexpected (PL/MP) and when it was expected (MP/MP)

	Unexpected MP (PL/MP)				Expected MP (MP/MP)			
	x	y	z	T	x	y	z	T
Frontal lobe								
Left inferior gyrus	−45	27	−13	3.59				NS
Left anterior cingulate				NS	−5	31	25	3.41
Occipital lobe								
Right lingual gyrus	19	−79	−9	4.51	11	−87	5	3.96
Left lingual gyrus	−7	−89	−9	4.23	−11	−89	5	4.78
Thalamus				NS	−11	−19	5	4.64
Cerebellum								
Right vermis	17	−63	−33	8.29	3	−63	−29	13.17
Left vermis	−15	−63	−33	6.78	−7	−63	−29	9.0

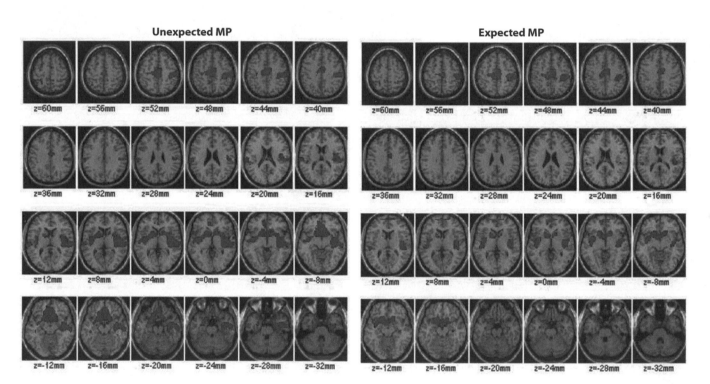

Figure 31.3. Brain maps obtained with SPM after normalization for the global metabolic increases to reveal the areas where MP induced relative decreases in metabolism for both unexpected and expected MP. Comparisons are with the "expected placebo received placebo" condition, and significance was set at p<0.005. Note the relative decreases for both conditions in limbic regions (NAc, Brodmann area 25, insula, amygdala) and in motor cortices.

and a larger area of activation for unexpected MP (PL/MP) when compared with expected MP (MP/MP) in left lateral OFC (Brodmann area 47) (11% vs. 0.5%; t=3.6; p<0.002) (Fig. 31.4).

The ROI analyses corroborated that the magnitude of the MP-induced increases in metabolism were significantly higher for expected than for unexpected MP in thalamus (12±11% vs. 19±14% increase in absolute metabolic measures; t=7.6; df=24; p<0.05) and in cerebellar vermis (11±7% vs. 19±16% increase in absolute metabolic measures; t=7.8; p<0.05).

Effects of Expectation on the Reinforcing Effects of MP and Correlation with the Metabolic Measures

MP increased self-reports of "drug liking," "high," "feel drug," and "restlessness" (Fig. 31.5). The self-reports of "high" were significantly greater for MP when expected (4.8) than unexpected (3.1) (Fig. 31.5). Indeed, the "high" was

Table 31.2.
Location of the center of the areas in which MP induced significant decreases ($p < 0.005$; cluster size > 100 pixels) in relative metabolic activity with respect to the x, y, z coordinates of the Talairach space and magnitude of the effects as assessed by the T values when MP was unexpected (PL/MP) and when it was expected (MP/MP)

	Unexpected MP (PL/MP)				Expected MP (MP/MP)			
	x	y	z	T	x	y	z	T
Frontal lobe								
Right medial gyrus	11	19	−17	3.53	13	11	−17	3.83
Left medial gyrus	−11	27	−17	3.46	−9	13	−17	4.84
Right rectal gyrus	3	37	−25	3.18				NS
Left rectal gyrus	−5	27	−21	2.96				NS
Right subcallosal gyrus	11	11	−13	5.13	11	11	−13	3.95
Left subcallosal gyrus	−5	7	−13	4.52	−9	11	−13	5.91
Right anterior cingulate	7	17	−9	3.77	5	15	−7	3.21
Left anterior cingulate	−7	19	−9	3.7	−3	11	−7	3.96
Right subgyral				NS	13	−15	43	3.59
Left subgyral				NS	−13	−23	43	3.34
Limbic lobe								
Right cingulate gyrus	5	−7	35	3.59	7	−11	41	4.72
Left cingulate gyrus	−1	−11	41	5.45				NS
Right insula	39	−7	−5	4.55	43	−15	3	5.81
Left insula	−39	−7	−5	3.8				NS
Right parahippocampal	31	−15	−20	4.35	35	−19	−15	3.14
Left parahippocampal	−25	−5	−20	3.26				NS
Right ventral striatum	15	11	−5	4.76	11	11	1	3.81
Left ventral striatum	−17	11	−5	3.66	−9	13	1	3.98
Temporal lobe								
Right middle temporal	43	−17	−9	5.09	43	−15	−9	3.33
Left middle temporal	−43	−9	−9	3.02	−37	−9	9	3.51

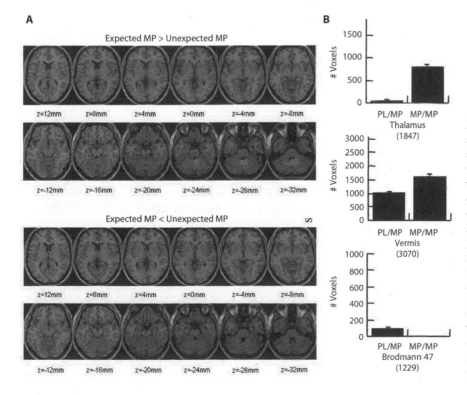

Figure 31.4. A, Brain maps obtained with SPM showing the areas where the increases were significantly larger for expected versus unexpected MP (top 2 rows of brain maps) and where they were significantly smaller for expected than unexpected MP (bottom 2 rows of brain maps). Significance was set at $p < 0.005$. B, Volumes of the areas of activation (number of pixels where activation was at the $p < 0.005$ level) for thalamus, vermis, and Brodmann area 47 for unexpected and expected MP. The volumes were significantly larger for expected MP in thalamus ($p < 0.001$) and vermis ($p < 0.05$) and for unexpected MP in Brodmann area 47 ($p < 0.002$). The numbers within the parentheses correspond to the total number of pixels for each region and were used to establish the scale in the ordinate axis.

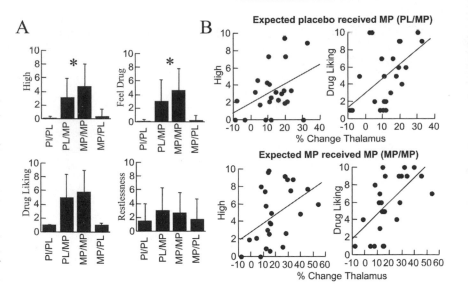

Figure 31.5. **A**, Self-reports of drug effects. MP (unexpected and expected) significantly increased self-report of "high" (repeated measures ANOVA; $F = 32$; $p < 0.0001$), "drug liking" ($F = 34$; $p < 0.0001$), "feel drug" ($F = 26$; $p < 0.0001$), and "restlessness" ($F = 4$; $p < 0.05$). Asterisk (*) indicates significant differences ($p < 0.05$) between MP when unexpected (PL/MP) versus when expected (MP/MP). **B**, Correlations between the changes in metabolism in thalamus and the increases in self-reports of "high" and "drug liking" after unexpected and expected MP.

~50% greater for expected than for unexpected MP. The "high" after placebo was low and did not differ whether subjects expected MP or not. A similar pattern occurred for the self-report of "feel drug."

The increases in self-reports of "high" and "drug liking" were significantly correlated with the increases in metabolism induced by MP (unexpected and expected) in thalamus (Fig. 31.5) but not in vermis (data not shown). The correlations between metabolic rates and "feel drug" ratings were not significant (data not shown).

Discussion

Effects of MP on Regional Brain Metabolism

Intravenous MP produced marked increases in whole-brain metabolism in cocaine abusers. This finding differs from a previous study that reported metabolic decreases after intravenous cocaine to cocaine abusers (London et al., 1990). Our design and methods may account for this difference. Both MP and cocaine have similar potencies in blocking DAT in the human brain (Volkow et al., 1999a), but they differ in their pharmacokinetics, with the half-life being much greater for MP than for cocaine (Volkow et al., 1995, 1996). Thus, during the 30 min uptake period of FDG, after cocaine the metabolic measures reflect the uptake and clearance from brain, whereas for MP they will reflect the uptake and plateau of the drug in brain.

The brain region most sensitive to MP effects regardless of condition was the cerebellum. We previously documented cerebellar activation after MP in controls (Volkow et al., 1997a) and in cocaine abusers (Volkow et al., 1999b). DAT density is low in cerebellum (Melchitzky and Lewis, 2000), so blockade of noradrenergic (norepinephrine [NE]) transporters by MP (Patrick et al., 1987) may have contributed to the metabolic increases in this brain region that receives a dense NE innervation (Reznikoff et al., 1986); however, it could also reflect downstream effects from DA stimulation of striatum, which sends projections to cerebellum (Hook

and Wise, 1995). Indeed, we showed previously that striatal DA D2 receptor availability predicted MP-induced increases in cerebellar metabolism (Volkow et al., 1997a,b). Although one could question why metabolic increases did not occur in striatum, this is likely to reflect the fact that metabolism predominantly reflects activity in nerve terminals and not cell bodies (Schwartz et al., 1979). MP by blocking DAT targets GABAergic cells in striatum, and thus metabolic changes are to be expected in regions where these projections terminate.

After controlling for "global" increases induced by MP, the SPM analyses revealed relative decreases in limbic regions that are part of brain reward circuits (ventral striatum, Brodmann area 25, insula, amygdala) (Schultz et al., 1998). This finding contrasts with increases in limbic regions reported after intravenous cocaine with functional MRI (fMRI) (Breiter et al., 1997), although more recent studies with fMRI have also reported decreases in limbic regions after intravenous MP (Dirckx et al., 2003). Nonetheless, extrapolation of fMRI and PET–FDG is difficult because the temporal resolution of these two techniques differs (30 min to measure metabolism with PET–FDG and 2–5 min to measure the peak blood oxygenation level dependent signal with fMRI) (Volkow et al. 1997b). The higher temporal resolution of fMRI than that of PET–FDG corresponds better to the short duration of the high (~10 min), and its ability to do continuous brain measurements allows one to assess the correspondence between the pharmacokinetics of the drug and the temporal course of its behavioral effects. Thus metabolic changes measured by PET–FDG reflect not only the neural changes associated with the high but also its aftereffects. Therefore, decreases in "relative metabolism" could reflect decreases, increases that were lower than those for the rest of the brain, or short-duration increases followed by decreases. Regardless, these results document that the reward circuit responds to intravenous MP differently than the rest of the brain.

For this study subjects were asked specifically to refrain from moving. Thus MP-induced relative decreases in motor cortex, an effect that has been documented previously by others (Devous et al., 2001), is likely to reflect the inhibitory control that subjects had to exert so that they did not move during the imaging procedure.

Effects of Expectation on MP-Induced Changes in Regional Brain Metabolism

When the subjects expected to receive MP and did (MP/MP), they had a significantly more intense and greater area of activation in cerebellum (vermis) and in thalamus than when they were not expecting it (PL/MP).

We hypothesized that expectation would enhance the pharmacological effects of MP, which amplifies DA and NE signals via blockade of DAT and norepinephrine transporters. Although we did not measure DA and NE changes in response to MP, the fact that the pattern of metabolic and behavioral effects induced by MP was similar although larger for expected than unexpected MP supports this hypothesis. Indeed, the notion that expectation can emulate the drug-induced brain effects may provide a neural basis for a "placebo" effect. For example, this was documented in a study of Parkinson's disease when a placebo resulted in DA increases that were equivalent to those induced by a DA agonist drug (de la Fuente-Fernández et al., 2001).

The enhanced activation of the thalamus when MP was expected (compared with unexpected MP) identifies this as a brain region involved with expectation effects in the response to the drug. This finding is consistent with that of a recent study in nonhuman primates, which showed that the largest difference between contingent versus noncontingent administration of cocaine were the increases in thalamic metabolism (Porrino et al., 2002). Metabolic activity in thalamus was also found to differ when rats received cocaine in a conditioned environment versus their home cage (Knapp et al., 2002). Using imaging we also reported that MP increased DA in thalamus in cocaine abusers but not in controls, which we postulated reflected a conditioned response from previous drug exposure (Volkow et al., 1997c). Thus the current findings provide further evidence in humans of thalamic involvement in conditioned reinforced responses (McAlonan et al., 1993). The ventral striatum is known to play a role in expectation (Cromwell and Schultz, 2003), and failure to document an effect in this study is likely to reflect the limited temporal resolution of PET–FDG. On the other hand, the fact that an expectation effect was observed in thalamus with a 30 min measurement suggests that thalamic involvement may be more sustained than that of other brain regions.

The significant association between MP-induced increases in thalamic metabolism and self-reports of "high" and "drug liking" suggests that it may modulate the reinforcing effects of MP. Indeed, the thalamus (mediodorsal nucleus) is neuroanatomically well situated to modulate reinforcing responses because it receives DA projections (Groenewegen, 1988) and is a relay between NAc and OFC (Nauta, 1971); however, correlations do not necessarily imply causal relationships, and more studies are required to establish whether the thalamus is involved with drug reinforcement.

The cerebellar vermis was the other region that differed between expected and unexpected MP. Unlike thalamic activation, however, the changes in vermis were not associated with the reinforcing effects of MP. Thus it is likely that the cerebellar response may reflect conditioned responses that are not linked with effects that are consciously perceived as rewarding. Animal studies have consistently documented the involvement of the cerebellum (including vermis) in conditioned responses (Supple and Leaton, 1990; Ghelarducci and Sebastiani, 1997; Fischer et al., 2000) and expectancy (Courtemanche et al., 2002). Imaging studies have reported cerebellar activation when cocaine abusers are exposed to cocaine cues, which also reflect a conditioned response (Grant et al., 1996).

It is notable that the opposite pattern was observed in left lateral OFC, where unexpected MP produced greater increases than expected MP. This effect is consistent with the recent literature on the impact of unexpected rewards on OFC (Schultz et al., 2000; Berns et al., 2001). In this study we were unable to show greater activation of OFC by expectation alone, which we reasoned was attributable to the poor temporal resolution of PET–FDG.

These results replicate previous findings showing that the reinforcing effects of drugs of abuse are greater when they are expected than when they are not (Kirk et al., 1998). The extent to which expectation affects natural reinforcers differently from drugs of abuse merits further investigation.

Study Limitations

Brain metabolic responses measured with PET–FDG reflect activity occurring over 30 min. Thus the short-lived duration of some of the behavioral effects were likely lost amid the metabolic responses. fMRI would have provided a better assessment of time course for the various drug effects; however, PET has the advantage of providing a measure that reflects absolute changes in activity.

Here we used MP instead of cocaine because its longer pharmacokinetics properties were advantageous for PET–FDG studies. However, subjects were told that the effects of MP would be very similar to those of cocaine, so it is possible that the effects of expectation may have been even stronger if they expected cocaine.

Metabolic measures are indirect measures of drug effects, and thus we cannot determine the extent to which the effects of expectation reflect an amplification of the effects of MP on DA and NE.

Summary

This study provides evidence that reinforcing effects of drugs of abuse are not just a function of their pharmacological effects but also of expectation of their effects. We documented an enhancement of MP-induced increases in thalamic and cerebellar metabolism and in its reinforcing effects when MP was expected versus when it was not. The thalamic activation with MP was associated with the subjective experience of "high" and "drug liking," suggesting that it reflects the expectation-induced enhancement of its reinforcing effects. A different pattern was documented for metabolic changes in OFC, which showed larger increases when MP was not expected than when it was expected, corroborating its role in unexpected reward.

REFERENCES

Bendriem B, Dewey SL, Schlyer DJ, Wolf AP, Volkow ND (1991) Quantitation of the human basal ganglia with positron emission tomography: a phantom study of the effect of contrast and axial positioning. IEEE Trans Med Imaging 10:216–222.

Berns GS, McClure SM, Pagnoni G, Montague PR (2001) Predictability modulates human brain response to reward. J Neurosci 21:2793–2798.

Breiter HC, Gollub RL, Weisskoff RM, et al. (1997) Acute effects of cocaine on human brain activity and emotion. Neuron 19:591–611.

Courtemanche R, Pellerin JP, Lamarre Y (2002) Local field potential oscillations in primate cerebellar cortex: modulation during active and passive expectancy. J Neurophysiol 88:771–782.

Cromwell HC, Schultz W (2003) Effects of expectations for different reward magnitudes on neuronal activity in primate striatum. J Neurophysiol 89:2823–2838.

de la Fuente-Fernández R, Ruth TJ, Sossi V, et al. (2001) Expectation and dopamine release: mechanism of the placebo effect in Parkinson's disease. Science 293:1164–1166.

Devous MD Sr., Trivedi MH, Rush AJ (2001) Regional cerebral blood flow response to oral amphetamine challenge in healthy volunteers. J Nucl Med 42:535–542.

Di Chiara GD, Imperato A (1988) Drugs abused by humans preferentially increase synaptic dopamine concentrations in the mesolimbic system of freely moving rats. Proc Natl Acad Sci USA 85:5274–5278.

Dirckx SG, Risinger RC, Ross TJ, et al. 2003 Comparing iv methylphenidate and cocaine in the human brain using fMRI. 9th International Conference on Functional Mapping of the Human Brain, New York, June.

Duvauchelle CL, Ikegami A, Asami S, et al. (2000) Effects of cocaine context on NAcc dopamine and behavioral activity after repeated intravenous cocaine administration. Brain Res 862:49–58.

Efron B (1982) The jackknife, the bootstrap, and other resampling plans. Philadelphia: Society for Industrial and Applied Mathematics.

Fischer H, Andersson JL, Furmark T, Fredrikson M (2000) Fear conditioning and brain activity: a positron emission tomography study in humans. Behav Neurosci 114:671–680.

Fischman MW, Foltin RW (1991) Utility of subjective-effects measurements in assessing abuse liability of drugs in humans. Br J Addict 86:1563–1570.

Friston KJ, Holmes AP, Worsley K, et al. (1995) Statistical parametric maps in functional brain imaging: a general linear approach. Hum Brain Mapp 2:189–210.

Ghelarducci B, Sebastiani L (1997) Classical heart rate conditioning and affective behavior: the role of the cerebellar vermis. Arch Ital Biol 135:369–384.

Graham J, Porrino LJ (1995) Neuroanatomical substrates of cocaine self-administration. In: Neurobiology of cocaine (Hammer R, ed.), pp. 3–14. Boca Raton, Fla.: CRC.

Grant S, London ED, Newlin DB, et al. (1996) Activation of memory circuits during cue-elicited cocaine craving. Proc Natl Acad Sci USA 93:12040–12045.

Groenewegen HJ (1988) Organization of the afferent connections of the mediodorsal thalamic nucleus in the rat, related to the mediodorsal-prefrontal topography. Neuroscience 24:379–431.

Hemby SE, Co C, Koves TR, Smith JE, Dworkin SI (1997) Differences in extracellular dopamine concentrations in the nucleus accumbens during response-dependent and response-independent cocaine administration in the rat. Psychopharmacology (Berl) 133:7–16.

Hook JC, Wise SP (1995) Distributed modular architecture linking basal ganglia, cerebellum and cerebral cortex: their role in planning and controlling action. Cereb Cortex 2:95–110.

Kirk JM, Doty P, De Wit H (1998) Effects of expectancies on subjective responses to oral delta 9-tetrahydrocannabinol. Pharmacol Biochem Behav 59:287–293.

Knapp CM, Printseva B, Cottam N, Kornetsky C (2002) Effects of cue exposure on brain glucose utilization 8 days after repeated cocaine administration. Brain Res 950:119–126.

Lancaster JL, Woldorff MG, Parsons LM, et al. (2000) Automated Talairach atlas labels for functional brain mapping. Hum Brain Mapp 10:120–131.

London ED, Cascella NG, Wong DF, et al. (1990) Cocaine-induced reduction of glucose utilization in human brain. A study using positron emission tomography and [fluorine18]-fluorodeoxyglucose. Arch Gen Psychiatry 47:567–574.

McAlonan GM, Robbins TW, Everitt BJ (1993) Effects of medial dorsal thalamic and ventral pallidal lesions on the acquisition of a conditioned place preference: further evidence for the involvement of the ventral striatopallidal system in reward-related processes. Neuroscience 52:605–620.

Melchitzky DS, Lewis DA (2000) Tyrosine hydroxylase- and dopamine transporter-immunoreactive axons in the primate cerebellum. Evidence for a lobular- and laminar-specific dopamine innervation. Neuropsychopharmacology 22:466–472.

Miller RG (1974) The jackknife—a review. Biometrika 61:1–15.

Mitchell SH, Laurent CL, De Wit H (1996) Interaction of expectancy and the pharmacological effects of d-amphetamine: subjective effects and self-administration. Psychopharmacology (Berl) 125:371–378.

Nauta WJH (1971) The problem of the frontal lobe: a reinterpretation. J Psychiatric Res 8:167–189.

Patrick KS, Caldwell RW, Ferris RM, Breese GR (1987) Pharmacology of the enantiomers of threo-methylphenidate. J Pharmacol Exp Ther 241:152–158.

Porrino LJ, Lyons D, Miller MD, et al. (2002) Metabolic mapping of the effects of cocaine during the initial phases of self-administration in the nonhuman primate. J Neurosci 22:7687–7694.

Quenouille MH (1956) Notes on bias in estimation. Biometrika 43:353–360.

Rademacher J, Morosan P, Schormann T, et al. (2001) Probabilistic mapping and volume measurement of human primary auditory cortex. NeuroImage 13:669–683.

Reznikoff GA, Manaker S, Rhodes CH, Winokur A, Rainbow TC (1986) Localization and quantification of beta-adrenergic receptors in human brain. Neurology 36:1067–1073.

Robinson TE, Berridge KC (1993) The neural basis of drug craving: an incentive-sensitization theory of addiction. Brain Res Rev 18:247–291.

Schultz W, Tremblay L, Hollerman JR (1998) Reward prediction in primate basal ganglia and frontal cortex. Neuropharmacology 37:421–429.

Schultz W, Tremblay L, Hollerman JR (2000) Reward processing in primate orbitofrontal cortex and basal ganglia. Cereb Cortex 10:272–284.

Schwartz WJ, Smith CB, Davidsen L, et al. (1979) Metabolic mapping of functional activity in the hypothalamo-neurohypophysial system of the rat. Science 205:723–725.

Sokoloff L, Reivich M, Kennedy C, et al. (1977) The ^{14}C-deoxyglucose method for the measurement of local cerebral glucose utilization: theory, procedure and normal values in the conscious and anesthetized albino rat. J Neurochem 28:897–916.

Srinivas NR, Hubbard JW, Quinn D, Korchinski ED, Midha K (1991) Extensive and enantioselective presystemic metabolism of

DL-threo-methylphenidate in humans. Prog Neuropsychopharmacol Biol Psychiatry 15:213–220.

Supple WF Jr., Leaton RN (1990) Lesions of the cerebellar vermis and cerebellar hemispheres: effects on heart rate conditioning in rats. Behav Neurosci 104:934–947.

Volkow ND, Ding Y-S, Fowler JS, et al. (1995) Is methylphenidate like cocaine? Studies on their pharmacokinetics and distribution in human brain. Arch Gen Psychiatry 52:456–463.

Volkow ND, Wang G-J, Gatley SJ, et al. (1996) Temporal relationships between the pharmacokinetics of methylphenidate in the human brain and its behavioral and cardiovascular effects. Psychopharmacology 123:26–33.

Volkow ND, Wang G-J, Fowler JS, et al. (1997a) Effects of methylphenidate on regional brain glucose metabolism in humans: relationship to dopamine D2 receptors. Am J Psychiatry 154:50–55.

Volkow ND, Rosen B, Farde L (1997b) Imaging the living human brain: magnetic resonance imaging and positron emission tomography. Proc Natl Acad Sci USA 94:2787–2788.

Volkow ND, Wang G-J, Fowler JS, et al. (1997c) Decreased striatal dopaminergic responsiveness in detoxified cocaine-dependent subjects. Nature 386:830–833.

Volkow ND, Wang G-J, Fowler JS, et al. (1999a) Methylphenidate and cocaine have a similar in vivo potency to block dopamine transporters in the human brain. Life Sci 65:7–12.

Volkow ND, Wang G-J, Fowler JS, et al. (1999b) Association of methylphenidate-induced craving with changes in right striato-orbitofrontal metabolism in cocaine abusers: implications in addiction. Am J Psychiatry 156:19–26.

Wang G-J, Volkow ND, Roque CT, et al. (1992) Functional significance of ventricular enlargement and cortical atrophy in normals and alcoholics as assessed by PET, MRI and neuropsychological testing. Radiology 186:59–65.

Wang G-J, Volkow ND, Hitzemann RJ, et al. (1997) Behavioral and cardiovascular effects of intravenous methylphenidate in normal subjects and cocaine abusers. Eur Addiction Res 3:49–54.

SECTION D. CONTEXTUAL FACTORS

32

Do Double-Blind Studies with Informed Consent Yield Externally Valid Results?

An Empirical Test

IRVING KIRSCH AND MICHAEL J. ROSADINO

Irving Kirsch and Michael J. Rosadino, "Do Double-Blind Studies with Informed Consent Yield Externally Valid Results? An Empirical Test," Psychopharmacology 1993;110:437–442.

The 1970s occasioned two important changes in biomedical research. One was the acceptance of double-blind, placebo-controlled trials as a prerequisite for the approval of new drugs (Rickels 1986). The second was the adoption of informed consent as an ethical standard in biomedical and psychological research (Faden and Beauchamp 1986). Because of the requirement of informed consent, subjects are told that they may be given a placebo and that neither they nor the experimenter will know which group they are in until the conclusion of the study.

Informing subjects that they may be given a placebo produces a cognitive set that is different from that of people who are ingesting drugs in nonexperimental settings. When people are given medication by a physician in clinical contexts, they are not told that the drug may be a placebo. Similarly, when they ingest drugs for recreational or social purposes, in most instances they have no reason to suspect that the agent they are ingesting might be a placebo. That informed consent is standard in drug evaluations implies a tacit assumption that this difference in cognitive set does not affect drug-placebo comparisons. The purpose of this study was to investigate whether this assumption is warranted.

Reasons for doubting the generalizability of double-blind studies with informed consent are suggested by the results of a study reported by Kirsch and Weixel (1988). Subjects in that study were given different apparent doses of a placebo (decaffeinated coffee) with different instructions about the content of the beverage they were ingesting. Half of the subjects were told that the coffee was caffeinated (deceptive instructions); the others were told that it might or might not be caffeinated (double-blind instructions). A theoretically predicted curvilinear effect on systolic blood pressure, alertness, tension, and certainty of having consumed caffeine was confirmed with deceptive instructions, but not with double-blind instructions, which produced curves in the opposite direction on each of these variables.

As noted by Kirsch and Weixel (1988), these data do not establish that double-blind comparisons with informed consent lack external validity. It is possible that the psychological and pharmacological effects of drug administration are additive, so that differences between drug and placebo are preserved as long as the same instructions are given to each group. Conversely, because of the surprising and unexplained effects of double-blind instructions, Kirsch and Weixel (1988) suggested that additivity be assessed rather than assumed. If psychological and pharmacological effects of drug administration are interactive, then double-blind studies may lead to spurious conclusions about the chemical effects of particular drugs in most non-research settings.

Instruction by drug interactions has been reported in studies of an appetite-depressing drug (phenmetrazine; Penick and Hinkle 1964) and epinephrine (Penick and Fisher 1965), although the instructional manipulations in those studies were different from those under consideration here. An instruction by drug interaction was also reported in an assessment of the effects of nicotine gum (Hughes et al. 1989). Subjects were given nicotine gum or placebo and were told that they were receiving nicotine, told that they were receiving placebo, or not told which gum they were receiving. Nicotine significantly increased abstinence among subjects given double-blind instructions, but not among subjects in the told nicotine or told placebo conditions.

The Hughes et al. (1989) study combined traditional double-blind methodology with the balanced placebo design described by Marlatt and Rohsenow (1980). In the balanced placebo design, an attempt is made to alter the cognitive set induced by informed consent. After consent is obtained for participation in a study in which some subjects will receive a placebo and others will receive the active drug, half of the subjects are told that they have been assigned to the active drug condition and half are told that they have been assigned to the control group. This information is veridical for half of the subjects and deceptive for the others. Thus, there are four groups in which subjects are (a) told they will receive the drug and in fact receive the drug, (b) told that they will receive the drug and are given a placebo, (c) told they will not receive the drug and are given the drug surreptitiously, or (d) told they will not receive the drug and are not given the drug. At the conclusion of the study, all subjects are debriefed with accurate information about the design of the study. The drug by instruction interaction reported by Hughes et al. (1989) suggests that these two experimental designs can lead to different conclusions about drug effectiveness.

In this study, we used the experimental design of the Hughes et al. (1989) study in a test of the effects of caffeine on mood, pulse rate, and blood pressure. The purpose of the study was to determine whether interactions similar to those found with nicotine could be found with another drug, since interactive effects of this sort challenge the validity of current methods of drug assessment.

Materials and Methods

Subjects

Subjects were 37 male and 63 female undergraduate students between 18 and 40 years of age (M = 19.52, SD = 2.39), who volunteered for participation in exchange for partial course credit in an introductory psychology class at the University of Connecticut. Participation was limited to students who reported compliance with a request to refrain from consuming caffeine for 24 h prior to the experimental session and who indicated an absence of heart disorders, hypertension, or anxiety-related disorders in themselves or their immediate families. Two potential subjects were excluded from participation. One was excluded after reporting caffeine consumption within 24 h of the experimental session, and the other was excluded because her arm was too large for the blood pressure assessment device.

Subjects were grouped into blocks of six subjects each and within each block were assigned randomly to experimental conditions. This resulted in six groups with nearly equal ns (16 or 17 subjects per group), with similar proportions of males and females and no significant differences in age.

Experimental Manipulations

INFORMED DOUBLE-BLIND CONDITIONS

Subjects in informed double-blind groups were shown two cans of ground coffee, one of which was labeled X and the other labeled Y. They were told that the coffee in only one of the cans was decaffeinated, and the container from which their coffee was brewed was determined by the last digit of their social security number. In fact, both cans contained decaffeinated coffee, but 300 mg caffeine citrate (150 mg caffeine) had previously been added to half of the cups into which the coffee was brewed.

BALANCED PLACEBO CONDITIONS

Subjects in the balanced placebo conditions were shown two cans of ground coffee, one of which was a commercial decaffeinated coffee can and the other a regular (not decaffeinated) commercial coffee can. They were told that they were assigned to the caffeine or no-caffeine group on the basis of the last digit of their social security number. For subjects in the Told Drug groups, coffee from the regular coffee can was brewed. For subjects in the Told Placebo groups, coffee from the decaffeinated coffee can was brewed. In fact, both cans contained decaffeinated coffee, but 300 mg caffeine citrate had previously been added to half of the cups into which the coffee was brewed.

Procedure

Subjects were tested between the hours of 8 a.m. and 5 p.m. Each subject was seen by two experimenters, neither of whom knew which beverages contained caffeine. The first experimenter asked subjects whether they had consumed coffee, tea, or chocolate in the 24 h prior to the session, and excused those who indicated that they had. He then administered the medical screening questionnaire, obtained informed consent, and asked subjects to complete baseline self-report measures of alertness and tension. In the consent form, subjects were informed that the purpose of the study was to determine various physiological and psychological effects of caffeine consumption, and that depending on group assignment they might or might not receive caffeine. Subjects were not told that they might be deceived.

Subjects were then escorted to a second room, to which they were accommodated by spending 5 min seated, reading a magazine prior to the initial physiological assessment. The room was a typical graduate student office in a university psychology department. Following the accommodation period, the second experimenter assessed baseline blood pressure and pulse rate, provided subjects with information or misinformation concerning the contents of the beverage, administered the beverage, and collected all subsequent physiological and self-report data. Subjects consumed a 12-oz cup of brewed, black, unsweetened, decaffeinated coffee over a 10 min period. Three scoops of coffee were used in brewing the beverage, and subjects were misinformed that this produced a beverage that was equivalent of three cups of coffee. This method of brewing produced a very strong flavor which disguised the flavor of the caffeine citrate.

Prior to the experimental session, 300 mg caffeine citrate (150 mg caffeine, equivalent to the average caffeine content of 1.5 cups of coffee) had been placed in half of the cups by a third experimenter, who also coded the bottom of the cups so that actual beverage content could later be determined. Blood pressure, pulse rate, alertness and tension were reassessed at 15, 30, and 45 min after ingestion. Subjects remained seated and read newspapers or magazines between assessments. After all other measures had been taken, subjects were asked to estimate the likelihood that the coffee they had consumed contained caffeine.

Measures

Physiological responses (blood pressure and pulse rate) were assessed on a Timex Healthcheck digital blood monitor. *Subjective mood* was assessed by asking subjects to rate the degree to which each of 15 adjectives described their current state on scales ranging from zero to ten. From these ratings, scores on the Alertness and Tension subscales developed by Kirsch and Weixel (1988) were calculated by summing the responses and dividing by the number of items in the subscale. Thus, both scales yielded scores with a potential range of zero to ten. Kirsch and Weixel reported high levels of internal reliability for each scale, and both have been shown to detect instruction-induced changes in mood (Kirsch and Weixel 1988; Fillmore and Vogel-Sprott 1992). *Likelihood that the coffee they had consumed contained caffeine* was assessed on a 7-point scale with the anchors: certainly decaffeinated, probably decaffeinated, possibly decaffeinated, do not know, possibly caffeinated, probably caffeinated, and certainly caffeinated. For ease of interpretation, these responses were then transformed into the following probabilities: 0, 0.17, 0.33, 0.50, 0.67, 0.83, and 1.00, respectively. At the conclusion of the study, subjects were debriefed as to the full design of the study and the condition to which they had been assigned.

Results

Subjects reported consuming a mean of 3.40 (SD = 2.22) cups of caffeinated coffee per day and a mean of 3.41 (SD = 2.69) daily servings of other caffeinated products (e.g., soda, tea, chocolate). Baseline mood ratings, blood pressure, and pulse rates are reported in Table 32.1. One-way analyses of variance failed to reveal any significance between group differences on baseline scores or on pre-study caffeine consumption.

Due to experimenter error, complete self-report data were not recorded for four subjects and physiological data for one of the assessments were missing for three subjects. An additional three subjects failed to complete all of the items on the alertness scale and three failed to complete all items on the tension scale. For these reasons, analyses were limited to the self-report data of 94 subjects and the physiological data of 97 subjects.

A $3 \times 2 \times 3$ (instructions $\times$ drug $\times$ time) analysis of covariance (ANACOVA), with baseline scores entered as the covariate, was run for each dependent variable except subjects' beliefs about the caffeine content of their beverages, for which a 3×2 (instructions $\times$ drug) analysis of variance (ANOVA) was run. When interactions involving time were found, these were supplemented by separate 3×2 (instructions $\times$ drug) ANACOVAs for each assessment. Post-hoc comparisons of instruction effects and instruction by drug interactions were performed using Tukey tests.

Alertness

Adjusted mean scores on the alertness scale are depicted in Fig. 32.1. The ANACOVA revealed a significant drug by time interaction ($F = 3.30$, $P < 0.04$), which was further analyzed by conducting separate 3×2 (instructions by drug) ANACOVAs for each assessment period. These indicated a significant drug effect only at 30 min after ingestion ($F = 4.07$, $P < 0.05$) and a significant instruction effect only at 15 min after ingestion, ($F = 4.77$, $P < 0.01$). Post-hoc analyses indicated that at 15 min after ingestion, subjects who had been told they were not receiving caffeine reported being significantly less alert than those who were told they were receiving caffeine ($P < 0.01$) or those who were given double-blind instructions ($P < 0.05$).

Tension

Adjusted mean scores on the tension scale are depicted in Fig. 32.2. The ANACOVA revealed a significant drug effect ($F = 5.16$, $P < 0.03$) and a significant drug by instruction interaction ($F = 3.65$, $P < 0.03$). A Tukey test revealed that subjects who were told they would receive caffeine and in fact did receive caffeine reported significantly greater tension than subjects in any of the other groups ($P < 0.01$).

Table 32.1.
Baseline mood ratings, blood pressure, and pulse

Caffeine		Alertness		Tension		Systolic BP mmHg		Diastolic BP mmHg		Pulse	
Told	Receive	Mean	SD	Mean	SD	Mean	SD	Mean	SD	Mean	SD
No	No	5.79	2.16	1.71	1.78	117.41	15.26	67.65	12.41	69.88	21.38
No	Yes	5.88	1.69	1.44	1.37	111.88	15.28	66.76	9.12	72.88	14.67
Yes	No	4.96	1.66	2.16	2.44	113.70	14.48	68.58	11.36	68.82	16.50
Yes	Yes	5.65	1.49	1.49	1.62	110.65	9.87	70.82	10.74	75.94	9.32
Maybe	No	5.61	2.01	1.03	0.86	110.87	13.80	70.70	15.75	62.19	16.08
Maybe	Yes	5.84	1.84	2.09	2.04	110.86	14.56	66.46	17.82	73.27	13.67

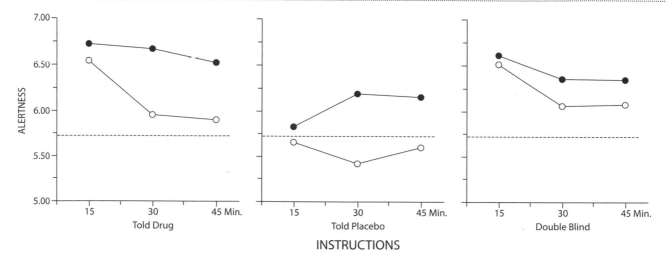

Figure. 32.1. Adjusted mean alertness scores at 15, 30, and 45 min after ingestion of caffeine or placebo. (—●—) Received drug; (—○—) received placebo; (- - -) baseline.

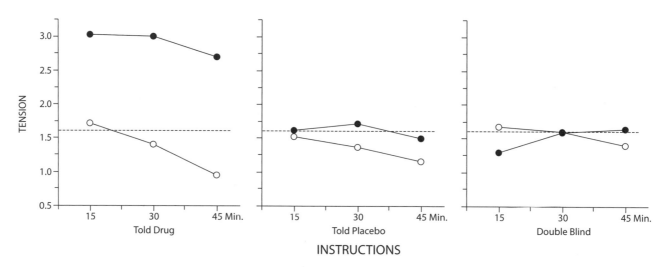

Figure. 32.2. Adjusted mean tension scores at 15, 30, and 45 min after ingestion of caffeine or placebo. For symbols, see legend of Fig. 32.1.

Systolic Blood Pressure

Adjusted mean systolic blood pressure scores are depicted in Fig. 32.3. The ANACOVA revealed a significant drug effect ($F = 10.46$, $P < 0.01$) and a significant drug by time interaction ($F = 3.85$, $P < 0.03$). Separate ANACOVAs for each assessment period indicated that the effect of caffeine on systolic blood pressure was significant at 30 min ($F = 9.75$, $P < 0.001$) and 45 min ($F = 14.35$, $P < 0.001$), but not at 15 min after ingestion.

Diastolic Blood Pressure

Adjusted mean diastolic blood pressure scores are depicted in Fig. 32.4. The ANACOVA revealed a significant instruction effect ($F = 3.66$, $P < 0.03$). Post-hoc tests revealed that subjects given double-blind instruction had significantly lower diastolic blood pressure than subjects who had either been informed or misinformed about the content of their beverages ($P < 0.05$).

Pulse

Adjusted mean pulse rates are depicted in Fig. 32.5. The ANACOVA did not reveal any significant main effects or interactions.

Subjects' Beliefs about Their Beverages

Subjects' ratings of the likelihood that their beverages contained caffeine are reported in Table 32.2. The ANOVA revealed a significant drug effect ($F = 9.12$, $P < 0.01$) and a significant instruction effect ($F = 9.29$, $P < 0.001$). A Tukey test indicated that the presence of caffeine was reliably discriminated only by subjects who had been given double-blind instructions.

Discussion

Significant increases in self-reported alertness have been reported as a function of both caffeine (Lane 1983; Lane and Williams 1987) and placebo (Kirsch and Weixel 1988; Fill-

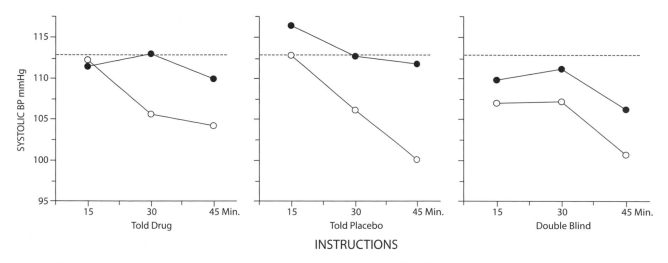

Figure. 32.3. Adjusted mean systolic blood pressure at 15, 30, and 45 min after ingestion of caffeine or placebo. For symbols, see legend of Fig. 32.1.

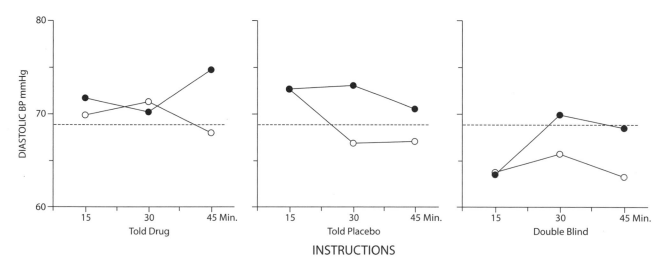

Figure. 32.4. Adjusted mean diastolic blood pressure at 15, 30, and 45 min after ingestion of caffeine or placebo. For symbols, see legend of Fig. 32.1.

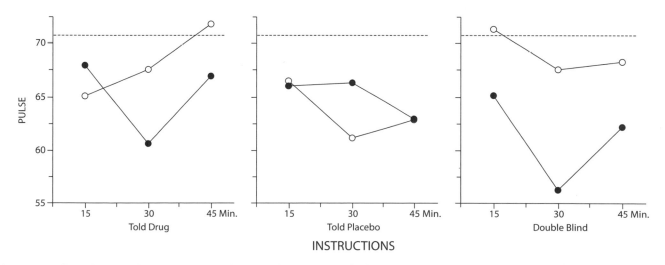

Figure. 32.5. Adjusted mean pulse rate at 15, 30, and 45 min after ingestion of caffeine or placebo. For symbols, see legend of Fig. 32.1.

Table 32.2.
Subjects' ratings of the likelihood that their beverages contained caffeine

Told caffeine	Receive caffeine	Mean	SD
No	No	0.33[b]	0.28
No	Yes	0.37[b]	0.32
Yes	No	0.59[a]	0.30
Yes	Yes	0.72[a]	0.22
Maybe	No	0.32[b]	0.29
Maybe	Yes	0.67[a]	0.30

Note: means sharing a common superscript do not differ significantly ($P < 0.05$).

more and Vogel-Sprott 1992). Our data replicate both effects. At 15 min after ingestion, subjects in the double-blind and told caffeine groups showed a small but significant increase in alertness relative to those in the told placebo groups. At 30 min after ingestion, subjects given caffeine reported slightly but significantly greater alertness than those whose beverages did not contain caffeine.

Increases in systolic and diastolic blood pressure have been reported following caffeine administration in double-blind studies (Robertson et al. 1978; Lane 1983; Lane and Williams 1987). We replicated the effect of caffeine on systolic blood pressure, but not on diastolic blood pressure. Robertson et al. (1978) also reported a decrease in heart rate at 30 and 45 min after ingestion, followed by an increase in heart rate. Consistent with the results reported by Lane (1983) and Lane and Williams (1987), we failed to replicate this effect. Note, however, that Robertson et al. (1978) reported peak effects of caffeine at 60 min after ingestion, whereas our last data were collected 45 min after ingestion.

The primary purpose of this study was to test the generalizability of standard double-blind methods, which would be challenged by significant drug by instruction interactions. A significant drug by instruction interaction was found for self-reported tension. Significant increases in tension were reported only by subjects who knowingly received caffeine. Consistent with previous double-blind research (Lane 1983), caffeine did not affect tension significantly among subjects given double-blind instructions.

The drug by instruction interaction on self-reported tension is consistent with Schachter and Singer's (1962) two factor theory of emotional states (also see Reinsenzein 1983). From this perspective, one can hypothesize that subjects receiving caffeine had detected some changes in arousal, but that these were interpreted as tension or irritability only when environmental cues unambiguously indicated that caffeine had been consumed. It is important to note that this is not a placebo effect, because instructions alone did not produce an increase in tension. Rather, it is a drug effect that is potentiated by knowledge of drug content. Effects of this sort suggest that current double-blind methods may fail to detect some genuine drug effects.

Both the design and the results of our study are similar to those of Hughes et al.'s (1989) study of the effect of nicotine gum, in that instructions and drugs produced additive effects on some variables and interactive effects on others. These data raise a number of questions: How extensive are interactive effects? With what drugs and on what responses can they be found? Why are drug effects and expectancy effects additive in some instances and interactive in others?

Answers to these questions have practical as well as theoretical importance. When different instructional sets yield differences in drug-placebo comparisons, on which results should decisions about drug use be based? When people consume coffee in real-life settings, they are generally aware of whether the coffee is caffeinated. Similarly, in clinical settings, medication is prescribed without any suggestion that it might be a placebo. Thus, comparisons involving subjects in the Told Drug condition of the balanced placebo design may provide the best indication of how people will respond in most non-research contexts. However, drugs are routinely tested with subjects knowing that they may be receiving a placebo. Therefore, the drug by instruction interactions reported by Hughes et al. (1989) and in this study constitute a challenge to the external validity of current double-blind methods.

It should be noted that double-blind and balanced placebo conditions differed in more than just verbal instructions. Subjects in the balanced placebo conditions were shown commercially labeled coffee cans, whereas those in double-blind groups were shown cans that were not commercially labeled. We do not know whether this had any impact apart from the accompanying verbal instructions. However, this is another respect in which balanced placebo methods provide a closer approximation to non-experimental settings in which caffeine is consumed. Our data suggest that greater attention to mimicking non-research conditions in drug research is warranted, a conclusion that is also supported by a recent study in which the setting in which a balanced placebo alcohol study was conducted (laboratory versus barroom) affected its outcome (Wigmore and Hinson 1991).

The addition of behavioral performance measures are warranted in future studies. Their use is complicated, however, by the presence of individual differences in beliefs about the effects of caffeine. Although some believe that it enhances performance, others expect it to degrade their performance on various behavioral tasks, and these beliefs alter the direction of the placebo effect on these responses (Kirsch and Weixel 1988; Fillmore and Vogel-Sprott 1992). Therefore, in assessing the interaction of caffeine and instructions on behavioral responses, it would be important to manipulate and/or evaluate subjects' beliefs.

REFERENCES

Faden RR, Beauchamp TL (1986) A history and theory of informed consent. Oxford University Press, New York.

Fillmore M, Vogel-Sprott M (1992) Expected effect of caffeine on motor performance predicts the type of response to placebo. Psychopharmacology 106: 209–214.

Hughes JR, Gulliver SB, Amori G, Mireault GC, Fenwick JF (1989) Effect of instructions and nicotine on smoking cessation, withdrawal symptoms and self-administration of nicotine gum. Psychopharmacology 99: 486–491.

Kirsch I, Weixel LJ (1988) Double-blind versus deceptive administration of a placebo. Behav Neurosci 102: 319–323.

Lane JD (1983) Caffeine and cardiovascular responses to stress. Psychosom Med 45: 447–451.

Lane JD, Williams RB (1987) Cardiovascular effects of caffeine and stress in regular coffee drinkers. Psychophysiology 24: 157–164.

Marlatt GA, Rohsenow DJ (1980) Cognitive processes in alcohol use: Expectancy and the balanced placebo design. In: Mello NK (ed.) Advances in substance abuse: behavioral and biological research. JAI Press, Greenwich, Conn., pp. 159–199.

Penick SB, Fisher S (1965) Drug-set interaction: Psychological and physiological effects of epinephrine under differential expectations. Psychosom Med 27: 177–182.

Penick SB, Hinkle LE (1964) The effect of expectation on response to phenmetrazine. Psychosom Med 26: 369–373.

Reinsenzein R (1983). The Schachter theory of emotion: two decades later. Psychol Bull 94: 239–264.

Rickels K (1986) Use of placebo in clinical trials. Psychopharmacol Bull 22: 19–24.

Robertson D, Frölich JC, Carr RK, et al. (1978) Effects of caffeine on plasma renin activity, catecholamines and blood pressure. N Engl J Med 298: 181–186.

Schachter S, Singer J (1962) Cognitive, social and physiological determinants of emotional state. Psychol Rev 69: 379–399.

Wigmore ST, Hinson RE (1991) The influence of setting on consumption in the balanced placebo design. Br J Addict 86: 205–215.

33

Response Expectancies in Placebo Analgesia and Their Clinical Relevance

ANTONELLA POLLO, MARTINA AMANZIO, ANNA ARSLANIAN, CATERINA CASADIO, GIULIANO MAGGI, AND FABRIZIO BENEDETTI

Antonella Pollo, Martina Amanzio, Anna Arslanian, Caterina Casadio, Giuliano Maggi, and Fabrizio Benedetti, "Response Expectancies in Placebo Analgesia and Their Clinical Relevance," Pain 2001;93:77–84.

1. Introduction

Several theories have been proposed to explain the placebo effect, and many of them are concerned with pain. The anxiety theory states that placebo analgesia is due to a reduction of anxiety (McGlashan et al., 1969; Evans, 1977). The conditioning theory assumes that the placebo effect is a conditioned response due to repeated associations between a conditioned stimulus (e.g. shape and colour of aspirin pills) and an unconditioned stimulus (the active substance of aspirin) (Gleidman et al., 1957; Herrnstein, 1962; Wickramasekera, 1980; Siegel, 1985; Voudouris et al., 1989, 1990; Ader, 1997). The cognitive theory proposes that expectations and beliefs of analgesia play an essential role (Bootzin, 1985; Kirsch, 1985, 1990; Montgomery and Kirsch, 1997; Price and Fields, 1997; Price et al., 1999), and the response-appropriate sensa-

tion hypothesis states that the global experience of pain results from a complex analysis of different brain states (Wall, 1993). These theories are not necessarily in conflict because each of them may represent a different aspect of the same phenomenon (Wall, 1992). In addition, many studies show that different placebo effects can be mediated by different mechanisms, like conditioning or expectation (Amanzio and Benedetti, 1999; Benedetti et al., 1999a,b; Price, 2000).

One of the most interesting mechanisms underlying the placebo effect is represented by response expectancies, that is, those expectations which an individual holds about his/ her emotional and physiological responses, such as anxiety and mood (Kirsch, 1985, 1990). These response expectancies appear to be space specific for they can be specifically obtained in different parts of the body (Montgomery and Kirsch, 1996; Benedetti et al., 1999b; Price et al., 1999). Interestingly, Kirsch and Weixel (1988) found that differences between double-blind and deceptive administration of placebos can produce different outcomes, and concluded that this is due to the different experimental designs which in turn produce different expectancies. In that study, coffee and decaffeinated coffee were administered following different verbal instructions. In one case, they were given according to the usual double-blind paradigm, in the other case decaffeinated coffee was deceptively presented as real coffee. The authors proposed that the deceptive administration would produce stronger effects than the double-blind protocol because in the double-blind administration expectations are uncertain. In fact, in the double-blind protocol the subject does not know whether the active substance or a placebo is being administered.

Taking into account all these considerations, we wanted to study the role of response expectancies in the clinical pharmacological setting, in order to compare placebo analgesia obtained through the classic double-blind design with placebo analgesia produced by the deceptive administration of a placebo.

2. Methods

A total of 38 patients participated in the study after they gave their informed consent to receive either a painkiller or a placebo and after approval by our local ethics committee. They underwent thoracic surgery for lung cancer and did not have any health problem other than those tightly related to the neoplasm. All patients with renal, hepatic, cardiovascular and metabolic problems had previously been excluded from the study. The operation was a standard posterolateral thoracotomy with the resection of at least three of the following muscles: latissimus dorsi, serratus anterior, trapezius and rhomboid. Anaesthesia was induced in all cases with fentanyl 150–250 mg i.v. and maintained with a combination of isoflurane and oxygen. Paralysis was achieved by means of atracurium 30–60 mg and reversed with 1 mg atropine and 2 mg neostigmine i.v. Ondansetron 4 mg was used as an antiemetic drug. All patients who required additional drugs or blood transfusions were excluded from the study.

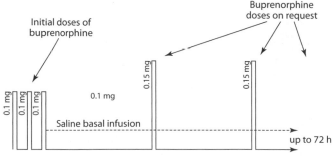

Figure. 33.1. Experimental paradigm and therapeutic protocol. Initial doses and doses on request of buprenorphine represent the real analgesic treatment of the postoperative patients of the present study (bold line). In addition, a basal infusion of saline solution was administered (broken line) by changing its symbolic meaning in three different groups of patients. The placebo analgesic effect was measured by recording the number of doses of buprenorphine for three consecutive days.

One hour after recovery from anaesthesia, the analgesic treatment was started. A first bolus of 0.1 mg of buprenorphine was given in about 3 min. After 15 min a second bolus of 0.1 mg was given with the same infusion time. Finally, a third bolus of 0.1 mg was administered after 15 min with the same infusion time of 3 min. At this point, a basal intravenous infusion of saline solution (NaCl 0.9%, 20 ml/h) was started and continued for three consecutive days. During this period the analgesic treatment was based on buprenorphine on verbal request, in which buprenorphine doses of 0.15 mg were administered when requested by the patients. The drug administrator was completely blind as to the treatment group to which the patient had been assigned. The therapeutic protocol is shown in Fig. 33.1, together with the subdivision of the patients into three groups. These groups differed only for the verbal instructions about the basal infusion.

The first group (Table 33.1) was used to furnish data about the natural history of analgesia. These patients were told nothing about any analgesic effect of the basal infusion. They simply knew that the infusion was a rehydrating solution.

The second group was studied according to the usual double-blind paradigm. The basal infusion was either buprenorphine (0.01 mg/h in NaCl 0.9%) or placebo (only NaCl 0.9%). According to the double-blind administration, these patients were told that the medication could be either a painkiller or a placebo. The double-blind protocol was run by administering buprenorphine to four patients and placebo to the remaining ten. Only the data of these ten patients will be shown (Table 33.1), since the other four were mainly used to allow the double-blind administration.

The patients of the third group received exactly the same double-blind treatment as the second group. However, the double-blind administration was slightly modified as far as the verbal instructions are concerned. In fact, the patients were told that the basal infusion was a powerful painkiller, even though they actually were receiving either buprenorphine or placebo. Therefore, those patients who actually were receiving the placebo were sure that the basal infusion was a painkiller. In this case also, the double-blind paradigm was run by giving buprenorphine to four patients and placebo to the other ten. Only the data of these ten patients will be shown (Table 33.1).

Thus the second and third groups differed for the verbal instructions. In fact, whereas the patients of Group 2 were uncertain about whether they actually were receiving a painkiller or a placebo (classic double-blind design), the patients of Group 3 were certain that a powerful analgesic drug was being administered (deceptive administration for those ten patients who actually were receiving the placebo).

The effects of these different verbal instructions were measured by recording the number of buprenorphine requests during the 3-day analgesic treatment. In addition, the

Table 33.1.
Characteristics of the patients of the three groups, including muscle resection during surgery

		First group (natural history)					Second group (double-blind design)					Third group (deceptive administration)		
Patient	Sex	Age (years)	Weight (kg)	Muscles resected	Patient	Sex	Age (years)	Weight (kg)	Muscles resected	Patient	Sex	Age (years)	Weight (kg)	Muscles resected
A	m	57	64	LD,SA,T	A	m	55	69	LD,SA,R	A	m	57	76	LD,T,R
B	f	58	73	LD,T,R	B	m	67	78	LD,SA,T	B	f	65	78	LD,T,R
C	f	58	54	LD,SA,T	C	f	54	51	LD,T,R	C	m	70	61	LD,SA,R
D	m	65	76	LD,SA,T	D	m	62	73	LD,SA,R	D	m	63	63	LD,SA,T
E	m	66	79	LD,SA,T	E	f	64	58	LD,SA,R	E	m	65	71	LD,SA,T
F	m	60	62	LD,SA,R	F	m	60	75	LD,T,R	F	m	56	67	LD,SA,T
G	f	57	77	LD,SA,R	G	m	65	50	LD,SA,T	G	f	55	64	LD,T,R
H	m	69	56	LD,T,R	H	f	68	70	LD,SA,R	H	m	59	57	LD,SA,R
I	m	63	67	LD,SA,R	I	m	57	60	LD,SA,T	I	f	54	58	LD,SA,T
J	m	60	54	LD,T,R	J	f	55	52	LD,T,R	J	m	60	53	LD,T,R
Mean±SD		61.3±4.22	66.2±9.7				60.7±5.25	63.6±10.64				60.4±5.21	64.8±8.22	

Note: LD, latissimus dorsi; SA, serratus anterior; T, trapezius; R, rhomboid.

patients were told to report their pain every hour according to a numerical rating scale (NRS) ranging from 0 = no pain to 10 = unbearable pain. This pain rating was assessed either by a doctor or by a relative during the night (when the patient was not sleeping) for three consecutive days. Sometimes, on the 2nd and 3rd day, the patient him/herself reported in a diary the NRS. The results were analysed by means of the analysis of variance (ANOVA) followed by the Newman-Keuls test for multiple comparisons. In addition, the data of each patient will be shown.

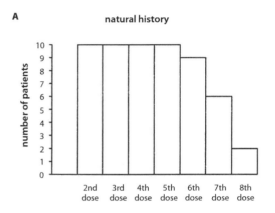

A natural history

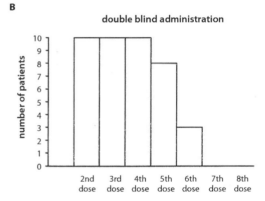

B double blind administration

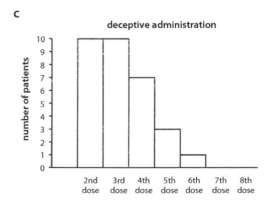

C deceptive administration

Figure. 33.2. Number of patients who requested different doses of buprenorphine. (**A**) Patients who did not receive any particular information about the saline basal infusion. They only knew it was a rehydrating solution. (**B**) Patients who underwent the classic double-blind administration of the saline basal infusion. They knew it could be either a painkiller or a placebo (**C**) Patients who received the deceptive administration of the saline basal infusion. They believed it was a painkiller.

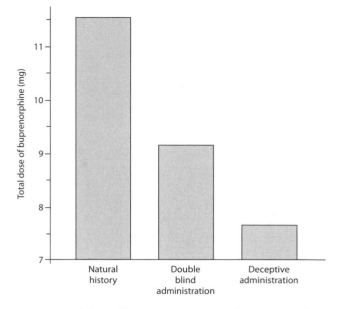

Figure. 33.3. Total dose of buprenorphine received at the end of the 3-day analgesic treatment in the three groups of patients. The three different verbal instructions about the saline basal infusion produced different buprenorphine intake.

3. Results

The three groups of patients did not differ for sex, age ($F_{(2,27)} = 0:09$, $P = 0.917$), weight ($F_{(2,27)} = 0:18$, $P = 0.832$) and type of surgery, as shown in Table 33.1. The number of buprenorphine doses received by the patients of the three groups during the 3-day treatment differed considerably, as shown in Fig. 33.2. It can be seen that there was a reduction of the doses of buprenorphine with the double-blind administration of the basal infusion compared to the natural history. This reduction was even larger with the deceptive administration of the basal infusion. Overall, the total dose of buprenorphine received at the end of the 3-day treatment was 11.55 mg in the natural history group, 9.15 mg in the double-blind group, which is a reduction of 20.8%, and 7.65 mg in the deceptive administration group, which represents a decrease of 33.8% with respect to natural history and of 16.4% compared with double-blind administration (Fig. 33.3).

These differences are statistically significant, as shown by the data of each patient in Table 33.2. Whereas the mean dose of buprenorphine received by the first group at the end of the three days was 1.15 ± 0.14 mg, the second group received a mean dose of 0.91 ± 0.11 mg and the third group 0.76 ± 0.15 mg ($F_{(2,27)} = 21.42$, $P < 0.001$). The Newman-Keuls test showed that the first group differed from the second ($q = 5.646$, $P < 0:01$), the second from the third ($q = 3.529$, $P < 0.01$), and the first from the third ($q = 9.175$, $P < 0:01$). Table 33.2 also shows the number of buprenorphine doses received by each patient.

Overall, the reduction of buprenorphine requests in the second group with respect to the first shows that a placebo analgesic effect of the saline basal infusion occurred. Like-

Table 33.2.

Number of doses and total dose of buprenorphine received at the end of the analgesic treatment for each patient

First group (natural history)			Second group (double-blind)			Third group (deceptive administration)		
Patient	Number of doses	Total dose (mg)	Patient	Number of doses	Total dose (mg)	Patient	Number of doses	Total dose (mg)
A	7	1.2	A	6	1.05	A	6	1.05
B	6	1.05	B	6	1.05	B	5	0.9
C	6	1.05	C	5	0.9	C	4	0.75
D	7	1.2	D	5	0.9	D	4	0.75
E	8	1.35	E	6	1.05	E	3	0.6
F	7	1.2	F	5	0.9	F	3	0.6
G	7	1.2	G	4	0.75	G	4	0.75
H	6	1.05	H	5	0.9	H	3	0.6
I	5	0.9	I	5	0.9	I	4	0.75
J	8	1.35	J	4	0.75	J	5	0.9
Mean±SD	6.7±0.95	1.15±0.14		5.1±0.74	0.91±0.11		4.1±0.99	0.76±0.15

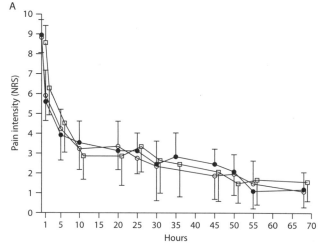

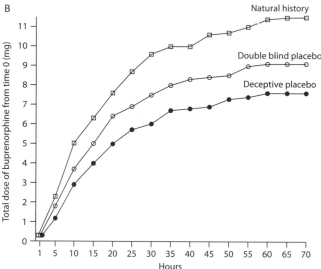

Figure. 33.4. Time course of pain (**A**) and total amount of buprenorphine received (**B**) in the three groups of patients. Empty squares: natural history. Empty circles: patients who received the placebo with the classic double-blind design. Black circles: patients who received the deceptive administration of the placebo. In (**A**) the missing circles mean that NRS could not be recorded because most of the patients were sleeping. In (**B**) each measure represents the total dose from time 0; therefore, the last measures on the right indicate the total doses at the end of the treatment. Note that the same analgesic effect (**A**) was obtained with different doses of buprenorphine (**B**).

wise, the larger reduction of buprenorphine requests in the third group relative to the second indicates that the placebo analgesic response was stronger in the former. This is also shown in Fig. 33.4, where it can be seen that the time course of pain was the same in the three groups of patients (A) in spite of the different doses of buprenorphine administered (B). In other words, the same analgesic effect was obtained with significantly different doses of buprenorphine, indicating that the larger the reduction of buprenorphine requests, the stronger the placebo analgesic effect.

We also considered the possibility that the patients of the second and third groups could have requested less doses of buprenorphine because they felt reassured by the supposed long-lasting effect of the continuous basal infusion. By contrast, the patients of the first group could have requested more buprenorphine doses simply because they were afraid of remaining without any painkiller, for example, during the night. If this was true, there should be differences between the three groups in pain rating at the time of the buprenorphine requests. However, that this was not the case is shown in detail in Table 33.3. It can be seen that there were no differences between the patients of the three groups (above), since in each case buprenorphine was requested when the NRS was around 4.5–5 (no statistically significant differences are present). Likewise, we found no significant differences when pain intensity was analysed for each buprenorphine dose request (Table 33.3). In addition, there were no differences in evening requests in the three groups. Thus the three groups showed exactly the same pain threshold for buprenorphine request, indicating that the request was triggered by the intensity of pain.

4. Discussion

The present study shows that different verbal instructions produced different outcomes, which, in turn, led to a significant change of behaviour and a significant reduction of opioid intake. In fact, the reduction of buprenorphine requests in the double-blind group was as large as 20.8% compared to the natural history group, and the reduction in the deceptive administration group was even larger, reaching

Table 33.3.
Mean pain intensity (NRS)±standard deviation at which buprenorphine was requested, in each patient (above) and for each dose (below)

First group (natural history)		Second group (double-blind)		Third group (deceptive administration)	
Patient	Pain intensity at which buprenorphine was requested (NRS)	Patient	Pain intensity at which buprenorphine was requested (NRS)	Patient	Pain intensity at which buprenorphine was requested (NRS)
A	5.4±0.65	A	5.1±0.48	A	5.38±1.25
B	4.7±0.67	B	4.72±1.02	B	5.5±0.71
C	4.7±0.67	C	5.45±0.88	C	5.17±1.04
D	4.42±0.97	D	5.28±1.05	D	5.1±0.42
E	5.33±1.47	E	5.17±0.96	E	5.17±1.04
F	5.08±0.58	F	4.9±0.75	F	5.5±0.71
G	5.5±1.46	G	5.1±0.9	G	4.5±0.71
H	5.17±0.88	H	5.3±1.1	H	4.9±1.24
I	5.25±1.04	I	4.62±1.12	I	5.1±0.74
J	4.9±0.65	J	5.23±0.87	J	5.1±0.82
First group (natural history)		Second group (double-blind)		Third group (deceptive administration)	
Dose	Pain intensity at which buprenorphine was requested (NRS)	Dose	Pain intensity at which buprenorphine was requested (NRS)	Dose	Pain intensity at which buprenorphine was requested (NRS)
2nd	5.65±0.67 (10 patients)	2nd	5.35±0.55 (10 patients)	2nd	5.65±0.47 (10 patients)
3rd	4.8±0.63 (10 patients)	3rd	5.1±0.7 (10 patients)	3rd	5.4±0.88 (10 patients)
4th	5.55±1.34 (10 patients)	4th	5.28±1.12 (10 patients)	4th	5.13±0.95 (7 patients)
5th	4.8±0.95 (10 patients)	5th	4.81±0.96 (8 patients)	5th	4.5±0.45 (3 patients)
6th	4.56±0.58 (9 patients)	6th	4.65±0.73 (3 patients)	6th	4.25±0.29 (1 patient)
7th	4.5±0.78 (6 patients)				
8th	4.3±0.56 (2 patients)				

Note: Therefore, the value of each patient is the mean of different doses, whereas the value for each dose is the mean of different patients.

33.8%. Despite this dose reduction of buprenorphine, the time course of pain was the same in the three groups over the 3-day period of treatment. This indicates that a strong placebo effect occurred, and that this was stronger in the deceptive administration group compared to the double-blind group.

We decided to measure the placebo effect in this way for ethical reasons. In fact, a procedure of this sort is not unethical for at least three reasons. First, the analgesic treatment with buprenorphine on request was exactly the same in the three groups of patients, and this therapeutic protocol is common practice in our ward. Second, the time course of pain was the same in all the three groups, so that analgesia was not reduced in any way. Third, we ran double-blind administrations after informed consent was obtained, so that the patients knew that they could receive either a painkiller or a placebo.

It is important to stress that the reduction of the requests of buprenorphine was due to a real analgesic placebo effect. In fact, the two placebo-treated groups could have requested fewer doses of buprenorphine because of factors which have nothing to do with pain intensity. We considered this possibility at the beginning of the study by recording the pain intensity every hour in order to see whether a true analgesic effect was present. For example, the placebo-treated patients were certainly more reassured than the natural history group, simply because the basal infusion made them confident of a continuous and constant analgesia. However, we ruled out the possibility that differences of this sort were present in the three groups. As shown in Fig. 33.4A, the analgesic effect was the same in the three groups and the pain thresholds for buprenorphine request were alike as well (Table 33.3). This indicates that the real trigger for the request of buprenorphine was pain intensity and not other factors, such as anxiety. All these data suggest that analgesia was the same in the three groups of patients.

The most interesting finding of the present study is concerned with the different outcomes obtained with the different experimental protocols. In a demonstration of the importance of response expectancies, Kirsch and Weixel (1988) compared the usual double-blind administration with a deceptive administration. These authors predicted that the deceptive administration would produce stronger effects than the double-blind administration because the latter induces less certain expectations about the outcome. In the present study we confirm these findings in the clinical pharmacological setting. In fact, our results indicate that the different placebo analgesic responses were due to the different verbal instructions which, in turn, induced different expectations. To be more specific, in the double-blind administration the patients were less certain about whether they actually were receiving a painkilling basal infusion, whereas in the deceptive administration the patients strongly believed that they were receiving an analgesic long-lasting basal infusion.

These findings are in agreement with those reported by the expectancy theorists, in particular by Kirsch and colleagues (Kirsch, 1985; Kirsch and Weixel, 1988; Wickless and Kirsch, 1989; Kirsch, 1990; Montgomery and Kirsch, 1997). Many other studies confirm that expectations about the outcome play a very important role in placebo analgesia (Bootzin, 1985; Gracely et al., 1985; Fields and Price, 1997; Price and Fields, 1997; Amanzio and Benedetti, 1999; Benedetti et al., 1999b; Price et al., 1999; Gracely, 2000; Price, 2000). However, it is worth pointing out that the explanatory mechanisms of response expectancies and conditioning are not mutually exclusive (Price, 2000). The modern interpretation of classical conditioning phenomena considers that conditioning itself leads to the acquisition of expectancies that certain events will follow other events (Rescorla, 1988). In addition, it should be stressed that either one mechanism or the other can be involved in different types of placebo effects. For example, some placebo responses can be explained on the basis of a pure conditioning mechanism (e.g. Siegel, 1985; Ader, 1997; Benedetti et al., 1999a).

It is worth emphasizing once again that the placebo protocol of the present study has important clinical implications. In fact, the use of the placebo basal infusion, and in particular the strong expectations induced by the deceptive administration, produced an important reduction of opioid intake. Therefore, the understanding of the placebo phenomenon and of its conditioning and expectancy mechanisms can also be harnessed to the patient's advantage.

REFERENCES

Ader R. The role of conditioning in pharmacotherapy. In: Harrington A, editor. The placebo effect: an interdisciplinary exploration, Cambridge, Mass.: Harvard University Press, 1997, pp. 138–165.

Amanzio M, Benedetti F. Neuropharmacological dissection of placebo analgesia: expectation-activated opioid systems versus conditioning-activated specific subsystems. J Neurosci 1999;19:484–494.

Benedetti F, Amanzio M, Baldi S, Casadio C, Maggi G. Inducing placebo respiratory depressant responses in humans via opioid receptors. Eur J Neurosci 1999a;11:625–631.

Benedetti F, Arduino C, Amanzio M. Somatotopic activation of opioid systems by target-directed expectations of analgesia. J Neurosci 1999b;19:3639–3648.

Bootzin RR. The role of expectancy in behaviour change. In: White L, Tursky B, Schwartz GE, editors. Placebo: theory, research, and mechanisms, New York: Guilford, 1985, pp. 196–210.

Evans FJ. The placebo control of pain: a paradigm for investigating nonspecific effects in psychotherapy. In: Brady JP, Mendels J, Reiger WR, Orne MT, editors. Psychiatry: areas of promise and advancement, New York: Plenum, 1977, pp. 249–271.

Fields HL, Price DD. Toward a neurobiology of placebo analgesia. In: Harrington A, editor. The placebo effect: an interdisciplinary exploration, Cambridge, Mass.: Harvard University Press, 1997, pp. 93–116.

Gleidman LH, Gantt WH, Teitelbaum HA. Some implications of conditional reflex studies for placebo research. Am J Psychiatry 1957;113:1103–1107.

Gracely RH. Charisma and the art of healing: can non-specific factors be enough? In: Devor M, Rowbotham MC, Wiesenfeld-Hallin Z, editors. Proceedings of the 9th World Congress of Pain, Seattle: IASP Press, 2000, pp. 1045–1067.

Gracely RH, Dubner R, Deeter WR, Wolskee PJ. Clinician's expectations influence placebo analgesia. Lancet 1985;1:8419–8423.

Herrnstein RJ. Placebo effect in the rat. Science 1962;138:677–678.

Kirsch I. Response expectancy as a determinant of experience and behaviour. Am Psychol 1985;40:1189–1202.

Kirsch I. Changing expectations: a key to effective psychotherapy. Pacific Grove, Calif.: Brooks-Cole, 1990.

Kirsch I, Weixel LJ. Double-blind versus deceptive administration of a placebo. Behav Neurosci 1988;102:319–323.

McGlashan TH, Evans FJ, Orne MT. The nature of hypnotic analgesia and placebo response to experimental pain. Psychosom Med 1969;31:227–246.

Montgomery GH, Kirsch I. Mechanisms of placebo pain reduction: an empirical investigation. Psychol Sci 1996;7:174–176.

Montgomery GH, Kirsch I. Classical conditioning and the placebo effect. Pain 1997;72:107–113.

Price DD. Factors that determine the magnitude and presence of placebo analgesia. In: Devor M, Rowbotham MC, Wiesenfeld-Hallin Z, editors. Proceedings of the 9th World Congress of Pain, Seattle: IASP Press, 2000, pp. 1085–1095.

Price DD, Fields HL. The contribution of desire and expectation to placebo analgesia: implications for new research strategies. In: Harrington A, editor. The placebo effect: an interdisciplinary exploration, Cambridge, Mass.: Harvard University Press, 1997, pp. 117–137.

Price DD, Milling LS, Kirsch I, et al. An analysis of factors that contribute to the magnitude of placebo analgesia in an experimental paradigm. Pain 1999;83:147–156.

Rescorla RA. Pavlovian conditioning: it is not what you think it is. Am Psychol 1988;43:151–160.

Siegel S. Drug-anticipatory responses in animals. In: White L, Tursky B, Schwartz GE, editors. Placebo: theory, research, and mechanisms, New York: Guilford, 1985, pp. 288–305.

Voudouris NJ, Peck CL, Coleman G. Conditioned response models of placebo phenomena: further support. Pain 1989;38:109–116.

Voudouris NJ, Peck CL, Coleman G. The role of conditioning and verbal expectancy in the placebo response. Pain 1990;43:121–128.

Wall PD. The placebo effect: an unpopular topic. Pain 1992;51:1–3.

Wall PD. Pain and the placebo response. Ciba Foundation Symposium 174. Experimental and theoretical studies of consciousness, New York: Wiley, 1993, pp. 187–216.

Wickless C, Kirsch I. The effects of verbal and experiential expectancy manipulations on hypnotic susceptibility. J Pers Soc Psychol 1989;57:762–768.

Wickramasekera I. A conditioned response model of the placebo effect: predictions from the model. Biofeedback Self-Regul 1980;5:5–18.

34
Placebos without Deception
A Randomized Controlled Trial in Irritable Bowel Syndrome

Ted J. Kaptchuk, Elizabeth Friedlander, John M. Kelley, Norma P. Sanchez, Efi Kokkotou, Joyce P. Singer, Magda Kowalczykowski, Franklin G. Miller, Irving Kirsch, and Anthony J. Lembo

Ted J. Kaptchuk, Elizabeth Friedlander, John M. Kelley, Norma P. Sanchez, Efi Kokkotou, Joyce P. Singer, Magda Kowalczykowski, Franklin G. Miller, Irving Kirsch, and Anthony J. Lembo, "Placebos without Deception: A Randomized Controlled Trial in Irritable Bowel Syndrome," PLoS ONE 2010;5(12):e15591.

Introduction

Placebo treatment can have a significant impact on subjective complaints [1]. Furthermore, recent studies have shown measurable physiological changes in response to placebo treatment that could explain how placebos alter symptoms [2]. A critical question is establishing how physicians and other providers can take optimal advantage of placebo effects consistent with their responsibility to foster patient trust and obtain informed consent. Directly harnessing placebo effects in a clinical setting has been problematic because of a widespread belief that beneficial responses to placebo treatment require concealment or deception [3]. This belief creates an ethical conundrum: to be beneficial in clinical practice placebos require deception but this violates the ethical principles of respect for patient autonomy and informed consent. In the clinical setting, prevalent ethical norms emphasize that "the use of a placebo without the patient's knowledge may undermine trust, compromise the patient-physician relationship, and result in medical harm to the patient" [4]. Nevertheless, a recent national survey of internists and rheumatologists in the U.S. found that while only small numbers of U.S. physicians surreptitiously use inert placebo pills and injections, approximately 50% prescribe medications that they consider to have no specific effect on patients' conditions and are used solely as placebos (sometimes called "impure placebos") [5]. Many other studies confirm this finding [6]. Given this situation, finding effective means of harnessing placebo responses in clinical practice without deception is a high priority.

Irritable bowel syndrome (IBS) is one of the top ten reasons for seeking primary care and with a world-wide prevalence of approximately 10 to 15% [7,8]. It is a chronic functional gastrointestinal disorder characterized by abdominal pain and discomfort associated with altered bowel habits [9]. The symptoms of IBS not only adversely affect a person's health-related quality of life (QOL) [10,11], but are associated with a substantial financial burden of reduced work productivity and an over 50% increase in the use of health-related resources [11,12]. While many therapies are commonly used to treat individual IBS symptoms such as constipation or diarrhea, few therapies have been shown to be effective and safe in relieving the global symptoms of IBS [11,13]. Previous research has demonstrated that placebo responses in IBS are substantial and clinically significant [14,15]. Furthermore, data from our previous qualitative study of IBS patients being treated single-blind with placebos indicated that patients can tolerate a high degree of ambiguity and uncertainty about placebo treatment and still benefit [16]. In view of these considerations, we selected IBS as a suitable condition to test the widespread belief that placebo responses are neutralized by awareness or knowledge that the treatment is a placebo.

The objectives of this study were to assess the feasibility of recruiting IBS patients to participate in a trial of open-label placebo and to assess whether an open-label placebo pill with a persuasive rationale was more effective than no treatment in relieving symptoms of IBS in the setting of matched patient-provider interactions.

Methods
Design

A three-week randomized controlled trial (RCT) comparing open-label placebo to no-treatment controls was conducted between August 2009 and April 2010 in a single academic medical center. Written informed consent was obtained from each patient prior to participation on the study. The Beth Israel Deaconess Medical Center Institutional Review Board approved the design and informed consent.

Patients who gave informed consent and fulfilled the inclusion and exclusion criteria were randomized into two groups: 1) placebo pill twice daily or 2) no treatment. Before randomization and during the screening, the placebo pills were truthfully described as inert or inactive pills, like sugar pills, without any medication in it. Additionally, patients were told that "placebo pills, something like sugar pills, have been shown in rigorous clinical testing to produce significant mind-body self-healing processes." The patient-provider relationship and contact time was similar in both groups. Study visits occurred at baseline (Day 1), midpoint (Day 11) and completion (Day 21). Assessment questionnaires were completed by patients with the assistance of a blinded assessor at study visits. (The protocol for this trial and supporting CONSORT checklist are available as supporting information; see Checklist S1 and Protocol S1 [available at: www.plosone.org—eds.].)

Patients

Participants were recruited from advertisements for "a novel mind-body management study of IBS" in newspapers and fliers and from referrals from healthcare professionals. During the telephone screening, potential enrollees were told that participants would receive "either placebo (inert) pills, which were like sugar pills which had been shown to have self-healing properties" or no treatment. Participants were adults (≥18 years old) meeting the Rome III criteria for IBS [17] with a score of ≥150 on the IBS Symptom Severity Scale (IBS-SSS) [18]. The diagnosis of IBS was based on typical symptoms and exclusion of patients with alarm symptoms [19,20] and was confirmed by a board certified gastroenterologist (AJL) or a nurse practitioner (EF) experienced in functional bowel disorders. Patients were excluded if they had any unexplained alarm features (i.e., weight loss >10% body weight, fevers, or blood in stools, or had family history of colon cancer, or inflammatory bowel disease). Patients with a history of pelvic floor dyssynergia, the need to use manual maneuvers in order to achieve a bowel movement, surgery of the colon at any time, abdominal surgery within 60 days prior to entry into the study, or laxative abuse were excluded from the study. Patients with other medical conditions (e.g., neurological disorders, metabolic disorders, or other significant disease), or pretreatment laboratory or ECG findings believed to impair their ability to participate in the study were also excluded. Any surgery within the past 30 days, pregnancy, breast-feeding, or participation in another clinical study within 30 days prior to the start of the study were also disqualifying factors.

Patients were allowed to continue IBS medications (e.g., fiber, anti-spasmodics, loperamide, etc.) as long as they had been on stable doses for at least 30 days prior to entering the study and agreed not to change medications or dosages during the trial. Patients were asked to refrain from making any major life-style changes (e.g., starting a new diet or changing their exercise pattern) during the study.

Interventions

Patients were randomly assigned either to open-label placebo treatment or to the no-treatment control. Prior to randomization, patients from both groups met either a physician (AJL) or nurse practitioner (EF) and were asked whether they had heard of the "placebo effect." Assignment was determined by practitioner availability. The provider clearly explained that the placebo pill was an inactive (i.e., "inert") substance like a sugar pill that contained no medication and then explained in an approximately fifteen minute *a priori* script the following "four discussion points": 1) the placebo effect is powerful, 2) the body can automatically respond to taking placebo pills like Pavlov's dogs who salivated when they heard a bell, 3) a positive attitude helps but is not necessary, and 4) taking the pills faithfully is critical. Patients were told that half would be assigned to an open-label placebo group and the other half to a no-treatment control group. Our rationale had a positive framing with the aim of optimizing placebo response. It was emphasized that each group was critical for the trial. All patients were told that they would receive educational recommendations for their IBS at the end of the study. After completion of the physical examination and assessments, patients were then randomized using sequentially numbered opaque sealed envelopes that contained treatment assignments drawn from a computer-generated random number sequence. Until this point, the patient-provider interaction—including delivering the persuasive rationale and the explanation of the importance of both groups—was similar for all participants. At this point, during the last moments of the interview, they were told their assignments. Patients randomized to the open-label placebo group were given a typical prescription medicine bottle of placebo pills with a label clearly marked "placebo pills" "take 2 pills twice daily." The placebo pills were blue and maroon gelatin capsules filled with Avicel, a common inert excipient for pharmaceuticals (Bird's Hill Pharmacy, Needham, MA). Patients in the no-treatment arm were reminded of the importance of the control arm. All visits were in the context of a warm supportive patient-practitioner relationship. The midpoint day 11 visit was brief (approximately 15 minutes) and included an opened question regarding adverse events, concomitant medications and a brief physical examination. After the examination, a treatment-blind researcher administered questionnaires. Patients receiving placebos received a short reminder regarding the "four discussion points." In the no-treatment arm, patients were encouraged and thanked for helping make a successful study.

Before the study began the providers practiced the trial procedures on simulated and real patients. Once a month, the two providers (AJL, EF) and a third researcher (TJK) met to discuss fidelity to the protocol and any other problems. AJL and EF consistently reported that they had no problem holding the entire initial interview process to approximately 30 minutes and the midpoint to 15 minutes.

Assessment

Our primary outcome measure was the IBS Global Improvement Scale (IBS-GIS) which asks participants: "Compared to the way you felt before you entered the study, have your IBS symptoms over the past seven days been: 1) Substantially Worse, 2) Moderately Worse, 3) Slightly Worse, 4) No Change, 5) Slightly Improved, 6) Moderately Improved or 7) Substantially Improved" [21,22]. Other measures included: the IBS-SSS measure, which contains five 100-point scales that assess the severity of abdominal pain, the frequency of abdominal pain, the severity of abdominal distention, dissatisfaction with bowel habits, and interference with quality of life [18]. All five components contribute to the score equally yielding a theoretical range of 0–500, with a higher score indicating greater symptom severity. The IBS-Adequate Relief (IBS-AR) is a single dichotomous (yes or no) item that asks participants "Over the past week have you had adequate relief of your IBS symptoms?" [23] The IBS-QOL is a 34-item measure assessing the degree to which IBS interferes with patient quality of life. Each item is rated on a 5-point Likert scale and a linear transformation yields a summed score with a theoretical range of 0 to 100, with a higher score indicating better quality of life [24]. Side effects were recorded at each assessment. A pill count was taken at visits two and three. Given the unprecedented na-

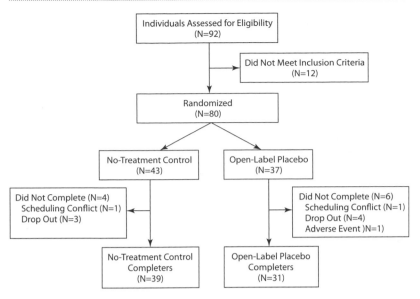

Figure 34.1. Enrollment flowchart.

ture of the study, at the completion of the trial patients were given a short qualitative open-ended check-out questionnaire and asked for written responses. The questions were different for each group. Those in the placebo treatment arm were asked four questions: What do you think about the idea of taking placebo? Did you expect it to work or were you skeptical? What did you think was in the placebo pills? Any further comments? Those in the no-treatment arm were asked three questions: Were you disappointed to be in the treatment-as-usual arm? What did you like most and least about the trial? Any further comments? All assessments were performed by a researcher who was blind to treatment assignment.

Statistical Analysis

All tests were two-tailed with alpha set at 0.05. All results are reported as mean ± SD unless otherwise noted. All analyses were intent-to-treat, and missing data were replaced using the last observation carried forward method. Since IBS-GIS and IBS-AR are change scores and are not assessed at baseline, we carried forward scores for patients who had at least one follow-up visit. For our main outcome measure (IBS-GIS at 21-day endpoint), we planned an independent samples t-test. We estimated a priori that a total sample size of 80 would provide 94% power to detect a large effect (d = 0.8) and 60% power to detect a medium effect (d = 0.5). For IBS-SSS and IBS-QOL, we computed change scores from baseline and then conducted independent samples t-tests. We used chi-square tests of independence for IBS-AR. Per protocol analyses were also conducted, but they produced no substantive differences from our planned intent-to-treat analyses and are not reported here.

Results

As shown in Figure 34.1, 92 patients were screened, and 80 eligible patients were randomized into the two arms (43 into

Table 34.1.
Demographics and baseline characteristics

Demographics and Baseline Characteristics	No Treatment (N=43)	Open Placebo (N=37)
Age	46±18	47±18
Female – no. (%)	32 (74)	24 (65)
White – no. (%)	36 (84)	26 (70)
IBS Type – no. (%)		
Diarrhea Predominant	16 (37)	10 (27)
Constipation Predominant	14 (33)	16 (43)
Mixed	13 (30)	11 (30)
IBS Duration in Years	13±11	16±12
Symptom Severity (IBS-SSS)	297±58	310±82
Quality of Life (IBS-QOL)	59±21	55±21
Upper GI Symptoms (GERD & Dyspepsia) – no. (%)	18 (42)	11 (30)
Taking Medications for IBS – no. (%)	15 (35)	20 (54)
Taking Antidepressants – no. (%)	7 (16)	9 (24)

Note: All values are means ± SD, unless otherwise noted. Group differences were examined using independent t-tests for continuous measures and chi square test for categorical measures. IBS=irritable bowel syndrome; IBS-SSS=IBS Symptom Severity Scale; IBS-QOL=IBS Quality of Life Scale; GI=Gastrointestinal; GERD=Gastroesophageal Reflux Disease.

no-treatment control and 37 into open-label placebo). There were missing outcome data for 13 patients at midpoint (16%; 6 no-treatment control, 7 open-label placebo), and for 10 patients at endpoint (13%; 4 no-treatment control, 6 open-label placebo). As noted above, missing data were replaced using the last observation carried forward method. Table 34.1 shows baseline data.

As shown in Figure 34.2 and Table 34.2, patients treated with open-label placebo had significantly greater scores

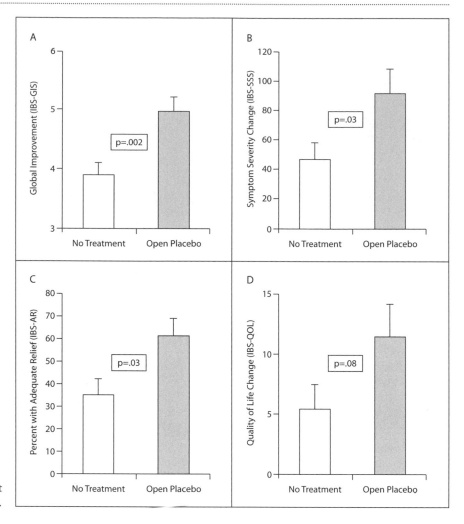

Figure 34.2. Outcomes at the 21-day endpoint by treatment group.

than the no-treatment control on the main outcome measure, Global Improvement Scale (IBS-GIS), at both the 11-day midpoint (5.2±1.0 vs. 4.0±1.1, p<.001, d=1.14) and the 21-day endpoint (5.0±1.5 vs. 3.9±1.3, p=.002, d=0.79). In addition, there were statistically significant differences at both time points on reduction in symptom severity (IBS-SSS) and adequate relief (IBS-AR), and a trend toward significance at the 21-day endpoint on improvement in quality of life (IBS-QOL).

Forty-three patients saw the male physician for all three visits, 20 patients saw the female nurse practitioner for all three visits, and 17 patients saw a combination of the two or missed a treatment session. Given that the two treatment providers differed by gender and discipline (MD vs. NP), we tested for differences in treatment outcomes. No significant differences were found between providers on the primary outcome measure, IBS-GIS (p=.57 at midpoint, and p=.51 at endpoint). Similarly, there were no significant differences between providers on any of the secondary outcome measures.

Adverse events were reported by only three placebo-treated patients (8%) at midpoint and five patients (14%) at endpoint. The most common adverse events that patients reported were upper respiratory infection (N=3) and pain

(N=2); other events included rash, runny stools, and a sty on the eye.

The detailed results of the qualitative check-out questionnaire will be reported elsewhere. However, responses to two questions seemed especially relevant to the interpretation of this quantitative report. Specifically, 1) did patients in the open-label arm understand that they were taking a placebo ("What did you think was in the placebo pills?") and 2) were patients in the no-treatment arm disappointed ("Were you disappointed to be in the treatment-as-usual arm?")? To answer these questions two researchers (TJK, MK) independently extracted the responses to these questions. A third researcher (JPS) compared these extracted responses and a discussion settled two occasions where handwriting was difficult to interpret. TJK categorized the data using the iterative and emergent methodology of grounded theory [25,26]. When participants in the placebo arm were asked: "What did you think was in the placebo pills?" of the 29 who responded, 16 wrote "sugar" (12), "flour" (3) or "calcium" (1), 6 responded "nothing," 5 responded "did not know," 1 responded "symbolic reminder," and 1 responded "possible test medication." When participants in the no-treatment arm were asked: "Were you disappointed to be in the treatment-as-usual arm?" of the 38 who responded, 29 said

Table 34.2.
Treatment outcomes

	No Treatment (N=43)	Open Placebo (N=37)	p-value
Midpoint (11 Days)			
Global Improvement (IBS-GIS)	4.0±1.1	5.2±1.0	<.001
Adequate Relief (IBS-AR) – no. (%)	10 (23)	18 (49)	.02
Symptom Severity Reduction (IBS-SSS)	28±66	75±87	.008
Quality of Life Improvement (IBS-QOL)	4.4±8.9	8.3±11.6	.10
Endpoint (3 Weeks)			
Global Improvement (IBS-GIS)	3.9±1.3	5.0±1.5	.002
Adequate Relief (IBS-AR) – no. (%)	15 (35)	22 (59)	.03
Symptom Severity Reduction (IBS-SSS)	46±74	92±99	.03
Quality of Life Improvement (IBS-QOL)	5.4±13.8	11.4±16.6	.08

Note: All values are means±SD except where noted. IBS=irritable bowel syndrome; IBS-GIS=IBS Global Improvement Scale; IBS-AR=IBS Adequate Relief; IBS-SSS=IBS Symptom Severity Scale; IBS-QOL=IBS Quality of Life Scale.

"no" and only 9 said "yes" or "a little." We then looked at the responses of the nine who expressed disappointment, to see how they responded to: "What did you like most and least about the trial?" All gave uniformly positive answers such as "I liked that my feeling about the intensity of the problem was validated and was taken seriously . . . and was able to discuss my IBS," "the doctor and the nurse were wonderful and accommodating," "I liked the one-on-one attention with the MD, able to ask questions about IBS with a person trained in the illness; this MD is <u>very</u> kind" (underling in the original). This qualitative data seems to indicate that, in general, patients understood they were taking placebo and were not overly disappointed in being in the no-treatment arm.

Discussion

We found that patients given open-label placebo in the context of a supportive patient-practitioner relationship and a persuasive rationale had clinically meaningful symptom improvement that was significantly better than a no-treatment control group with matched patient-provider interaction. To our knowledge, this is the first RCT comparing open-label placebo to a no-treatment control. Previous studies of the effects of open-label placebo treatment either failed to include no-treatment controls [27] or combined it with active drug treatment [28]. Our study suggests that openly described inert interventions when delivered with a plausible rationale can produce placebo responses reflecting symptomatic improvements without deception or concealment.

Our results challenge "the conventional wisdom" that placebo effects require "intentional ignorance" [29]. Our data suggest that harnessing placebo effects without deception is possible in the context of 1) an accurate description of what is known about placebo effects, 2) encouragement to suspend disbelief, 3) instructions that foster a positive but realistic expectancy, and 4) directions to adhere to the medical ritual of pill taking. It is likely our study also benefited from ongoing media attention giving credence to powerful placebo effects.

Both treatment arms were given in a context of a warm patient-provider relationship. It is possible that this relationship had a positive benefit for the patients, and indeed, the no-treatment arm showed improvement. Given that patients in both treatment arms experienced the same frequency and duration of contact time and the content of the interaction was very similar, we believe that the incremental improvement in our open-label arm was due to the addition of open-label placebo treatment. The magnitude of improvement reported by those on open-label placebo treatment was not only statistically significant but also clinically meaningful. The effect size for the primary outcome, calculated as the standardized mean difference (d) between the open-label placebo and no-treatment groups, was 0.79 at endpoint, which is conventionally interpreted as a large effect [30]. At endpoint, we also observed medium-sized effects for the differences between placebo and control groups on symptom severity (d=0.53) and quality of life (d=0.40). An improvement from baseline of 50 points on the IBS-SSS reliably indicates meaningful symptomatic improvement [18]. The open-label group improved by 92 points on this measure; in addition, the improvement shown by the open-label placebo group exceeded that shown by the no-treatment group by 46 points. Similarly, an increase of 10 points on the IBS-QOL indicates a clinically meaningful improvement, and we observed an increase of 11 points on this measure for the open-label group [24]. Finally, the percentage of patients reporting adequate relief during the preceding seven days at the 21-day endpoint (59%) is comparable with the responder rates in clinical trials of drugs currently used in IBS [31,32]. A recent meta-analysis of double-blind, placebo-controlled trials of alosetron in IBS estimated that 51% of patients treated with alosetron had adequate relief as compared to 38% of patients treated with placebo [33]. Our results were remarkably similar (59% for open-label placebo; 35% for no-treatment control), suggesting that open-label placebo in the context of a persuasive rationale may show comparable efficacy to established IBS treatments.

The placebo response in this trial (59% on IBS-AR) was substantially higher than typical reported placebo responses of 30–40% in double-blind IBS pharmaceutical studies [15]. This finding seems counterintuitive. We speculate that it is an indication of the credibility of our open-label rationale. Patients in our study accepted that they were receiving an active treatment, albeit not a pharmacological one, whereas patients in double-blind trials understand that they have only a 50% chance of receiving active treatment. It may be that one hundred percent certainty that one is receiving the "treatment of interest" (in this case open-label placebo) is more placebogenic than a fifty percent probability of receiving an inactive control.

It may be worthwhile to interpret our study in light of the 2001 landmark meta-analysis of placebo effects and its 2010 expanded and updated version [34,35]. In the recent analysis, the authors found 202 randomized trials in 60 medical conditions that included placebo and no-treatment groups. When meta-analytically combined, in general, little evidence of clinically meaningful effects of placebo beyond no treatment was found. The meta-analysis, however, demonstrated a significantly larger placebo effect for a subset of 28 studies with a specific aim of investigating the placebo effect. Perhaps this subset is most relevant to our study which also specifically examined placebo effects. Further prospective research will be necessary to clarify under what circumstances and in what conditions one can expect or not expect to find robust placebo responses.

There are intimations in the placebo literature that providers with greater perceived expertise or authority (e.g., physician versus nurse, dentist versus technician) will elicit greater placebo responses [36,37]. In our study, we found no evidence for significant differences between male physician and female nurse practitioner.

In addition to its clinical significance, our study has important ethical implications. As mentioned above, evidence indicates that physicians continue to use placebo treatment without transparent disclosure to patients [5,6]. Our results suggest that the placebo response is not necessarily neutralized when placebos are administered openly. Thus our study points to a potential novel strategy that might allow the ethical use of placebos consistent with evidence-based medicine. Minimally, open-label placebo may have potential as a "wait and watch" strategy before prescription drugs are prescribed. Further studies of open-label placebo are merited not only for IBS but for illnesses primarily diagnosed by subjective symptoms and introspective self-appraisal. In sum, our study suggests that for some disorders it may be appropriate for clinicians to recommend that patients try an inexpensive and safe placebo accompanied by careful monitoring before and after prescribing medication. Clearly, replication and further research is essential before such a practice could be implemented.

Limitations

This RCT has several limitations. Most important, our sample size was relatively small and the trial duration was too short to obtain estimates of long-term effects. Therefore, the trial could be described as a "proof-of-principle" pilot study. Obviously, replication with a larger sample size and a longer follow-up is needed before clear clinical decisions could be made based on our data.

Other potential limitations of our study may be the issue of report bias (e.g., "wishing to please the experimenter"). However, given the impossibility of double-blind assessment of open-label placebo versus no-treatment control, the effects of report bias cannot be eliminated. Another related limitation is that patients assigned to no treatment may have been disappointed, thus inflating the differences between open-label placebo and no-treatment control groups. Importantly, our qualitative check-out data found the no-treatment group experiencing positive support, with 76% of them reporting that they were not disappointed with their assignment. This argues against disappointment being a significant factor. A further possible limitation is that our results are not generalizable because our trial may have selectively attracted IBS patients who were attracted by an advertisement for "a novel mind-body" intervention. Obviously, we cannot rule out this possibility. However, selective attraction to the advertised treatment is a possibility in virtually all clinical trials. In any case, patients in clinical practice are ultimately given choices and it may turn out that open-label placebo will be helpful only for those who elect to try this option. Finally, it could be argued that IBS is a poor illness to study placebo effects because it lacks objective measures. However, there are many serious conditions for which primary outcomes are primarily subjective (e.g. depression, anxiety and chronic pain), and the preponderance of evidence indicates that placebo treatments are most effective for such patient-centered complaints [1].

In summary, our study suggests that patients are willing to take open-label placebos and that such a treatment may have salubrious effects. Further research is warranted in IBS and perhaps other illnesses to confirm that placebo treatments can be beneficial when provided openly and to determine the best methods for administering such treatments.

REFERENCES

1. Miller FG, Colloca L, Kaptchuk TJ (2009) The placebo effect: illness and interpersonal healing. Perspectives in Biology and Medicine 52: 518–539.
2. Finniss DG, Kaptchuk TJ, Miller FG, Benedetti F (2010) Placebo effects: biological, clinical and ethical advances. Lancet 375: 686–695.
3. Miller FG, Colloca L (2009) The legitimacy of placebo treatments in clinical practice: evidence and ethics. American Journal of Bioethics 9(12): 39–47.
4. American Medical Association (2006) Placebo Use in Clinical Practice. CEJA Report 2-I-2006. Available at: http://www.ama-assn.org/ama1/pub/upload/mm/369/ceja_recs_2i06.pdf.
5. Tilburt JC, Emanuel EJ, Kaptchuk TJ, Curlin FA, Miller FG (2008) Prescribing "placebo treatments": results of national survey of US internists and rheumatologists. BMJ 337: a1938.
6. Fässler M, Meissner K, Schneider A, Linde K (2010) Frequency and circumstances of placebo use in clinical practice—a systematic review of empirical studies. BMC Medicine 8: 15.
7. Saito YA, Schoenfeld P, Locke GR 3rd (2002) The epidemiology of irritable bowel syndrome in North American: a systematic review. American Journal of Gastroenterology 97: 1910–1915.
8. Drossman DA, Camilleri M, Mayer EA, Whitehead WE (2002) AGA technical review on irritable bowel syndrome. Gastroenterology 123: 2108–2131.

9. Longstreth GF, Thompson WG, Chey WD, et al. (2006) Functional bowel disorders. Gastroenterology 130: 1480–1491.

10. Gralnek IM, Hays RD, Kilbourne A, Naliboff B, Mayer EA (2000) The impact of irritable bowel syndrome on health-related quality of life. Gastroenterology 119: 654–660.

11. Drossman DA, Morris CB, Schneck S, et al. (2009) International survey of patients with IBS: symptom features and their severity, health status, treatments, and risk taking to achieve clinical benefit. Journal of Clinical Gastroenterology 43: 541–550.

12. Paré P, Gray J, Lam S, et al. (2006) Health-related quality of life, work productivity, and health care resource utilization of subjects with irritable bowel syndrome: baseline results from LOGIC (Longitudinal Outcomes Study of Gastrointestinal Symptoms in Canada), a naturalistic study. Clinical Therapeutics 28: 1726–1735.

13. American College of Gastroenterology Task Force on Irritable Bowel Syndrome (Brandt LJ, Chey WD, Foxx-Orenstein AE, et al.) (2009) An evidence-based position statement on the management of irritable bowel syndrome. American Journal of Gastroenterology 104 (Suppl.1): S1–S35.

14. Kaptchuk TJ, Kelley JM, Conboy LA, et al. (2008) Components of placebo effect: randomised controlled trial in patients with irritable bowel syndrome. BMJ 336: 999–1003.

15. Patel SM, Stason WB, Legedza A, et al. (2005) The placebo effect in irritable bowel syndrome (IBS) trials—a meta-analysis. Neurogastroenterology & Motility 17: 332–340.

16. Kaptchuk TJ, Shaw J, Kerr CE, et al. (2009) "Maybe I made up the whole thing": Placebos and patients' experiences in a randomized controlled trial. Culture, Medicine and Psychiatry 33: 382–411.

17. Thompson WG, Longstreth GF, Drossman DA, et al. (1999) Functional bowel disorders and functional abdominal pain. Gut 45 (Suppl.2): II43–II47.

18. Francis CY, Morris J, Whorwell PJ (1997) The irritable bowel severity scoring system: a simple method of monitoring irritable bowel syndrome and its progress. Alimentary Pharmacology & Therapeutics 11: 395–402.

19. Hammer J, Eslick GD, Howell SC, Altiparmak E, Talley NJ (2004) Diagnostic yield of alarm features in irritable bowel syndrome and functional dyspepsia. Gut 53: 666–672.

20. Vanner SJ, Depew WT, Paterson WG, et al. (1999) Predictive value of the Rome criteria for diagnosing the irritable bowel syndrome. American Journal of Gastroenterology 94: 2912–2917.

21. Lembo AJ, Wright RA, Bagby B (2001) Alosetron controls bowel urgency and provides global symptom improvement in women with diarrhea-predominant irritable bowel syndrome. American Journal of Gastroenterology 96: 2662–2670.

22. Gordon S, Ameen V, Bagby B, et al. (2003) Validation of irritable bowel syndrome Global Improvement Scale: an integrated symptom end point for assessing treatment efficacy. Digestive Disease Science 48: 1317–1323.

23. Mangel AW, Hahn BA, Heath AT, et al. (1998) Adequate relief as an endpoint in clinical trials in irritable bowel syndrome. Journal of International Medical Research 26: 76–81.

24. Drossman DA, Patrick DL, Whitehead WE, et al. (2000) Further validation of the IBS-QOL: a disease-specific quality-of-life questionnaire. American Journal of Gastroenterology 95: 999–1007.

25. Glaser BG, Strauss A (1967) Discovery of Grounded Theory: Strategies for Qualitative Research. Edison, N.J.: Aldine Transactions.

26. Denzin NK, Lincoln YS, eds. (2003) Collecting and Interpreting Qualitative Materials. Thousand Oaks, Calif.: Sage Publications.

27. Park LC, Covi L (1965) Nonblind placebo trial. Archives of General Psychiatry 12: 336–345.

28. Sandler AD, Bodfish JW (2008) Open-label use of placebos in the treatment of ADHD: a pilot study. Child: Care, Health and Development 34: 104–110.

29. Kaptchuk TJ (1998) Intentional ignorance: a history of blind assessment and placebo controls. Bulletin of the History of Medicine 72: 389–433.

30. Cohen J (1992) A power primer. Psychological Bulletin 112: 155–159.

31. Camilleri M, Northcutt AR, Kong S, et al. (2000) Efficacy and safety of alosetron in women with irritable bowel syndrome: a randomized, placebo-controlled trial. Lancet 355: 1034–1040.

32. Novick J, Miner P, Krause R, et al. (2002) A randomized, double-blind, placebo-controlled trial of tegaserod in female patients suffering from irritable bowel syndrome with constipation. Alimentary Pharmacology & Therapeutics 16: 1877–1888.

33. Rahimi R, Nikfar S, Abdollahi M (2008) Efficacy and tolerability of alosetron for the treatment of irritable bowel syndrome in women and men: A meta-analysis of eight randomized, placebo-controlled, 12-week trials. Clinical Therapeutics 30: 884–901.

34. Hróbjartsson A, Gøtzsche PC (2001) Is the placebo powerless? An analysis of clinical trials comparing placebo with no treatment. New England Journal of Medicine 344: 1594–1602 [erratum: New England Journal of Medicine 2001; 345: 304].

35. Hróbjartsson A, Gøtzsche PC (2010) Placebo interventions for all clinical conditions. Cochrane Database of Systematic Reviews. 2010; 1: CD003974. doi: 10.1002/14651858.CD003974.pub3.

36. Gryll SL, Katahn M (1978) Situational factors contributing to the placebo effect. Psychopharmacology 57: 253–261.

37. Spiro HM (1986) Doctors, Patients, and Placebos. New Haven, Conn.: Yale University Press.

35

Finasteride 5 mg and Sexual Side Effects

How Many of These Are Related to a Nocebo Phenomenon?

Nicola Mondaini, Paolo Gontero, Gianluca Giubilei, Giuseppe Lombardi, Tommaso Cai, Andrea Gavazzi, and Riccardo Bartoletti

Nicola Mondaini, Paolo Gontero, Gianluca Giubilei, Giuseppe Lombardi, Tommaso Cai, Andrea Gavazzi, and Riccardo Bartoletti, "Finasteride 5 mg and Sexual Side Effects: How Many of These Are Related to a Nocebo Phenomenon?," Journal of Sexual Medicine 2007;4:1708–1712.

Introduction

Sexuality is an essential aspect of a couple's relationship and has a significant impact on life satisfaction. Benign prostatic hyperplasia (BPH) is a condition that commonly affects older men and is often associated with lower urinary tract symptoms (LUTS) and sexual dysfunction [1]. Men with moderate-to-severe LUTS are at increased risk for sexual dysfunction, including moderate-to-severe erectile dysfunction (ED), ejaculatory dysfunction (EjD), and hypoactive desire [1]. The results of several recent large-scale studies have shown a consistent and strong relationship between LUTS and both ED and EjD [2]. It appears that the pathophysiological mechanisms of LUTS and the related prostatic enlargement of BPH, as well as certain treatments for this condition, may have an impact on both the erection and ejaculation components of the sexual response [3,4]. Finasteride is the first

5-alphareductase inhibitor that received clinical approval for the treatment of human BPH and androgenetic alopecia (male pattern hair loss) [5]. A large randomized trial has also shown that finasteride can decrease the incidence of prostate cancer [6]. These clinical applications are based on the ability of finasteride to inhibit the type II isoform of the 5-alpha-reductase enzyme, which is the predominant form in human prostate and hair follicles, and the concomitant reduction of testosterone to dihydrotestosterone [5]. Sexual adverse experiences such as ED, loss of libido, and ejaculation disorders have been consistent side effects of finasteride in a maximum percentage of 15% after one year of therapy as reported in the PLESS study [7]. Following a low dose (1 mg) administration of finasteride for androgenic alopecia, none of 186 young patients (age range between 19–43 years; mean age, 28.3 years) scored abnormal values for the sexual health inventory for men questionnaire [8]. Such data could be seen as far from reality, if compared to a higher percentage that seems perceived in clinical practice. A. R. Zlotta et al. reported 38.6% of patients treated with finasteride considered their sexual function as deteriorated after six months of therapy for BPH [9]. The current study aims to assess whether counseling on sexual side effects may generate a higher rate of sexual dysfunction than no counseling, thus relating the dichotomy between literature's data and clinical practice data to a nocebo effect (an adverse side effect that is not a direct result of the specific pharmacological action of the drug) as reported by A. Silvestri et al. for beta-blockers [10].

Materials and Methods

A consecutive series of men with an age range between 45 and 65 complaining of LUTS underwent prostate-specific antigen (PSA) and total testosterone testing, digital rectal examination (DRE), transrectal ultrasound sonography, medical history, international prostate symptoms score (IPSS), and uroflowmetry. The patients were requested to complete the International Index of Erectile Function (IIEF) [11] and the male sexual function-4 (MSF-4 Item) [12,13] questionnaires. The MSF-4 is a psychometrically validated questionnaire with good reproducibility and clinical validity, which allows easy and appropriate assessment of male sexual function in the clinical setting ([i] interest in sex; [ii] quality of erection; [iii] achievement of orgasm; and [iv] achievement of ejaculation.) MSF-4 scoring comprises a global score (from 0 to 20 with higher scores indicating more sexual disorders) and subscores from zero (normality for the relative item) to five (maximal dysfunction for the relative item) for each of the item. The patients were eligible for the study for a total score of < 8 and/or for individual item scores not exceeding two.

The patients were enrolled if they met the following inclusion criteria: (i) a clinical diagnosis of BPH (defined as follows: IPSS > 7; uroflowmetry maximal urinary flow rate [Qmax] between >4 and <15 mL/s; PSA between >1.5 and <4 ng/mL; DRE nonsuspicious for prostate cancer, ultrasound prostate volume > 40 cc); (ii) age ranging between 45 and 65; (iii) being sexually active with no sexual dysfunction (defined as an erectile function [EF] domain score of the IIEF > 25 and a score of < 2 for each question of the MSF-4) and in a stable relationship for at least six months; (iv) testosterone level within the normal range; (v) never on previous BPH medications; (vi) anamnesis and objective check up negative for genital pathologies; and (vii) having signed the study informed consent. The exclusion criteria included any medical therapy for pathologies considered at risk for sexual disorders.

One hundred twenty patients out of a total number of 265 that were screened in the period June–December 2005 were eligible and randomized to receive finasteride 5 mg concealed as an "X compound of proven efficacy for the treatment of BPH" with two different modes of counseling on sexual side effects. Group 1: In this group, the patients knew the "X molecule" had proven efficacy for the treatment of BPH, but were kept blinded to its potential sexual side effect. Group 2: In this group, the patients received counseling on the "X molecule" efficacy for the treatment of BPH as well as on its potential risk of sexual side effects. The phrase used to inform the patients regarding the possible occurrence of sexual problems was ". . . it may cause erectile dysfunction, decrease libido, problems of ejaculation but it is uncommon."

At six and twelve months follow-up, the patients were asked to complete the MFS-4 as well as a self-administered nonvalidated questionnaire that investigated changes in sexual function by answering yes or no to the following four items:

1. Was your overall sexual function affected in the last few months?
2. Did you notice any impairment in your erectile function?
3. Did you notice any change in your ejaculatory function?
4. Has your sexual drive been affected in the last few months?

Sexual dysfunction was defined as a total MSF-4 score ≥ 8 together or as a score > 2 in any individual item and at least one positive answer to the self-administered questionnaire.

In patients who discontinued prematurely for sexual side effects, follow-up information was obtained six months after discontinuation to determine whether their sexual side effect had been resolved.

The patients who reported to have still ED used sildenafil 50 mg tablet on demand. We used sildenafil because it has a positive impact on men with mild to moderate LUTS [14].

This randomized observational study was approved by the ethics committee of our institution.

Statistical Analysis

The difference in distribution among the groups of patients was calculated at one year by using the Mann-Whitney U-test. Statistical significance was achieved if P was < 0.05. All reported P values are two sides.

Results

Data are referred to 107 patients who completed the study. Thirteen were lost during a follow-up. Baseline clinical features of study patients are reported in Table 35.1, and did not significantly differ among the two groups.

At six months follow-up, the overall incidence of sexual dysfunction in patients from both groups was 24.3%, ED 15.8%, decreased libido 11.2%, and ejaculation disorders 8.4%. In group 1 (52 patients), 11.5% (six patients) reported sexual dysfunction. The incidence of ED was 5.7% (three patients), decreased libido 3.8% (two patients), and ejaculation disorders 5.7% (three patients). In group 2 (55 patients), 36.3% (20 patients) reported sexual dysfunction. The incidence of ED was 25.4% (14 patients), decreased libido 18.1% (10 patients), and ejaculation disorders 10.9% (six patients).

At one year, the incidence of sexual dysfunction in all patients was 29.9%, ED was 20.5%, decreased libido 15.8%, and ejaculation disorders 11.2%. In group 1 (52 patients), 15.3% (eight patients) reported sexual dysfunction. The incidence of ED was 9.6% (five patients), decreased libido 7.7% (four patients), and ejaculation disorders 5.7% (three patients). In group 2 (55 patients), 43.6% (24 patients) reported sexual dysfunction. The incidence of ED was 30.9% (17 patients), decreased libido 23.6% (13 patients), and ejaculation disorders 16.3% (nine patients) (Table 35.2).

Table 35.3 shows the evolution in the subscoring for each of the four-item MSF-4 questionnaire at six and twelve months in the patients who reported sexual side effects (8 in group 1 and 24 in group 2).

Table 35.1.
Demographics of the study

Characteristic	Group 1	Group 2
Mean age (year)	60 (range 52–65)	61 (range 51–65)
Main PSA (ng/mL)	2.9	2.7
Mean IPSS	14.3	15.4
Mean Qmax (mL/s)	10.7	11.2
Median prostate volume (g)	45	45.7
Mean IIEF	27	26.8
Mean testosterone (ng/DL)	425	434

Note: PSA = prostate-specific antigen; IPSS = international prostate symptoms score; Qmax = maximal urinary flow rate; IIEF = International Index of Erectile Function.

Table 35.2.
Side effects at one year reported by patients + MSF-4

	Side effects			
	Any sexual adverse experience (%)	ED (%)	Decreased libido (%)	Ejaculation disorders (%)
All patients	29.90	20.50	15.80	11.20
Group 1	15.30	9.60	7.70	5.70
Group 2	43.60	30.90	23.60	16.30

Note: MSF-4 = male sexual function-4; ED = erectile dysfunction.

The patients were reevaluated six months later for sexual side effects. Only three patients were reported to still have ED, which was resolved with sildenafil 50 mg on demand.

Discussion and Conclusion

LUTS and male sexual dysfunction are highly prevalent and strongly linked in aging men. ED risk factors are very prevalent among patients with LUTS [15]. Various treatment strategies for BPH/LUTS may affect sexuality, with differences between drug classes and between drugs within the same class. The 5-alpha-reductase inhibitors finasteride and dutasteride are associated with a greater risk of ED, EjD, and decreased libido than placebo. The main objective of our study was to assess whether a discrepancy exists in finasteride-related sexual side effects between double-blind trials and clinical practice, and if the difference might be partially related to a nocebo effect.

To address these questions, a selected series of BPH patients with no sexual dysfunction was randomized to receive an "X compound" corresponding to the molecule finasteride in two groups that differed in the mode of counseling on treatment side effects. While group 1 patients were kept blinded on the potential side effects of the X compound in a similar way to a "single blind" trial design, information regarding the drug's sexual side effects was disclosed to group 2 patients in a manner closer to a clinical scenario. The significantly higher rate of sexual disturbances among the patients aware of the drug side effects compared to those blinded to the drug side effects is consistent with a nocebo effect [16].

Notably, the incidence of sexual side effects detected by the MSF-4 in our "blinded" arm was similar to the incidence reported at one year in the treatment arm of randomized double-blind studies such as the PLESS study [7]. A cumulative one-year sexual side effect rate as high as 29.9% in all patients (group 1 + group 2) is likely to represent a more reliable estimation of the burden of sexual complaints encountered in clinical practice than that suggested by clinical trials. As previously reported, the maximum incidence of side effects is present after one year of therapy [7]. This observation is further supported by our results because a considerable proportion of patients from both arms developed side effects in the treatment period between six and twelve months.

Patients who are taking active medications frequently experience adverse side effects, which are not a direct result of

Table 35.3.
Changes in MSF-4 global score at 6–12 months of therapy

	Interest (SLQ1)	Erection (SLQ2)	Orgasm (SLQ3)	Ejaculation (SLQ4)
6 months	1.2	2	1	0.8
12 months	1.7	2.2	1.2	1

Note: SLQ1 asked respondents about their interest in sex; SLQ2, the quality of their erection; SLQ3, achieving orgasm; and SLQ4, achieving ejaculation.

the specific pharmacological action of the drug. Although this phenomenon is common, distressing, and costly, it is rarely studied and poorly understood. Our data confirm that the nocebo effect occurs frequently in clinical practice. These have a high prevalence in erectile disease where placebo has good results in 30–35% patients [17]. In managing adverse drug reactions through oral assumption, the nocebo effect is mandatory to recognize false positive responses. Some mechanisms have been postulated, which might be associated with the development of nocebo effects: the patient's expectations of adverse effects at the outset of treatment; a process of conditioning in which the patient learns from prior experiences to associate medication-taking with somatic symptoms; certain psychological characteristics such as anxiety, depression, and the tendency to somatize; and situational and contextual factors [18].

Recent experimental evidence indicates that negative verbal suggestions induce anticipatory anxiety about the impending pain increase, and this verbally induced anxiety triggers the activation of cholecystokinin (CCK), which, in turn, facilitates pain transmission. CCK-antagonists have been found to block this anxiety-induced hyperalgesia, thus opening up the possibility of new therapeutic strategies whenever pain has an important anxiety component [19]. Physicians and other health care personnel can attempt to ameliorate nonspecific side effects to active medications by identifying in advance those patients most at risk for developing them, and by using a collaborative relationship with the patient to explain and help the patient to understand and tolerate these bothersome but nonharmful symptoms.

In conclusion, because finasteride has different effects on sexuality, the sexual dimension should be considered when assessing patients' expectations. The physician relationship with his/her patients is fundamental for an excellent result in terms of a low incidence of sexual side effects.

REFERENCES
[1] Rosen RC, Giuliano F, Carson CC. Sexual dysfunction and lower urinary tract symptoms (LUTS) associated with benign prostatic hyperplasia (BPH). Eur Urol 2005;47:824–837.
[2] Costabile RA, Steers WD. How can we best characterize the relationship between erectile dysfunction and benign prostatic hyperplasia? J Sex Med 2006;3:676–681.
[3] Giuliano F. Impact of medical treatments for benign prostatic hyperplasia on sexual function. BJU Int 2006;97(2 suppl.):34–38, discussion 44–45.
[4] Kassabian VS. Sexual function in patients treated for being prostatic hyperplasia. Lancet 2003;361:60–62.
[5] Finn DA, Beadles Bohling AS, et al. A new look at the 5-alpha-reductase inhibitor finasteride. CNS Drug Rev 2006;12:53–76.
[6] Thompson IM, Goodman PJ, Tangen CM, et al. The influence of finasteride on the development of prostate cancer. N Engl J Med 2003;349:215–224.
[7] Wessells H, Roy J, Bannow J, et al. Incidence and severity of sexual adverse experiences in finasteride and placebo treated men with benign prostatic hyperplasia. Urology 2003;61:579–584.
[8] Tosti A, Pazzaglia M, Soli M, et al. Evaluation of sexual function with an international index of erectile function in subjects taking finasteride for androgenetic alopecia. Arch Dermatol 2004;140:857–858.
[9] Zlotta AR, Teillac P, Raynaud JP, Schulman CC. Evaluation of male sexual function in patients with lower urinary tract symptoms (LUTS) associated with benign prostatic hyperplasia (BPH) treated with a phytotherapeutic agent (permixon), tamsulosin or finasteride. Eur Urol 2005;48:269–276.
[10] Silvestri A, Galetta P, Cerquetani E, et al. Report of erectile dysfunction after therapy with beta-blockers is related to patient knowledge of side effect and is reversed by placebo. Eur Heart J 2003;24:1928–1932.
[11] Rosen RC, Riley A, Wagner G, et al. The International Index of Erectile Function (IIEF): A multidimensional scale for assessment of erectile dysfunction. Urology 1997;49:822–830.
[12] Marquis P, Marrel A. Reproducibility and clinical and concurrent validity of the MSF-4: A four-item male sexual function questionnaire for patients with benign prostatic hyperplasia. Value Health 2001;4:335–343.
[13] Kaplan SA. Reproducibility and clinical and concurrent validity of the MSF-4: A four-item male sexual function questionnaire for patients with benign prostatic hyperplasia. J Urol 2002;168:1661–1662.
[14] Mulhall JP, Guhring P, Parker M, Hopps C. Assessment of the impact of sildenafil citrate on lower urinary tract symptoms in men with erectile dysfunction. J Sex Med 2006;3:662–667.
[15] El Sakka AI. Lower urinary tract symptoms in patients with erectile dysfunction: Analysis of risk factors. J Sex Med 2006;3:144–149.
[16] Hahn RA. The nocebo phenomenon: Concept, evidence, and implications for public health. Prev Med 1997;26:607–611.
[17] Montorsi F, Padma-Nathan H, Glina S. Erectile function and assessments of erection hardness correlate positively with measures of emotional well-being, sexual satisfaction, and treatment satisfaction in men with erectile dysfunction treated with sildenafil citrate (Viagra). Urology 2006;68(3 suppl.):26–37.
[18] Barsky AJ, Saintfort R, Rogers MP, Borus JF. Nonspecific medication side effects and the nocebo phenomenon. J Am Med Assoc 2002;287:622–627.
[19] Benedetti F, Lanotte M, Lopiano L, Colloca L. When words are painful: Unraveling the mechanisms of the nocebo effect. Neuroscience 2007;147:260–271.

36

Overt versus Covert Treatment for Pain, Anxiety, and Parkinson's Disease

LUANA COLLOCA, LEONARDO LOPIANO, MICHELE LANOTTE, AND FABRIZIO BENEDETTI

Luana Colloca, Leonardo Lopiano, Michele Lanotte, and Fabrizio Benedetti, "Overt Versus Covert Treatment for Pain, Anxiety, and Parkinson's Disease," *Lancet Neurology* 2004; 3: 679–684.

Benefits of standard medical treatments have two components, the specific effects of the treatment itself and the perception that the therapy is being given (figure 36.1). The latter is better known as the placebo, or non-specific, effect. In order to study the placebo component of a treatment and to eliminate the specific effects of the treatment, a dummy treatment (the placebo) is administered. This approach is common in clinical trials and has also shown the underlying

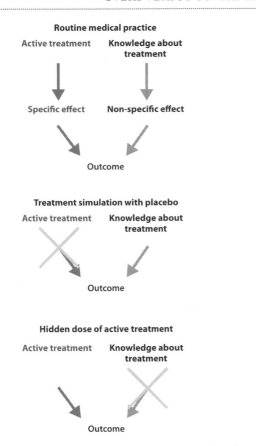

Figure 36.1. Every treatment in clinical practice has a specific and a non-specific effect. The non-specific effect comes from the knowledge that a treatment is being given. The effectiveness of the active treatment can be assessed either by eliminating its specific effect (placebo study) or by eliminating the non-specific effects (hidden treatment).

biological mechanisms of the placebo effect in disorders like Parkinson's disease[1,2] and pain.[3–5]

A radically different approach to the analysis of placebo effects has been implemented, in which placebo effects are assessed without placebo groups.[6,7] In this experimental approach, the placebo component is eliminated and the specific effects of the treatment are maintained (figure 36.1). In order to eliminate the placebo component, patients must not be aware that a treatment is being given. The difference between outcomes on hidden treatment and on open treatment is the placebo component.

All of the studies done with the covert closing method were on disorders that involve the nervous system, such as pain, anxiety, and Parkinson's disease. We review the therapeutic outcomes of treatments given covertly and discuss the implications of this treatment method.

Informed Consent

Informed consent is an important issue in open versus hidden treatment methods. Different approaches are used to obtain full, informed consent and there is no general rule. Most study participants are told that they could receive either an active drug, a placebo, or nothing, thus giving their informed consent to receive different treatments. When drug administration is hidden, participants believe that nothing is being given. For example, postoperative patients are told that they could receive either a painkiller or nothing depending on their postoperative state and that they will not necessarily be informed when any analgesic treatment will be started. In this way, patients do not know if or when the treatment will be given. This is what happens sometimes in routine clinical practice; patients agree to receive a painkiller but they do not know when the infusion machine will start delivering the drug. The patients with Parkinson's disease who come to our department, at various times after surgical implantation of chronic electrodes, for checks of the stimulation variables provide another example. They give full, informed consent to manipulation of stimulus intensity, but are not necessarily told the type of stimulus intensity manipulation (an increase or decrease) and when it is done.

One approach is an unknown time sequence of drug administration. The patients give informed consent for the administration of a medical procedure but they do not know when it will be given. For example, the patient is in a bed with an intravenous line attached to a preprogrammed infusion machine and the drug can be delivered at the first, fourth, or tenth hour without the patient's knowledge. If the drug is really effective, symptom reduction should be temporally correlated with drug administration. We also use this approach for hidden interruptions of drugs. The patients know that the medical procedure will be stopped but they do not know when.

Open versus Hidden Injections of Analgesic and Antianxiety Drugs

In the 1980s and 1990s, some studies were done in which analgesic drugs were delivered by machines through hidden infusions.[8–11] Infusion of a drug can be hidden by use of a computer-controlled infusion pump that is preprogrammed to deliver the drug at the desired time. Importantly, the patient does not know that any drug is being injected. This hidden procedure is done easily in the postoperative phase; the computer-controlled infusion pump delivers the painkiller automatically, without any doctor or nurse in the room, and with the patient completely unaware that an analgesic treatment has been started. Levine and colleagues[8] and Levine and Gordon[10] found that, for postoperative pain after extraction of the third molar, telling the patients that a painkiller is being injected and actually giving a saline solution is as potent as a 6–8 mg dose of morphine. The researchers concluded that an open injection of morphine, which represents usual medical practice, is more effective than a hidden one because in the latter the placebo component is absent.

Our group has studied the differences between open and hidden injections of analgesics.[6] We analysed the effects of four widely used painkillers—buprenorphine, tramadol, ketorolac, and metamizol—in the postoperative setting with open and hidden dosing. A doctor gave the open drug at the

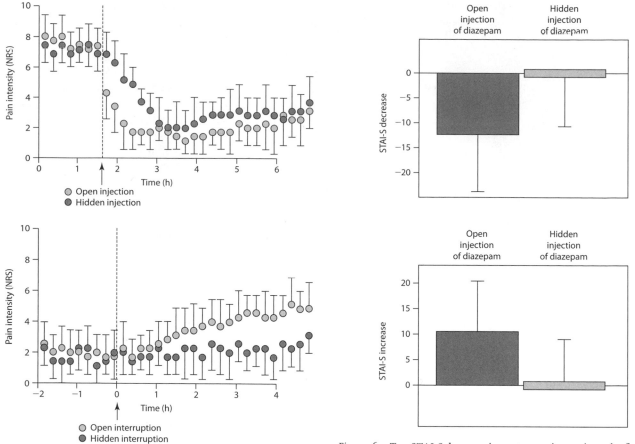

Figure 36.2. Top: Open versus hidden administration of morphine treatment (10 mg) for postoperative pain. The broken line indicates time of injection. Whereas the open group knew when they received their morphine, the hidden group did not know when morphine was given. Note the slower decrease in pain intensity in the hidden group compared with the open one, suggesting that most of the initial benefit in the open group is attributable to a placebo effect. *Bottom:* Open versus hidden interruption of a morphine treatment. The broken line shows the time of morphine interruption. Note the early relapse of pain in the open group but not in the hidden one. NRS = numerical rating scale.

Figure 36.3. Top: STAI-S decrease in postoperative anxiety 2 h after open and hidden doses of diazepam (10 mg). Note that a hidden injection is completely ineffective in reducing anxiety. *Bottom:* Score (STAI-S) increase 8 h after open and hidden interruption of a diazepam therapy. A hidden interruption did not induce any relapse of anxiety.

bedside, telling the patient that the injection was a powerful analgesic and that the pain was going to subside in a few minutes. By contrast, an automatic infusion machine delivered the hidden injection of the same analgesic dose without any doctor or nurse in the room; these patients were completely unaware that an analgesic therapy had been started. We found that the analgesic dose needed to reduce pain by 50% was much higher with hidden infusions of the four painkillers than with open infusions. Similarly, the time course of pain after surgery with open and hidden infusions was substantially different. During the first hour after the injection, pain ratings were much higher with a hidden injection than with an open one.

We confirmed these findings in a study with morphine in which we assessed not only open and hidden giving of a painkiller but also open and hidden interruption of morphine therapy (figure 36.2).[12] We found that relapse of pain

happened faster and pain intensity was greater when patients were told morphine was being stopped than when treatment interruption was hidden; this suggests that hidden interruption prolonged the analgesia. The faster relapse of pain after the open compared with the hidden interruption could be attributed to a "nocebo" effect, in which knowledge that the treatment has been stopped leads to an increase in anxiety. In other words, the fear of pain relapse (because analgesics are no longer provided) might have a hyperalgesic effect.

We did another study in patients with high anxiety scores, measured by the state anxiety scale of the State–Trait Anxiety Inventory (STAI-S), after surgery (figure 36.3).[12] To reduce anxiety, some patients were treated with open doses of diazepam whereas other patients were given hidden infusions of the drug. The open and hidden doses were given with the same procedures as those described above for pain. Likewise, the same procedure was used to interrupt the diazepam therapy overtly and covertly. The difference between the open and the hidden administration of diazepam was highly significant 2 h after the injection. In the open group there was a clear decrease in state anxiety whereas in the hidden group diazepam was ineffective, suggesting that anxiety

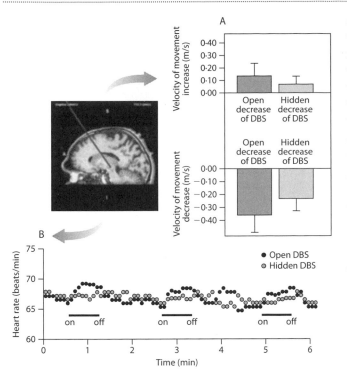

Figure 36.4. The effects of open and hidden DBS on the velocity of hand movement. In all cases, hidden DBS is less effective than open DBS (**A**). Heart rate responses of a patient with Parkinson's disease receiving three sequential stimulations (horizontal bars) of the ventral limbic portion of the subthalamic region overtly and covertly. The hidden stimulations are ineffective (there is no matching between stimulus on–off and heart rate changes), suggesting that heart rate increases after the open stimulations do not result from the stimulation itself but other factors, such as attention, arousal, and expectation (**B**).

reduction after the open diazepam administration was a placebo effect. When diazepam was openly interrupted, anxiety increased significantly after 4 h and 8 h; however, when it was covertly interrupted anxiety did not change. The anxiety relapse after the open interruption of diazepam could be attributed to a nocebo effect.

Open Versus Hidden Deep Brain Stimulation in Parkinson's Disease

We have applied the open–hidden method of study to the treatment of Parkinson's disease, specifically deep brain stimulation (DBS) of the subthalamic nucleus (STN). Two types of evidence suggest that hidden DBS is less effective than open treatment: study of stimulation with macroelectrodes in the postoperative phase[13,14] and study of autonomic and emotional responses to intraoperative stimulation with microelectrodes (figure 36.4).[15]

Firstly, we studied ten patients with idiopathic Parkinson's disease with open and hidden bilateral stimulations of the STN.[13,14] A hand movement analyser assessed bradykinesia as these patients did a visual directional-choice task in which the right index finger was positioned on a central sensor and moved towards a target when a light was turned on. Each patient was tested twice, once with overt and once with covert stimulation, on different days. With overt stimulation, the stimulus intensity was reduced to 20% of the optimal stimulation, and the patient was told that motor function was going to worsen. After 2 h, the stimulus intensity was increased to optimal stimulation overtly, and the patients were told that motor performance was going to return to normal. By contrast, with covert stimulation, the 20% reduction in stimulation and the subsequent increase to optimal stimulation were hidden, with the patients completely unaware that such changes were being done. The open interruption of STN stimulation was associated with a greater decrease in movement velocity at 30 min than the hidden one. Likewise, when the stimulation returned to normal, after 10 min the open procedure was more effective than the hidden one. Therefore, the hidden interruption was associated with the least deterioration of motor function, and the hidden stimulus increase was associated with the least improvement.

Secondly, study of autonomic and emotional responses to intraoperative stimulation of the most dorsal part of the subthalamic region, which includes the zona incerta and the dorsal pole of the STN, with microelectrodes produced the same autonomic responses in the hidden and the open conditions.[15] By contrast, stimulation of the most ventral region, which includes the ventral pole of the STN and the substantia nigra pars reticulata, produced autonomic and emotional responses that varied over time and in accordance with open or hidden conditions of stimulation (figure 36.4). In fact, the mean minimum stimulus intensity to produce a response increased from 2.25 V (SD 1.4) in the open condition to 4.1 V (SD 0.9) in the hidden condition. In other words, the hidden stimulation was less effective than open stimulation, such that an increase of the stimulus intensity was needed to induce an autonomic response. Interestingly, the most ventral part of the subthalamic region is probably involved in limbic-associative functions.[16–20] In our study[15] two patients reported no sensation when stimulation of the ventral subthalamic region was hidden, whereas a pleasant sensation was reported during the open stimulation of the same area. The fact that these differences between open and hidden stimulations were not observed in the most dorsal part of the subthalamic region suggests that these effects are specific, and limited, to the most ventral limbic region.

Clinical Implications

Although the evidence for differential effects of open and hidden treatments is limited to disorders involving the nervous system, and thus is not generalisable to all medical and surgical treatments, these provocative studies have two major findings. First, although many factors and variables may contribute to the differences between the outcomes of covert and overt treatments, certainly the awareness of the treatment, the presence of the therapist, and the expectation of the outcome are likely to be very important. Because all these factors are strongly influenced by the doctor-patient interaction, the patients' knowledge about a therapy seems to be fundamental to the production of optimum therapeutic effects.

Second, interestingly and paradoxically, patients' awareness of a treatment is advantageous only when the therapy is being given. If the therapy has to be interrupted, such awareness might be deleterious for the patient. In fact, open interruption of morphine, diazepam, and STN stimulation produces a greater worsening of the symptoms than hidden interruption (figures 36.2, 36.3, and 36.4).

In clinical practice, all efforts should be made to make the patient aware of what is going on, why a procedure is being done, and the expected outcome. Although many clinicians have long known the power of their words and attitudes, and indeed many studies show the powerful effect of the psychosocial context on the patient,[21–29] the differences in outcome between open and hidden therapy should alert doctors, nurses, psychologists, and all other medical and paramedical personnel of the importance of their interaction with patients. Even when a treatment has to be stopped, the relationship between the medical professional and patient is essential. The way in which drugs and brain stimulation are delivered or interrupted has an effect on treatment outcome. Although we cannot recommend withholding information about a treatment interruption, even though it is beneficial, appropriate words and attitudes should be adopted in order to reduce the potentially negative effects of fear of treatment interruption.

Ethical Considerations for Clinical Trials

The ethics of the open–hidden methods are relevant beyond routine medical practice and involve many parts of biomedical research. The use of placebos in clinical trials is still the focus of a hot debate and lively discussion. Critics of placebo-controlled trials have condemned the use of placebos because withholding proven, effective treatment results in suboptimum treatment. In other words, placebo groups do not receive the best treatment available. The World Medical Association (WMA) Declaration of Helsinki states that it is unethical to allow patients to receive a placebo when effective treatment exists (paragraph 29),[30] although in October 2001 a clarification deeming placebos to be ethically acceptable in some circumstances was added.[31] The positions of official organisations, such as the U.S. Food and Drug Administration (FDA), the American Medical Association (AMA), the European Committee for Proprietary Medicinal Products (CPMP) and WHO, differ.[32] The FDA has always demanded and defended placebo-controlled studies for the development of new pharmaceuticals, even if effective therapy exists.[33] Whereas the AMA generally supports the FDA's position, WHO affirms that placebos are not justified if there is already an approved and accepted drug for the disorder that a candidate drug is designed to treat.[34] The CPMP takes a somewhat ambiguous position because, regarding schizophrenia, it states that in principle placebo-controlled trials will be required to show the efficacy of a new product but recognises that suitable alternative designs may be developed.[34]

Although the debate on the use of placebos in clinical practice is not as lively as that in the clinical-trial setting, the same arguments for and against the use of placebos can be applied. The use of a placebo is sometimes seen as an unethical procedure because some degree of deception is needed, thus damaging the institution of medicine and contributing to the erosion of confidence and trust in medical staff and carers.[35,36] Rawlinson[37] justifies deception by invoking the concept of paternalism and benevolent deception—in which the physician's purpose is not actually to deceive but to cure—and further asserts that one of the effects of illness is an undermining of the patient's autonomy. According to Rawlinson it is the physician who must restore this loss, even through the use of benevolent paternalism and deception.

Several approaches for overcoming the ethical problems related to placebo administration and deception have been proposed. For example, if the purpose of the study must be withheld, participants could be informed that the nature of the study will not be described accurately but that they will be fully informed at the conclusion of the research.[38] Alternatively, the patients could be informed that they may experience symptomatic worsening as a result of being given a placebo.[39]

We believe the open–hidden method in clinical trials is worth pursuing because the use of placebos can be avoided. Hidden dosing of a painkiller is less effective than open dosing, thus the placebo component of the treatment is represented by the difference between responses to the open and the hidden injection: the larger the difference between the open and the hidden delivery, the larger the placebo component and the smaller the effect of the active treatment. For example, the open–hidden difference for diazepam is notable (figure 36.3) and for movement velocity during STN stimulation is small (figure 36.4), suggesting that with diazepam much of the benefit can be attributed to a placebo effect whereas with STN stimulation the active treatment is very effective on motor responses.

The open–hidden method enables provision of the best available therapy and avoidance of placebos in accordance with the Declaration of Helsinki. In fact, when either hidden analgesic injection or DBS is done the optimum treatment is given. We are aware that a hidden procedure is not always easy to do and can be used only in some circumstances; it needs to be conducted in a hospital through an intravenous line and a computer-controlled infusion pump, because a hidden oral dosing is difficult to devise. Some complex ethical issues, such as the use of sham surgery in trials of cell transplantation in Parkinson's disease, will almost certainly not be resolved by use of open–hidden therapy methods.[40] Despite these limitations, a first and important step will be to define the range of treatments for which the open–hidden design might serve as a substitute for the use of placebo controls.

Conclusions

We believe that the open–hidden approach can be used to address many unanswered questions, including nature of the placebo effect. When we measure the difference between open and hidden treatments, the term placebo effect is misleading because no placebo has been given. Therefore, the difference could be better described as the psychosocial component of treatment that comes from patient knowledge that they are receiving treatment. Our research shows that administration of drugs or brain stimulation happens in a complex psychobiological context that is capable of modulating the effect of the treatment. We believe that open–hidden methods of study and future research of this topic will answer many questions on various subjects, from the doctor-patient relationship to the nature of the placebo effect, and from the role of the psychosocial context in treatment outcome to the design of clinical trials.

We also believe that research using the open–hidden method will improve our understanding of the neurobiological mechanisms of the placebo effect. For example, recent research has shown that placebo administration to patients with Parkinson's disease induces dopamine release in the striatum[1] and modifies the activity of STN neurons.[2] It will be interesting to study these effects not only after placebo administration, but also after hidden administrations of anti-Parkinson agents.

REFERENCES

1 de la Fuente-Fernández R, Ruth TJ, Sossi V, et al. Expectation and dopamine release: mechanism of the placebo effect in Parkinson's disease. *Science* 2001; 293: 1164–1166.

2 Benedetti F, Colloca L, Torre E, et al. Placebo-responsive Parkinson patients show decreased activity in single neurons of subthalamic nucleus. *Nat Neurosci* 2004; 7: 587–588.

3 Amanzio M, Benedetti F. Neuropharmacological dissection of placebo analgesia: expectation-activated opioid systems versus conditioning-activated specific sub-systems. *J Neurosci* 1999; 19: 484–494.

4 Petrovic P, Kalso E, Petersson KM, Ingvar M. Placebo and opioid analgesia—imaging a shared neuronal network. *Science* 2002; 295: 1737–1740.

5 Wager TD, Rilling JK, Smith EE, et al. Placebo-induced changes in fMRI in the anticipation and experience of pain. *Science* 2004; 303: 1162–1167.

6 Amanzio M, Pollo A, Maggi G, Benedetti F. Response variability to analgesics: a role for nonspecific activation of endogenous opioids. *Pain* 2001; 90: 205–215.

7 Price DD. Assessing placebo effects without placebo groups: an untapped possibility? *Pain* 2001; 90: 201–203.

8 Levine JD, Gordon NC, Smith R, Fields HL. Analgesic responses to morphine and placebo in individuals with postoperative pain. *Pain* 1981; 10: 379–389.

9 Gracely RH, Dubner R, Wolskee PJ, Deeter WR. Placebo and naloxone can alter postsurgical pain by separate mechanisms. *Nature* 1983; 306: 264–265.

10 Levine JD, Gordon NC. Influence of the method of drug administration on analgesic response. *Nature* 1984; 312: 755–756.

11 Benedetti F, Amanzio M, Maggi G. Potentiation of placebo analgesia by proglumide. *Lancet* 1995; 346: 1231.

12 Benedetti F, Maggi G, Lopiano L, et al. Open versus hidden medical treatments: the patient's knowledge about a therapy affects the therapy outcome. *Prevention & Treatment* 2003; 6(1): 1a. Available at: http://psycnet.apa.org/journals/pre/6/1/1a/.

13 Pollo A, Torre E, Lopiano L, et al. Expectation modulates the response to subthalamic nucleus stimulation in Parkinsonian patients. *NeuroReport* 2002; 13: 1383–1386.

14 Benedetti F, Pollo A, Lopiano L, et al. Conscious expectation and unconscious conditioning in analgesic, motor and hormonal placebo/nocebo responses. *J Neurosci* 2003; 23: 4315–4323.

15 Benedetti F, Colloca L, Lanotte M, et al. Autonomic and emotional responses to open and hidden stimulations of the human subthalamic region. *Brain Res Bull* 2004; 63: 203–211.

16 Alexander GE, DeLong MR, Strick PL. Parallel organization of functionally segregated circuits linking basal ganglia and cortex. *Annu Rev Neurosci* 1986; 9: 357–381.

17 Alexander GE, Crutcher MD, DeLong MR. Basal ganglia-thalamocortical circuits: parallel substrates for motor, oculomotor, "prefrontal" and "limbic" functions. *Prog Brain Res* 1990; 85: 119–146.

18 Limousin P, Greene J, Pollak P, et al. Changes in cerebral activity pattern due to subthalamic nucleus or internal pallidum stimulation in Parkinson's disease. *Ann Neurol* 1997; 42: 283–291.

19 Bejjani BP, Damier P, Arnulf I, et al. Transient acute depression induced by high-frequency deep-brain stimulation. *N Engl J Med* 1999; 340: 1476–1480.

20 Krack P, Kumar R, Ardouin C, et al. Mirthful laughter induced by subthalamic nucleus stimulation. *Mov Disord* 2001; 16: 867–875.

21 Stewart MA, McWhinney IR, Buck CW. The doctor-patient relationship and its effect upon outcome. *J R Coll Gen Pract* 1979; 29: 77–82.

22 Starfield B, Wray C, Hess K, et al. The influence of patient-practitioner agreement on outcome of care. *Am J Pub Health* 1981; 71: 127–132.

23 Gracely RH, Dubner R, Deeter WR, Wolskee PJ. Clinicians' expectations influence placebo analgesia. *Lancet* 1985; 325(8419): 43.

24 Greenfield S, Kaplan S, Ware JE. Expanding patient involvement in care. *Ann Int Med* 1985; 102: 520–528.

25 Bass MJ, Buck C, Turner L, et al. The physician's actions and the outcome of illness in family practice. *J Fam Pract* 1986; 23: 43–47.

26 Thomas KB. General practice consultations: is there any point in being positive? *BMJ* 1987; 294: 1200–1202.

27 Kaplan SH, Greenfield S, Ware JE. Assessing the effects of physician-patient interactions on the outcomes of chronic disease. *Med Care* 1989; 27 (Suppl. 3): S110–S127.

28 Stewart MA. Effective physician-patient communication and health outcomes: a review. *CMAJ* 1995; 152: 1423–1433.

29 Di Blasi Z, Harkness E, Ernst E, Georgiou A, Kleijnen J. Influence of context effects on health outcomes: a systematic review. *Lancet* 2001; 357: 757–762.

30 World Medical Association. Declaration of Helsinki. Amended by the 52nd WMA General Assembly, Edinburgh, Scotland, October 2000. *JAMA* 2000; 284: 3043–3045.

31 Word Medical Association. Declaration of Helsinki. Note of clarification on paragraph 29.

32 Rothman KJ, Michels KB. The continuing unethical use of placebo controls. *N Engl J Med* 1994; 331: 394–398.

33 Temple RJ. Placebo controlled trials and active controlled trials: ethics and inference. In: Guess HA, Kleinman A, Kusek JW, Engel LW, eds. The science of the placebo: toward an interdisciplinary research agenda. London: BMJ Books, 2002: 209–226.

34 Michels KB, Rothman KJ. Update on unethical use of placebos in randomised trials. *Bioethics* 2003; 17: 188–204.

35 Bok S. The ethics of giving placebos. *Sci Am* 1974; 231(5): 17–23.

36 Bok S. Ethical issues in use of placebo in medical practise and clinical trials. In: Guess HA, Kleinman A, Kusek JW, Engel LW, eds. The science of the placebo: toward an interdisciplinary research agenda. London: BMJ Books, 2002: 63–73.

37 Rawlinson MC. Truth-telling and paternalism in the clinic: philosophical reflection on the use of placebo in medical practice. In: White L, Tursky B, Schwartz GE, eds. Placebo: theory, research, and mechanisms. Guilford: New York, 1985: 403–416.

38 Wendler D, Miller FG. Deception in the pursuit of science. Arch Int Med 2004; 164: 597–600.

39 Emanuel EJ, Miller FG. The ethics of placebo-controlled trials—a middle ground. N Engl J Med 2001; 345: 915–919.

40 Freed CR, Greene PE, Breeze RE, et al. Transplantation of embryonic dopamine neurons for severe Parkinson's disease. N Engl J Med 2001; 344: 710–719.

37
Components of Placebo Effect

Randomised Controlled Trial in Patients with Irritable Bowel Syndrome

TED J. KAPTCHUK, JOHN M. KELLEY, LISA A. CONBOY, ROGER B. DAVIS, CATHERINE E. KERR, ERIC E. JACOBSON, IRVING KIRSCH, ROSA N. SCHNYER, BONG HYUN NAM, LONG T. NGUYEN, MIN PARK, ANDREA L. RIVERS, CLAIRE A. MCMANUS, EFI KOKKOTOU, DOUGLAS A. DROSSMAN, PETER GOLDMAN, AND ANTHONY J. LEMBO

Ted J. Kaptchuk, John M. Kelley, Lisa A. Conboy, Roger B. Davis, Catherine E. Kerr, Eric E. Jacobson, Irving Kirsch, Rosa N. Schnyer, Bong Hyun Nam, Long T. Nguyen, Min Park, Andrea L. Rivers, Claire A. McManus, Efi Kokkotou, Douglas A. Drossman, Peter Goldman, and Anthony J. Lembo, "Components of Placebo Effect: Randomised Controlled Trial in Patients with Irritable Bowel Syndrome," BMJ 2008;336:999–1003.

Introduction

Aside from the provision of a specific therapeutic regimen, a medical encounter might elicit non-specific or contextual benefits or what are most often called placebo effects. Experimental settings seek to contain these "nuisance" effects with placebo controls. Such non-specific effects in a clinical setting can theoretically be separated into three components: a patient's response to observation and assessment (Hawthorne effects), the patient's response to the administration of a therapeutic ritual (placebo treatment), and the patient's response to the patient-practitioner interaction.[1–3] We tested this by determining whether these distinct potential contributions to clinical care can be separated and then combined incrementally under controlled conditions to produce progressive improvement in clinical outcomes in a manner resembling a graded dose escalation of component parts. We also quantified the extent to which the patient-practitioner relationship enhances the effects of a placebo treatment alone and whether a placebo intervention is more effective than no treatment/natural course of the illness alone.

We carried out the trial on patients with irritable bowel syndrome. This is a chronic, functional gastrointestinal disorder characterised by recurrent abdominal pain and disturbed bowel function—that is, diarrhoea, constipation, or alternation between the two.[4] Irritable bowel syndrome is one of the top ten reasons for seeking primary care and is the reason for nearly a third of all consultations with gastroenterologists,[5] with an estimated direct and indirect cost in the eight major industrial countries of over $41bn (£20bn, €27bn).[6] Irritable bowel syndrome seemed a suitable disease to study because previous randomised controlled trials of treatments have shown a large positive response (about 40%) in placebo groups.[7] This also suggests that it might be possible to show a graded response when the three hypothetical non-specific components of the clinical encounter were added individually or in combinations.

Methods

Study Design

We conducted this randomised controlled trial in a single centre in 262 participants over two study periods of three weeks (Figure 37.1) For the first three-week period, participants were randomised to one of three groups: a "waiting list" that controlled for any effects of assessment and observation (Hawthorne effects) as well as the effects of the natural course of the illness and regression to the mean; "limited interaction," providing placebo treatment with minimal interaction with the practitioner; or "augmented interaction," providing placebo treatment with a defined positive patient-practitioner relationship. Our placebo treatment was delivered with a validated sham acupuncture device. We therefore assumed that the three study groups represented the successive addition of the three postulated elements of the non-specific clinical interactions: group 1 (waiting list) having only observation alone, group 2 (limited) adding a dummy treatment, and group 3 (augmented) adding a warm, empathetic, and confident patient-practitioner relationship. All participants were evaluated at entry to the trial and after three and six weeks.

At the end of the first three-week period, participants in groups 2 (limited) and 3 (augmented) were, without their knowledge, randomised a second time in equal numbers either to continue with sham acupuncture or to receive genuine acupuncture. Patient-practitioner relationships for these groups, however, remained the same. (Results of this nested secondary study, comparing acupuncture and sham acupuncture, in the second three-week period will be reported elsewhere.) Data from patients in groups 2 and 3 who remained on placebo for the second period, however, again as planned prospectively, are included in this report. Participants in group 1 (waiting list) remained on the list for the second three-week period. Results at three weeks provided data for the primary end point; those who remained on placebo for the additional three weeks served to provide observations on non-specific effects over time.

We randomly assigned participants to the three study arms using permuted block randomisation with variable block sizes and assignments provided in sequentially num-

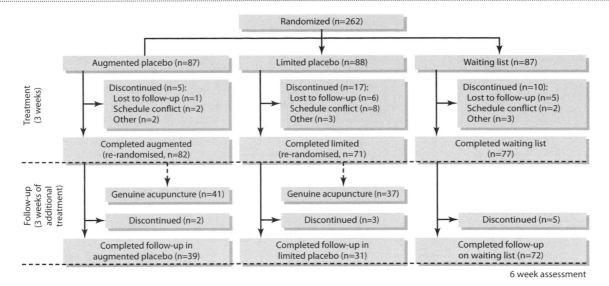

Figure. 37.1. Flow of participants through study.

bered opaque sealed envelopes. An administrative assistant, not otherwise involved in the study, opened the assignment envelopes and recorded the assignment of each participant in a confidential log. At three weeks, we used similar methods to randomise patients in the sham acupuncture groups to continue sham acupuncture or to switch to genuine acupuncture. This randomisation was stratified by the level of abdominal pain at the three week visit (<30 vs. ≥30 on a 100-point visual analogue scale).

Recruitment

Participants were recruited from advertisements in the media, fliers, and referrals from health professionals, were all at least 18 years old, and met the Rome II criteria for irritable bowel syndrome[8] with a score of ≥150 on the symptom severity scale.[9] We excluded patients if they had unexplained findings such as weight loss >10% body weight, fever, blood in stools, family history of colon cancer, or inflammatory bowel disease; they were also excluded if they had previously received acupuncture. The diagnosis of irritable bowel syndrome was based on typical symptoms and confirmed by a board certified gastroenterologist experienced in functional bowel disorders (AL) who also judged the exclusion of patients with alarm symptoms.[10,11] Participants were allowed to continue medications for irritable bowel syndrome taken before entering the study (such as fibre, anti-spasmodics, and loperamide) if this therapeutic regimen had remained constant for at least the previous 30 days and they agreed to keep the regimen constant during the trial.

Intervention Components

GROUP 1 (WAITING LIST)

Participants had neither placebo treatment nor interaction with a healthcare practitioner but, like other participants, were assessed at baseline and at three and six weeks.

GROUP 2 (LIMITED INTERACTION)

Participants received a placebo intervention and "limited" interaction with a practitioner (see below).

We chose dummy acupuncture for our placebo because the evidence is that acupuncture has high placebo effects.[12] The validated sham acupuncture is indistinguishable from acupuncture itself.[13] (The shaft of the sham device does not actually pierce the skin but creates the illusion of doing so because it retracts into a hollow handle; a small plastic mount and surgical tape hold the sham needle in place.) Placebo treatments were performed twice a week, a schedule similar to that used by many acupuncturists. At each session, six to eight dummy needles were placed for 20 minutes over predetermined non-acupuncture points on the arms, legs, and abdomen; this intervention was the same for groups 2 (limited) and 3 (augmented).

The limited patient-practitioner relationship was established at the initial visit (duration <5 minutes) during which practitioners introduced themselves and stated they had reviewed the patient's questionnaire and "knew what to do." They then explained that this was "a scientific study" for which they had been "instructed not to converse with patients." The placebo needles were then placed, and the patient left alone in a quiet room for 20 minutes, a common acupuncture practice, after which the practitioner returned to remove the "needles." Subsequent visits were scheduled twice a week for 20 minutes. At week three, participants completed assessments and those randomised to continue the placebo treatment received an additional six sham treatments.

GROUP 3 (AUGMENTED INTERACTION)

Participants in group 3 (augmented) also received six sessions of placebo acupuncture under the same conditions and in the same room(s) as group 2. Unlike participants in group

2 (limited), however, they received an augmented patient-practitioner relationship that began at the initial visit (45 minutes' duration) and was structured with respect to both content (four primary discussions) and style (five primary points). Content included questions concerning symptoms, how irritable bowel syndrome related to relationships and lifestyle, possible non-gastrointestinal symptoms, and how the patient understood the "cause" and "meaning" of his or her condition. The interviewer incorporated at least five primary behaviours including: a warm, friendly manner; active listening (such as repeating patient's words, asking for clarifications); empathy (such as saying "I can understand how difficult IBS must be for you"); 20 seconds of thoughtful silence while feeling the pulse or pondering the treatment plan; and communication of confidence and positive expectation ("I have had much positive experience treating IBS and look forward to demonstrating that acupuncture is a valuable treatment in this trial."). We based this intervention model on research concerning an optimal patient-practitioner relationship.[14,15] Only after completing this nine-item agenda did the acupuncturist place the placebo needles and leave the participant in a quiet room for 20 minutes. On returning, the practitioner "removed" the placebo needles and exchanged a few words of encouragement. Specific cognitive and behavioural interventions that might be beneficial for irritable bowel syndrome (such as relaxation,[16] cognitive behavioural therapy,[17] or education/counselling[18]) were not allowed.

PRACTITIONERS FOR GROUP 2 AND 3

The practitioners in this study consisted of four licensed acupuncturists, all of whom had participated in previous randomised placebo-controlled trials on acupuncture. The practitioners' training followed methods described in earlier studies of structured patient-physician interactions.[19] Practitioners received 20 hours of training to ensure they were able to create the two different clinical contexts. They were instructed in advance on the "scripts" for their interactions with the two treated groups by means of a training manual, a video of model sessions, and by role playing with both simulated and real patients. During the trial, practitioners also received routine feedback from the videotaping of all sessions, which was used to score adherence to protocol (see below). Practitioners never had contact with participants in group 1 (waiting list).

Informed Consent and Blinding

All participants gave written informed consent, but the consent disclosure omitted certain descriptors of the trial to protect the study's scientific validity. Thus, participants were told that the trial was a placebo controlled study of acupuncture for irritable bowel syndrome and were completely unaware of the study's primary aim to examine placebo effects.

Although the trial was prospectively designed to investigate non-specific effects in irritable bowel syndrome, its design included a nested acupuncture substudy that allowed potential participants in the "treatment" arms to be told, truthfully, that they had a 50% chance of receiving genuine acupuncture during the trial. When the study ended, a letter was sent to all participants explaining the exact purpose of the study and offering them the opportunity to withdraw their original consent to use their data. All study personnel, except the practitioners, were blinded to participant assignment. Blinded registered nurses who were otherwise unconnected to the study conducted assessments.

Adherence to Treatment

We evaluated the adherence of practitioners to protocols by videotaping all treatment sessions, of which 102 (10% of the sample) were randomly selected for evaluation. We used a well-established procedure.[19,20] Two research assistants otherwise unconnected with the trial separately rated each session. Reliability between raters was high ($\kappa = 0.92$), and 97% of sessions were rated as adherent.

Outcome Assessments

Following validated procedures in research on irritable bowel syndrome, our a priori primary outcome was a change from baseline at three weeks in the global improvement scale, which asks participants, "Compared to the way you felt before you entered the study, have your IBS symptoms over the past seven days been: (1)=substantially worse, (2)=moderately worse, (3)=slightly worse, (4)=no change, (5)=slightly improved, (6)=moderately improved, or (7)=substantially improved."[21,22] Our other main outcome was adequate relief, which is a single dichotomous categorisation that asks participants "Over the past week have you had adequate relief of your IBS symptoms?"[23,24] Neither of these primary outcomes were measured at baseline. Our other two outcomes were the symptom severity scale and the quality of life scale. The symptom severity scale is a questionnaire that measures the sum of the participant's evaluation on a 100 point scale of each of five items: severity of abdominal pain, frequency of abdominal pain, severity of abdominal distension, dissatisfaction with bowel habits, and interference with quality of life.[9] All five components contribute equally to the score, yielding a theoretical range of 0–500, in which a higher score indicates a more severe condition. The quality of life scale is a 34-item assessment of the degree to which the condition interferes with a patient's quality of life. Each item is rated on a five-point Likert scale and a linear transformation yields a summed score with a theoretical range of 0 to 100, a higher score indicating better quality of life.[25] Side effects were recorded at each assessment.

Statistical Analysis

We estimated a priori that a sample size of 262 would provide 95% power for finding a significant difference in scores on the global improvement scale at three weeks if the augmented, limited, and waiting list groups reported improvements of 50%, 40%, and 25%, respectively. Even if the rates were only 20%, 15%, and 10%, respectively, however, a sample size of 87 per group would afford a power of 55%. We replaced missing data from dropouts using the last observation carried forward method. We did not, however, carry forward a baseline observation to week six if a participant missed assessments at both three and six weeks.

The primary test for each outcome measure was a test of trend examining the ordered alternative hypothesis, waiting list (group 1) < limited (group 2) < augmented (group 3). For dichotomous measures, we used Cochran-Armitage tests. For continuous measures, we used a Wald test from ordinary least squares regression models with two independent variables: a treatment group variable (coded waiting list = 1; limited = 2; augmented = 3) and the baseline (before treatment) value of the outcome variable. Using a Bonferroni correction, we considered $P < 0.0125$ (two sided) to be significant for each test of trend. To better describe the association between group and outcome, if the trend test was significant we conducted pairwise comparisons of the groups—that is, augmented vs. limited and limited vs. waiting list. For the dichotomous outcomes we used Pearson χ^2 tests, and for the continuous outcomes we used Tukey tests from analysis of covariance (ANCOVA), again using the baseline measures of the outcome variables as the covariate. All analyses were carried out on an intention to treat basis.

Results

Study Population

Between December 2003 and February 2006, we screened 350 prospective participants of whom 289 were eligible. We randomised 262 people into the three groups. (Simultaneously, we randomly selected an additional 27 patients to participate in a parallel qualitative study of identical assessments and treatments that also included a series of interviews on their experiences. Prospectively, these participants were considered a separate study.) At baseline the three groups were well balanced with regard to demographics, psychiatric symptoms (as measured by the Beck anxiety index and the Maier subscale of the Carroll depression scale), type of irritable bowel syndrome, and quality of life score (Table 37.1), though the limited group had lower symptom severity scale scores. Our data analysis plan included the use of analysis of covariance for continuous measures such as the symptom severity scale. This adjusts for baseline differences between individuals and thus provides a statistical control for group differences when randomisation does not succeed in producing completely balanced groups on baseline measures.

Outcomes at Three Weeks

The observed values for all outcome measures were consistent with our prediction of a progressive improvement in

Table 37.1.

Demographics and baseline symptoms in participants with irritable bowel syndrome

Characteristic	Waiting list (n=87)	Limited (n=88)	Augmented (n=87)
Demographics			
Mean (SD) age (years)	39 (14)	38 (14)	38 (14)
Women	65 (75)	65 (74)	69 (79)
White	78 (90)	71 (81)	80 (92)
Married/living together	34 (39)	40 (46)	43 (49)
Graduated high school	85 (98)	84 (95)	86 (99)
Employed	71 (82)	63 (72)	74 (85)
Type and duration of irritable bowel syndrome			
Constipation	23 (26)	21 (24)	15 (17)
Diarrhoea	22 (25)	18 (21)	29 (33)
Alternating	43 (49)	48 (55)	44 (51)
>1 year	83 (95)	82 (93)	82 (94)
Baseline symptoms			
Mean (SD) symptom severity scale	281 (67)	255 (75)	280 (74)
Mean (SD) quality of life	86 (25)	80 (25)	85 (26)
Psychiatric symptoms			
Anxiety (SD)	11.6 (9.6)	11.7 (8.8)	13.6 (11.0)
Depression (SD)	3.8 (3.8)	3.2 (3.3)	4.0 (3.9)

Note: Figures are number (percentages) unless stated otherwise.

symptoms among the three groups such that waiting list was less effective than limited, which was less effective than augmented. As indicated in Table 37.2 and Figure 37.2 the test of trend for each of the outcome measures was significant ($P < 0.001$). For the global improvement scale and the adequate relief of symptoms, each of the pairwise comparisons (augmented vs. limited and limited vs. waiting list) was significant ($P < 0.001$). For the symptom severity score, the augmented group improved significantly more than the limited group ($P = 0.007$), but the limited and waiting list groups were not significantly different ($P = 0.20$). We observed the same pattern for quality of life ($P = 0.01$ and $P = 0.58$). The proportions of patients reporting moderate or substantial improvement on the global improvement scale were 3% (waiting list), 20% (limited), and 37% (augmented) ($P < 0.001$).

Outcomes at Six Weeks

For participants in the augmented and limited groups, the follow-up evaluation was limited to those who were randomised to continue placebo treatments. As can be seen in Table 37.2 and Figure 37.3, each of the tests for trend at week six was significant. Moreover, except for quality of life where improvement in the waiting list group was similar to that in the limited group, the observed values for all outcome measures were consistent with our a priori prediction of order of improvement.

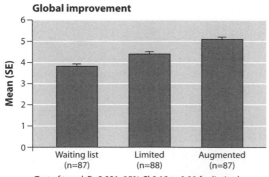

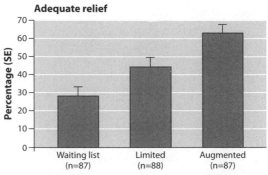

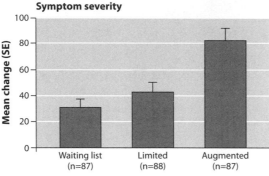

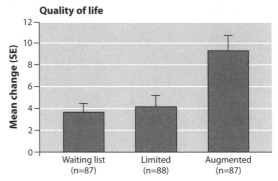

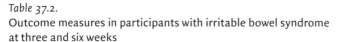

Figure. 37.2. Outcomes at three-week end point.

Table 37.2.
Outcome measures in participants with irritable bowel syndrome at three and six weeks

Outcome measure	Waiting list (n=87)	Limited (n=88)	Augmented (n=87)	P value for trend
At 3 weeks				
Global improvement scale	3.8 (1.0)	4.3 (1.4)	5.0 (1.3)	<0.001
% with adequate relief of symptoms	28	44	62	<0.001
Change in symptom severity score	30 (63)	42 (67)	82 (89)	<0.001
Change in quality of life	3.6 (8.1)	4.1 (9.4)	9.3 (14.0)	0.001
At 6 weeks				
Global improvement scale	3.7 (1.0)	4.6 (1.2)	5.1 (1.5)	<0.001
% with adequate relief of symptoms	35	53	61	0.005
Change in symptom severity score	35 (80)	53 (80)	108 (91)	<0.001
Change in quality of life	5.5 (10.8)	5.4 (9.9)	12.4 (15.1)	0.002

Note: Figures are mean (SD) unless stated otherwise.

Adverse Effects

More than 80% of patients reported no side effects. The most common side effects included pain during needle placement (10%) and redness or swelling (6%) or pain (5%) after needle removal. At the three-week assessment, 2% of patients reported that they considered increased constipation, increased diarrhoea, and dry mouth as probably caused by the treatment. Also, up to 1% of patients reported bad dreams, loss of appetite, sleepiness, fatigue, insomnia, nausea, giddiness, weakness, dizziness, and headache as possibly related to their treatment.

Blinding

At the three-week end point 76% of the limited group and 84% of the augmented group thought that they had been treated with genuine acupuncture. This difference was not significant (P=0.21), suggesting that blinding was successful. In contrast, at the six-week follow-up, 56% of the limited group and 84% of the augmented group thought that they had been treated with genuine acupuncture. This difference was significant (P=0.02). We could not ask any questions about participants' beliefs about their different group assignment because they were never told that the study included different patient-practitioner relationships until the study was over.

Discussion

In this large prospective study of placebo effects we found that such effects can be disentangled into three components that can then be recombined to produce incremental improvement in symptoms in a manner resembling a graded dose escalation of component parts. In the pairwise com-

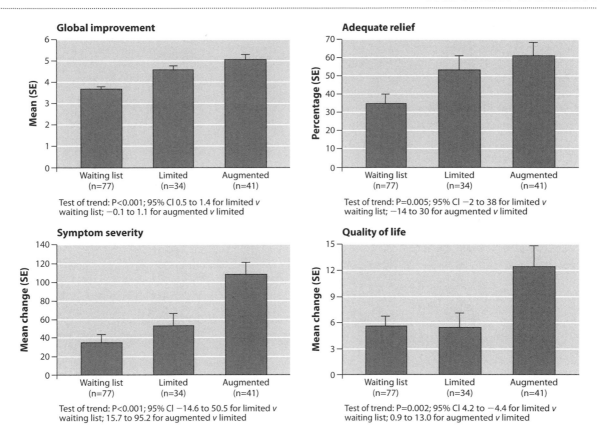

Figure. 37.3. Outcomes at six-week follow-up.

parisons, we also found that an enhanced relationship with a practitioner, together with the placebo treatment, provides the most robust effect in terms of the four measures we used. Placebo treatment with only limited interaction with practitioners was superior to staying on a waiting list with respect to only two of the four measures, suggesting that the supportive interaction with a practitioner is the most potent component of non-specific effects.

The magnitude of non-specific effects in the augmented arm is not only statistically significant but also clearly clinically significant in the management of irritable bowel syndrome. A decrease in the symptom severity score of 50 reliably indicates improvement in symptoms,[9] and our study indicates that 61% and 59% of patients in the augmented arm achieved this level of improvement at three and six weeks, respectively. Likewise, the changes we observed in quality of life indicate at least moderate clinical improvement in symptoms.[25] Finally, the percentage of patients reporting adequate relief (62% and 61% at three and six weeks, respectively) is comparable with the responder rate in clinical trials of drugs currently used in the treatment of irritable bowel syndrome.[26,27] These results indicate that such factors as warmth, empathy, duration of interaction, and the communication of positive expectation might indeed significantly affect clinical outcome. Future investigations will have to determine the relative importance of each of these elements of the patient-practitioner relationship.

Limitations

One limitation of our study is that we could not separate the effects of observation and assessment (and related issues like reporting bias). Thus, an additional control might have been a waiting list group in which participants were followed without their knowledge. As setting up such a control group would have been operationally and ethically difficult to arrange, we believe that our waiting list group is the only feasible and best baseline control for estimating the effects of placebo treatment.

Our outcome measures were subjective rather than objective. Nonetheless, these measures, including the global improvement scale and adequate relief of symptoms are consistent with the recommendations by the Rome committees for use in trials of irritable bowel syndrome because no objective measures of severity are currently available.[28] We chose irritable bowel syndrome for this study because we suspected that non-specific effects are most likely to be demonstrable in disorders defined by subjective symptoms rather than more objective measures of disease.[29] Whether our findings apply to other illnesses, including those with biochemical or other objective outcome measures, awaits further study. Nonetheless, our study has important implications for routine clinical care and suggests that routine medical care would be less efficient if patient-practitioner interactions were reduced. Based on the results of the present study, a positive patient-practitioner relationship can make a difference.

Additionally in terms of limitations, it is unclear whether our placebo outcomes correspond to biological changes in irritable bowel syndrome or have any of the biochemical, neuroendocrine, or neuroanatomical correlates of placebo response found in recent laboratory experiments[30,31] or whether our outcomes are mainly related to shifts in selective attention to diffuse symptoms.[32] In either case, our study represents an incremental step in placebo studies and shows that non-specific effects have a considerable clinical impact.

REFERENCES

1 Kaptchuk TJ. Powerful placebo: the dark side of the randomized controlled trial. *Lancet* 1998;351:1722–1725.

2 Hróbjartsson A. What are the main methodological problems in the estimation of placebo effects. *J Clin Epidemiol* 2002;55:430–435.

3 Miller FG, Kaptchuk TJ. The power of context: reconceptualizing the placebo effect. *J Roy Soc Med* 2008;101:222–225.

4 Longstreth GF, Thompson WG, Chey WD, et al. Functional bowel disorders. *Gastroenterology* 2006;130:1480–1491.

5 Mitchell CM, Drossman DA. Survey of the AGA membership relating to patients with functional gastrointestinal disorders. *Gastroenterology* 1987;92:1282–1284.

6 Inadomi JM, Fennerty MB, Bjorkman D. Systematic review: the economic impact of irritable bowel syndrome. *Aliment Pharmacol Ther* 2003;18:671–682.

7 Patel SM, Stason WB, Legedza A, et al. The placebo effect in irritable bowel syndrome trials: a meta-analysis. *Neurogastroenterol Motil* 2005;17:332–340.

8 Thompson WG, Longstreth GF, Drossman DA, et al. Functional bowel disorders and functional abdominal pain. *Gut* 1999;45(suppl. 2):II43–II47.

9 Francis CY, J. Morris J, Whorwell PJ. The irritable bowel severity scoring system: a simple method of monitoring irritable bowel syndrome and its progress. *Aliment Pharmacol Ther* 1997;11:395–402.

10 Hammer J, Eslick GD, Howell SC, et al. Diagnostic yield of alarm features in irritable bowel syndrome and functional dyspepsia. *Gut* 2004;253:666–672.

11 Vanner SJ, Depew WT, Paterson WG, et al. Predictive value of the Rome criteria for diagnosing the irritable bowel syndrome. *Am J Gastroenterol* 1999;94:2912–2917.

12 Kaptchuk TJ, Stason WB, Davis RB, et al. Sham device *v* inert pill: randomised controlled trial of two placebo treatments. *BMJ* 2006;332:391–397.

13 Kleinhenz J, Streitberger KJ. Randomised clinical trial comparing the effects of acupuncture and a newly designed placebo needle in rotator cuff tendonitis. *Pain* 1999;83:235–241.

14 Owens DM, Nelson DK, Talley NJ. The irritable bowel syndrome: long-term prognosis and the physician-patient interaction. *Ann Intern Med* 1995;122:107–112.

15 Chaput de Saintonge DM, Herxheimer A. Harnessing placebo effects in healthcare. *Lancet* 1994;344:995–998.

16 Keefer L, Blanchard EB. The effects of relaxation response meditation on the symptoms of irritable bowel syndrome: results of a controlled treatment study. *Behav Res Ther* 2001;39:801–811.

17 Drossman DA, Toner BB, Whitehead WE, et al. Cognitive-behavioral therapy versus education and desipramine versus placebo for moderate to severe functional bowel disorders. *Gastroenterology* 2003;125:19–31.

18 Bengtsson M, Ulander K, Borgdal EB, Christensson AC, Ohlsson B. A course of instruction for women with irritable bowel syndrome. *Patient Educ Couns* 2006;62:118–125.

19 Lang EV, Benotsch EG, Fick LJ, et al. Adjunctive non-pharmacological analgesia for invasive medical procedures: a randomised trial. *Lancet* 2000;355:1486–1490.

20 Moncher FJ, Prinz FJ. Treatment fidelity in outcomes studies. *Clin Psych Rev* 1991;11:247–266.

21 Mangel AW, Hahn BA, Heath AT, et al. Adequate relief as an endpoint in clinical trials in irritable bowel syndrome. *J Int Med Res* 1998;26:76–81.

22 Mangel AW. Personal view: adequate relief as a primary endpoint in irritable bowel syndrome. *Aliment Pharmacol Ther* 2006;23:879–881.

23 Lembo T, Wright RA, Bagby B, et al. Alosetron controls bowel urgency and provides global symptom improvement in women with diarrhea-predominant irritable bowel syndrome. *Am J Gastroenterol* 2001;96:2662–2670.

24 Gordon S, Ameen V, Bagby B, et al. Validation of irritable bowel syndrome Global Improvement Scale: an integrated symptom end point for assessing treatment efficacy. *Dig Dis Sci* 2003;48:1317–1323.

25 Drossman DA, Patrick DL, Whitehead WE, et al. Further validation of the IBS-QOL: a disease-specific quality-of-life questionnaire. *Am J Gastroenterol* 2000;95:999–1007.

26 Camilleri M, Northcutt AR, Kong S, et al. Efficacy and safety of alosetron in women with irritable bowel syndrome: a randomised, placebo-controlled trial. *Lancet* 2000;355:1035–1040.

27 Novick J, Miner P, Krause R, et al. A randomized, double-blind, placebo-controlled trial of tegaserod in female patients suffering from irritable bowel syndrome with constipation. *Aliment Pharmacol Ther* 2002;16:1877–1888.

28 Camilleri M, Mangel AW, Fehnel SE, et al. Primary endpoints for irritable bowel syndrome trials: a review of performance of endpoints. *Clin Gastroenterol Hepatol* 2007;5:534–540.

29 Kaptchuk TJ. The placebo effect in alternative medicine: can the performance of a healing ritual have clinical significance? *Ann Intern Med* 2002;136:817–825.

30 Benedetti F, Mayberg HS, Wager TD, Stohler CS, Zubieta JK. Neurobiological mechanisms of the placebo effect. *J Neurosci* 2005;25:10390–10402.

31 Pacheco-López, G, Engler H, Niemi MB, Schedlowski M. Expectations and associations that heal: immunomodulatory placebo effects and its neurobiology. *Brain Behav Immun* 2006:20:430–446.

32 Allan LG, Siegel S. A signal detection theory analysis of the placebo effect. *Eval Health Prof* 2002;25:410–420.

38
Conditioned Pharmacotherapeutic Effects

A Preliminary Study

Robert Ader, Mary Gail Mercurio, James R. Walton, Deborra James, Michael Davis, Valerie E. Ojha, Alexa Boer Kimball, and David Fiorentino

Robert Ader, Mary Gail Mercurio, James R. Walton, Deborra James, Michael Davis, Valerie E. Ojha, Alexa Boer Kimball, and David Fiorentino, "Conditioned Pharmacotherapeutic Effects: A Preliminary Study," *Psychosomatic Medicine* 2010:72:192–197.

Introduction

Clinical research and drug evaluation studies have adhered to the model in which a drug or placebo is administered to evaluate the efficacy of pharmacotherapies or to define the pharmacological (as opposed to the psychological) action of a drug (1). There have been repeated but unanswered calls for studies of the placebo effect as a phenomenon that may have important clinical implications in its own right (2). Still, it is only the initial, nonspecific response to a placebo that is studied in the majority of placebo research. Here, we address placebo effects as they apply to chronic drug treatment conditions.

The response to a placebo "looks like" the response to a conditioned stimulus. In behavioral terms, physiological effects elicited by pharmacologic agents are unconditioned responses, the drug itself being the unconditioned stimulus (UCS). Events or stimuli that are coincidentally or purposely associated with and reliably predict the voluntary or involuntary receipt of drug—but are neutral with respect to eliciting the unconditioned effects of the active drug—are conditioned stimuli (CSs). These could include the environment in which medication is taken or administered (and by whom) and characteristics of the "pill" or injection, itself. Repeated associations of CS and UCS eventually enable the CS to elicit a conditioned response—an approximation of the response unconditionally elicited by the UCS. Thus, the response to an inert or therapeutically irrelevant substance or placebo has been described as a conditioned response.

There is a substantial literature in humans and lower animals supporting the proposition that the response to a placebo is a learned response (3) and one that is specific rather than nonspecific (4). The substitution of CSs for a proportion of active immunosuppressive drug treatments delayed the onset of proteinuria and mortality in lupus-prone mice, using a cumulative amount of drug that was not, by itself, sufficient to influence progression of the autoimmune disorder (5), suggesting that there might be some heuristic value in viewing pharmacotherapeutic protocols as a series of conditioning trials. This strategy was also effective in the treatment of a child with systemic lupus erythematosus (6). Other studies have also shown the salutary effects of exposure to CSs previously paired with therapeutic agents in animals (7–11) and in humans (12). The response to a placebo is influenced by the sequence in which drug and placebo are administered (13–15), and relapse is delayed among patients who are given placebos on withdrawal of active medication (16). Also, conditioning is a parsimonious explanation of the delayed relapse that occurs among patients treated with drug and then switched to placebo (CSs) in double-blind crossover studies (17,18).

The role of conditioning in placebo responding has been questioned on the grounds that some conditioned pharmacologic responses, compensatory or paradoxical conditioned responses, are opposite in direction to the effects of the drug used as the UCS (19). However, there is an operational difference between conditioned pharmacologic and conditioned pharmacotherapeutic responses (3). In the former, the UCS delivered to normal subjects elicits a physiological response that represents some deviation from some homeostatic level, and there are occasions when the UCS elicits a compensatory response. In the case of conditioned pharmacotherapeutic responses, a therapeutic agent delivered to a subject (patient) is calculated to correct a naturally occurring or experimentally induced physiologic imbalance. We are unaware of any direct evidence of compensatory, conditioned, pharmacotherapeutic responses.

Currently, research designed to evaluate drug effects involves two distinct groups: an experimental group that receives active drug and a control group that does not—receiving, instead, an inert or chemically irrelevant substance (the placebo). In all other respects, the stimuli that attend drug or placebo administration are, presumably, "identical." Experimental subjects receive medication that is invariably followed (reinforced) by the unconditioned effects of the drug (in behavioral terms, a continuous or 100% reinforcement schedule). In contrast, control subjects who engage in the same behaviors, are subject to the same environmental conditions, and receive placebo medications that are never therapeutically reinforced; they are on a 0% reinforcement schedule. One is, therefore, prompted to ask about schedules of reinforcement between 0% and 100%. There is an alternative to evaluating drug effects by administering drug or placebo: one can administer drug and placebo. One can introduce partial schedules of reinforcement in which "medication" and the attendant environmental cues are therapeutically reinforced on some occasions but not on others. Thus, by capitalizing on conditioning effects, it might be possible to approximate the therapeutic effects of a continuous schedule of reinforcement, that is, suppress symptoms or maintain some homeostatic limits, using lower cumulative amounts of drug.

We explore this possibility by attempting to reduce the amount of corticosteroid medication required for the maintenance of patients with mild-to-moderate psoriasis. Psoriasis is not a fatal disease, but usually requires lifelong treatment and can become a source of significant morbidity. There is strong evidence that immune regulation plays a pathophysiologic role in the development of this disease (20), and there is striking evidence for the involvement of neurogenic inflammation as well (21,22). There is also literature implicating neuroendocrine factors in the inflammatory and proliferate processes of psoriasis (23,24). It is not surprising, then, that affective states and stressful life experiences have been associated with the appearance or exacerbation of psoriasis (25,26), and it would not, therefore, be unlikely that conditioned pharmacotherapeutic responses could affect the course of disease.

We propose, then, to capitalize on conditioned pharmacotherapeutic responses to reduce the cumulative amount of corticosteroid medication used in the treatment of psoriasis. Specifically, we will test the prediction derived from a conditioning model of pharmacotherapy (3) that patients treated under an intermittent schedule of corticosteroid medication will have a lower occurrence rate of relapse and less severe symptoms of disease compared with patients treated with that same (reduced) amount of drug administered under a continuous schedule of reinforcement.

Methods

Participants

Patients with mild-to-moderate psoriasis, 19 years to 70 years of age, were recruited from newspaper and television advertisements and paid for their participation. Patients reported that they had not been treated with topical or systemic psoriasis medication in the previous two months and agreed to refrain from using any other psoriasis treatments during the course of the study. A total of 251 subjects were screened and 139 satisfied inclusion criteria. Of these, 58 failed to meet baseline period criteria, 27 withdrew from the study (17 before completing the baseline period) for a variety of personal reasons or, most often (70%), without providing reasons, and eight were victims of protocol errors (e.g., remained under baseline conditions after attaining the inclusion criterion), providing a population of 46 patients (83% were white and 56% were male) for analysis (Fig. 38.1). Approximately half the patients were studied at the University of Rochester School of Medicine and Dentistry and half at the Stanford University Medical School throughout the calendar year between 2001 and 2006. The protocol was approved by the Institutional Review Board of both universities. Patients signed a consent form, indicating that this study was an attempt to determine if their psoriasis could be managed with smaller amounts of corticosteroid and, at some point in the course of the study, we

might reduce the amount of medication they were receiving and that the chance of being in such a group was completely random.

Procedures

During an initial screening, two comparable psoriatic plaques were selected and clinically evaluated with respect to erythema, induration, and scaling on a 9-point modified Psoriasis Severity Scale (PSS) (27). Only patients with a PSS score of ≥7 were enrolled. The majority of lesions (approximately 70%) were on elbows or knees, and the target and control lesions were on contralateral sides. There were no group differences in the location of lesions. At this same time, participants also completed several brief questionnaires: the Psoriasis Life Stress Inventory (28,29), Hassle Scale (30), an Impact of Events Scale (31), and the Interpersonal Support Evaluation List (32).

For the next 3 weeks to 6 weeks, each patient applied his or her distinctively fragrant and colored medication, 0.1% triamcinolone acetonide in aquaphor (Aristocort A), twice daily, to the randomly selected "target" lesion. A commercial moisturizing cream was applied to the "control" lesion. Medication was packaged in a connected strip of daily application syringes sufficient for one week. Evaluations of the psoriatic lesions were made weekly throughout the maintenance (conditioning) and experimental periods by a dermatologist blinded to the group to which patients belonged. Patients who did not show evidence of improvement within six weeks (a ≥3-point decline in PSS score) or showed an equal PSS decline in the target and control lesions were excused from further participation in the study.

After the baseline period, patients were randomly assigned to one of three groups (Table 38.1):

Standard Therapy patients continued to receive a full dose of medication on the same continuous (100%) reinforcement schedule received during the baseline (maintenance) period. Corticosteroid was applied to the selected lesion twice daily for as many as eight additional weeks. This is a continuation of their standard pharmacotherapeutic regimen.

Partial Reinforcement patients, the experimental group, were treated under a partial schedule of reinforcement. That

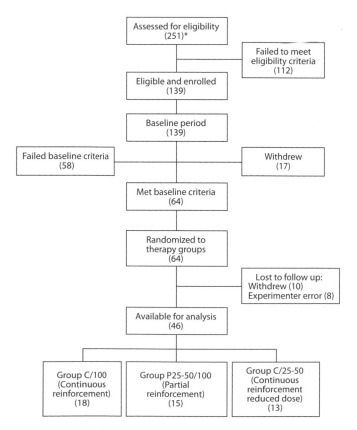

Figure 38.1. Flow of participants through each stage of the study. Asterisk indicates number.

Table 38.1.

Experimental protocol

Group	Baseline Period (3–6 Weeks)		Experimental Period (8 Weeks)	
	Drug Dose[a]	Reinforcement Schedule[b]	Drug Dose	Reinforcement Schedule
Standard Therapy (n=18)	100	100	100	100
Partial Reinforcement (n=15)	100	100	100	25–50
Dose Control (n=13)	100	100	25–50	100

[a] Percentage of 0.1% Aristocort A.

[b] Percentage of treatment occasions when active drug is received.

is, patients received the same 0.1% dose of Aristocort A, but only a portion of the syringes contained active drug; the remaining syringes contained a placebo ointment (aquaphor with the same embellished fragrance and color as the corticosteroid ointment, absent the corticosteroid)—a CS. Initially, patients in the Partial Reinforcement ($n = 6$) and Dose Control ($n = 4$) groups were treated under a 50% reinforcement schedule or dose of triamcinolone acetonide. It seemed, however, that the prevalence of relapse might be insufficient to discriminate among the groups, so the protocol was amended and the reinforcement schedule was reduced to 25% for the remaining experimental patients ($n = 9$) and adjusted accordingly in the Dose Control group ($n = 9$). The sequence of medication was random with the restriction that one of every two or four randomly selected applications of salve contained active drug.

Dose Control patients served as a control for the cumulative amount of drug received. They were treated twice daily under a continuous reinforcement schedule, but each syringe contained only 25% or 50% of the dose of corticosteroid received during the baseline period. Thus, patients in the Partial Reinforcement and Dose Control groups treated under different schedules of pharmacologic reinforcement received the same cumulative amount of active drug.

The primary outcome measures were based on PSS scores. "Relapse," defined a priori as a return to a PSS score within 2 PSS units of the individual patient's initial score is an arbitrary criterion but does signify an inability to maintain the therapeutic effects achieved during the standard pharmacotherapeutic regimen imposed during the baseline period. Additionally, we analyzed changes in PSS scores over time. Per-protocol analyses were limited to participants who met the baseline criteria and provided at least 4 data points during the 8-week treatment period.

It was considered possible that a noncontinuous or intermittent schedule of pharmacologic reinforcement (and the concomitant reduced amount of active drug) could exert effects indistinguishable from a continuous (standard) regimen of pharmacotherapy (a higher cumulative amount of drug). That outcome or comparison, however, is not critical for evaluating the role of conditioning in the pharmacotherapy of psoriasis. Specifically, we tested the prediction that patients treated under a partial schedule of corticosteroid medication would show a greater amelioration of symptoms and a reduced prevalence and rate of relapse than that achieved by patients treated with that same (reduced) amount of drug administered under a continuous schedule of reinforcement.

Statistical Methods

The prevalence of relapse was analyzed with nonparametric tests and a repeated-measures analysis of variance (Group × Week × Site) was applied to the PSS data. Based on the specificity of the a priori hypothesis, the available n for these preliminary observations and the significant effects

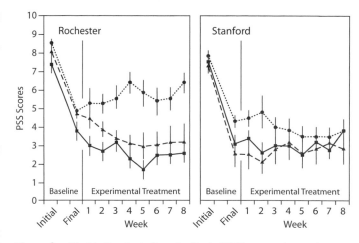

Figure 38.2. Weekly Psoriasis Severity Scale (PSS) scores (mean ± standard error) as a function of reinforcement schedule and amount of drug at each of the study sites. ■ = Standard Therapy (Rochester $n = 5$; Stanford $n = 13$); ▲ = Partial Reinforcement (Rochester $n = 8$; Stanford $n = 7$); ● = Dose Control (Rochester $n = 7$; Stanford $n = 6$).

found in a preliminary unpublished experiment, we used post hoc one-tailed tests for the planned comparisons of the prevalence of relapse of the Standard Therapy versus the Dose Control group (a dose effect) and the Partial Reinforcement versus the Dose Control group (the predicted experimental effect).

Results

There were no differences in initial PSS scores or between the target and control lesions of the groups of patients who did and did not remain in the study, and neither age nor sex were related to either PSS scores or relapse. Furthermore, neither group comparisons nor correlation analyses uncovered any associations between any of the psychometric instruments used to gauge the level or manner of dealing with the life stressors accompanying psoriasis at the time of enrollment and either subsequent relapse or PSS scores.

PSS scores (including the final baseline values) yielded a significant Group × Week × Site interaction ($F(16,320) = 2.47$, $p = .002$). Differences among treatment groups varied at the two study sites (Fig. 38.2). At Stanford, PSS scores remained at the approximate level of the final baseline scores and there were no group differences ($F(16,184) = 1.14$, $p = .33$). In Rochester, there was no difference between the final baseline PSS values of the Partial Reinforcement and Dose Control groups. Under these circumstances, partial reinforcement effected a greater reduction in lesion severity during the experimental period than continuous reinforcement with the same cumulative amount of drug ($F(16,136) = 2.29$, $p = .005$). The Partial Reinforcement Group did not differ from the Standard Therapy group that received two to four times more drug.

With respect to relapse, there were no differences between the 25% and 50% reinforcement schedules or between patients studied in New York and California. These groups

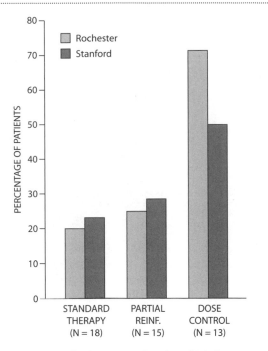

Figure 38.3. Incidence of "relapse" as a function of reinforcement schedule and amount of drug. Planned comparisons showed incidence of relapse in the Partial Reinforcement group to be lower than in Dose Control patients treated with the same amount of corticosteroid.

were therefore combined. The incidence of relapse is shown in Figure 38.3. An overall χ^2 analysis revealed differences in the frequency with which relapse occurred in the three differentially treated groups ($\chi2 = 5.81$, $p < .05$, one tail). Among those treated under a standard regimen of corticosteroid therapy, four (22.2%) of 18 patients relapsed within the 8-week experimental period. Among patients treated under a partial schedule of reinforcement, four (26.7%) of 15 relapsed. In contrast, eight (61.5%) of the 13 dose control patients who received the same reduced amount of drug relapsed in the same period of time. Planned comparisons showed that the frequency of relapse in the Partial Reinforcement group was lower than in Dose Control patients treated with the same amount of corticosteroid ($\chi^2 = 3.45$, $p < .05$) and did not differ from patients receiving a full dose of drug all the time ($\chi^2 = 0.09$, $p > .10$).

The control lesion, which defines the effects of emollient alone, provides an approximation of a within-subject control for the natural history of disease. Therefore, we compared the difference between the PSS scores of the target and control lesions for each patient to determine the effect of treatment over and above the effects of emollient. There were group differences ($F(2,43) = 3.94$, $p = .027$), but there were no interaction effects. Overall, the difference between target and control lesions among patients in the Dose Control group was significantly (44%) less (i.e., the severity of the psoriatic lesions was greater) than among patients in the Partial Reinforcement Group (protected least significant difference Critical Difference = 1.23, $p = .014$). There was no difference between the Partial Reinforcement and the Standard

Therapy groups ($p = .39$). Again, however, these differences paralleled differences seen at the final baseline week and cannot be used to support the hypothesis.

Discussion

Based on a learning model of placebo effects under chronic drug treatment conditions (3), the hypothesis that psoriasis patients treated under a partial schedule of pharmacologic reinforcement would show greater amelioration of symptoms and less relapse than patients treated with the same cumulative amount of drug under a standard pharmacotherapeutic regimen—a continuous schedule of pharmacologic reinforcement—was confirmed. These observations are consistent with the results obtained in the animal research (3,5,7–10) from which the present study was derived. At one of the study sites, however, there were no group differences in PSS scores that could be attributed to the different treatments. This may have been related to the (not to be expected) high baseline values in the randomly selected Dose Control subjects. It might even reflect the amount of sunshine available in Stanford relative to Rochester. This subset of data for this outcome measure, then, neither supports nor refutes the hypothesis. The elevated PSS baseline in the Dose Control group cannot, however, explain the difference in the prevalence of relapse between the Partial Reinforcement and Dose Control groups, as the higher frequency of relapse occurred in Dose Control subjects in Rochester where there was no difference in baseline PSS scores.

Among psoriasis patients who showed comparable levels of improvement under standard treatment conditions, the subsequent imposition of a partial schedule of pharmacologic reinforcement enabled these patients to be maintained with a cumulative amount of topical corticosteroid that was, under standard treatment regimens, relatively ineffective in treating the disease. The fact that there were no differences between patients treated under a schedule of partial reinforcement and those treated under a standard treatment regimen who received two to four times more drug is another interesting feature of these results. We cannot conclude, however, that the partial and continuous reinforcement treatments were equivalent. Nonetheless, these results suggest that a parametric examination of the interactions among drug dose, frequency, and schedule of reinforcement would yield interesting results with important implications for the design of pharmacotherapeutic regimens.

Although the feasibility of incorporating a behavioral strategy in the titration of prescribed medications has been established here, we can only infer, based on the operations performed, that conditioning processes were responsible for the observed effects. In this initial study, we did not have an independent measure of conditioned physiological responses relevant to the amelioration of symptoms of psoriasis. Also, other predictions that can be derived from the model have yet to be tested. For example, would preexposure to the CS or UCS attenuate learning and would reinforcement schedule predict resistance to extinction (the partial reinforcement effect)?

Similarly, alternative hypotheses need to be addressed. Multiple doses of 0.025% or 0.05% Aristocort A may not be pharmacodynamically equivalent to 0.1% Aristocort A and, although repeated low doses are relatively ineffective, a bolus of corticosteroid once every other day or every four days (without intervening CS) may be sufficient to maintain reduced symptoms of psoriasis. If true, however, the standard q day or bid dosing regimen for treating psoriasis may be prescribing two to four times more corticosteroid than necessary. One might (should) consider a comparison group maintained on a continuous schedule of reinforcement that receives only a full dose of drug once every two or four days. Experimentally, the data from such a group would be suspect, however, because, unlike all other study subjects, these patients could not be blinded. Even so, such a group will need to be studied.

Another variable to consider is that the "side" effects of drug treatments could be reduced under a partial schedule of reinforcement (less drug is being administered), resulting in greater adherence to the treatment regimen than occurs under a continuous, full dose regimen. This beneficial side effect may play some role in the therapeutic equation in humans. But, it could not explain the comparable results obtained in lupus-prone mice treated under the same conditions described here (5).

It has been shown that, even in the case of an autoimmune disorder, animals behave in their biological interests. For example, unlike normal mice that develop an aversion to flavors associated with the effects of cyclophosphamide, lupus-prone mice do not display an aversion to a novel taste associated with the immunosuppressive drug (33). The possibility that a conditioned compensatory response could emerge in a pharmacotherapeutic situation, a biologically maladaptive outcome seems unlikely, but could be examined in subhuman animals, using a pharmacologic agent that reliably elicits a compensatory response in normal animals and has therapeutic effects in animals with a spontaneously occurring or experimentally induced pathologic condition.

There are, in addition, several methodological issues that will need to be addressed. Thus far, the selection of reinforcement schedule has been essentially arbitrary and will need to be established (and is likely to be different) for different medical conditions. The duration of the baseline period—the period during which conditioning occurs—has yet to be examined. Given a sufficient number of treatment trials (each medication instance constituting a single trial), we would predict that all patients (not just a subgroup of placebo "responders") would eventually acquire the conditioned pharmacotherapeutic response.

Psoriasis was chosen for this first study because neither the disease nor treatment with topical corticosteroid was considered a major health risk, there were measurable clinical outcomes and, presumably, a sufficient number of qualified participants. This model, however, was not ideal for examining possible biological mechanisms. Corticosteroids are assumed to influence the expression of psoriasis through their immunosuppressive and anti-inflammatory actions, but which specific aspects of immune function are responsible for the alleviation of symptoms of psoriasis and which of these are capable of being conditioned remains to be determined. It seems unlikely that a single biological mechanism will be found to explain conditioned pharmacotherapeutic effects. Hypothetically, an elaboration of the biological mechanisms underlying conditioned pharmacotherapeutic responses will depend on the ability to condition those effects of specific drugs that are directly or indirectly responsible for alleviating the symptoms of specific disease processes.

Although there are several research strategies that need to be pursued, these initial data, limited by a smaller than expected or planned number of patients, may reasonably be construed as providing a proof-of-principle in illustrating the feasibility and potential clinical impact of designing drug treatment protocols that consider a behavioral dimension that is an inherent component of many pharmacotherapeutic regimens. Operationally, it is not possible to administer a therapeutic agent that is not accompanied by conditioned stimuli. One can choose to ignore the learning component of pharmacotherapies. Alternatively, one can explore ways to exploit conditioning in designing drug treatment regimens that consider both the behavioral and the pharmacologic components of the response to medications. Although these strategies would not apply in the case of replacement therapies, the adoption of a conditioning perspective suggests testable hypotheses and innovative strategies for the experimental analysis of drug and placebo effects and for the design of pharmacotherapeutic regimens in a variety of other disorders. The present results support the proposition, based on principles of learning, that the imposition of partial schedules of reinforcement in a pharmacotherapeutic protocol might: 1) reduce the total amount of drug required for the treatment of some pathophysiological conditions, thereby maximizing benefits and reducing risks; 2) reduce (deleterious or noxious) side effects (and thereby increase adherence to a treatment protocol); 3) extend the effects of pharmacotherapy (i.e., increase resistance to extinction); and last, but by no means least, 4) reduce substantially the cost of long-term drug treatments.

REFERENCES

1. Tilburt JC, Emanuel EJ, Kaptchuk TJ, et al. Prescribing "placebo treatments": results of national survey of US internists and rheumatologists. BMJ 2008;337:a1938.
2. Guess HA, Kleinman A, Kusel JW, Engel LW, editors. The Science of the Placebo. London: BMJ Books; 2002.
3. Ader R. The role of conditioning in pharmacotherapy. In: Harrington A, editor. The Placebo Effect: An Interdisciplinary Exploration. Cambridge, Mass.: Harvard University Press; 1997.
4. Amanzio M, Benedetti F. Neuropharmacological dissection of placebo analgesia: expectation-activated upload systems versus conditioning-activated specific subsystems. J Neurosci 1999;19:484–494.

5. Ader R, Cohen N. Behaviorally conditioned immunosuppression and murine systemic lupus erythematosus. Science 1982;215:1534–1536.

6. Olness K, Ader R. Conditioning as an adjunct in the pharmacotherapy of lupus erythematosus. J Dev Behav Pediatr 1992;13:124–125.

7. Klosterhalfen W, Klosterhalfen S. Pavlovian conditioning of immunosuppression modifies adjuvant arthritis in rats. Behav Neurosci 1983;97:663–666.

8. Gorczynski RM. Conditioned enhancement of skin allografts in mice. Brain Behav Immun 1990;4:85–92.

9. Grochowicz PM, Schedlowski M, Husband AJ, et al. Behavioral conditioning prolongs heart allograft survival in rats. Brain Behav Immun 1991;5:349–356.

10. Exton MS, von Hörsten SB, Schultz M, et al. Behaviourally conditioned immunosuppression using cyclosporine A: central nervous system reduces IL-2 production via splenic innervation. J Neuroimmunol 1998;88:182–191.

11. Jones RE, Moes NM, Zwickey H, et al. Treatment of experimental autoimmune encephalomyelitis with alpha lipoic acid and associative conditioning. Brain Behav Immun 2008;22:538–543.

12. Castes M, Palenque M, Canelones P, et al. Classic conditioning and placebo effects in the bronchodilator response of asthmatic children. Neuroimmunomodulation 1998;5:70.

13. Batterman RC. Methodology of analgesic evaluation: experience with orphenadrine citrate compound. Curr Ther Res Clin Exp 1965;7:639–647.

14. Sunshine A, Laska, E, Meisner M, Morgan, S. Analgesic studies of indomethacin as analyzed by computer techniques. Clin Pharmacol Ther 1964;5:699–707.

15. Moertel CG, Taylor WF, Roth A, Tyce FA. Who responds to sugar pills? Mayo Clin Proc 1976;51:96–100.

16. Greenberg LM, Roth S. Differential effects of abrupt versus gradual withdrawal of chlorpromazine in hospitalized chronic schizophrenic patients. Am J Psychiatry 1966;123:221–226.

17. Ader R. Conditioning effects in pharmacotherapy and the incompleteness of the double-blind, crossover design. Integ Psychiatry 1989;6:165–170.

18. Suchman AL, Ader R. Classic conditioning and placebo effects in crossover studies. Clin Pharmacol Ther 1992;52:372–377.

19. Kirsch I. Specifying nonspecifics: psychological mechanisms of placebo effects. In: Harrington A, editor. The Placebo Effect: An Interdisciplinary Exploration. Cambridge, Mass.: Harvard University Press; 1997.

20. Farber EM, Lanigan SW, Boer J. The role of cutaneous sensory nerves in the maintenance of psoriasis. Int J Dermatol 1990;29:418–420.

21. Raychaudhuri SP, Farber EM. Are sensory nerves essential for the development of psoriatic lesions? J Am Acad Dermatol 1993;28:488–489.

22. Raychaudhuri SP, Farber EM. Neuroendocrine influences on the pathogenesis of psoriasis. In: Ader R, Cohen N, Felten D, editors. Psychoneuroimmunology. 3rd ed. New York: Academic Press; 2000.

23. Farber EM, Nickoloff BJ, Recht B, Fraki JE. Stress, symmetry, and psoriasis: possible role of neuropeptides. J Am Acad Dermatol 1986;114:305–311.

24. Fava GA, Perini GI, Santonastaso P, Fornasa CV. Life events and psychological distress in dermatologic disorders: psoriasis, chronic urticaria and fungal infections. Br J Med Psychol 1980;53:277–282.

25. Seville RH. Psoriasis and stress. Br J Dermatol 1977;97:297–302.

26. Raychaudhuri SP, Gross J. Psoriasis risk factors: role of lifestyle practices. Cutis 2000;66:348–352.

27. Emtestam L, Bergland L, Angelin B, et al. Tinproroporphyrin and long wave length ultraviolet light in treatment of psoriasis. Lancet 1989;1:1231–1233.

28. Gupta MA, Gupta AK. The psoriasis life stress inventory: a preliminary index of psoriasis-related stress. Arch Dermatol Venerol (Stockh) 1995;75:240–243.

29. Fortune D, Main CJ, O'Sullivan TM, Griffiths CE. Assessing illness-related stress in psoriasis: the psychometric properties of the psoriasis life stress inventory. J Psychosom Res 1997;42:467–475.

30. Kanner D, Coyne JHC, Schaefer C, Lazarus RS. Comparison of two modes of stress measurement: daily hassles and uplifts versus major life events. J Behav Med 1981;4:1–39.

31. Horowitz M, Wilner N, Alvarez W. Impact of event scale: a measure of subjective stress. Psychosom Med 1979;41:209–218.

32. Cohen S, Mermelstein R, Kamarack T, Hoberman HM. Measuring the functional components of social support. In: Sarason G, Sarason BR, editors. Social Support: Theory, Research and Applications. The Hague: Martinus Nijhoff; 1985.

33. Ader R, Grota LJ, Moynihan JA, Cohen N. Behavioral adaptations in autoimmune disease-susceptible mice. In: Ader R, Felten DL, Cohen N, editors. Psychoneuroimmunology. 2nd ed. San Diego: Academic Press; 1991.

Ethical Issues Raised by the Use of Placebos in Research and Clinical Practice

Ethical concerns relating to the use of placebos arise in a number of contexts. These include placebo-controlled clinical trials, research on the placebo effect, and the use of placebos and interventions aimed at promoting placebo responses in clinical practice. Some of the key ethical issues at stake are highlighted here as background to the landmark articles in Part III. Also included is a brief discussion of ethical issues relating to nocebo effects, which have received scant attention.

Placebo-Controlled Trials

Randomized, double-blind, placebo-controlled trials are widely considered to be the "gold standard" for rigorous scientific evaluation of treatment efficacy. Pharmaceutical regulatory agencies frequently require them as a precondition for licensing new drugs in a wide range of medical conditions. Use of placebo, masked to appear indistinguishable from treatment under investigation, permits researchers to experimentally control for a variety of factors that can confound judgments of treatment efficacy. These include regression to the mean and/or spontaneous improvement (patients typically enter clinical trials when their symptoms are at a high level, which are likely to diminish when evaluated at a subsequent point in time); biased assessment of outcomes by patient-subjects or investigators (especially problematic for subjective, patient-centered outcomes such as pain or mood); and the placebo effect associated with patients believing that they are receiving an effective treatment and expecting benefit, so-called response expectancies. Superiority to placebo in a randomized, double-blind trial constitutes an important minimal evidentiary threshold for treatment efficacy, suggesting that the inherent properties (or "characteristic factors," as Adolf Grünbaum put it [Grünbaum 1986]) of the treatment under investigation are causally responsible for improved patient outcomes.

Despite promoting methodological rigor, the use of placebo controls is ethically controversial under two conditions: (1) when trials withhold proven effective treatment to patients randomized to placebo, and (2) when the placebo intervention consists of an invasive (and, thus, harmful) sham procedure. Ethical concerns with withholding proven effective treatment became prominent in the 1990s after an article in the *New England Journal of Medicine* sparked debate (Rothman and Michels 1994). Kenneth Rothman and Karin

Michels, whose paper we include here as chapter 39, argue that many placebo-controlled trials were unethical because they withheld proven effective treatment and thereby violated the Declaration of Helsinki, the leading international guidance on the ethics of clinical research. The 1989 version of the Declaration (the extant version at the time Rothman and Michels wrote) states: "In any medical study, every patient—including those of a control group, if any—should be assured of the best proven diagnostic and therapeutic method." As they note, a straightforward reading of this statement and acceptance of its normative force would have prohibited the conduct of many placebo-controlled trials that were nonetheless being conducted and later published in top medical journals. Rothman and Michels argue against the ethical justifiability of such trials, and they call on investigators to explicitly justify the need for placebo controls in their studies. Moreover, they call on institutional review boards, research sponsors, journal editors, and especially regulatory agencies to demand that investigators provide such justifications. This article brought to the foreground the issue of placebo controls in medical research and launched a lively debate in the literature that continues today.

In addition to their arguable violation of the Declaration of Helsinki, many placebo-controlled trials have been criticized as contravening *clinical equipoise*—widely considered a fundamental moral requirement of research ethics that stipulates that randomized trials are ethical only when a state of genuine uncertainty regarding the comparative merits of the therapies proposed for study exists within the appropriate clinical community (Freedman 1987; Freedman et al. 1996b). In their chapter, Benjamin Freedman and his colleagues claim that, although the controversial statement from the Declaration of Helsinki (quoted above) is badly worded, the normative principle underlying this statement is "clear and noncontroversial," namely, clinical equipoise. As they argue, clinical equipoise prohibits trials that employ treatments known to be inferior to the evidence-based standard of care, thus ruling out the use of placebo controls that withhold proven effective treatment. In recent years, however, some bioethics scholars have criticized the ethical grounding and force of clinical equipoise (Gifford 2007; Miller and Brody 2003; Miller and Joffe 2011; Veatch 2007). Part of the criticism of clinical equipoise has been that it conflates the ethics of clinical research with the ethics of medical care; put differently, those who defend clinical equipoise adopt a problematic therapeutic orientation to clinical research that should be dispensed with (Miller and Brody 2003; Miller and Rosenstein 2003). Among critics of clinical equipoise, placebo-controlled trials that withhold proven effective treatment from those enrolled have been defended provided that there are sound scientific reasons for using placebo controls and that patient-subjects are not exposed to excessive risks of harm. The contributions in this anthology by Robert Temple and Susan Ellenberg (Temple and Ellenberg 2000) and by Ezekiel Emanuel and Franklin Miller (Emanuel and Miller 2001) develop these lines of thought. The ethical debate regarding the use of placebos in clinical research is complex and encompasses issues of scientific validity, the clinical value of different trial designs (for example, active-control equivalence or noninferiority trials), risk-benefit assessment, and the duties of physician-investigators to patient-subjects (Ellenberg and Temple 2000; Freedman et al. 1996a; Miller and Weijer 2007).

A related controversy erupted in 1997 over the issue of placebo controls in international research designed to test a feasible and inexpensive intervention with the aim of preventing transmission of HIV from pregnant women to their children in poor countries. Antiretroviral treatment in a relatively complex and expensive regimen tested in the United States and France had been proven effective in reducing transmission of HIV by two-thirds (Connor et al. 1994). Because this regimen was neither logistically feasible nor affordable in many poor countries, it seemed desirable to investigate an alternative treatment regimen that might be effective, easier to implement, and affordable. The use of placebo-controlled trials, sponsored by U.S. government agencies, was criticized for unjustly applying a double standard, as investigators would never be permitted to enroll pregnant women with HIV in developed countries in such trials in view of the availability of a highly effective treatment regimen (Angell 1997). Others defended the placebo-controlled trials as both scientifically necessary and ethically appropriate to the aim of seeking a feasible and affordable treatment for use in poor countries (Crouch and Arras 1998; Varmus and Satcher 1997). The ethical debate has centered in part on the appropriate *standard of care* for international clinical trials (Hawkins and Emanuel 2008; London 2000). As a matter of principle, should control groups in trials to test new interventions be provided with the best proven effective treatment for their condition that is available anywhere in the world? Or is it ethical for them to receive treatment comparable to what they otherwise would be entitled to in their local setting (which may be no treatment, thus legitimating the use of placebo controls)? Consensus has not been reached on this complex issue of global justice and the responsibility of physician-investigators to patient-subjects, but those who take up the question of using placebo controls in international research cannot ignore them.

Over time, established ethical guidance with respect to placebo-controlled trials has shifted, as reflected in the revisions to the Declaration of Helsinki. In 2000 the Declaration was substantially revised. The principle relating to use of placebo controls was modified to make it clear that when proven effective treatment exists, new treatments should be tested against "the best current" treatment, thus ruling out placebo controls in this situation. However, a "Note of Clarification" was inserted into the Declaration in 2002 to permit placebo controls *despite* proven effective treatment under some conditions, and this was codified in the revised version of 2008:

> The benefits, risks, burdens and effectiveness of a new intervention must be tested against those of the best current proven intervention, except in the following circumstances:
> - The use of placebo, or no treatment, is acceptable in studies where no current proven intervention exists; or
> - Where for compelling and scientifically sound methodological reasons the use of placebo is necessary to determine the efficacy or safety of an intervention and the patients who receive placebo or no treatment will not be subject to any risk of serious or irreversible harm.
>
> Extreme care must be taken to avoid abuse of this option.
> (World Medical Association 2008)

The exact interpretation of this provision of the Declaration remains open to question. Should *any* risk of serious or irreversible harm be taken literally, or should the principle be understood as permitting sufficiently low risk of such harm? What is the appropriate standard of care baseline—that in the developed or developing world?—in international trials for determining the risks of withholding treatment connected with placebo assignment?

Placebo controls also pose ethical issues when they are used to evaluate invasive procedures. It may seem intuitively obvious that physician-investigators should not expose patient-subjects to fake surgeries in clinical trials. Unlike pharmacology trials, in which those receiving placebo bear no (or very little) risk from the placebo intervention itself, sham surgery interventions directly subject recipients to risks of harm, a fact some critics claim contributes to the ethical unjustifiability of such surgeries (Macklin 1999). Consequently, sham surgery trials have rarely been conducted. Nevertheless, some surgical techniques are sufficiently low risk to make it seem legitimate to consider use of minimally invasive masked sham interventions as a rigorous control for trials that evaluate these surgical procedures with respect to subjective outcomes, such as relief of pain. A landmark sham-controlled surgery trial demonstrated that the widely used procedure of arthroscopic surgery for osteoarthritis of the knee was no more effective than a sham control involving skin incision without manipulation of the knee (Moseley et al. 2002). We include here the commentary that accompanied the publication of this trial in the *New England Journal of Medicine* (Horng and Miller 2002). In it, Sam Horng and

Franklin Miller argue that the risks posed by the sham surgery intervention in the osteoarthritis trial were justifiable when one considers the value of the knowledge to be gained by the study and given that there was no reason to be concerned about the validity of the consent given by the participants. Although Horng and Miller restrict the bulk of their analysis to the osteoarthritis study, the analytic framework they articulate and employ is applicable to any trial that involves a sham-surgery control group.

In addition to concerns about the ethics of trial design, placebo-controlled trials also raise issues relating to informed consent. Placebo-controlled trials conceal the treatment received, but they typically are not deceptive because patient-subjects are clearly informed that they will receive either the treatment under investigation or a masked placebo control. However, some placebo-controlled trials have been deceptive in the way that the control group intervention has been described to research participants. For example, many recent acupuncture trials have randomized patients with various conditions to either acupuncture performed according to traditional methods or to a sham acupuncture intervention, consisting either of superficial needling at non-acupuncture points or merely the appearance of needling without skin penetration. The sham controls have often been described to research subjects as a non-traditional form of acupuncture, rather than as a fake intervention designed to be a placebo control. This approach is deceptive, making it contrary to the moral requirements of informed consent; moreover, it is methodologically unnecessary (Miller and Kaptchuk 2007). Another form of deception is the use of a single-blind placebo lead-in phase in placebo-controlled pharmaceutical trials, under which all participants receive placebo for a period of time prior to being randomized to either the study drug or a placebo control. The major ostensible purpose of the placebo lead-in is to reduce the number of placebo responders. Although subjects are informed that they will receive either the study treatment or placebo, they typically are not informed that they *all* will receive placebo at some point during the trial. The deceptive placebo lead-in has been criticized as unethical and methodologically unnecessary (Evans 2000; Mann 2007).

Finally, consent to placebo-controlled trials may be compromised by a phenomenon known as the *therapeutic misconception*. Survey research has indicated that, despite accurate disclosure about basic elements of trial design and conduct, many patient-subjects believe that they will receive treatment in the clinical trial based on a personalized judgment of what is considered medically best for them. In other words, they confuse trial participation with routine clinical care. "To maintain a therapeutic misconception," as Paul Appelbaum and his colleagues argue in their chapter in this anthology, "is to deny the possibility that there may be major disadvantages to participating in clinical research that stem from the nature of the research process itself" (Appelbaum et al. 1987, 20). The therapeutic misconception was originally discovered and characterized in the context of survey research relating to informed consent for placebo-controlled psychiatric trials, but evidence for its existence has been seen in a wide range of clinical trials and is not limited to those that involve placebo controls (Appelbaum et al. 2004). The extent to which it compromises informed consent, however, is a matter of debate (Miller and Joffe 2006). Appelbaum and his colleagues found that a discussion with a neutral professional focused on the differences between trial participation and clinical care prior to trial enrollment improves the comprehension of patient-subjects (Appelbaum et al. 1987).

Research on the Placebo Effect

Laboratory investigation of the placebo effect, aimed at understanding its psychological and neurobiological mechanisms, typically involves administering inert placebos to research subjects deceptively described to them as real interventions. For example, in experiments on placebo analgesia, as described in many of the articles in Part II of this volume, placebo pills or creams are presented to subjects as powerful pain-relieving agents. Subjects also are typically deceived, or not accurately informed, about the purpose of the study to investigate placebo effects. Such deception is necessary to promote scientific validity but contravenes informed consent. Franklin Miller and colleagues have recommended *authorized deception* as an approach aimed at improving the consent process without compromising the scientific validity of the research (Miller et al. 2005; Wendler and Miller 2004). Using this approach, prospective subjects are informed that aspects of the research have not been described accurately; that this deception is necessary to obtain valid results; that the use of deception has been approved by a research ethics committee; and that they will be accurately informed about the purpose of the study and procedures employed after the conclusion of research participation. In contrast to the usual approach, which does not alert prospective subjects to the use of deception, authorized deception respects the autonomy of research subjects by giving them the opportunity to decide whether they are willing to participate in research that involves deception.

However, given that many outcomes in studies of the placebo response are subjective and open to the vagaries of perception, Miller and colleagues recognized that the use of authorized deception might yield biased results by, say, influencing the magnitude and direction of the placebo response. They thus recommended that the authorized deception methodology be experimentally validated. Recently, a placebo analgesia experiment was undertaken with the purpose of investigating the effects of authorized deception on recruitment, retention, and study results. We include it here (Martin and Katz 2010). Healthy subjects were randomized to either the standard (non-authorized) deception or authorized deception consent procedures, then enrolled in a validated protocol investigating the effect of placebo cream on experimentally induced pain. No differences in study outcomes between the two groups were observed. Although further experimental testing is needed, involving various groups of patient-subjects and different types of placebo interventions, authorized deception appears to be a sound method for conducting deceptive research while respecting subject autonomy. A recent investigation of placebo-induced dopamine release in Parkinson's disease adopted the authorized deception consent procedure (Lidstone et al. 2010), thus suggesting that this approach may become more widely used in both psychological and neurobiological research on the placebo effect (Miller and Kaptchuk 2008).

Use of Placebo Treatments in Clinical Practice

Traditionally, deliberate use of placebo treatments in clinical practice was thought to be appropriate, and was likely a common practice. It came under attack, however, in the wake of the critique of medical paternalism and emphasis on patient autonomy that gathered force in the second half of the twentieth century. Ethicists criticized prescription of placebo treatments as deceptive, and thus contrary to informed consent; as potentially deleterious to the physician-patient relationship by promoting distrust when discovered by patients; and as unnecessary, since empathetic communication and fostering positive expectations for medically indicated treatments can be effective in promoting therapeutically valuable placebo responses. In their chapters in this anthology, Sissela Bok and Howard Brody examine arguments for and against the use of placebos in clinical practice (Bok 1974; Brody 1982). While Bok sees the use of placebos in clinical practice as deceptive and thus morally problematic, Brody argues that physicians can elicit beneficial placebo effects from their patients using non-deceptive means and without resorting to inert pills, thus making non-deceptively induce placebo *effects* (rather than placebos *per se*) of potential clinical value.

Apart from these objections to placebo use, one might suspect that the use of placebo treatments would have died out owing simply to the growing armamentarium of effective treatments available to contemporary physicians, reinforced by professional commitment to evidence-based medicine. Nevertheless, recent surveys of physicians in Europe and the United States have indicated that use of placebo treatments remains common in clinical practice (Fässler et al. 2010; Hróbjartsson and Norup 2003; Tilburt et al. 2008). Although physicians rarely recommend or administer "inert" interventions, such as sugar pills or saline injections, they frequently recommend what some have called "impure placebos"—treatments that contain active medication but that is not thought to be effective for the patient's condition. As Jon Tilburt and his colleagues report, these include antibiotics for viral infections, vitamins, sedatives, and over-the-counter analgesics (Tilburt et al. 2008). Clinicians stated that they recommended such placebo treatments because, among other reasons, they wanted to satisfy patient expectations of receiving a prescribed treatment (that is, they wanted to avoid confrontations with patients) and in order to promote a beneficial placebo response (Hróbjartsson and Norup 2003).

The two major empirical issues relevant to the ethical use of placebo treatments in clinical practice are whether there is adequate evidence supporting the ability of placebo interventions to promote a clinically meaningful placebo response and whether placebo treatments can be effective in producing a beneficial placebo response without the use of deception. Franklin Miller and Luana Colloca discuss these issues in their paper in this anthology (Miller and Colloca 2009). Although some, like Walter Brown in his paper we include here, have recommended the prescription of honestly described inert placebo pills, for example, as a first line treatment for depression (Brown 1994), it seems intuitively implausible that patients would derive therapeutic benefit from treatment with a pill known to contain no pharmacological ingredients at all (or, at least, none targeted to their condition). Nevertheless, two psychiatric investigators found that a small group of patients with various anxiety disorders reported meaningful symptomatic improvement after receiving placebos described as "sugar pills" with "no medication at all" but given with a positive expectation for benefit (Park and Covi 1965). The study, however, was methodologically weak because it lacked a no-treatment control group. Recently, open placebo was tested in a pilot randomized trial enrolling patients with irritable bowel syndrome (Kaptchuk et al. 2010). Patients were randomized to open placebo described as containing no medication, like a sugar pill, and to no treatment, in the context of positive information regarding the potential for beneficial placebo responses. Those receiving placebo reported greater improvement in symptoms—differences that were statistically and clinically significant. It appears that placebo responses can be obtained from receiving pill placebos without deception.

A rather different method of using placebos in clinical practice is in the context of deliberate conditioning involving partial substitution of placebo for drug treatment aimed at maintaining a therapeutic response with lower side effects. Recently, pioneering experiments with psoriasis and ADHD patients have suggested promising results (Ader et al. 2010; Sandler et al. 2010). There is no need for deception in trials of conditioned placebo substitution. The placebo either can be presented to the patient in an open-label fashion, for example, described as a "dose extender" containing no medication (Sandler et al. 2010), or in a masked form indistinguishable from the drug with which it is paired, with patients told that at some point in the course of the conditioning trial the amount of medication received will be reduced by substituting placebo (Ader et al. 2010).

Alternative medicine treatments, such as herbal treatments and acupuncture, may be promising interventions for the purpose of promoting placebo responses. For example, well-designed trials of glucosamine for low back pain and lumbar arthritis and saw palmetto for male prostate and lower urinary tract symptoms have indicated that they are no better than placebos (Bent et al. 2006; Wilkens et al. 2010). These low-risk treatments, however, may promote placebo responses, but this has never been tested in trials including a no-treatment control group. In contrast, large-scale acupuncture trials for low back pain have demonstrated that while acupuncture is no better than a sham acupuncture intervention, both are superior to wait-list control groups and to usual medical care (Brinkhaus et al. 2006; Cherkin et al. 2009; Haake et al. 2007). These studies strongly suggest (but do not prove) that acupuncture relieves low back pain by means of a placebo response. Whether meaningful clinical benefit can be obtained if patients are informed transparently that these types of treatment are being recommended for the purpose of promoting a placebo response has not been demonstrated. In addition, if placebo treatments can be effective without being deceptive, it will be important to devote attention to the level of risk from a placebo intervention that might be acceptable to promote a placebo response (Miller et al. 2011).

Further clinically oriented placebo research and ethical inquiry are needed to assess the legitimacy of inert placebos and treatment interventions for the purpose of promoting placebo responses in clinical practice. There is, however, a flip-side to the issue of producing beneficial placebo effects in the clinic, namely, the inadvertent production of nocebo effects by the way in which clinicians communicate with patients. Clinicians are responsible for informing patients about the side effects of treatments as part of obtaining informed consent. However, research has demonstrated that informing patients about side effects may create expectations that produce or augment the experience of side effects (Barsky et al. 2002; Mondaini et al. 2007). How can clinicians minimize nocebo effects consistent with securing valid consent?

Are patients manipulated in an ethically problematic manner if physicians communicate side effect risk information truthfully but in a way that takes into account framing effects? A study of patients appropriate for influenza immunization randomized them to logically equivalent information disclosures relating to side effects that were framed in positive and negative ways (O'Connor et al. 1996). In the positive framing, subjects were told the percentage of patients free of vaccine side effects based on available data; in the negative framing, they were told the percentage who report side effects. Even though the framing did not influence patients' decisions about whether or not to be vaccinated, those receiving the positive framing reported significantly lower incidence of side effects and work absenteeism following immunization. As long as relevant side effect information is not withheld and is disclosed truthfully, framing in a way that minimizes nocebo effects appears desirable (Miller and Colloca 2011).

A potentially more controversial strategy for minimizing nocebo effects is to adopt an *authorized concealment* approach, analogous to authorized deception in the context of research on the placebo effect. Would it be ethical for physicians to inform their patients about the nocebo phenomenon and then ask them if they would prefer not to be informed about potential treatment side effects, such as nausea or headaches, that are psychologically bothersome but do not pose serious risks of harm to health? By agreeing to the withholding of such side effect information, patients would voluntarily waive a standard element of informed consent. Although this would not constitute *informed* consent, it arguably would be sufficiently informed and valid consent that respects autonomy. In addition to critical thinking, ethics-related empirical research evaluating this strategy would be needed before it could be considered appropriate in clinical practice (Miller and Colloca 2011).

REFERENCES

Ader R, Mercurio MG, Walton J, et al. Conditioned pharmacotherapeutic effects: A preliminary study. *Psychosomatic Medicine* 2010;72:192–197.

Angel M. The ethics of clinical research in the third world. *New England Journal of Medicine* 1997;337:847–849.

Appelbaum PS, Lidz CW, Grisso T. Therapeutic misconception in clinical research: Frequency and risk factors. *IRB: Ethics and Human Research* 2004;26(2):1–8.

Appelbaum PS, Roth LH, Lidz CW, et al. False hopes and best data: Consent to research and the therapeutic misconception. *Hastings Center Report* 17(2):20–24.

Barsky AJ, Saintfort R, Rogers MP, Borus JF. Nonspecific medication side effects and the nocebo phenomenon. *JAMA* 2002;287:622–627.

Bent S, Kane C, Shinohara K, et al. Saw palmetto for benign prostatic hyperplasia. *New England Journal of Medicine* 2006;354:557–566.

Bok S. The ethics of giving placebos. *Scientific American* 1974;231(5):17–23.

Brinkhaus B, Witt CM, Jena S, et al. Acupuncture in patients with chronic low back pain: A randomized controlled trial. *Archives of Internal Medicine* 2006;166:450–457.

Brody H. The lie that heals: The ethics of giving placebos. *Annals of Internal Medicine* 1982;97:112–118.

Brown WA. Placebo as a treatment for depression. *Neuropsychopharmacology* 1994;10:265–269.

Cherkin DC, Sherman KJ, Avins AL, et al. A randomized trial comparing acupuncture, simulated acupuncture, and usual care for chronic low back pain. *Archives of Internal Medicine* 2009;169:858–866.

Connor EM, Sperling RS, Gelber R, et al. Reduction of maternal-infant transmission of human immunodeficiency virus type 1 with zidovudine treatment. *New England Journal of Medicine* 1994;331:1173–1180.

Crouch RA, Arras JD. AZT trials and tribulations. *Hastings Center Report* 1998;28(6):26–34.

Ellenberg SS, Temple R. Placebo-controlled trials and active-control trials in the evaluation of new treatments. Part 2: Practical issues and specific cases. *Annals of Internal Medicine* 2000;133:464–470.

Emanuel EJ, Miller FG. The ethics of placebo-controlled trials—a middle ground. *New England Journal of Medicine* 2001;345:915–919.

Evans M. Justified deception? The single blind placebo in drug research. *Journal of Medical Ethics* 2000;26:188–193.

Fässler M, Meissner K, Schneider A, Linde K. Frequency and circumstances of placebo use in clinical practice—a systematic review of empirical studies. *BMC Medicine* 2010;8:15.

Freedman B. Equipoise and the ethics of clinical research. *New England Journal of Medicine* 1987;317:141–145.

Freedman B, Weijer C, Glass KC. Placebo orthodoxy in clinical research I: Empirical and methodological myths. *Journal of Law, Medicine, and Ethics* 1996a;24:243–251.

Freedman B, Glass KC, Weijer C. Placebo orthodoxy in clinical research II: Ethical, legal and regulatory myths. *Journal of Law, Medicine, and Ethics* 1996b;24:252–259.

Gifford F. So-called "clinical equipoise" and the argument from design. *Journal of Medicine and Philosophy* 2007;32:135–150.

Grünbaum A. The placebo concept in medicine and psychiatry. *Psychological Medicine* 1986;16:19–38.

Haake M, Müller H-H, Schade-Brittinger C, et al. German acupuncture trials (GERAC) for chronic low back pain: Randomized, multicenter, blinded, parallel-group trial with 3 groups. *Archives of Internal Medicine* 2007;167:1892–1898.

Hawkins JS, Emanuel EJ (eds.). *Exploitation and Developing Countries: The Ethics of Clinical Research.* Princeton, N.J.: Princeton University Press, 2008.

Horng S, Miller FG. Is placebo surgery unethical? *New England Journal of Medicine* 2002;347:137–139.

Hróbjartsson A, Norup M. The use of placebo interventions in medical practice: A national questionnaire survey of Danish clinicians. *Evaluation and the Health Professions* 2003;26:153–165.

Kaptchuk TJ, Friedlander E, Kelley JM, et al. Placebos without deception: A randomized controlled trial in irritable bowel syndrome. *PLoS ONE* 2010;5(12):e15591.

Lidstone SC, Schulzer M, Dinelle K, et al. Effects of expectation on placebo-induced dopamine release in Parkinson disease. *Archives of General Psychiatry* 2010;67:857–865.

London AJ. The ambiguity and the exigency: Clarifying "standard of care" arguments in international research. *Journal of Medicine and Philosophy* 2000;25:379–397.

Macklin R. The ethical problems with sham surgery in clinical research. *New England Journal of Medicine* 1999;341:992–996.

Mann H. Deception in the single-blind run-in phase of clinical trials. *IRB: Ethics and Human Research* 2007;29(2):14–17.

Martin AL, Katz J. Inclusion of authorized deception in the informed consent process does not affect the magnitude of the placebo effect for experimentally induced pain. *Pain* 2010;149:208–215.

Miller FG, Brody H. A critique of clinical equipoise: Therapeutic misconception in the ethics of clinical trials. *Hastings Center Report* 2003;33(3):19–28.

Miller FG, Colloca L. The legitimacy of placebo treatments in clinical practice: Evidence and ethics. *American Journal of Bioethics* 2009;9(12):39–47.

Miller FG, Colloca L. The placebo phenomenon and medical ethics: Rethinking the relationship between informed consent and risk-benefit assessment. *Theoretical Medicine and Bioethics* 2011;32:229–243.

Miller FG, Joffe S. Evaluating the therapeutic misconception. *Kennedy Institute of Ethics Journal* 2006;16:353–366.

Miller FG, Joffe S. Equipoise and the randomized clinical trial dilemma. *New England Journal of Medicine* 2011;364:476–480.

Miller FG, Kallmes DF, Buchbinder R. Vertebroplasty and the placebo response. *Radiology* 2011;259:621–625.

Miller FG, Kaptchuk TJ. Acupuncture trials and informed consent. *Journal of Medical Ethics* 2007;33:43–44.

Miller FG, Kaptchuk TJ. Deception of subjects in neuroscience: An ethical analysis. *Journal of Neuroscience* 2008;28:4841–4843.

Miller FG, Rosenstein DL. The therapeutic orientation to clinical trials. *New England Journal of Medicine* 2003;348:1383–1386.

Miller FG, Wendler D, Swartzman LC. Deception in research on the placebo effect. *PLoS Medicine* 2005;2(9):e262.

Miller PB, Weijer C. Equipoise and the duty of care in clinical research. *Journal of Medicine and Philosophy* 2007;32:117–133.

Mondaini N, Gontero P, Giubilei G, et al. Finasteride 5 mg and sexual side effects: How many of these are related to a nocebo phenomenon? *Journal of Sexual Medicine* 2007;4:1708–1712.

Moseley JB, O'Malley K, Petersen NJ, et al. A controlled trial of arthroscopic surgery for osteoarthritis of the knee. *New England Journal of Medicine* 2002;347:81–88.

O'Connor AM, Pennie RA, Dales RE. Framing effects on expectations, decisions, and side effects experienced: The case of influenza immunization. *Journal of Clinical Epidemiology* 1996;49:1271–1276. [Erratum: *Journal of Clinical Epidemiology* 1997;50:747–748.]

Park LC, Covi L. Nonblind placebo trial: An exploration of neurotic patients' responses to placebo when its inert content is disclosed. *Archives of General Psychiatry* 1965;12:336–345.

Sandler AD, Glesne CE, Bodfish JW. Conditioned placebo dose reduction: A new treatment in attention-deficit disorder? *Journal of Development and Behavioral Pediatrics* 2010;31:369–375.

Temple R, Ellenberg SS. Placebo-controlled trials and active-control trials in the evaluation of new treatments. Part 1: Ethical and scientific issues. *Annals of Internal Medicine* 2000;133:455–463.

Tilburt JC, Emanuel EJ, Kaptchuk TJ, et al. Prescribing "placebo treatments": Results of national survey of U.S. internists and rheumatologists. *BMJ* 2008;337:a1938.

Varmus H, Satcher D. Ethical complexities of conducting research in developing countries. *New England Journal of Medicine* 1997;337:1003–1005.

Veatch R. The irrelevance of equipoise. *Journal of Medicine and Philosophy* 2007;32:167–183.

Wendler D, Miller FG. Deception in the pursuit of science. *Archives of Internal Medicine* 2004;164:597–600.

Wilkens P, Scheel IB, Grundnes O, et al. Effect of glucosamine on pain-related disability in patients with chronic low back pain and degenerative lumbar osteoarthritis: A randomized controlled trial. *JAMA* 2010;304:45–52.

World Medical Association. Declaration of Helsinki—Ethical Principles for Medical Research Involving Human Subjects (2008). Available online: www.wma.net/en/30publications/10policies/b3/.

39
The Continuing Unethical Use of Placebo Controls

KENNETH J. ROTHMAN AND KARIN B. MICHELS

Kenneth J. Rothman and Karin B. Michels, "The Continuing Unethical Use of Placebo Controls," *New England Journal of Medicine* 1994;331:394–398.

Is it ethical to use a placebo? The answer to this question will depend, I suggest, upon whether there is already available an orthodox treatment of proved or accepted value. If there is such an orthodox treatment the question will hardly arise, for the doctor will wish to know whether a new treatment is more, or less, effective than the old, not that it is more effective than nothing.

—A. Bradford Hill[1]

Unaccountably, in these times of raised ethical consciousness, placebo treatments are still commonly used in medical research in circumstances in which their use is unethical. We refer not to the deceptive use of placebo, but to studies in which patients are informed that they may receive a placebo and then give their consent. Even so, such studies are unethical if patients are assigned a placebo instead of a therapy effective in treating their condition. Here we examine why this ethical breach persists and suggest ways to reduce it.

The Ethics of Placebo Controls

The Nuremberg Code, "the cornerstone of modern human experimentation ethics,"[2] was formulated shortly after World War II in response to Nazi atrocities. The World Health Organization adopted a version of the code in 1964 as the Declaration of Helsinki.[3] The declaration elevates concern for the health and rights of individual patients in a study over concern for society, for future patients, or for science. "In any medical study," it asserts "every patient—including those of a control group, if any—should be assured of the best proven diagnostic and therapeutic method."[4] This statement effectively proscribes the use of a placebo as control when a "proven" therapeutic method exists. The declaration also directs that a study that violates its precepts should not be accepted for publication.

Nevertheless, studies that breach this provision of the Declaration of Helsinki are still commonly conducted, with the full knowledge of regulatory agencies and institutional review boards. Although some are published in peer-reviewed medical journals, the declaration notwithstanding, many trials that are conducted in order to gain regulatory approval for new drugs or devices never reach libraries. Thus, there is no straightforward way to estimate how many trials are undertaken that involve the unethical use of placebos.

Below are a few examples from among those that have actually been published. Some of these examples might be challenged by specialists in the disciplines involved, who might argue that the use of placebo was justifiable in the case under discussion. In the aggregate, however, the examples indicate that patients in trials are often denied "best proven" treatments.

Ivermectin Trial

In 1985 a group of investigators reported the efficacy of ivermectin to treat onchocerciasis, or river blindness.[5] The investigators assigned some of the study participants to placebo when, according to the investigators themselves, the drug diethylcarbamazine had been "the standard therapy . . . for over three decades." The study participants were illiterate Liberian seamen, some of whom indicated their "informed consent" by thumbprint.

Rheumatoid Arthritis Trials

In recent years there have been numerous placebo-controlled trials of secondary treatments for rheumatoid arthritis. In many of these trials,[6–9] some enduring for years, all the patients were assigned to receive a primary therapy, such as a nonsteroidal anti-inflammatory agent, and were then randomly assigned to receive either a new secondary treatment or a placebo in addition. New placebo trials of secondary treatments for arthritis continue to be proposed and conducted, even though many such trials have shown various secondary treatments to be more effective than placebo.[10] Participants who receive placebo in these studies are at risk for serious and irreversible degenerative changes that can, to some extent, be prevented.

Antidepressant-Drug Trials

A 1992 report of a randomized trial of treatment for major depression began with the statement "Effective antidepressant compounds have been available for over 30 years."[11] Nevertheless, the investigators in that study assigned half the seriously depressed patients in the trial to receive placebo and the other half to receive paroxetine. Placebo controls are commonplace in trials of antidepressant drugs, despite the availability of therapies whose success is acknowledged.[12–18]

Ondansetron Trials

Considerable advances have been made in controlling chemotherapy-induced emesis in recent years.[19] Several drugs are available for use singly or in combination; they include metoclopramide, phenothiazines, substituted benzamides, corticosteroids, and benzodiazepines.[20–22] Nevertheless, when a new agent, ondansetron, was tested, it was compared with placebo in several trials.[23–25] (This use of placebo was criticized in an editorial accompanying the published report of one of the trials.[26])

Trials of Drugs for Congestive Heart Failure

Angiotensin-converting-enzyme inhibitors are accepted as a standard treatment for congestive heart failure.[27] Although a number of these drugs have been approved, new ones, as well as other drugs for congestive heart failure, are commonly evaluated against placebo.[28–30]

Antihypertensive-Drug Trials

Trials of new drugs for mild-to-moderate hypertension typically use placebo controls, despite the established efficacy of many agents in treating mild-to-moderate hypertension.[31–33] For example, in the introduction to a "dose-ranging" study of the calcium antagonist verapamil,[33] verapamil was described as "an effective antihypertensive drug, which is dose dependent, superior to placebo, comparable to or more effective than propranolol, and comparable with nifedipine." Despite these assertions, the investigators assigned some patients in the study to receive placebo.

Placebo Controls and Drug Approval

In the United States, many drug studies are conducted to meet the requirements of the Food and Drug Administration (FDA) so that the drug can be marketed. The Code of Federal Regulations under which the FDA operates is ambiguous about the acceptability of placebo controls. In one place it suggests that they should be avoided: "The test drug is compared with known effective therapy; for example, where the condition treated is such that administration of placebo or no treatment would be contrary to the interest of the patient."[34] The regulations go on, however, to suggest including both placebo controls and active-treatment controls in a study: "An active treatment study may include additional treatment groups, however, such as a placebo control . . ."[34]

In practice, FDA officials consider placebo controls the "gold standard." Agency guidelines specify the study designs required to obtain approval for new drugs. Placebo controls are, in effect, required for disorders of moderate severity and pain, even when an alternative treatment is available. For example, in its "Guidelines for the Clinical Evaluation of Anti-Inflammatory and Antirheumatic Drugs,"[35] the FDA demands the inclusion of a placebo group when new-drug applications are submitted for fixed-dose combinations of nonsteroidal anti-inflammatory drugs (NSAIDs) with codeine: "The combination must be shown to be superior to each component and the NSAID must be superior to placebo in order for the study to be persuasive." For the clinical evaluation of disease-modifying antirheumatic drugs (DMARDs), placebo controls also appear necessary: "In order to develop the body of information necessary for approval of a DMARD, studies using the following different control groups should generally be conducted: Comparison of the drug with a placebo . . ."

In at least one instance, the FDA refused to approve a new drug, a beta-blocker for use in angina pectoris, even though the application showed that the new drug had an effect similar to that of propranolol, an already approved drug. The application was rejected because the drug had not been tested against placebo,[36] even though a placebo-controlled trial would have violated the Declaration of Helsinki.

Is There a Scientific Rationale for Placebos?

The FDA is not alone in pushing for placebo controls. For example, a recent textbook on clinical drug trials advocates using them because "if a new drug has only been compared to an active control (without a placebo-controlled trial), this is not a convincing proof of efficacy (even if equivalence can be demonstrated)."[37] Without justification, such statements confer on placebo control a stature that ranks it with double blinding and randomization as a hallmark of good science.

The randomized, controlled trial is well recognized as the most desirable type of study in which to evaluate a new treatment. This recognition acknowledges the essential role of comparison and the importance of randomization in enhancing the comparability of two or more treatment groups. Using a placebo for comparison controls for the psychological effects of receiving some treatment and also permits blinding. No scientific principle, however, requires the comparison in a trial to involve a placebo instead of, or in addition to, an active treatment. Why, then, are placebo controls considered important? Three arguments have been advanced, none of which withstands scrutiny.

Establishing a Reference Point

By allowing the investigator to determine whether a new treatment is better than nothing (beyond the psychological benefits of treatment), a placebo control offers a clear benchmark. After all, even if a new treatment is worse than an existing one, it may still be "effective" in that it is better than no treatment. On the other hand, as Hill pointed out in 1963, the essential medical question at issue is how the new treatment compares with the old one, not whether the new treatment is better than nothing.[1]

Avoiding Difficult Decisions about Comparison Treatments

Determining whether one treatment is better than another is not always a straightforward matter. Beyond the question of efficacy, one can and should take into account unintended effects, interactions, costs, routes of administration, and other factors. Thus, it may appear simplistic to demand that the best proven treatment be chosen as the standard for comparison, if "best proven" refers only to efficacy. For some patients there may be advantages to a treatment that is inferior to a current standard with regard to efficacy but better with respect to cost or quality of life. For example, the adverse effects of some accepted treatments might offset the therapeutic benefits for some patients sufficiently that a placebo control would be ethically justified. This reasoning involves a complex decision that should be defended in submitted research proposals and published reports. It is not justifiable, however, to assign placebo controls simply to avoid the complex decision of which treatment should be used as a standard. Investigators are ethically obliged to make such decisions.

Bolstering Statistical Significance

One FDA scientist contends that placebo-controlled trials are superior to studies using an active treatment as the control because it is much easier to demonstrate a statistically significant effect in the former case.[36] The FDA relies heavily on statistical significance in judging the efficacy of new drugs.[36] Despite its popularity, however, this tool is not a good one for measuring efficacy.[38–42] The significance of an association depends on two characteristics—the strength of the association and its statistical variability. A weak effect can be "significant" if there is little statistical variability in its measurement, whereas a strong effect may not be "significant" if there is substantial variability in its measurement. Of the two characteristics, only the strength of the effect should be fundamental to the decision about approval of the drug. Ideally, statistical variability should be reduced nearly to zero when the magnitude of a drug effect is assessed, so that random error does not influence the assessment.

Unfortunately, the main way to reduce statistical variability is to conduct large studies, which are expensive. Statistical significance, on the other hand, can be obtained even in small studies, if the effect estimate is strong enough. When a placebo control is used instead of an effective treatment, the effect of a new drug appears large and may be statistically significant even in a small study. The scientific benefit, however, is illusory. Because the study is small, the measurement of the effect is subject to considerable statistical error. Thus, the actual size of the effect, even when a new drug is compared with placebo, remains obscure, and the study does not address the question of the effectiveness of the new treatment as compared with currently accepted treatments.

The small placebo-controlled studies fostered by the FDA benefit drug companies, which can more easily obtain approval of an inferior drug by comparing it with placebo than they can by testing it against a serious competitor. Smaller studies are also cheaper. Unfortunately, the costs saved by the drug company are borne by patients, who receive placebos instead of effective treatments, and by the public at large, which is supplied with a drug of undetermined efficacy.

There is no sound scientific basis for these arguments on behalf of placebo controls. Furthermore, regardless of any apparent merit these arguments have, scientific considerations should not take precedence over ethical ones, even if the use of active controls requires more difficult decisions about study design, more costly studies, and more complicated analyses.

Ethical Counterarguments

Two ethical arguments are sometimes advanced to justify the use of placebos when effective therapies exist. First, one can argue that withholding an accepted treatment may not lead to serious harm. For example, treating pain or nausea with a placebo may cause no long-term adverse effects, and the patient can call attention to any treatment failure or even choose to drop out of the study. Nevertheless, although withholding an accepted treatment may occasionally seem innocuous, allowing investigators to do so runs counter to the ethical principle that every patient, including those in a control group, should receive either the best available treatment or a new treatment thought to be as good or better. Instead, it concedes to individual investigators and to institutional review boards the right to determine how much discomfort or temporary disability patients should endure for the purpose of research. Ethical codes in medical experimentation have been developed expressly to shield patients from such vulnerability.

The second justification offered is that of informed consent. This argument says that if patients are fully informed about the risks of entering a trial and still agree to participate, there is no reason to prevent them from doing so. The ethical burden is passed directly to the patients. Informed consent is always desirable, but investigators should not put patients in a position in which their health and well-being could be compromised, even if the patients agree. There are several reasons. Despite the best efforts to inform patients, they will rarely if ever be as well informed about their treatment options as their physicians.[43] Moreover, even informed patients may not be disinterested enough to decide rationally whether it is tolerable to be deprived of an accepted treatment. Finally, patients are given the choice of participating in a trial or not, but they are given no choice about which treatments will be studied. It may be more desirable to a patient to be a part of the trial than to decline to participate, but it might have been preferable to be in a different trial that did not have a placebo arm.

Recommendations

Placebo is likely to continue to be used in place of an effective control until all parties to such studies are held strictly accountable for the ethical conduct of the research. We recognize that in some situations an accepted treatment may not be better than placebo for a given indication and that arguments can be made to justify the use of placebo instead of an existing treatment. The burden of justification, however, should fall not on critics but on those responsible for the research, including investigators, regulatory agencies, research sponsors, institutional review boards, and journal editors. All these parties should adhere to the precept that patients ought not to face unnecessary pain or disease on account of a medical experiment, and they should question the ethical legitimacy of using placebos in any experiment. Investigators should be routinely required by regulatory agencies, institutional review boards, and funding agencies to justify in writing the use of placebos in any study that uses them. This explanation should be part of all proposals, protocols, and published papers. Editors should be vigilant about questioning the use of placebos in experiments involving humans; regardless of assertions authors make about institutional review, editors should always require authors to justify in their manuscripts any use of placebo controls.

The change needed most is the enforcement of ethical guidelines at regulatory agencies, such as the FDA, which review research that may never be published. The FDA should conduct an ethical review of every study submitted to it. Any study proposing to use placebos in place of effective treatments without making a persuasive ethical justification should be disapproved. Studies involving unethical use of placebos should be ignored in the drug-approval process. Above all, scientific imperatives should never be weighed against established ethical canons.

REFERENCES

1. Hill AB. Medical ethics and controlled trials. BMJ 1963;1:1043–1049.
2. Grodin MA. Historical origins of the Nuremberg Code. In: Annas GJ, Grodin MA, eds. The Nazi doctors and the Nuremberg Code: human rights in human experimentation. New York: Oxford University Press, 1992:121–144.
3. Appendix 3. In: Annas GJ, Grodin MA, eds. The Nazi doctors and the Nuremberg Code: human rights in human experimentation. New York: Oxford University Press, 1992:331–342.
4. Declaration of Helsinki IV, World Medical Association, 41st World Medical Assembly, Hong Kong, September 1989. In: Annas GJ, Grodin MA, eds. The Nazi doctors and the Nuremberg Code: human rights in human experimentation. New York: Oxford University Press, 1992:339–342.
5. Greene BM, Taylor HR, Cupp EW, et al. Comparison of ivermectin and diethylcarbamazine in the treatment of onchocerciasis. N Engl J Med 1985;313:133–138.
6. Tugwell P, Bombardier C, Gent M, et al. Low-dose cyclosporin versus placebo in patients with rheumatoid arthritis. Lancet 1990;335:1051–1055.
7. Johnsen V, Borg G, Trang LE, et al. Auranofin (SK&F) in early rheumatoid arthritis: results from a 24-month double-blind, placebo-controlled study: effect on clinical and biochemical assessments. Scand J Rheumatol 1989;18:251–260.
8. Williams HJ, Ward JR, Dahl SL, et al. A controlled trial comparing sulfasalazine, gold sodium thiomalate, and placebo in rheumatoid arthritis. Arthritis Rheum 1988;31:702–713.
9. Trentham DE, Dynesius-Trentham RA, Orav EJ, et al. Effects of oral administration of type II collagen on rheumatoid arthritis. Science 1993;261:1727–1730.
10. Felson DT, Anderson JJ, Meenan RF. The comparative efficacy and toxicity of second-line drugs in rheumatoid arthritis: results of two meta-analyses. Arthritis Rheum 1990;33:1449–1461.
11. Rickels K, Amsterdam J, Clary C, et al. The efficacy and safety of paroxetine compared with placebo in outpatients with major depression. J Clin Psychiatry 1992;53(Suppl):30–32.
12. Kiev A. A double-blind, placebo-controlled study of paroxetine in depressed outpatients. J Clin Psychiatry 1992;53(Suppl):27–29.
13. Smith WT, Glaudin V. A placebo-controlled trial of paroxetine in the treatment of major depression. J Clin Psychiatry 1991;53(Suppl):36–39.
14. Fabre LF. Buspirone in the management of major depression: a placebo-controlled comparison. J Clin Psychiatry 1990;51(Suppl):55–61.
15. Amsterdam JD, Dunner DL, Fabre LF, et al. Double-blind placebo-controlled, fixed dose trial of minaprine in patients with major depression. Pharmacopsychiatry 1989;22:137–143.
16. Silverstone T. Moclobemide—placebo-controlled trials. Int Clin Psychopharmacol 1993;7:133–136.
17. Fabre LF. Double-blind multicenter study comparing the safety and efficacy of sertraline with placebo in major depression [abstract]. Presented at the Fifth World Congress of Biological Psychiatry, Florence, Italy, June 1991.
18. Bowden CL, Brugger AM, Swann AC, et al. Efficacy of divalproex vs lithium and placebo in the treatment of mania. JAMA 1994;271:918–924.
19. Gralla RJ, Tyson LB, Kris MG, Clark RA. The management of chemotherapy-induced nausea and vomiting. Med Clin North Am 1987;71:289–301.
20. Cunningham D, Evans C, Gazet J-C, et al. Comparison of antiemetic efficacy of domperidone, metoclopramide, and dexamethasone in patients receiving outpatient chemotherapy regimens. BMJ (Clin Res Ed) 1987;295:250.
21. Cox R, Newman CE, Leyland MJ. Metoclopramide in the reduction of nausea and vomiting associated with combined chemotherapy. Cancer Chemother Pharmacol 1982;8:133–135.
22. Edge SB, Funkhouser WK, Berman A, et al. High-dose oral and intravenous metoclopramide in doxorubicin/cyclophosphamide-induced emesis: a randomized double-blind study. Am J Clin Oncol 1987;10:257–263.
23. Beck TM, Ciociola AA, Jones SE, et al. Efficacy of oral ondansetron in the prevention of emesis in outpatients receiving cyclophosphamide-based chemotherapy. Ann Intern Med 1993;118:407–413.
24. Gandara DR, Harvey WH, Monaghan GG, et al. The delayed-emesis syndrome from cisplatin: phase III evaluation of ondansetron versus placebo. Semin Oncol 1992;19 (Suppl.):67–71.
25. Cubeddu LX, Hoffmann IS, Fuenmayor NT, Finn AL. Efficacy of ondansetron (GR 38032F) and the role of serotonin in cisplatin-induced nausea and vomiting. N Engl J Med 1990;322:810–816.
26. Citron ML. Placebos and principles: a trial of ondansetron. Ann Intern Med 1993;118:470–471.
27. Braunwald E. ACE inhibitors—a cornerstone of the treatment of heart failure. N Engl J Med 1991;325:351–353.
28. Kelbaek H, Agner E, Wroblewski H, et al. Angiotensin converting enzyme inhibition at rest and during exercise in congestive heart failure. Eur Heart J 1993;14:692–695.
29. Packer M, Narahara KA, Elkayam U, et al. Double-blind, placebo-controlled study of the efficacy of flosequinan in patients with chronic heart failure. J Am Coll Cardiol 1993;22:65–72.
30. Cowley AJ, McEntegart DJ. Placebo-controlled trial of flosequinan in moderate heart failure: the possible importance of aetiology and method of analysis in the interpretation of the results of heart failure trials. Int J Cardiol 1993;38:167–175.
31. Svetkey LP, Brobyn R, Deedwania P, et al. Double-blind comparison of doxazosin, nadolol, and placebo in patients with mild-to-moderate hypertension. Curr Ther Res 1988;43:969–978.
32. Torvik D, Madsbu HP. Multicentre 12-week double-blind comparison of doxazosin, prazosin and placebo in patients with mild to moderate essential hypertension. Br J Clin Pharmacol 1986;21:Suppl 1:69S–75S.
33. Carr AA, Bottini PB, Prisant LM, et al. Once-daily verapamil in the treatment of mild-to-moderate hypertension: a double-blind placebo-controlled dose-ranging study. J Clin Pharmacol 1991;31:144–150.
34. Code of Federal Regulations, Food and Drugs, 21. Parts 300 to 499. Revised as of April 1, 1993. Section 314.126. Washington, D.C.: Government Printing Office, 1987.
35. Guidelines for the clinical evaluation of anti-inflammatory and antirheumatic drugs. Washington, D.C.: Department of Health and Human Services, 1988.
36. Temple R. Government viewpoint of clinical trials. Drug Inf J 1982:10–17.

37. Spriet A, Dupin-Spriet T, Simon P. Choice of the comparator: placebo or active drug? In: Methodology of clinical drug trials. 2nd ed. New York: Karger, 1994:75–87.

38. Salsburg DS. The religion of statistics as practiced in medical journals. Am Stat 1985;39:220–223.

39. Gardner MJ, Altman DG. Confidence intervals rather than P values: estimation rather than hypothesis testing. BMJ 1986;292:746–750.

40. Rothman KJ. Significance questing. Ann Intern Med 1986;105:445–447.

41. Walker AM. Reporting the results of epidemiologic studies. Am J Public Health 1986;76:556–558.

42. Savitz DA. Is statistical significance testing useful in interpreting data? Reprod Toxicol 1993;7:95–100.

43. Cassileth BR, Zupkis RV, Sutton-Smith K, March V. Informed consent—why are its goals imperfectly realized? N Engl J Med 1980;302:896–900.

40

Placebo Orthodoxy in Clinical Research II

Ethical, Legal, and Regulatory Myths

BENJAMIN FREEDMAN, KATHLEEN CRANLEY GLASS, AND CHARLES WEIJER

Benjamin Freedman, Kathleen Cranley Glass, and Charles Weijer, "Placebo Orthodoxy in Clinical Research II: Ethical, Legal, and Regulatory Myths," Journal of Law, Medicine, and Ethics 1996;24:252–259.

Placebo-controlled trials are held by many, including regulators at agencies like the United States Food and Drug Administration (FDA), to be the gold standard in the assessment of new medical interventions. Yet the use of placebo controls in clinical trials has been the focus of considerable controversy.[1] In this two-part article, we challenge a number of common beliefs concerning the value of placebo controls. [Part I not included in this volume—eds.] Part I critiques statistical and other scientific justifications for the use of placebo controls in clinical research. The continued use of placebo controls in clinical trials on diseases for which accepted treatment exists raises equally important ethical, legal, and regulatory issues for which various justifications have been given. Defense of this practice relies on normative as well as empirical myths.

Myth I: The Real Problem Is the Helsinki Declaration

In their attack on the prevailing use of placebo controls, Kenneth Rothman and Karin Michels[2] emphasize that this practice stands in violation of the World Medical Association's guidelines on the ethics of human experimentation, most commonly known as the Helsinki Declaration. These guidelines, the document with probably the greatest international authority in the history of human experimentation, state without equivocation, "In any medical study, every patient—including those of a control group, if any—should be assured of the best proven diagnostic and therapeutic method."[3]

This statement seems incompatible with the relegation of any proportion of subjects in a clinical trial to placebo as long as the illness under study is one for which a proven therapy exists. This is an unwelcome message for those who support the prevailing placebo orthodoxy. Their response: shoot—or, at any rate, amend—the messenger. Louis Lasagna takes this tack in an article whose title tips his hand: "The Helsinki Declaration: Timeless Guide or Irrelevant Anachronism?"[4] Noting that the declaration has been frequently amended, Lasagna suggests that the above statement is ripe for reexamination.

The gist of the argument against the Helsinki statement is that, taken literally, it would prohibit all controlled research except where a condition has no proven treatment whatsoever. In most cases, just as a placebo arm is excluded because placebo is not "the best proven . . . therapeutic method," so, too, are the experimental arms; for until a research study has validated a new treatment's safety and efficacy, it cannot be considered the best proven approach. This is the interpretation adopted by the Council for International Organizations of Medical Sciences (CIOMS), which on those grounds considered placebos to be an exception to the Helsinki statement.[5]

The Helsinki statement is badly worded, when considered as a statement of medical science or of ethics. It seems to rest on dubious assumptions: that at some defined point treatments are proven, and that for a given population we can scientifically identify a single best diagnostic and therapeutic method. In fact, however, throughout the process of introducing and disseminating a new treatment, its therapeutic index (including both its efficacy and safety) varies along the lines of "more-or-less well confirmed," rather than suddenly "proven" at one decisive moment, or through the means of one crucial experiment. Associated with that is the fact that, considering the uncertainties of medical science and the heterogeneity of patient populations, it is rare for the medical community to be in accord as to which treatment approach is best.

That said, however, the principle underlying the Helsinki statement is clear and noncontroversial. Rather than assume, as Lasagna and (apparently) CIOMS have, that the Declaration was simply a blunder unnoticed and uncorrected by the international research community, we may see it as a poorly worded effort at expressing a widely accepted principle of research ethics. That principle can be put into normative or scientific language. As a normative matter, it defines ethical trial design as prohibiting any compromise of a patient's right to medical treatment by enrolling in a study. The same concern is often stated scientifically when we assert that a study must start with an honest null hypothesis, genuine medical uncertainty concerning the relative merits of the various treatment arms included in the trial's design. These principles allow for testing new agents when sufficient information has accumulated to create a state of clinical equipoise vis-à-vis established methods of treatment.[6] At the same time, they foreclose the use of placebos in the face of established treatment, because enrolling in a trial would imply that a proportion of enrollees will receive medical attention currently considered inferior by the expert clinical community.

Underlying the Helsinki statement, then, is the view that persons, by enrolling in a trial, should not be agreeing to medical attention that is known to be inferior to current medical practice. The survival of the Helsinki statement through two revisions may attest to the fact that despite its poor wording, this underlying principle is not easily dismissed nor amended out of existence. The same principle, though expressed differently, can be found in other statements on the ethics of clinical research, such as in Canada's Medical Research Council's Guidelines[7] and in the American Medical Association's 1966 Ethical Guidelines for Clinical Investigation.[8]

Myth II: Placebo-Controlled Trials Do Not Result in Real Harm to Subjects

If, as we argued in Part I, the heart of the present placebo debate is an issue of risk/benefit, it is natural to ask how harmful the current reliance on placebos is to subjects. Defenders of the practice insist that in current research, subjects assigned to a placebo group do not experience real or serious harm. They argue that trials are relatively short, that subjects are carefully monitored and withdrawn from the trial if their condition deteriorates,[9] and that the number of subjects exposed to placebo is often limited[10] (for example, by restricting the placebo arm to 33 percent or 25 percent of the trial population, rather than 50 percent). Along these same lines, some argue that placebos may not be ethically justifiable in drug trials whose primary end points are death or permanent disability,[11] or where irreversible harm could result from denial of therapeutic benefit from conventional therapy,[12] or even where existing treatment can prevent "serious morbidity";[13] but, in other circumstances, they argue that placebos are acceptable provided the benefits to society are sufficiently great.[14]

Without a central registry, it is difficult to generalize about the effects of placebo-controlled trials; many are performed to gain regulatory approval for drugs and so the results are never published.[15] Occasionally, though, placebo-controlled studies are on their face so dangerous that critical commentary will appear in the professional literature. The testing of thrombolytic agents (drugs or biological products designed to dissolve blood clots in coronary arteries) on patients experiencing myocardial infarction provides one notable example. After one of these agents, streptokinase, had been shown to be effective in preventing reinfarction (with its associated morbidity and mortality), placebo-controlled testing of new drugs continued by at least two major international study groups.[16]

Few, however, defend placebos where there is an accepted therapy in the presence of end points of mortality and per-manent disability. But how much harm to subjects, short of these end points, should be cause for concern? One group studied patients with chronic schizophrenia who had been enrolled in a placebo-controlled trial of fluphenazine decanoate, to detect any long-term deleterious effects on the cohort who had received placebo.[17] During this nine-month trial, 66 percent of the placebo group relapsed, compared with 8 percent of the treatment group. In this follow-up study, however, done seven years after the trial, investigators found no consistent difference between the two groups in clinical or social outcome. The authors state: "This negative finding has implications for the debate on the risk of placebo controlled trials of maintenance treatment in chronic schizophrenia."[18]

It is worth asking what sort of "implications" this "negative study" could have. Because it is very likely that schizophrenics will deteriorate over time, it becomes increasingly difficult as time passes to find any difference between the two groups that might be attributable to their experience in the study. Seven years after the fact, they found "80% of the patients had deteriorated . . . as assessed by social measures,"[19] a proportion comparable in each group.

Yet a fundamental problem exists here. In the original study, 66 percent of the placebo group relapsed compared with 8 percent of the treatment group. That is, in the course of the trial, those assigned to the placebo group were eight times more likely to suffer more seriously from schizophrenia than those who received active treatment. Does a drug company, regulator, investigator, or institutional review board (IRB) have the right to judge that the direct harm suffered by the placebo group during the course of the trial period is not serious? In some cases, the point should be clear: many sufferers of schizophrenia or depression consider their malady a fate worse than death. The Office for Protection from Research Risks IRB Guidebook describes a placebo control as unacceptable if there is an acceptable therapy for relief of "severe symptoms or amelioration of a serious condition."[20] The question becomes one of defining "seriousness" and "severity." Discounting the psychological pain, the disruption of relationships, and the heavy burden on families during a period of nontreatment as not being serious or severe enough to mandate treatment demonstrates an unacceptable disregard for the well-being of psychiatric patients and those responsible for their care.

In other cases of placebo-controlled trials, for example, of allergy medication, the harm is incomparably less. Yet even then, consider that many subjects are enrolled when they seek treatment at a health facility. Does the mere fact that the patient is sufficiently troubled to seek medical attention not indicate that, *from the subject's own point of view*, these symptoms should be treated?

Finally, attempting to justify a study by saying that it does not cause too much harm to too many people fails to take account of the physician's or investigator's responsibility to each individual patient or subject. This is clarified when we consider placebo-controlled trials through the legal prism of negligence and malpractice, which is the legal means for defining harm and assessing compensation. Principles of civil liability apply to health care[21] and medical research[22] as they do to other matters. It is well established that doctors owe a duty of care to their patients. To determine whether that duty has been breached, a doctor's actions will be measured against the accepted standard of practice as set by professional norms. Those whose treatment falls below the professional standard and causes harm to patients may be held civilly liable for that failure. Although no court case directly addresses the issue of placebo-controlled trials, legal interpretation based on the principles established in medical judgments is instructive.

The weight of legal commentary is that an investigator's chief concern should be the health and well-being of subjects.[23] A number of writers have commented that, in the specific context of placebo-controlled trials, it is both legally and morally questionable to withhold a recognized treatment believed to be safe and effective for a subject's condition.[24] New drugs should be tested against the known standard.[25] Courts have already established a higher standard for disclosure of information for research than for clinical practice.[26] It is not unreasonable to expect courts to take a very hard look at the use of placebo controls in cases where effective standard treatment exists, and to find that an investigator enrolling sick patients who may be assigned to placebo has, by definition, fallen below the existing clinical standard of practice.

Having established that failing to treat with available standard therapy constitutes negligence, a court would entertain legal excuses. The ethical problems with excusing this failure by appealing to subject consent are discussed below. Legal difficulties arise as well. Although the law allows for the voluntary assumption of risk whereby the duty owed by a defendant to observe the required standard of care is waived, this defense is quite restricted.[27] A patient may freely assume the risks of competently practiced medical interventions, but a physician cannot escape the professional duty to practice competent medicine by eliciting patient consent.[28] Nor will consent legitimate intervention that is contrary to public policy, public order, or good morals.[29] The basis for the argument is simple: Should, for example, an inept surgeon be free to continue to butcher patients because he has disclosed his deficiencies to patients? The notion of informed consent would likewise be irrelevant in the case of a known breach of fiduciary duty by a physician inappropriately relinquishing authority over a patient out of self-interest.[30]

Withdrawal of indicated therapeutic treatment in order to conduct a placebo-controlled clinical trial has received very little legal analysis. However, the principles of law noted above imply that such an action would constitute negligence. When specific legal commentary addresses use of placebo controls in trials where effective standard therapy exists,

controls have been described as "improper"[31] and "clearly contra legem artis et bonos mores."[32]

Myth III: Informed Consent to Placebo-Controlled Trials Makes Them Ethically Acceptable

Some defenders of placebo trials believe that all ethical objections become moot with the subject's consent. Robert Temple, one of the architects of the FDAs rationale for requiring placebo controls, is quoted as saying that "IRBs and patient consent forms, which tell patients exactly what they might be getting into, can assure the ethical nature of drug trials."[33] As long as a subject enrolls in a study in a free and informed manner, why should any outside party complain?

This powerful appeal to the claims of liberty fails on theoretical and practical grounds. As a theoretical matter, every major code of ethics for human experimentation, from the Nuremberg Code to the present, has recognized that adequate subject consent and an acceptable risk/benefit ratio are two independent preconditions for clinical research. For example, although placing great emphasis on adequate consent, Department of Health and Human Services regulations also require that, for protocol approval, an IRB must find that the risks subjects will face "are reasonable in relation to anticipated benefits."[34] As independent and necessary preconditions, issues of consent and of risk/benefit must each be resolved in a satisfactory manner before a trial can be approved. As a rule, a poor risk/benefit ratio cannot be compensated for by consent, just as an absence of consent cannot be justified by appealing to a highly favorable risk/benefit ratio. The point applies to all clinical trials, including those using active-treatment controls; but only in the case of placebo-controlled studies is there systematic reason to suspect an unacceptable risk/benefit ratio.

Beyond a theoretical response, other points should be noticed. Those who support the current routine reliance on placebos tend to emphasize one aspect of valid consent, namely, information. But valid consent must also be freely obtained[35] from a competent subject.[36] A very large number of objectionable placebo-controlled trials are performed on populations where the assumptions of competence and voluntariness should be carefully examined. Notably, the continuing reliance on placebo controls in the introduction of new drugs for the treatment of schizophrenia, major depression, and other serious psychiatric disorders raises such questions. Are subjects enrolling reluctantly, in a state of confusion, or because they rely on an unwarranted belief in the therapeutic intention of the clinician inviting them to participate in a placebo-controlled trial?

Skepticism concerning the ability of all these subjects to make an informed choice may be justified. Despite what many outside the field would expect, placebo-controlled studies of anti-psychotic medication do not uniformly restrict the population to outpatients who have not received benefit from available medication. Rather, they frequently involve the use of institutionalized patients, including individuals whose symptoms have improved on standard medication that must be stopped in the placebo group for the duration of the trial. Why would these patients agree to such a bad bargain?

There are a number of possible answers to this question. Studies have demonstrated that patients in such circumstances have substantial difficulty distinguishing research from treatment, and they find it hard to understand that staff would not act in their best interests in all circumstances.[37] Institutionalized patients frequently include incompetent or questionably competent individuals as well as many who are passive and willing to comply with instructions.[38] Any recruitment situation presents the potential for duress, coercion, and misrepresentation.[39] Beyond outright duress, coercion, or misrepresentation, an improper show of authority[40] or an imbalance or obvious disadvantage in bargaining power[41] can affect the voluntariness, and therefore the validity, of consent. Because the fiduciary nature of the patient-physician relationship imposes an affirmative obligation to inform a patient adequately, any silence or concealment of relevant facts may be interpreted as fraudulent,[42] invalidating consent.

As a final practical matter, we question the adequacy of the information provided at present to participants in placebo-controlled trials. IRBs commonly require that consent forms be amended because they have obfuscated the fact and implications of the trial's placebo arm. An adequate statement on many current two-arm placebo-controlled trials, in plain language, could say something like this:

> You suffer from a condition for which therapy exists that is currently accepted by physicians as sufficiently safe and effective to be considered standard treatment. If you went to a physician with your symptoms, he/she would in all likelihood prescribe this treatment for your condition. In the study that we are asking you to join, however, you will not receive this treatment. Rather, for the trial's duration, you will randomly be assigned either a new treatment or a placebo, that is, a substance that looks identical with the new treatment but which has been chosen because it is thought to have no biological effect on your condition at all. In enrolling in this trial, you should understand that standard, accepted, and routine medical treatment will be withheld from you for the duration of the trial. Thus, a major risk associated with enrolling in this trial is that you are denied the benefit of accepted medical treatment for as long as the trial runs.

Nothing short of such a blunt statement fully informs a prospective subject of what is at stake when enrolling in a two-arm placebo study for which accepted treatment exists. We have never encountered any drug trials that proposed comparably clear language in the consent form originally submitted for IRB approval. Further study is needed on what effect this statement would have on subject recruitment in placebo studies.

Myth IV: The Law Compels FDA to Predicate Drug Approval on Satisfactory Placebo-Controlled Trials

As we saw earlier, at the heart of the current debate over placebos are two competing approaches to demonstrating the effectiveness of new drugs when accepted treatments exist for the relevant medical conditions. Current FDA guidelines state that, for some studies, drug companies should test new drugs against placebo and repeatedly demonstrate that the drugs are superior to placebo. The alternative approach would test the new drug against accepted forms of treatment, and would require the drug company to demonstrate why the drug should be added to the therapeutic armamentarium. This might be done by showing that the new drug is comparably effective to current treatment, or that, despite being less effective, it has fewer side-effects, attains better compliance, or is effective in patients who do not respond to standard treatment.

In addition to the ethical and legal difficulties posed by the FDA approach (and discussed above), an obvious practical deficiency arises; that is, it allows for the approval of new drugs that are inferior in every way to current accepted treatment, provided only that those new drugs are reliably shown superior to placebo. When a new drug with no demonstrable advantage over existing treatments is proposed, current practice invests enormous sums of money toward the clinically uninteresting proof that the drug is better than nothing, an exercise that helps nobody except the applicant drug company.

What is the basis for this approach, and is it really required? Originally, the federal drug regulator's role was limited to requiring that new drug applications demonstrate safety. In 1962, the Kefauver-Harris amendments to the Food and Drug Act expanded FDA's mandate to include an evaluation of a drug's effectiveness by requiring "substantial evidence that the drug will have the effect it purports or is represented to have under the conditions of use prescribed . . ." It then went on to describe "substantial evidence" as consisting of

> adequate and well-controlled investigations, including clinical investigations, by experts qualified by scientific training and experience to evaluate the effectiveness of the drug involved, on the basis of which it could fairly and responsibly be concluded by such experts that the drug will have the effect it purports or is represented to have under the conditions of use prescribed, recommended, or suggested in the labelling or proposed labelling thereof.[43]

FDA's requirements for Good Clinical Practice, in the U.S. Code of Federal Regulations, describe "adequate and well-controlled studies" as those using a design that permits a valid comparison with a control to provide a "quantitative assessment of drug effects." The following types of possible control are cited: (1) placebo concurrent control; (2) dose-comparison concurrent control; (3) no treatment concurrent control; (4) active-treatment concurrent control; and (5) historical control.[44]

With the assistance of experts from government, academia, and industry, FDA has published a number of guidelines for the conduct of clinical trials,[45] including guidelines for the clinical evaluation of psychotropic drugs.[46] These latter guidelines are meant "to provide investigators in the field with sound principles of methodology to ensure the safety and efficacy of psychotropic drugs according to the latest state-of-the-art and highest ethical standards."[47] The guidelines suggest that "[i]n at least some studies, the investigational drug should be compared to matching placebo control to establish its efficacy. Other studies may include only active treatment control or both." These guidelines were designed to improve the "quality and meaningfulness of clinical trials designed to evaluate new psychotropic drugs."[48] They are not legal requirements. An investigator may "choose to use alternative procedures or standards for which there is scientific rationale, even though they are not provided for in the guideline."[49]

Draft guidelines for psychotropic drugs published in 1974 raised the ethical question whether placebo could be justified in trials of medication for depression, anxiety, or psychosis. The authors decided that for conditions such as depression and anxiety, "the superiority of standard existing drugs over placebo" was *at that time* of "sufficiently modest extent to make the administration of placebo to some patients entirely justifiable." However, the issue of acutely ill schizophrenic patients was considered different, given the "substantial superiority of available antipsychotic drugs over placebo." It was therefore recommended that initial placebo-controlled studies be undertaken in chronically hospitalized patients who failed to benefit from existing treatments,[50] an approach that does not deny ill patients potentially effective treatment.

As noted above, FDA's own regulations describe research designs that can serve as alternatives to concurrent placebo controls, including an active-treatment control. Moreover, the use of placebo controls when a standard accepted treatment exists is arguably contrary to other federal regulatory requirements, which state that active controls are to be used "when the condition treated is such that administration of placebo or no treatment would be contrary to the interest of the patient . . ."[51]

The commonly accepted legal interpretation of FDA's mandate is that it may only require a demonstration of *absolute* effectiveness (better than nothing) rather than *relative* effectiveness (comparable to or better than the standard). If this is so, FDA cannot require anything more rigorous or clinically relevant than placebo controls. Yet in the face of some of the absurd implications of allowing provably inferior treatments to compete in the marketplace, FDA has found creative ways to go beyond the straitjacket of absolute effectiveness. In some cases, drugs that have passed that test have nonetheless been disallowed because they are relatively less safe than other approved drugs.[52] Another approach has been to require that the label of the less effective drug specify that there is another preferred drug.[53] A more direct approach has been to argue that to be found effective a drug has to be shown to have a clinically significant effect.[54]

The fundamental debate over placebos should not rest on the interpretation of statutes, but over the propriety of policies. The real question is ethical in nature. It concerns what the law *should* allow or require, not what the law *does* allow or require. At present, FDA not only permits unethical placebo-controlled studies, but also refuses to license new drugs unless the applicant performs such studies.

Myth V: Placebo Controls Are Always Justified When Accepted Treatment Has Not Been Scientifically Validated

This final normative myth is different from those discussed previously. Both critics of current practice and its defenders may agree with this statement; where they will disagree is, perhaps, over what is meant by "scientifically validated." The myth is one of reification. It lies in believing that there is a single, definable, unequivocal measure of scientifically validating a treatment; and that until that has been done, the treatment in question should not be the standard against which new drugs are tested.

Those seeking reform of current placebo policy and practice may differ as to whether and when an accepted medical practice must serve as the reference standard for the introduction of new treatments, instead of placebos serving this purpose. A hard position may maintain that, as a general rule, first-generation treatments should only be accepted as the reference when they have been shown superior to placebo in a sound and scientifically rigorous trial; and second-generation treatments need to be shown at least equivalent to those of the first generation by similarly fastidious studies. A soft position may hold that there are many ways in which treatments may justifiably enter clinical practice. For this view, the crucial question for determining a reference treatment is whether it is in fact the standard form of treatment for the condition under study.

Before discussing these alternatives, we should note that however this dispute is resolved, current practice and policy on placebos, which are in the above terms harder than hard, will remain deficient. For example, numerous drugs have been proven superior to placebo in the treatment of depression and schizophrenia, yet drug regulators continue to require at least the inclusion of a placebo group in studies of new drugs. Recognition that current practice needs reform need not await a definitive resolution of this question, and should not be held hostage to that resolution. But a resolution is required on behalf of IRBs that must make decisions on that basis.

It is our view that the soft position is not only preferable, but is also often ethically and legally mandatory. Two observations lead to this conclusion. First, it is almost trivial to note that many medical and surgical treatments in common practice have never been scientifically validated by means of a rigorous placebo-controlled study, and yet it would be unthinkable to test any of their proposed replacements by means of a placebo control. Consider the case of the first-generation treatment for appendicitis—appendectomy—which has never been proven to beat the placebo. Should a medical treatment for early appendicitis prove promising enough to be worth clinical study, can anyone imagine that it should be tested against a placebo, rather than surgery?

Second, several of the objections we have presented are not neutral between the hard and soft positions; they would remain telling against a reform of current practice that would allow for placebo controls in studies of all those conditions for which no treatment had been proven superior to placebo. Ethically, we have seen, numerous codes demand that the physician exercise his/her best clinical judgment for subjects of studies. Legal principles require the same. Although it would be preferable for clinicians to be more skeptical of the claimed efficacy of treatments, clinical judgment will often entail prescription of treatments whose previous studies have lacked desirable rigor. Legally, too, we have argued that current placebo practice runs afoul of malpractice law, and could arguably be said to constitute professional negligence. The same would be true under a hard reform. The law expects physicians to meet the practice of the profession, to provide the same treatment any other reasonable colleague would prescribe to someone in the patient's condition. As long as the medical profession as a whole has not adopted the stance that no first-generation treatment should be accepted if it has not beaten the placebo, then it would be negligent, on that basis, to withhold accepted treatment from one cohort while providing that cohort with placebo.

We do not pretend the approach we have outlined is free of all difficulty. Certain borderline questions are particularly difficult. It is easy to say in the abstract that because effective treatments with serious side effects have an unfavorable therapeutic index, therefore placebo-controlled studies of their associated conditions are justifiable. In practice, though, it is hard to know where to draw the line. Penile erectory dysfunction may be effectively treated by local injection. Certain oral preparations are currently under study. Is it ethical to test these drugs against placebo, on the grounds that the discomfort of penile injection renders it an unacceptable treatment? A more common example: too often, cancer treatments that have been proven effective have only marginal benefits—survival advantages measured in weeks rather than months—at the cost of substantial side effects. Do such treatments have an unfavorable therapeutic index? Is the question settled by seeing what proportion of practitioners recommend such treatments?—Or, perhaps, what proportion of patients agree to them?

Another borderline question concerns the definition of *refractory population*. If a patient, for example, refuses to accept a certain standard treatment because of its side effects, may he be considered refractory to that treatment and hence

an appropriate subject for a placebo-controlled trial (assuming there is no other standard treatment he would not accept)? If enough men suffering from erectile dysfunction accept penile injection, to take the above example, we may well say that patients have voted with their feet, and this treatment is standard treatment. At that point, though, we need to ask whether the population that refuses this modality is for that reason refractory to current standard treatment, and hence may be legitimately enrolled in placebo-controlled studies of oral medication.

No bioethical theory is self-interpreting; none resolves all doubts. Our approach raises new questions, even as it settles others. But the new questions being raised are, in our view, the ones we should have been arguing about all along. For example: How good does a new drug have to be before it is good enough to be added to the therapeutic armamentarium? What is the role of practitioners and of patients in determining when a drug is standard treatment?

Conclusion

The question of placebo-controlled trials is multifaceted, partaking of scientific, statistical, legal, and ethical issues. Our discussion would be incomplete without including one final consideration: perhaps above all, placebos pose a political question.

When, in 1962, the U.S. Congress extended FDA's mandate to ascertain effectiveness as well as safety of drugs, what exactly was it requiring? The undisputed legal interpretation of effectiveness has been absolute effectiveness—better than nothing—rather than a more useful measure, such as clinical effectiveness. For this reason, FDA has required placebo controls rather than active controls.

And yet, to understand effectiveness in this way is absurd; by this measure, flinging a glass of water at a burning building is an effective fire-fighting strategy because it is better than nothing. The public knows that FDA represents a massive, expensive bureaucracy, needed to fulfill its role as a gatekeeper of new drugs. But how many health care professionals or lay members of the public are aware that FDA understands its role as ensuring that new drugs are better than nothing, rather than comparable to existing drugs? How many are aware that because of its reliance on placebo controls, the normal operation of FDA may result in the licensure of a new drug inferior in every way to presently available treatment? And how many are aware that to fulfill this mandate, FDA will not license new drugs unless the manufacturer runs trials that are contrary to numerous authoritative pronouncements on research ethics, both national and international?

We have advanced one means of rationally reforming the current system, by requiring new drugs to prove comparability to existing treatment before licensure. We think the added expense is justified by the amount of public benefit, in the form of clinically relevant information that would ensue. Other possible approaches exist; one deregulatory approach could focus, for example, on labelling rather than licensure. But current placebo practice, which spends immense sums of money to run unethical trials that will produce clinically useless information, certainly needs to change. And the first step to changing placebo practice must be the rejection of current placebo orthodoxy.

REFERENCES

1. K.J. Rothman and K.B. Michels, "The Continuing Unethical Use of Placebo Controls," *N. Engl. J. Med.*, 331 (1994): 394–398.
2. *Id.*
3. *Declaration of Helsinki* (Helsinki: 18th World Medical Assembly, 1964; rev., Tokyo: 29th World Medical Assembly, 1975; rev., Venice, 35th World Medical Assembly, 1983; rev., Hong Kong: 41st World Medical Assembly, 1989; rev., Somerset West, South Africa: 48th General Assembly, 1996): II.3. The 1996 revision added the following sentence to II.3. "This does not exclude the use of inert placebo in studies where no proven diagnostic or therapeutic method exists."
4. L. Lasagna, "The Helsinki Declaration: Timeless Guide or Irrelevant Anachronism?" *Journal of Clinical Psychopharmacology*, 2 (1995): 96–98.
5. Council for International Organizations of Medical Sciences, *International Ethical Guidelines for Biomedical Research Involving Human Subjects* (Geneva: World Health Organization, 1993): 52.
6. B. Freedman, "Placebo Controlled Trials and the Logic of Clinical Purpose," *IRB: A Review of Human Subjects Research*, 12, no. 6 (1990): 1–6.
7. Medical Research Council of Canada, *Guidelines on Research Involving Human Subjects* (Ottawa: Minister of Supply and Services, 1987).
8. American Medical Association, "Ethical Guidelines for Clinical Investigation, 1966," in W.T. Reich, ed., *Encyclopedia of Bioethics* (New York: Free Press, 1978): 1773–1774.
9. K. Rickels, "Use of Placebo in Clinical Trials?," *Psychopharmacology Bulletin*, 22, no. 1 (1986): 19–24; and G.L. Klerman, "Scientific and Ethical Considerations in the Use of Placebo Controls in Clinical Trials in Psychopharmacology," *Psychopharmacology Bulletin*, 22, no. 1 (1986): 25–29.
10. R. Pohl and R. Baron, letter; comment; discussion, "The Use of Placebo Controls," *N. Engl. J. Med.*, 332 (1995): 61–62.
11. R. Levine, oral comment, Public Responsibility in Medicine and Research Conference, Nov. 1, 1994.
12. Lasagna, *supra* note 4.
13. R. Temple, "Government Viewpoint of Clinical Trials," *Drug Information Journal*, 16 (1982): 10–17.
14. R.J. Levine, "The Use of Placebos in Randomized Clinical Trials," *IRB: A Review of Human Subjects Research*, 7, no. 2 (1985): 1–4.
15. D. Clery, "Use of Placebo Controls in Clinical Trials Disputed," *Science*, 267 (1995): 25–26.
16. B. Freedman, "Ethics and Placebo-Controlled Thrombolytic Trials: The Future," *Coronary Artery Disease*, 2 (1991): 849–852; E. Geraci, "Enrolment in Trials of Thrombolysis," *Lancet*, 336 (1990): 1069–1070; and B.A. Brody, *Ethical Issues in Drug Testing, Approval, and Pricing* (New York: Oxford University Press, 1995): ch. 2.
17. D.A. Curson et al., "Does Short Term Placebo Treatment of Chronic Schizophrenia Produce Long Term Harm?" *British Medical Journal (Clinical Research Edition)*, 293 (1986): 726–728.
18. *Id.*
19. *Id.*
20. National Institutes of Health, Office for Protection from Research Risks, *Protecting Human Subjects: Institutional Review Board Handbook* (Washington, D.C.: U.S. Government Printing Office, 1993): 4–23.
21. E. Picard, *Legal Liability of Doctors and Hospitals in Canada* (Toronto: Carswell, 2nd ed., 1994); and W. Prosser and W. Keaton, *The Law of Torts* (St. Paul, Minn.: West, 5th ed., 1984).
22. *Halushka v. University of Saskatchewan* (1965) 93 D.L.R. 2d 436; and *Kus v. Sherman Hospital*, 644 N.E.2d 1214 (Ill. App. 1995).
23. J.K. Mason and R.A. McCall-Smith, *Law and Medical Ethics* (London: Butterworth, 2nd ed., 1987); D. Giesen, *International Medical Malpractice Law* (Dordrecht: Nijhoff, 1988): §48, para. 1200; and J.-L. Baudouin, "L'expérimentation sur les humains: un conflit de valeurs," *McGill Law Journal*, 26 (1986): 809–846.
24. L. Simmons, "Problems in Deceptive Medical Procedures: An Ethical and Legal Analysis of the Administration of Placebos," *Journal of Medical Ethics*, 4 (1978): 172–181; M.B. Kapp, "Placebo Therapy and the Law: Prescribe with Care," *American Journal of Law and Medicine*, 8 (1983): 371–405; Mason and McCall-Smith, *supra* note 23; Giesen, *supra* note 23; and Baudouin, *supra* note 23.
25. Mason and McCall Smith, *supra* note 23; and Giesen, *supra* note 23.
26. *Halushka*, 93 D.L.R. 2d, 436; and *Sherman Hospital*, 644 N.E.2d, 1214.
27. Prosser and Keaton, *supra* note 21, §68.
28. I. Kennedy and I. Grubb, *Medical Law: Text and Materials* (London: Butterworth, 1989): 452; and C.B. Perry, "Conflicts of Interest and the Physician's Duty to Inform," *American Journal of Medicine*, 96 (1994): 375–380.
29. Giesen, *supra* note 23, §46, para. 1200.
30. Prosser and Keaton, *supra* note 21, §§106–07; and Perry, *supra* note 28.
31. Mason and McCall-Smith, *supra* note 23.
32. Giesen, *supra* note 23.
33. Clery, *supra* note 15.
34. 45 C.F.R. §46.111(a)(2) (1991).
35. P.S. Appelbaum, C.W. Lidz, and A. Meisel, *Informed Consent: Legal Theory and Clinical Practice* (New York: Oxford University Press, 1987): 60–62.
36. R. Faden and T. Beauchamp, *A History and Theory of Informed Consent* (New York: Oxford University Press, 1986): 274, 287–294.
37. C.W. Lidz, et al., *Informed Consent: A Study of Decisionmaking in Psychiatry* (New York: Guilford Press, 1984): 235.
38. National Commission for the Protection of Human Subjects of Biomedical and Behavioral Research, "The Belmont Report: Ethical Principles and Guidelines for the Protection of Human Subjects of Research," *OPRR Reports*, Apr. 18 (1979): 1–8; and R. Ratzan, "Being Old Makes You Different: The Ethics of Research with Elderly Subjects," *Hastings Center Report*, 10, no. 5 (1980): 32–46.
39. Picard, *supra* note 21, 61, 119.
40. C.D. Baker, *Tort* (London: Sweet and Maxwell, 2nd ed., 1976): 52; and Kennedy and Grubb, *supra* note 28, 279.
41. Prosser and Keaton, *supra* note 21, §68.
42. Kapp, *supra* note 24.
43. Food, Drug, and Cosmetic Act of 1938, 52 Stat. 1040, 21 U.S.C. §§301 *et seq.*, §505(d) (as amended 1962).
44. 21 C.F.R. §314.26(b)(2) (1991).
45. "Investigation of Drugs in Humans; Availability of Guidelines," 44 Fed. Reg. 20796 (1979).
46. "Guidelines for the Conduct of Clinical Trials: FDA Guidelines for Psychotropic Drugs," *Psychopharmacology Bulletin*, 10, no. 4 (1974): 70–91; and "FDA Guidelines for the Clinical Evaluation of Psychotropic Drugs—Antidepressant and Antianxiety Drugs," *Psychopharmacology Bulletin*, 14, no. 2 (1978): 45–63.
47. "FDA Guidelines," *supra* note 46.
48. "Guidelines for the Conduct of Clinical Trials," *supra* note 46.
49. "Investigation of Drugs in Humans," *supra* note 45.
50. "Guidelines for the Conduct of Clinical Trials," *supra* note 46.
51. 21 C.F.R. §314.26(b)(2)(iv) (1991).
52. J.C. Ballin, "Who Makes the Therapeutic Decisions?" *JAMA*, 242 (1979): 2875.
53. P.B. Hutt and R.A. Merrill, *Food and Drug Law* (Westbury, N.Y.: Foundation Press: 1991): 528n.
54. 44 Fed. Reg. 51512 (Aug. 31, 1979).

41

Placebo-Controlled Trials and Active-Control Trials in the Evaluation of New Treatments

Part 1. Ethical and Scientific Issues

ROBERT TEMPLE AND SUSAN S. ELLENBERG

Robert Temple and Susan S. Ellenberg, "Placebo-Controlled Trials and Active-Control Trials in the Evaluation of New Treatments: Part 1. Ethical and Scientific Issues," *Annals of Internal Medicine* 2000;133:455–463.

Placebo-controlled trials are used extensively in the development of new pharmaceuticals. They are sometimes challenged as unethical in settings in which patients could be treated with an existing therapy (1–7). The issues of when placebo controls are ethically acceptable and when they are scientifically necessary are important and worthy of discussion.

The Ethics of Placebo Controls

The Declaration of Helsinki

The Declaration of Helsinki (8) is an international document that describes ethical principles for clinical investigation. Those who contend that placebo controls are unethical whenever known effective therapy exists for a condition usually cite the following sentence in the Declaration as support for that position: "In any medical study, every patient—including those of a control group, if any—should be assured of the best proven diagnostic and therapeutic method."

We believe that an interpretation of this sentence as barring placebo controls whenever an effective treatment exists is untenable. First, the requirement that all patients receive the "best proven diagnostic and therapeutic method" would bar not only placebo-controlled trials but also active-control and historically controlled trials. When effective treatment exists, the patient receiving the investigational treatment instead of the established therapy is clearly not getting the best proven treatment.

Second, it does not seem reasonable to consider as equivalent all failures to use known effective therapy. Historically, concerns about placebo use have usually arisen in the context of serious illness. There is universal agreement that use of placebo or otherwise untreated controls is almost always unethical when therapy shown to improve survival or decrease serious morbidity is available. But in cases in which the treatment does not affect the patient's long-term health, an ethical imperative to use existing therapy is not plausible. Can it be, for example, that because topical minoxidil or oral finasteride can grow hair, a placebo-controlled trial of a new remedy for baldness is unethical? Is it really unethical to use placebos in short-term studies of drugs for allergic rhinitis, insomnia, anxiety, dermatoses, heartburn, or headaches in

fully informed patients? We do not believe that there is a reasonable basis for arguing that such studies and many other placebo-controlled studies of symptom relief are unethical and that an informed patient cannot properly be asked to participate in them.

Third, there is good reason to doubt that the cited phrase was intended to discourage placebo-controlled trials. The phrase under discussion was not part of the original 1964 Declaration but was added in 1975 to reinforce the idea that the physician-patient relationship "must be respected just as it would be in a purely therapeutic situation not involving research objectives" (8). In the explanation accompanying the 1975 change, the issue of placebo-controlled trials was not even mentioned (9). The American Medical Association (10), the World Health Organization (11), and the Council for International Organizations of Medical Sciences (12) have rejected the position that the Declaration uniformly bars placebo-controlled trials when proven therapy is available.

Informed Consent in Placebo-Controlled Trials

Patients asked to participate in a placebo-controlled trial must be informed of the existence of any effective therapy, must be able to explore the consequences of deferring such therapy with the investigator, and must provide fully informed consent. Concern about whether consent to participate in trials is as informed as we would like to believe is valid, but these concerns apply as much to the patient's decision to forgo known effective treatment and risk exposure to a potentially ineffective or even harmful new agent in an active-control trial as to a decision to accept possible persistence of symptoms in a placebo-controlled trial. Thus, this problem is not unique to placebo-controlled trials.

For the above reasons, we conclude that placebo-controlled trials may be ethically conducted even when effective therapy exists, as long as patients will not be harmed by participation and are fully informed about their alternatives. Although in many cases application of this standard will be fairly straightforward, in others it will not, and there may be debate about the consequences of deferring treatment (13).

Assessment of Effectiveness with Active-Control Trials

Clinical trials that, because of deficiencies in study design or conduct, are unlikely to provide scientifically valid and clinically meaningful results raise their own ethical concerns (12,14). The remainder of this paper will address the inability of commonly proposed alternatives to placebo-controlled trials to evaluate the effectiveness of new treatments in many medical settings.

Active-Control Equivalence Trials (Noninferiority Trials)

The ability to conduct a placebo-controlled trial ethically in a given situation does not necessarily mean that placebo-controlled trials should be carried out when effective therapy exists. Patients and physicians might still prefer a trial in which every participant is given an active treatment. What remains to be examined is why placebo-controlled trials (or, more generally, trials intended to show an advantage of one treatment over another) are frequently needed to demonstrate the effectiveness of new treatments and often cannot be replaced by active-control trials showing that a new drug is equivalent or noninferior to a known effective agent. The limitations of active-control equivalence trials (ACETs) that are intended to show the effectiveness of a new drug have long been recognized and are well described (15–33) but are perhaps not as widely appreciated as they should be. A recent proposed international guideline on choice of control group addresses this issue in detail (33).

The Fundamental Problem: Need for Assay Sensitivity

There are two distinct ways to show that a new therapy is effective. One can show that the new therapy is superior to a control treatment, or one can show that the new therapy is equivalent to or not worse by some defined amount than a known effective treatment. Each method can be valid, but each requires entirely different inferential approaches. A well-designed study that shows superiority of a treatment to a control (placebo or active therapy) provides strong evidence of the effectiveness of the new treatment, limited only by the statistical uncertainty of the result. No information external to the trial is needed to support the conclusion of effectiveness. In contrast, a study that successfully shows "equivalence"—that is, little difference between a new drug and known active treatment—does not by itself demonstrate that the new treatment is effective. "Equivalence" could mean that the treatments were both effective in the study, but it could also mean that both treatments were ineffective in the study. To conclude from an ACET that a new treatment is effective on the basis of its similarity to the active control, one must make the critical (and untestable within the study) assumption that the active control had an effect in that particular study. In other words, one must assume that if a placebo group had been included, the placebo would have been inferior to the active control (15–33). Support for this assumption must come from sources external to the trial. Although it might appear reasonable to expect a known active agent to be superior to placebo in any given appropriately designed trial, experience has shown that this is not the case for many types of drugs.

The ability of a study to distinguish between active and inactive treatments is termed *assay sensitivity*. If assay sensitivity cannot be assumed, then even if the new and standard treatments appear virtually identical and the confidence interval for their comparison is exquisitely narrow, the study cannot demonstrate effectiveness of the new drug. (Note that in practice, ACETs are not designed simply to show lack of a statistically significant difference between treatments. Rather, such trials are designed to show noninferiority—that the new treatment is not inferior to the control by more than a specified margin. This approach is described in the Appendix.)

The best evidence that an active drug would have an effect superior to that of placebo in a given study would be a series of trials of similar design in which the active drug has reliably outperformed placebo. The ACET thus requires information external to the trial (the information about past placebo-controlled studies of the active control) to interpret the results. In this respect, an ACET is similar to a historically controlled trial. In some settings, such as highly responsive cancers, most infectious diseases, and some cardiovascular conditions, such external information is available and ACETs can and do provide a valid and reliable basis for evaluating new treatments. In many cases, however, the historically based assumption of assay sensitivity cannot be made; for many types of effective drugs, studies of apparently adequate size and design do not regularly distinguish drugs from placebo (16–18,25,34). More than 20 years ago, Lasagna (19) described this difficulty particularly well (reflecting long recognition of the problem among analgesiologists):

> . . . a comparison between new drug and standard . . . is convincing only when the new remedy is superior to standard treatment. If it is inferior, or even indistinguishable from a standard remedy, the results are not readily interpretable. In the absence of placebo controls, one does not know if the "inferior" new medicine has any efficacy at all, and "equivalent" performance may reflect simply a patient population that cannot distinguish between two active treatments that differ considerably from each other, or between active drug and placebo. Certain clinical conditions, such as serious depressive states, are notoriously difficult to evaluate because of the delay in drug effects and the high rate of spontaneous improvement, and even known remedies are not readily distinguished from placebo in controlled trials.

The problem is well recognized in studies of antidepressant drugs (18,32). In practice, many such studies include three arms—new drug, active control, and placebo—to provide clear evidence of effectiveness (new drug vs. placebo) and an internal standard (active control vs. placebo). This design allows a clear distinction (particularly valuable to a drug manufacturer) between a *drug* that does not work (the standard agent is superior to placebo but the new drug is not) and a *study* that does not work (neither the standard drug nor the new drug is superior to placebo).

The assay sensitivity problem was illustrated by Leber (18), who examined the results of all three-arm studies comparing nomifensine (an effective but toxic antidepressant), imipramine (a standard tricyclic antidepressant shown to be superior to placebo in dozens of clinical trials), and placebo. The results of the studies are shown in Table 41.1. No study found a difference between nomifensine and imipramine on the Hamilton depression scale (a standard measure of depression), but the changes from baseline with both drugs were substantial and seemed clinically meaningful. Examination of the placebo results, however, shows similar changes. Only one of the six studies—the smallest one—

Table 41.1.
Results of six trials comparing nomifensine, imipramine, and placebo*

Study	Common Baseline Score on the Hamilton Depression Scale	Four-Week Adjusted Score on the Hamilton Depression Scale (Number of Participants)			P Value[†]
		Nomifensine	Imipramine	Placebo	
R301	23.9	13.4 (33)	12.8 (33)	14.8 (36)	0.78
G305	26.0	13.0 (39)	13.4 (30)	13.9 (36)	0.86
C311(1)	28.1	19.4 (11)	20.3 (11)	18.9 (13)	0.81
V311(2)	29.6	7.3 (7)	9.5 (8)	23.5 (7)	0.63[‡]
F313	37.6	21.9 (7)	21.9 (8)	22.0 (8)	1.0
K317	26.1	11.2 (37)	10.8 (32)	10.5 (36)	0.85

* Results shown are those reported in the review by Leber (18).
[†] Two-tailed P value for nomifensine versus imipramine.
[‡] P < 0.001 for nomifensine versus placebo and imipramine versus placebo.

found any significant difference between either of the two active drugs and placebo. None of the other five studies showed even a trend favoring either drug. These five studies appear to have lacked assay sensitivity; they could not distinguish active from inactive treatments. Although some of these studies were small, three studies with 30 or more patients per group were typical of studies that often did show effectiveness of imipramine or other antidepressants.

Although we cannot be certain of the reason for these outcomes, the most likely explanation is that differences in study samples, study designs, or study conduct affected the response to these antidepressants and thus the ability of the studies to identify effective therapy. It does not seem to be merely a matter of study size, however; many studies with 10 to 30 patients per group (including one of the six shown) detect effects of antidepressant drug effects, and many much larger studies of essentially the same design do not show even a favorable trend. Similar patterns, although not as extreme, have been seen with many recently developed antidepressants, such as fluoxetine (34). Overall, in recent experience at the U.S. Food and Drug Administration, about one third to one half of modern antidepressant trials do not distinguish a known effective drug from placebo (Laughren T. Unpublished observations).

One might speculate that variable results of trials of antidepressants are simply the consequence of modest effect sizes coupled with samples too small to overcome the inherent variability of the condition studied. Results, however, are consistent with effect sizes that vary greatly and unpredictably from study to study. With current knowledge, one cannot specify a particular study population, treatment protocol, or sample size that will regularly identify active agents.

Antidepressants are only one of many classes of drugs with assay sensitivity problems. Analgesics (35), anxiolytics, antihypertensives, hypnotics, antianginal agents, angiotensin- converting enzyme inhibitors for heart failure, postinfarction β-blockers (36), antihistamines, nonsteroidal asthma prophylaxis, motility-modifying drugs for gastroesophageal reflux disease, and many other effective agents are often indistinguishable from placebo in well-designed and well-conducted trials.

A recently published overview by Tramèr and coworkers (37) of studies of ondansetron, a widely used and very effective antiemetic, provides a further example of this phenomenon. Although the totality of data clearly supports the efficacy of this agent, many placebo-ondansetron comparisons show no effect of the drug. It is notable that the incidence of nausea and vomiting varied greatly among the trials and in some cases was so low that it precluded any demonstration of efficacy. In a placebo-controlled study of an antiemetic, a low rate of nausea and vomiting in the placebo group would lead to a negative outcome—the drug could not appear superior to placebo, and the trial could not provide evidence of effectiveness. In contrast, an ACET (new drug vs. ondansetron) with a low rate of nausea and vomiting in both arms would not be unambiguously interpretable. If one assumed that the low rate in the active-control group reflected the known ability of ondansetron to reduce a rate of nausea and vomiting that would have been high in the absence of treatment, one would conclude that the new drug was also effective. But the article by Tramèr and coworkers shows that such an assumption cannot be supported in many situations. Clearly, if many placebo-controlled studies of ondansetron showed no effect, a trial showing "equivalence" of a new agent to ondansetron could not be considered reliable evidence that the new agent was effective, unless one could identify a treatment setting (for example, a setting defined by the chemotherapy administered) in which ondansetron was regularly distinguishable from placebo.

In the cases described, the effectiveness of drugs that sometimes (or even often) fail to be proven superior to placebo is not in doubt; even if a drug is statistically significantly superior to placebo in only 50% of well-designed and well-conducted studies, that proportion is still vastly greater than the small fraction that would be expected to occur by chance if the drugs were ineffective. The problem may be a generally small response that varies among populations, insufficient adherence to therapy or use of concomitant medication, study samples that improve spontaneously (leaving no room for drug-induced improvement) or that are unresponsive to the drug, or some other reason not yet recognized. What all of these influences have in common is that they reduce or eliminate the drug-placebo difference, so that a study design and size adequate to detect a larger effect will not detect the reduced effect. In each case, however, the problem is not identifiable a priori by examining the study; it is recognized only by the observed failure of the trial to distinguish the drug and placebo treatments.

INCENTIVE TO MINIMIZE ERRORS IS REDUCED IN ACETs

Active-control equivalence trials present another problem that is difficult to quantitate or assess in any given study. Most imperfections in a clinical trial—patient non-adherence to treatment, use of concomitant therapy potentially affecting study outcome, inclusion of inappropriate patients (for example, those who lack the disease or those who experience spontaneous improvement), or administering the wrong treatments—tend to reduce observable differences between treatment groups, promoting the conclusion that the two treatments are indistinguishable. Study organizers seeking to demonstrate a difference between treatments have a powerful incentive to minimize such imperfections and to identify a population in which an effect could be demonstrated. This incentive is absent when the intent is to demonstrate lack of difference (17,32). This is not to suggest that trial organizers deliberately make less of an effort to maintain study quality in ACETs than in placebo-controlled trials, any more than the practice of blinding investigators to treatment suggests that investigators are not to be trusted. It is important, however, to recognize the possible influence of the desired outcome on the conduct of clinical trials.

It is difficult in any given ACET to determine the extent to which the ability to show potential treatment differences has been diminished by deficiencies in study design and conduct. In such areas as treatment of depression, however, even placebo-controlled trials, in which the incentive to conduct an excellent study capable of showing a difference between treatments is maximal, often cannot distinguish effects of active drugs from those of placebo. Results of ACETs would be expected to be at least as variable as those of placebo-controlled trials in their ability to detect treatment differences. In considering how to conduct ACETs, this issue needs to be recognized. In addition, approaches to study interpretation usually thought of as conservative, such as intention-to-treat analyses, are no longer conservative when the objective of a trial is to show no difference between treatments (17,24,32).

USE OF ACTIVE CONTROLS

Active-control equivalence trials can be informative and have been used successfully and appropriately in many therapeutic areas in which assay sensitivity is not in doubt. These trials are often credible and have been widely used in such areas as treatment of cancer, infectious disease, and some cardiovascular conditions (for example, acute myocardial infarction treated with thrombolysis). In general, the larger the effect size, the less study-to-study variability in outcomes, and the fewer the instances of unexplained failure of the control agent to show superiority to placebo in well-controlled studies, the more persuasive is the case for using this design. Investigators who intend to perform an ACET will therefore need to review previous placebo-controlled trials of the control agent to see whether it can be persuasively shown that such information exists. The ACET should be as similar as possible to the past placebo-controlled trials with regard to patient selection, dose, end points, assessment procedures, use of concomitant therapy, and other pertinent study design characteristics (17,20).

Given the inevitable residual uncertainty about the assay sensitivity of a trial that does not contain an internal standard, reliance on ACETs may also require more evidence of replicability than would be needed for trials intended to show differences. It should be appreciated, however, that even if assay sensitivity can be assumed, the effect that the active control can be presumed to have had under the study conditions will often be relatively small. In such cases, large sample sizes will be needed to provide the narrow confidence interval needed to ensure that the new drug is not inferior to the control by more than that amount. This issue is considered further in the Appendix.

STUDYING RELATIVE EFFECTIVENESS

In some cases, a study may be intended to evaluate the comparative effectiveness of two known active treatments. In that case, too, the presence of assay sensitivity is essential to interpretation of the trial. If one cannot be confident that the trial could have distinguished active drug from placebo, one cannot be confident that it could have distinguished a more effective drug from a less effective drug. A three-arm study (new drug, placebo, and active control) is optimal because it can 1) assess assay sensitivity and, if assay sensitivity is confirmed, 2) measure the effect of the new drug and 3) compare the effects of the two active treatments.

Alternative Approaches

Not all placebo-controlled studies leave patients untreated. It is frequently possible to provide standard therapy while carrying out a superiority study—that is, a study intending to demonstrate an advantage of a treatment regimen over the control. Sometimes a new agent can be assessed by using an "add-on" study design in which all patients are given standard therapy and are randomly assigned to also receive either new agent or placebo. This design is common in trials of therapy for cancer, heart failure, and epilepsy, in which omitting standard therapy would generally be unacceptable. Such studies are not directly informative about a drug as monotherapy, but they do provide interpretable evidence of effectiveness in a well-defined setting and are particularly appropriate where clinical use of the new agent will largely be as added treatment. Moreover, if successful, they demonstrate the ability to provide benefit greater than the standard therapy alone, in contrast to the (usually) less clinically interesting demonstration that a new therapy is not worse than the standard. This design is not useful, however, if the new drug and standard therapy are pharmacologically similar.

Although we have argued that an informed patient may choose to accept pain or discomfort or to defer needed long-term therapy for a short time to participate in a placebo-controlled trial, we do not mean to suggest that indifference to patient discomfort is appropriate. Some study designs limit the duration of placebo exposure without compromising the rigor of the study. These include "early escape" designs and randomized withdrawal studies (31, 38). In an "early escape" study, patients are randomly assigned to receive new drug or placebo, but a well-defined treatment failure end point (such as persistence of symptoms or maintenance of elevated blood pressure at a specified time) is used as the basis for changing therapy in patients who are not benefiting from their initially assigned treatment. In a randomized withdrawal study, apparently responsive patients are given an investigational therapy for a period and are randomly assigned to receive placebo or to continue active therapy. The randomly assigned groups can be compared for a defined period or by using an "early escape" approach. This design was initially proposed by Amery (39) as a way of avoiding extended placebo treatment of patients with angina pectoris. A particular value of the randomized withdrawal study is that it demonstrates a persistent effect for durations that would be difficult to study in placebo-controlled trials.

Regulatory Status of Study Designs

Critics of placebo-controlled trials have often attributed their use to Food and Drug Administration practices that favor the smallest possible trials, seek to assess absolute efficacy, and ignore what they consider the more important clinical question of how a new drug compares with standard therapy (1–6). Although a broad range of trial designs can be used to demonstrate the effectiveness of a new drug (15), regulations describing adequate and well-controlled studies have since 1985 indicated concerns about the interpretation of ACETs, reflecting views expressed since the 1950s by numerous clinical and statistical researchers (15–33). Thus, where assay sensitivity cannot be established for an ACET, trials that show a difference between treatments (a placebo-controlled trial is only one such example) would be needed to demonstrate effectiveness. The basis for this requirement is not a preference for small trials (although efficiency is not a trivial matter) nor indifference to comparisons (although under law, a drug need not be superior to or even as good as other therapy to be approved), but rather the fundamental need for evidence of assay sensitivity to interpret an ACET as showing effectiveness of a new drug.

Conclusions

Placebo controls are clearly inappropriate for conditions in which delay or omission of available treatments would increase mortality or irreversible morbidity in the population to be studied. For conditions in which forgoing therapy imposes no important risk, however, the participation of patients in placebo-controlled trials seems appropriate and ethical, as long as patients are fully informed. Arguments to the contrary are not based on established ethical principles but rather rely on a literal reading of one passage in the Declaration of Helsinki that would also preclude the conduct of active-control trials, and even historically controlled trials, whenever effective treatment exists. It seems inconceivable that the authors of the 1975 revision intended such an outcome, and nothing in their explanation of the revision suggests they did (8). We therefore believe this interpretation is untenable.

If ACETs were always adequate substitutes for placebo-controlled trials, the ethical issue might not arise. Unfortunately, ACETs are often uninformative. They can neither demonstrate the effectiveness of a new agent nor provide a valid comparison to control therapy unless assay sensitivity can be assured, which often cannot be accomplished without inclusion of a concurrent placebo group.

APPENDIX

Blackwelder (40) and others (20,22,24,31) have pointed out that equivalence testing can be better described in most cases as a test of a one-sided hypothesis that the test drug is not inferior to the control by a defined amount, the "equivalence margin," also called the noninferiority margin. The null and alternate hypotheses H_o and H_a then become:

$$H_o = E_S - E_T \geq \Delta$$
$$H_a = E_S - E_T < \Delta$$

where E_S and E_T are the effects of the standard and test drugs, respectively, and Δ is the equivalence or noninferiority margin of interest. The null hypothesis is rejected if the upper bound of the confidence interval for the difference between the treatment being tested and control is smaller than the specified margin. In this case, the new agent is considered effective. A confidence interval that cannot exclude a difference greater than the margin would not permit rejection of the null hypothesis, and noninferiority would not be supported.

Choice of the margin is critical and depends on both knowledge of the effect of the control drug and clinical judgment. The margin chosen must be no larger than the smallest difference between control drug and placebo that could regularly be demonstrated in controlled trials. Exclusion of a difference greater than that margin would therefore mean that at least some part of the effect of the control agent was

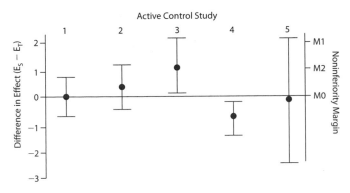

Figure 41.1. Interpretation of equivalence margins in active-control trials. Hypothetical results of five studies are shown. The result of each study is shown on the y-axis as the difference between treatments ($E_S–E_T$), where E_S represents the control and E_T represents the test drug. A positive difference favors the standard drug. Error bars show hypothetical 95% confidence intervals for these differences. Three possible noninferiority margins are shown (M0, M1, M2). For more explanation, see the Appendix.

preserved for the test drug and that the test drug therefore had at least some effect. If it were thought medically compelling to assure preservation of a specific fraction of the control drug effect, the specified margin would have to be made smaller than the largest possible noninferiority margin. If the control drug has not regularly shown superiority to placebo in trials of adequate size and design, the noninferiority margin must be set at zero: that is, only superiority to the control could be interpreted as evidence of effectiveness of the new drug. The ability to choose a margin representing the "guaranteed" effect of the control agent thus becomes functionally equivalent to saying that the trial has "assay sensitivity," an ability to distinguish active from inactive treatments.

The use of equivalence margins is shown in Figure 41.1. The hypothetical results of five different active-control studies are presented. The result of each study is shown on the y-axis as the difference between treatments ($E_S – E_T$, the difference between the standard drug control and test drug, with a positive difference favoring the standard drug) and confidence intervals for these differences. Three possible noninferiority margins are shown. M1 is the smallest effect the standard drug can be presumed to have in the study compared to a placebo treatment. M2 is a fraction of M1, chosen because it is considered essential to ensure that the new drug retains some substantial fraction of the effect of the standard drug. M0 is the margin that must be used when the standard drug is not regularly superior to placebo: that is, only superiority of the new drug is acceptable evidence of effectiveness.

The results of studies 1 through 5 (Figure 41.1) are summarized in the following paragraphs.

Study 1: Where an effectiveness margin M1 can be defined, effectiveness is shown because the confidence inter-

val of the difference favoring the standard drug excludes inferiority greater than M1. Moreover, the study shows that more than 50% of the standard drug effect is preserved. If, however, assay sensitivity cannot be assumed (that is, there is no assurance that the standard drug had any effect in the study so that the noninferiority margin is M0), the study would not show effectiveness of the new drug.

Study 2: Effectiveness would be shown by noninferiority of the new drug based on the M1 margin but not if the more stringent M2 margin were used.

Study 3: Effectiveness is not demonstrated because noninferiority to the standard drug based on the effectiveness margin M1 is not demonstrated; the test drug may have no effect at all.

Study 4: Effectiveness of the test drug is demonstrated for any choice of margin by a showing of superiority of the test drug to the standard drug.

Study 5: Effectiveness is not demonstrated, despite the favorable point estimate of the effect of the test drug, because the wide confidence interval does not exclude inferiority to the standard drug greater than the M1 margin.

REFERENCES

1. Rothman KJ, Michels KB. The continuing unethical use of placebo controls. N Engl J Med. 1994;331:394–398.
2. Agostini A. Placebo and EU Guidelines. Lancet. 1995;310:1710.
3. Aspinall RL, Goodman NW. Denial of effective treatment and poor quality of clinical information in placebo controlled trials of ondansetron for postoperative nausea and vomiting: a review of published trials. BMJ. 1995; 311:844–846.
4. Henry D, Hill S. Comparing treatments. BMJ. 1995;310:1279.
5. Freedman B, Weijer C, Glass KC. Placebo orthodoxy in clinical research. I: Empirical and methodological myths. J Law Med Ethics. 1996;24:243–251.
6. Freedman B, Glass KC, Weijer C. Placebo orthodoxy in clinical research. II: Ethical, legal, and regulatory myths. J Law Med Ethics. 1996;24:252–259.
7. Angell M. The ethics of clinical research in the Third World. N Engl J Med. 1997;337:847–849.
8. World Medical Association. Declaration of Helsinki. Recommendations guiding physicians in biomedical research involving human subjects. JAMA. 1997;277:925–926.
9. World Medical Association. Summary History of the World Medical Association Declaration of Helsinki. Ferney-Voltaire, France: World Medical Association; 1985.
10. American Medical Association Council on Ethical and Judicial Affairs. The use of placebo controls in clinical trials. Report 2-A-1996. Chicago: American Medical Association; 1996.
11. Grof P, Akhter MI, Campbell M, et al. Clinical Evaluation of Psychotropic Drugs for Psychiatric Disorders: Principles and Proposed Guidelines. WHO Expert Series on Biological Psychiatry. Vol. 2. Seattle: Hogrefe & Huber; 1993:28–29.
12. Council for International Organizations of Medical Sciences. International Ethical Guidelines for Biomedical Research Involving Human Subjects. Geneva: Council for International Organizations of Medical Sciences; 1993.
13. Ellenberg SS, Temple R. Placebo-controlled trials and active control trials in the evaluation of new treatments. Part 2: Practical issues and specific cases. Ann Intern Med. 2000;133:464–470.

14. Levine RJ. Ethics and Regulation of Clinical Research. 2nd ed. New Haven, Conn.: Yale Univ Pr; 1986.

15. Adequate and well-controlled studies. Code of Federal Regulations, 21 Part 314.126. Revised as of 1 April 2000. Washington, D.C.: U.S. Government Printing Office; 2000.

16. Temple R. Government viewpoint of clinical trials. Drug Information Journal. 1982;16:10–17.

17. Temple R. Difficulties in evaluating positive control trials. Proceedings of the American Statistical Association. 1983:1–7.

18. Leber P. Hazards of inference: the active control investigation. Epilepsia. 1989;30(Suppl.1):S57–S63.

19. Lasagna L. Placebos and controlled trials under attack. Eur J Clin Pharmacol. 1979;15:373–374.

20. Makuch R, Johnson M. Issues in planning and interpreting active control equivalence studies. J Clin Epidemiol. 1989;42:503–511.

21. Modell W, Houde RW. Factors influencing clinical evaluation of drugs: with special reference to the double-blind technique. JAMA. 1958;167:2190–2199.

22. Fleming TR. Treatment evaluation in active control studies. Cancer Treat Rep. 1987;71:1061–1065.

23. Fleming TR. Evaluation of active control trials in AIDS. J Acquired Immune Defic Syndr. 1990;3(Suppl.2):S82–S87.

24. Jones B, Jarvis P, Lewis JA, Ebbutt AF. Trials to assess equivalence: the importance of rigorous methods. BMJ. 1996;313:36–39.

25. Temple R. Problems in interpreting active control equivalence trials. Accountability in Research. 1996;4:267–275.

26. Dollery CT. A bleak outlook for placebos (and for science). Eur J Clin Pharmacol. 1979;15:219–221.

27. Smith JL. Placebos in clinical trials of peptic ulcer. ACG Committee on FDA-Related Matters. Am J Gastroenterol. 1989;84:469–474.

28. Freston JW. Dose-ranging in clinical trials: rationale and proposed use with placebo or positive controls. Am J Gastroenterology. 1986;81:307–311.

29. Prien RF. Methods and models for placebo use in pharmacotherapeutic trials. Psychopharmacol Bull. 1988;24:4–8.

30. Sachar DB. Placebo-controlled trials clinical trials in gastroenterology. A position paper of the American College of Gastroenterology. Am J Gastroenterology. 1984;79:913–917.

31. Laska EM, Klein DF, Lavori PW, et al. Design issues for the clinical evaluation of psychotropic drugs. In: Prien RF, Robinson DS, eds. Clinical Evaluation of Psychotropic Drugs: Principles and Guidelines. New York: Raven Pr; 1994:29–35.

32. Pledger G, Hall DB. Active control equivalence studies: do they address the efficacy issue? In: Peace KE, ed. Statistical Issues in Drug Research and Development. New York: Marcel Dekker; 1990:226–238.

33. International Conference on Harmonization: choice of control group in clinical trials. Federal Register. 1999;64:51767–51780.

34. Sramek JJ, Cutler NR. The use of placebo controls. N Engl J Med. 1995;332:62.

35. Max MB. Divergent traditions in analgesic clinical trials. Clin Pharmacol Ther. 1994;56:237–241.

36. Yusuf S, Peto R, Lewis J, et al. Beta blockade during and after myocardial infarction: an overview of the randomized trials. Prog Cardiovasc Dis. 1985;27:335–371.

37. Tramèr MR, Reynolds DJ, Moore RA, McQuay HJ. When placebo controlled trials are essential and equivalence trials are inadequate. BMJ. 1998;317:875–880.

38. Temple R. Special study designs: early escape, enrichment, studies in non-responders. Communications in Statistics. 1994;23:499–531.

39. Amery W, Dony J. A clinical trial design avoiding undue placebo treatment. J Clin Pharmacol. 1975;15:674–679.

40. Blackwelder WC. "Proving the null hypothesis" in clinical trials. Control Clin Trials. 1982;3:345–353.

42

The Ethics of Placebo-Controlled Trials
A Middle Ground

EZEKIEL J. EMANUEL AND FRANKLIN G. MILLER

Ezekiel J. Emanuel and Franklin G. Miller, "The Ethics of Placebo-Controlled Trials—A Middle Ground," *New England Journal of Medicine* 2001;345:915–919.

The first placebo-controlled trial was probably conducted in 1931, when sanocrysin was compared with distilled water for the treatment of tuberculosis.[1] Ever since then, placebo-controlled trials have been controversial, especially when patients randomly assigned to receive placebo have forgone effective treatments.[2–5] Recently, the debate has become polarized. One view, dubbed "placebo orthodoxy" by its opponents, is that methodologic considerations make placebo-controlled trials necessary.[6–11] The other view, which might be called "active-control orthodoxy," is that placebo orthodoxy sacrifices ethics and the rights and welfare of patients to presumed scientific rigor.[10–14] The latest revision of the Declaration of Helsinki, although controversial,[15,16] embraces the active-control orthodoxy.[17] Both views discount the ethical and methodologic complexities of clinical research. In this essay, we argue that placebo-controlled trials are permissible when proven therapies exist, but only if certain ethical and methodologic criteria are met.

Placebo Orthodoxy

Advocates of placebo-controlled studies argue that it is ethical to conduct such trials even in the case of medical conditions for which there are interventions known to be effective, because of the methodologic limitations of trials in which active treatment is used as the control.[6–9] Sometimes therapies that are known to be effective are no better than placebo in particular trials because of variable responses to drugs in particular populations, unpredictable and small effects, and high rates of spontaneous improvement in patients. Consequently, without a placebo group to ensure validity, the finding that there is no difference between the investigational and standard treatments can be misleading or uninterpretable.[8,9] New treatments that are no better than existing treatments may still be clinically valuable if they have fewer side effects or are more effective for particular subgroups of patients.[18] However, no drug should be approved for use in patients unless it is clearly superior to placebo or no treatment. Despite the methodologic rigor of placebo-controlled trials, commentators acknowledge that they are unethical in some circumstances, especially when withholding an effective treatment might be life-threatening or might cause serious morbidity.[8,9]

There are serious problems with placebo orthodoxy. First, in our opinion, the criteria for ethical use of placebo controls are never precisely stated. In a recent review, for instance, Temple and Ellenberg[8,9] claimed that the use of placebo controls is ethical if the research participants who receive placebo will experience "no permanent adverse consequence," if there is a risk of "only temporary discomforts," or if they "will not be harmed." We think that these formulations are not equivalent. Since patients may be harmed by temporary but reversible conditions, the criterion of no harm would exclude many placebo-controlled trials that meet the criterion of no permanent adverse consequence.

Second, the criteria permit intolerable suffering on the part of study participants. This point is illustrated by trials of the antinausea medication ondansetron.[8] In 1981, research demonstrated clinically and statistically significant differences between metoclopramide and placebo for the treatment of vomiting induced by chemotherapy.[19] In the early 1990s, placebo-controlled trials of ondansetron for chemotherapy-induced vomiting, some of which involved patients who had not previously received chemotherapy, were reported.[20–22] These trials were unethical.[23,24] Although vomiting induced by chemotherapy, especially with highly emetic drugs such as cisplatin, is not life threatening and does not cause irreversible disability, it causes serious, avoidable harm that is more than mere discomfort. Indeed, the need for better antiemetic medication had been justified in the first place by the argument that "uncontrolled nausea and vomiting [from chemotherapy] frequently results in poor nutritional intake, metabolic derangements, deterioration of physical and mental condition, as well as the possible rejection of potentially beneficial treatment."[22] Even in 1990, patients receiving the chemotherapeutic drugs evaluated in the ondansetron trials were routinely given antiemetic prophylaxis. Other trials conducted at the time used active controls.[25,26]

Finally, the proponents of placebo controls seem to focus on physical harm. In arguing for placebo-controlled trials of antidepressants, Temple and Ellenberg suggest that the only relevant harm is depression-induced suicide.[8,9] Psychological and social harms caused by depression—such as mental anguish, loss of employment, and disruption of relationships—are either not considered or dismissed. Yet psychological and social harms are invoked to justify the value of the research. This is contradictory. In evaluating the risk–benefit ratio, psychological and social harms must be addressed.

Active-Control Orthodoxy

Because of these problems, commentators have attacked placebo orthodoxy as unethical.[10–14] Proponents of active controls contend that whenever an effective intervention for a condition exists, it must be used in the control group. Furthermore, they argue that placebo controls are inappropriate because the clinically relevant question is not whether a new

drug is better than nothing but whether it is better than standard treatments. To justify this approach, they cite the Declaration of Helsinki,[13,14,17] the most recent version of which states, "The benefits, risks, burdens and effectiveness of a new method should be tested against those of the best current prophylactic, diagnostic, and therapeutic methods. This does not exclude the use of placebo, or no treatment, in studies where no proven prophylactic, diagnostic or therapeutic method exists."[27] Advocates of active controls criticize placebo orthodoxy for placing the demands of science ahead of the rights and well-being of study participants.

Active-control orthodoxy also has several problems. First, the dichotomy between rigorous science and ethical protections is false. Scientific validity constitutes a fundamental ethical protection.[24] Scientifically invalid research cannot be ethical no matter how favorable the risk–benefit ratio for study participants.[24,28] If placebo controls are necessary or desirable for scientific reasons, that constitutes an ethical reason to use them, although it may not be a sufficient reason.

Second, in some cases, the harm and discomfort associated with the use of placebo controls are nonexistent or are so small that there can be no reasonable ethical requirement for new treatments to be tested only against standard treatments. Who could persuasively argue that for trials involving conditions such as baldness or some types of headaches, it is unethical to withhold effective treatments from some study participants and give them placebo instead?[29] There is no meaningful harm that stringent ethicists should worry about in letting a person who has given informed consent continue to suffer temporarily from a headache or untreated baldness as part of a clinical trial. Some critics of placebo controls contend that such trials are unethical because physicians owe medical care to patients who are seeking treatment for these ailments.[11] This argument conflates clinical research with clinical care. Clinicians frequently do not treat such ailments and patients often forgo treatment, indicating that there can be no ethical necessity to provide it.[9] The absolute prohibition against the use of placebo controls in every case in which an effective treatment exists is too broad; the magnitude of harm likely to be caused by using placebo must be part of the ethical consideration.

Third, opponents of placebo-controlled trials pay insufficient attention to the power of the placebo response. Substantial proportions of patients receiving placebo have measurable and clinically meaningful improvements—for example, 30 to 50 percent of patients with depression[30] and 30 to 80 percent of those with chronic stable angina.[31] A recent meta-analysis of randomized clinical trials with both placebo and no-treatment groups found little evidence of the therapeutic benefits of placebo over no treatment.[32] However, the patients given no treatment received clinical attention that may have contributed to observed improvements. This clinical attention may account for the placebo effect. Placebo-controlled trials in which patients receive potentially therapeutic clinical attention test whether an investigational treatment is better than this attention, not whether it is better than nothing.[33]

Most important, trials with active controls may expose more patients to harm than placebo-controlled trials. Equivalence trials, which evaluate the hypothesis that one drug is equivalent to another, typically require larger samples to achieve sufficient power, because the delta, or difference between the rates of response to the two drugs, is likely to be smaller than that between the rates of response to an investigational treatment and placebo.[18,34] Consider an equivalence trial in which an investigational drug is compared with a standard drug that is known to have a 60 percent response rate. With a delta of 10 percent (if they were equivalent, the difference between the standard and investigational drugs would be less than 10 percent) and a one-sided statistical test to show equivalence, each group must contain 297 participants. Conversely, if a placebo is hypothesized to have a 30 percent response rate and the investigational drug a 60 percent response rate, then only 48 participants are needed in each group.

With the sample required for the equivalence trial—larger by a factor of six than the sample required for the placebo-controlled trial—many more subjects will be exposed to an investigational drug that may be ineffective or even more toxic than the standard drug. Moreover, if it turns out that the rate of response to the investigational drug is 53 percent—still within the 10 percent range for equivalence—more participants will actually be harmed by not receiving the standard treatment than if a placebo-controlled trial were conducted instead. That is, in an equivalence trial of an investigational drug with a response rate of 53 percent, there will be 21 more subjects without a response in the group of 297 receiving the investigational drug than in the group of 297 receiving the standard drug with a known response rate of 60 percent. Conversely, consider a placebo-controlled trial with a 30 percent rate of response to placebo and a 53 percent rate of response to the investigational drug. Then, there will be 18 more subjects without a response in the group of 96 patients participating in the trial than if all 96 patients had received the standard drug. Indeed, the lower the rate of response to the investigational drug, the larger the number of participants in an equivalence trial who will be exposed to the harms associated with nonresponse. It is therefore simplistic to argue that placebo-controlled trials involving conditions for which the existing interventions are only partly effective necessarily sacrifice the well-being of patients.

A Middle Ground

For clinical research to be ethical, it must fulfill several universal requirements. Among other requirements, it must be scientifically valid and must minimize the risks to which the research participants are exposed.[24] When these requirements conflict, advocates of placebo controls opt for maintaining scientific validity, whereas advocates of active controls opt for minimizing risks. We believe these absolute positions are neither tenable nor defensible.

There is a middle ground. First, both sides agree that certain placebo-controlled trials are clearly unethical. If effective, life-saving, or at least life-prolonging treatment is available, and if patients assigned to receive placebo would be substantially more likely to suffer serious harm than those assigned to receive the investigational drug, a placebo-controlled trial should be prohibited. The efficacy of streptokinase in reducing morbidity and mortality after myocardial infarction made it unethical to conduct placebo-controlled trials of tissue plasminogen activator.[35]

Second, advocates of active controls should agree that for ailments that are not serious, if there is only a minimal chance that patients randomly assigned to receive placebo will suffer harm or even severe discomfort, the use of placebo controls is ethical.[36] A placebo-controlled trial of a new treatment for allergic rhinitis would be ethical because the moderate discomfort associated with allergic rhinitis typically does not impair health or cause severe discomfort.[29] Indeed, the risks associated with such trials are no greater than those deemed acceptable in natural-history and epidemiologic studies in which blood samples are obtained solely for research purposes and in pharmacokinetic studies in which medications are administered to healthy volunteers and blood samples obtained from them even though there is no prospect of a benefit to the study participants.

The disagreements center on whether it is ethical to use placebo controls when there is a treatment known to be effective and there is some potential for harm to participants receiving placebo. In this context, it is important to recognize that placebo-controlled trials and those in which active treatment is used as the control frequently have distinct objectives, and each type of trial may have a role in a sequential approach to evaluating new interventions. Whenever the risks of research with placebos are similar to the risks in these other types of studies, the use of placebo should be ethically justifiable. Placebo-controlled trials are often deemed important to determine the efficacy of a new treatment and to facilitate the design of larger trials in which the new treatment is compared with standard interventions. In addition, a trial comparing standard and new interventions may include a placebo group for internal validity when high placebo-response rates are anticipated.[32] However, proponents of active controls deem even these initial efficacy and three-group trials unethical when effective standard therapies exist. Placebo-controlled trials of treatments for angina and depression have been the focus of this disagreement, as have short-term trials designed to establish the efficacy of new treatments for asthma and hypertension before large, randomized trials are conducted to compare the new intervention with standard therapies.

When effective treatments exist, there must be compelling methodologic reasons to conduct a placebo-controlled trial. Proving that a new treatment has sufficient efficacy before large-scale equivalence trials are conducted is such a reason, whereas conducting a scientifically valid study with a smaller sample is not. A placebo-controlled trial has a sound scientific rationale if the following criteria are met: there is a high placebo-response rate; the condition is typically characterized by a waxing-and-waning course, frequent spontaneous remissions, or both; and existing therapies are only partly effective or have very serious side effects; or the low frequency of the condition means that an equivalence trial would have to be so large that it would reasonably prevent adequate enrollment and completion of the study.

If these methodologic criteria are met, then the risk of using a placebo control should be evaluated according to several criteria. Research participants in the placebo group should not be substantially more likely than those in the active-treatment group to die; to have irreversible morbidity or disability or to suffer other harm; to suffer reversible but serious harm; or to experience severe discomfort. There is no way of removing qualifying words such as "serious" or "severe" from these criteria, since ethical evaluation necessarily calls for contextualized judgments. Just as courts are empowered to make contextualized judgments about the standard of a separation between church and state, federal regulations empower institutional review boards to determine the levels of risk and severity of harm associated with research.

Although placebo-controlled trials that meet these methodologic and ethical criteria may be justifiable even though the participants forgo therapies known to be effective, they remain worrisome because of the potential to cause suffering. Consequently, standard precautions must be scrupulously implemented for these trials. When such a trial is proposed, the institutional review board must ensure that the following safeguards are instituted to minimize harm: participants at increased risk of harm from nonresponse are excluded; the placebo period is limited to the minimum required for scientific validity; subjects will be carefully monitored, with inpatient observation when appropriate; rescue medications will be administered if serious symptoms develop; and there are explicit and specific criteria for the withdrawal of subjects who have adverse events. In addition, as part of the informed-consent process, the investigators must clearly disclose the rationale for using placebo, explain that subjects who are randomly assigned to the placebo group will not receive standard effective treatments, and state the risks associated with forgoing such treatments. The protocol should include provisions to ensure optimal treatment for participants who withdraw early or who remain symptomatic at the conclusion of the trial.

A Case Example

Chronic stable angina can cause substantial functional impairment and suffering. It is associated with a placebo-response rate of 30 to 80 percent.[31] Patients with chronic stable angina typically have fluctuating courses with sponta-

neous remissions, and for some patients, current therapies are partly effective at best. The long history of positive findings from open trials of cardiovascular treatments that have subsequently been disproved by blinded, placebo-controlled trials—including ligation of the internal mammary artery for angina,[37,38] chelation for claudication,[39] encainide and flecainide for arrhythmias,[40] and most recently, laser systems that create holes in cardiac tissue[41]—provides good scientific reasons for conducting placebo-controlled trials of treatments for chronic angina.

Even if it is methodologically sound, a placebo-controlled trial of a new treatment for chronic angina should satisfy the ethical criteria for an acceptable level of risk—that is, participation in the trial would not cause death, irreversible disability, reversible but serious harm, or severe discomfort. There is no evidence that medical management of chronic angina prolongs survival. Furthermore, a comprehensive review of double-blind, placebo-controlled, randomized trials of treatment for chronic angina showed that the risk of adverse events did not differ significantly between the drug and placebo groups.[42] The authors concluded that "withholding active treatment does not increase the risk of serious cardiac events." Nonetheless, patients at high risk for myocardial infarction and other cardiac events should be excluded from such trials, nitroglycerin should be provided for breakthrough anginal pain, and the period of treatment with placebo should be brief, usually less than 10 weeks. Patients should be contacted frequently to ensure careful monitoring of their condition, and those whose symptoms exceed an explicit threshold should be withdrawn from the trial. The informed-consent process must make it clear to patients that their angina may worsen and that they are free to withdraw from the trial at any time.

Conclusions

Placebo-controlled trials are caught in a battle between two orthodoxies. One is that placebo should be used as a control unless there is an increased risk of death or irreversible morbidity associated with its use. The other view is that if an effective therapy exists, the use of a placebo should be prohibited. These two positions are both absolute and indefensible. We propose a middle ground in which placebo-controlled trials are permitted but only when the methodologic reasons for their use are compelling, a strict ethical evaluation has made it clear that patients who receive placebo will not be subject to serious harm, and provisions have been made to minimize the risks associated with the receipt of placebo. This framework provides a basis for deliberation in difficult cases, with the recognition that reasonable people might make divergent judgments in a particular case.

REFERENCES

1. Lilienfeld AM. The Fielding H. Garrison Lecture: Ceteris paribus: the evolution of the clinical trial. Bull Hist Med 1982;56:1–18.

2. Lasagna L, Mosteller F, von Felsinger JM, Beecher HK. A study of the placebo response. Am J Med 1954;16:770–779.

3. Lasagna L. Placebos and controlled trials under attack. Eur J Clin Pharmacol 1979;15:373–374.

4. Feinstein AR. Should placebo-controlled trials be abolished? Eur J Clin Pharmacol 1980;17:1–4.

5. Way WL. Placebo controls. N Engl J Med 1984;311:413–414.

6. Temple R. Government viewpoint of clinical trials. Drug Inform J 1982;16:10–17.

7. Temple R. Problems in interpreting active control equivalence trials. In: Accountability in research. Vol. 4. New York: Gordon and Breach, 1996:267–275.

8. Temple R, Ellenberg SS. Placebo-controlled trials and active-control trials in the evaluation of new treatments. I. Ethical and scientific issues. Ann Intern Med 2000;133:455–463.

9. Ellenberg SS, Temple R. Placebo-controlled trials and active-control trials in the evaluation of new treatments. II. Practical issues and specific cases. Ann Intern Med 2000;133:464–470.

10. Freedman B, Weijer C, Glass KC. Placebo orthodoxy in clinical research. I. Empirical and methodological myths. J Law Med Ethics 1996; 24:243–251.

11. Freedman B, Glass KC, Weijer C. Placebo orthodoxy in clinical research. II. Ethical, legal, and regulatory myths. J Law Med Ethics 1996; 24:252–259.

12. Freedman B. Placebo-controlled trials and the logic of clinical purpose. IRB 1990;12(6):1–6.

13. Rothman KJ, Michels KB. The continuing unethical use of placebo controls. N Engl J Med 1994;331:394–398.

14. Rothman KJ. Declaration of Helsinki should be strengthened. BMJ 2000;321:442–445.

15. Shapiro HT, Meslin EM. Ethical issues in the design and conduct of clinical trials in developing countries. N Engl J Med 2001;345:139–142.

16. Koski G, Nightingale SL. Research involving human subjects in developing countries. N Engl J Med 2001;345:136–138.

17. Enserink M. Helsinki's new clinical rules: fewer placebos, more disclosure. Science 2000;290:418–419.

18. Senn S. Active control equivalence studies. In: Senn S. Statistical issues in drug development. Chichester, England: John Wiley, 1997:207–217.

19. Gralla RJ, Itri LM, Pisko SE, et al. Antiemetic efficacy of high-dose metoclopramide: randomized trials with placebo and prochlorpera-zine in patients with chemotherapy-induced nausea and vomiting. N Engl J Med 1981;305:905–909.

20. Cubeddu LX, Hoffmann IS, Fuenmayor NT, Finn AL. Efficacy of ondansetron (GR 38032F) and the role of serotonin in cisplatin-induced nausea and vomiting. N Engl J Med 1990;322:810–816.

21. Gandara DR, Harvey WH, Monaghan GG, et al. The delayed-emesis syndrome from cisplatin: phase III evaluation of ondansetron versus placebo. Semin Oncol 1992;19:67–71.

22. Beck TM, Ciociola AA, Jones SE, et al. Efficacy of oral ondansetron in the prevention of emesis in outpatients receiving cyclophosphamide-based chemotherapy. Ann Intern Med 1993;118:407–413.

23. Hait WN. Ondansetron and cisplatin-induced nausea and vomiting. N Engl J Med 1990;323:1485–1486.

24. Emanuel EJ, Wendler D, Grady C. What makes clinical research ethical? JAMA 2000;283:2701–2711.

25. Marty M, Pouillart P, Scholl S, et al. Comparison of the 5-hydroxytryptamine₃ (serotonin) antagonist ondansetron (GR 38032F) with high-dose metoclopramide in the control of cisplatin-induced emesis. N Engl J Med 1990;322:816–821.

26. Hainsworth J, Harvey W, Pendergrass K, et al. A single-blind comparison of intravenous ondansetron, a selective serotonin antagonist, with intravenous metoclopramide in the prevention of nausea and vomiting associated with high-dose cisplatin chemother-apy. J Clin Oncol 1991;9:721–728.

27. World Medical Association. Declaration of Helsinki: ethical principles for medical research involving human subjects. Edinburgh, Scotland: World Medical Association, October 2000.

28. Rutstein DD. The ethical design of human experiments. In: Freund PA, ed. Experimentation with human subjects. New York: George Braziller, 1970:383–401.

29. Senn S. The misunderstood placebo. Appl Clin Trials 2001;10(5):40–46.

30. Khan A, Warner HA, Brown WA. Symptom reduction and suicide risk in patients treated with placebo in antidepressant clinical trials: an analysis of the Food and Drug Administration database. Arch Gen Psychiatry 2000; 57:311–317.

31. Bienenfeld L, Frishman W, Glasser SP. The placebo effect in cardiovas-cular disease. Am Heart J 1996;132:1207–1221.

32. Hróbjartsson A, Gøtzsche PC. Is the placebo powerless? An analysis of clinical trials comparing placebo with no treatment. N Engl J Med 2001;344:1594–1602.

33. Miller FG. Placebo-controlled trials in psychiatric research: an ethical perspective. Biol Psychiatry 2000;47:707–716.

34. Leon AC. Placebo protects subjects from nonresponse: a paradox of power. Arch Gen Psychiatry 2000;57:329–330.

35. Brody BA. When are placebo-controlled trials no longer appropriate? Control Clin Trials 1997;18:602–612.

36. Vastag B. Helsinki discord? A controversial declaration. JAMA 2000; 284:2983–2985.

37. Dimond EG, Kittle CF, Crockett JE. Evaluation of internal mammary artery ligation and sham procedure in angina pectoris. Circulation 1958; 18:712–713.

38. Cobb LA, Thomas GI, Dillard DH, Merendino KA, Bruce RA. An evaluation of internal-mammary-artery ligation by a double-blind technic. N Engl J Med 1959;260:1115–1118.

39. van Rij AM, Solomon C, Packer SGK, Hopkins WG. Chelation therapy for intermittent claudication: a double-blind, randomised, controlled trial. Circulation 1994;90:1194–1199.

40. The Cardiac Arrhythmia Suppression Trial (CAST) Investigators. Preliminary report: effect of encainide and flecainide on mortality in a randomized trial of arrhythmia suppression after myocardial infarction. N Engl J Med 1989;321:406–412.

41. Winslow R. Placebo study questions effectiveness of laser heart treatment. Wall Street Journal. October 19, 2000:B14.

42. Glasser SP, Clark PI, Lipicky RJ, Hubbard JM, Yusuf S. Exposing patients with chronic, stable, exertional angina to placebo periods in drug trials. JAMA 1991;265:1550–1554.

43
Is Placebo Surgery Unethical?

Sam Horng and Franklin G. Miller

Sam Horng and Franklin G. Miller, "Is Placebo Surgery Unethical?" *New England Journal of Medicine* 2002;347:137–139.

Surgical procedures are often introduced into practice with-out rigorous evaluation. Moreover, clinical trials of surgery have seldom included placebo surgery as a control, owing to ethical concerns. In 1959, the *New England Journal of Medicine* published the results of a placebo-controlled trial of ligation of the internal thoracic artery for the treatment of angina.[1] [In a more recent issue of the same journal], Moseley et al. report on a placebo-controlled trial of arthroscopic surgery for osteoarthritis of the knee.[2] In both studies, the surgical interventions were no more effective than placebo operations. A major difference between the use of placebo surgery [in 1959] and its use now, however, is the degree of attention to the ethical aspects of conducting clinical research.

The Ethics of Clinical Research

The idea of using placebo surgery is apt to elicit an immediate negative judgment, because it appears to violate the fundamental ethical principles of beneficence and nonmaleficence.[3] Doctors should not expose patients to risks if there is no prospect of possible benefits. With respect to surgery, this means that surgeons should not invade the body except for the purpose of cure or amelioration. In a recent ethical critique of placebo surgery for Parkinson's disease, Clark asserted, "The researcher has an ethical responsibility to act in the best interest of subjects."[4]

Although this statement reflects a commonly articulated moral stance with regard to clinical research, it confounds the ethics of clinical research with the ethics of clinical care. The randomized, controlled trial is not a form of individualized medical therapy; it is a scientific tool for evaluating treatments in groups of research participants, with the aim of improving the care of patients in the future. Clinical trials are not designed to promote the medical best interests of enrolled patients and often expose them to risks that are not outweighed by known potential medical benefits. Accordingly, the use of placebo surgery must be evaluated in terms of the ethical principles appropriate to clinical research, which are not identical to the ethical principles of clinical practice.[5]

Clinical research involves an inherent tension between the ethical values of pursuing rigorous science and protecting participants from harm.[6] To avoid exploiting research subjects, clinical trials must satisfy several ethical requirements.[5] Clinical trials are unethical if they are not designed to answer valuable scientific questions with the use of valid research methods. In addition to having scientific merit, clinical trials must present a favorable risk-benefit ratio: the risks to participants must be minimized and justifiable by the benefits to them, if any, and the potential value of the scientific knowledge to be gained from the study. Finally, investigators must obtain informed consent from participants.

Use of an invasive procedure as a placebo control poses risks to research subjects assigned to the control group, without the prospect of a benefit from their participation, and the burden of proof is therefore on those who argue that placebo surgery is warranted as a means of evaluating the efficacy of surgical procedures. The use of placebo surgery in clinical trials raises three key ethical questions. First, is placebo surgery compatible with the ethical requirement to minimize risks? Second, are the risks associated with placebo surgery reasonable and justifiable in relation to the potential value of the scientific knowledge to be gained from its use? Third, can informed consent be obtained for a trial that randomly assigns patients to undergo genuine or placebo surgery?

Placebo Surgery
Minimizing Risks

Placebo-controlled trials of medical agents involve the administration of inert substances disguised as active medication. Trial participants do not incur risks by taking the placebo pill, but they may be at risk for clinical deterioration or lack of improvement because they are not receiving an active therapeutic agent. In contrast, participants in a placebo-controlled trial of surgery are exposed to risks from the placebo procedure itself.

Macklin argued that placebo surgery violates "an essential standard for research: the requirement to minimize the risk of harm to subjects."[7] The ethical requirement to minimize risks in randomized, controlled trials must be considered in the context of alternative study designs for answering scientific questions about the efficacy of treatment. Can a valid evaluation of a given surgical intervention be conducted without the use of a placebo control, thus minimizing risks without compromising scientific rigor?

In the trial of arthroscopic knee surgery reported by Moseley et al., the primary outcome measure was pain, an inherently subjective phenomenon. It is doubtful that valid data could be obtained from a randomized clinical trial that compared a group of patients assigned to undergo arthroscopic surgery with a control group that received no treatment. Because patients enrolled in such a trial would obviously know whether or not they had undergone surgery, their reports of pain might be biased. In reporting the degree of knee pain and function, patients might be influenced by their expectation of improvement after surgery and postoperative care. Furthermore, assessment of the outcome without knowledge of the treatment assignments would require that patients not disclose the treatment they had received—an unlikely prospect.

In addition to the possibility of biased evaluations of outcomes, a trial that compares surgery with no treatment or with standard medical treatment does not control for the placebo effect of surgery.[8] Reduced pain and improved function may result from the invasiveness of the procedure and the belief that one is undergoing surgery, rather than from any specific effects of surgery. A recent meta-analysis called into question the power of the placebo effect,[9] but that analysis did not include trials of surgery. Furthermore, the outcome variable that was most suggestive of a true placebo effect was pain. There is reason to believe that the invasiveness of surgery may be associated with a pronounced placebo effect.[10-13]

These methodologic considerations lead to the conclusion that a placebo control is required for a rigorous scientific evaluation of surgery when the primary outcome is a subjective phenomenon such as pain or the quality of life.[14] If a placebo control is necessary for a valid test of the efficacy of a surgical procedure, then use of placebo surgery does not contravene the requirement of minimizing risks. In this case, there is no alternative to a placebo control; no other sufficiently rigorous study design poses less risk.

In addressing the issue of minimizing risks, one must consider not only the question of whether placebo surgery is methodologically necessary but also the question of whether the risks of placebo surgery can be reduced. Moseley et al. reduced the risks of the placebo surgery in their trial by using a short-acting tranquilizer combined with an opioid for anesthesia, which is less risky than general anesthesia with endotracheal intubation, the standard form of anesthesia used in patients undergoing arthroscopic surgery.

Justifying Risks

Even if the risks of a scientifically valuable and valid clinical trial have been minimized, it does not follow that they are justified. Critics of placebo surgery have argued that it exceeds an acceptable threshold of risk for subjects who are randomly assigned to undergo the invasive intervention merely as a scientific control.[4,15] These subjects are exposed to substantial risks without the prospect of possible benefits.

Can the potential value of the knowledge to be gained from a well-controlled trial involving the use of placebo surgery justify the risks to the participants? It is clearly unethical to jeopardize severely the health and well-being of research subjects only for the good of future patients. In the trial of arthroscopic surgery reported by Moseley et al., the risks for subjects who were randomly assigned to the placebo group included potential harm from three skin incisions and from anesthesia. These risks are certainly greater than minimal, but they do not substantially exceed the risks of other generally accepted research interventions, such as muscle biopsy, bronchoscopy, and phase 1 testing of experimental drugs in healthy volunteers, which do not offer participants a prospect of direct benefits. The trial of arthroscopic surgery posed considerably less risk to participants in the placebo group than did the controversial placebo-controlled trial of a cellular-based treatment for Parkinson's disease, which involved the drilling of burr holes in the skull and the administration of general anesthesia, intravenous antibiotics, and low doses of cyclosporine.[16]

Informed Consent

Why would subjects volunteer for a clinical trial if they understood that they might undergo placebo surgery? Empirical studies of informed consent in clinical trials involving patients with psychiatric disorders and those with cancer have shown evidence of a "therapeutic misconception" about research.[17,18] Many research participants appear to confuse treatment in the scientific context of clinical trials with individualized medical care. There is also evidence that they overestimate the benefits of participation in a trial and underestimate the risks.[18] These deficits in understanding make it difficult to obtain meaningful informed consent.

Problems with informed consent are of particular concern in studies involving interventions that depart substantially from standard clinical practice, especially if the risks of these interventions, such as placebo surgery, are substantial.[4,7] There is also concern about the enrollment of "vulnerable" subjects—those who may have an impaired capacity to give informed consent or who may be susceptible to "undue inducement" to participate in research.[19]

We see no reason for special concern about informed consent in the trial conducted by Moseley et al. Osteoarthritis of the knee is a painful and potentially debilitating condition, but it is not life threatening. Nor is it associated with impaired decision-making capacity. Moseley et al. report that enrolled patients were required to write in their charts that they understood that they might undergo an invasive placebo procedure that would not involve potentially beneficial treatment of their arthritis. The fact that 44 percent of the eligible patients declined participation indicates that the enrolled subjects decided to participate in the trial without undue inducement or coercion.

An additional ethical concern about obtaining informed consent for participation in trials that involve placebo surgery is the use of communication and actions designed to give the false impression that subjects randomly assigned to placebo surgery have undergone a real surgical procedure.[7] Because of the possibility that some patients might remain conscious during the placebo surgical procedure in the study by Moseley et al., it was performed to resemble arthroscopic débridement. The report does not state whether the plan to use a placebo intervention that mimicked arthroscopic débridement was disclosed to prospective subjects as part of the informed-consent process. Such a practice can be ethical if investigators inform prospective participants that it will be used to maintain the blinded condition and if they reveal the nature of the deception at the end of the study.[20]

Conclusions

Reasonable people are bound to differ over the ethics of a controversial practice such as the use of placebo surgery in clinical trials. Ethical objections—based on the requirements to minimize risks, limit the level of risks that are not offset by the potential benefits to participants, and obtain informed consent—do not support an absolute prohibition against the use of placebo surgery when its use is methodologically necessary to answer clinically important questions. Indeed, we suggest that the trial conducted by Moseley et al. exemplifies the ethically justified use of placebo surgery. Each proposed trial involving placebo surgery must be evaluated carefully in the light of these ethical considerations.

A full ethical assessment must include consideration of the consequences of not conducting rigorous trials of surgery. Arthroscopic surgery has become a common treatment for osteoarthritis of the knee in the absence of rigorous scientific evaluation of its efficacy. According to data cited by Moseley et al., the costs of this intervention are approximately $3.25 billion per year. Yet the results of this important study demonstrate that two methods of arthroscopic surgery are no more effective than a placebo operation. Thus, patients have been exposed to risks and third-party payers have incurred substantial costs for a treatment that offers no benefit to the patient. Trials of surgical procedures that include the use of placebo surgery should be conducted before the procedures become standard treatments, provided that these trials meet the ethical requirements that are appropriate for clinical research.

REFERENCES

1. Cobb LA, Thomas GI, Dillard DH, Merendino KA, Bruce RA. An evaluation of internal-mammary-artery ligation by a double-blind technic. N Engl J Med 1959;260:1115–1118.

2. Moseley JB, O'Malley K, Petersen NJ, et al. A controlled trial of arthroscopic surgery for osteoarthritis of the knee. N Engl J Med 2002;347:81–88.

3. Beauchamp TL, Childress JF. Principles of biomedical ethics. 5th ed. New York: Oxford University Press, 2001.

4. Clark PA. Placebo surgery for Parkinson's disease: do the benefits outweigh the risks? J Law Med Ethics 2002;30:58–68.

5. Emanuel EJ, Wendler D, Grady C. What makes clinical research ethical? JAMA 2000;283:2701–2711.

6. Miller FG, Rosenstein DL, DeRenzo EG. Professional integrity in clinical research. JAMA 1998;280:1449–1454.

7. Macklin R. The ethical problems with sham surgery in clinical research. N Engl J Med 1999;341:992–996.

8. Johnson AG. Surgery as a placebo. Lancet 1994;344:1140–1142.

9. Hróbjartsson A, Gøtzsche PC. Is the placebo powerless? An analysis of clinical trials comparing placebo with no treatment. N Engl J Med 2001; 344:1594–1602.

10. Beecher HK. Surgery as placebo: a quantitative study of bias. JAMA 1961;176:1102–1107.

11. Kaptchuk TJ, Goldman P, Stone DA, Stason WB. Do medical devices have enhanced placebo effects? J Clin Epidemiol 2000;53:786–792.

12. Moseley JB Jr, Wray NP, Kuykendall D, Willis K, Landon G. Arthroscopic treatment of osteoarthritis of the knee: a prospective, randomized, placebo-controlled trial. Results of a pilot study. Am J Sports Med 1996;24:28–34.

13. Moerman DE, Jonas WB. Deconstructing the placebo effect and finding the meaning response. Ann Intern Med 2002;136:471–476.

14. Gillett GR. Unnecessary holes in the head. IRB Ethics Hum Res 2001;23(6):1–6.

15. Weijer C. I need a placebo like I need a hole in the head. J Law Med Ethics 2002;30:69–72.

16. Freeman TB, Vawter DE, Leaverton PE, et al. Use of placebo surgery in controlled trials of a cellular-based therapy for Parkinson's disease. N Engl J Med 1999;341:988–992.

17. Appelbaum PS, Roth LH, Lidz CW, Benson P, Winslade W. False hopes and best data: consent to research and the therapeutic misconception. Hastings Cent Rep 1987;17(2):20–24.

18. Joffe S, Cook EF, Cleary PD, Clark JW, Weeks JC. Quality of informed consent in cancer clinical trials: a cross-sectional survey. Lancet 2001;358:1772–1777.

19. Levine RJ. Ethics and regulation of clinical research. 2nd ed. Baltimore: Urban & Schwarzenberg, 1986:72–93.

20. Wendler D. Deception in medical and behavioral research: is it ever acceptable? Milbank Q 1996;74:87–114.

44
Deception in Research on the Placebo Effect

Franklin G. Miller, David Wendler, and Leora C. Swartzman

Franklin G. Miller, David Wendler, and Leora C. Swartzman, "Deception in Research on the Placebo Effect," PLoS Medicine 2005;2(9):e262.

The placebo effect is a fascinating yet puzzling phenomenon, which has challenged investigators over the past 50 years. Recently, it has been defined as the "positive physiological or psychological changes associated with the use of inert medications, sham procedures, or therapeutic symbols within a healthcare encounter" [1]. Increasing scientific inquiry has been aimed at elucidating the mechanisms responsible for placebo effects and determining how inert interventions can lead to positive changes in patients [1,2]. The majority of placebo mechanism research has been done within the context of experimental and clinical pain.

Patients' expectations for improvement, also referred to as "response expectancies," are thought to be one of the central mechanisms responsible for placebo effects [3–5]. Brain imaging techniques are being used to explore both the neurophysiological correlates of these expectations and the mechanisms underlying placebo effects in a variety of contexts, including pain relief in healthy participants, relief of symptoms of depression, and motor functioning in patients with Parkinson disease [6–8]. Understanding these mechanisms is an important step in harnessing the placebo effect in patient care. In the words of a National Institutes of Health request for applications, "understanding how to enhance the therapeutic benefits of placebo effect in clinical practice has the potential to significantly improve healthcare" [9]. Toward that end, the National Institutes of Health invited submissions for systematic studies aimed at discerning the psychosocial factors (including expectancy) in the patient-clinician relationship and/or in the health-care environment that can potentiate healing.

A common feature of research investigating the placebo effect is deception of research participants about the nature of the research. This use of deception is considered necessary to understanding the placebo effect, but has received little systematic ethical attention. In this article, we examine ethical issues relating to deception in research on the placebo effect, with a particular focus on experiments involving patients in clinical settings. We propose a method of informing participants about the use of deception that can reconcile the scientific need for deceptive research designs with the ethical requirements for clinical research.

Altering Expectations to Examine Placebo Mechanisms

Response expectancy is seen to be a major driving force behind the placebo effect. Therefore, a common (and some

Table 44.1.
The balanced placebo design

What Participants Are Told	What Participants Receive	
	Participants Given Drug	Participants Given Placebo
Participants told they will receive drug	True (no deception)	False (deception)
Participants told they will receive placebo	False (deception)	True (no deception)

would argue, necessary) feature of research aimed at elucidating placebo mechanisms is the use of deception in experimental manipulation of participants' expectations (e.g., about whether or not they will receive a "powerful pain killer" or a "sugar pill"), while holding constant the pharmacological (or other) properties of the administered intervention. This research has clearly shown (across a wide range of clinical conditions) that altering expectancies for improvement has an impact on therapeutic outcomes [8,10–13].

The tension between scientific methods for elucidating the placebo effect and ethical norms for conducting research involving human participants is illustrated most clearly by "the balanced placebo design," an approach designed to disentangle the relative effects of pharmacology and response expectancy. Table 44.1 displays the balanced placebo design in a way that highlights the deception of participants that occurs in two of the four arms of the design.

In the balanced placebo design, investigators manipulate both expectancies (e.g., informing participants that they will receive a drug versus informing them that they will receive placebo) and the pharmacological agent (giving a drug versus giving a placebo). As reviewed by Swartzman and Burkell, researchers using this paradigm with healthy volunteers have shown that expectation plays a role in the subjective and behavioral effects of a range of psychoactive substances [14]. These substances include dexamfetamine, alcohol, caffeine, nicotine, and tetrahydrocannabinol [15–19].

The balanced placebo design offers a powerful and elegant approach to evaluate drug versus expectancy effects and their interactions. As Kirsch notes, this design yields information that cannot be obtained from conventional clinical trials [20]. It provides a direct assessment of the drug effect, independent of expectancy, and the nondeceptive arms are more ecologically valid than the double-blind administration in conventional randomized trials (i.e., they mimic what goes on in the real world of clinical practice). Thus, it is not surprising that Caspi recently suggested that the balanced placebo design "be used more often in clinical trials of drug efficacy" [21]. Despite the methodological virtues of the balanced placebo design, and its prior use in healthy volunteers, we are unaware of any trials that have employed this approach with patients. Clinical investigators likely have avoided use of the balanced placebo design out of concern for the ethical acceptability of deceiving patients.

An often-cited article on the balanced placebo design characterized the deception in the following way: "Although deception is involved, it is no greater than is involved in any study using placebos" [22]. However, this defense of the balanced placebo design confuses the ethical issues it raises. Placebo-controlled trials aimed at evaluating the efficacy of treatments may be regarded as having an element of deception, since the placebo control is designed to appear indistinguishable from the active treatment under investigation. Nevertheless, when these studies are conducted under effective double-blind conditions, participants are told that they will receive either a drug or a placebo, and neither the investigators nor the research participants know which intervention is received by any of the participants. Accordingly, administering the study interventions, unlike the situation of the balanced placebo design, does not involve intentionally false communication; it requires investigators to withhold information, but not to lie to participants about the interventions they will receive.

Research designed to understand the placebo effect by deceptively manipulating the expectations of participants holds great promise for understanding the psychological and neurobiological dimensions of healing. However, to pursue this research while respecting participants, it is necessary to develop an approach that reconciles the outright deception involved in placebo research, including the balanced placebo design, with the ethical norms governing clinical research.

What Makes Deception in Scientific Investigation Ethically Problematic?

At the outset, it is useful to appreciate the conflict between the ethos of science and the use of deceptive techniques. Science aims to discover and communicate the truth about the natural world and human conduct. There are sound methodological reasons for using deception to probe for the truth about human attitudes and beliefs and their effects on behavior. It follows, however, that when deception is used, a conflict between the means and ends of scientific investigation ensues: the end of discovering the truth is pursued by the means of deliberate untruth.

It might be argued that deception in scientific investigation is no more problematic than the pervasive and accepted use of deception in daily life and in social contexts [23]. In a recent news article reporting advances in the design of computers to simulate human responsiveness, Clifford Nass, a professor of communication at Stanford University, endorses the deception involved in this project: "We spend enormous amounts of time teaching children to deceive—it's called being polite or social. The history of all advertising is about deceiving. In education, it's often important to deceive people—sometimes you say, 'Boy you are really doing good,' not because you meant it but because you thought it would be helpful" [24].

Deception in ordinary life typically is justified on the grounds that it is for the benefit of the individual who is being deceived. For instance, the polite and social deception that Nass cites is justified on the grounds that it is better to deceive someone slightly than to criticize the person or to hurt the person's feelings. Notice, however, that this condition is not relevant to placebo research, including the balanced placebo design. In placebo research, participants are not deceived for their own benefit. Rather, they are deceived for the benefit of science and society in general, through the development of generalizable knowledge.

Deception of research participants also clearly conflicts with the ethical norms governing clinical research [25,26]. First, it violates the principle of respect for persons by infringing on the right of prospective research participants to choose whether to participate in research based on full disclosure of relevant information. Second, it may manipulate individuals to volunteer when they otherwise would not have chosen to do so had they been informed accurately about the nature of the research, including its use of deception. For these reasons, deception, as it is currently practiced in the conduct of research on the placebo effect, is incompatible with informed consent.

Third, although scant systematic data have been collected on the effects of deception on clinical research participants, some available evidence indicates that when the deception is revealed, as in the debriefing process that often accompanies deceptive research, it causes distress to at least some participants [27]. The adverse impact of deception in psychological research, and whether it can be reversed adequately through a debriefing process, is a subject of debate [28–31]. Furthermore, deception in research involving patients in clinical settings may prove more upsetting. This is because participants in deceptive psychological research are, for the most part, psychology undergraduates who often are aware that deception is sometimes used in psychological research [32]. Patients, in contrast, legitimately expect to be able to trust in, and receive truthful communication from, clinicians and clinical investigators. This trust is violated by the use of deception. Especially problematic is the use of deception in experiments conducted by clinicians who have a prior clinician-patient relationship with the patients enrolled in the study. When patients learn about the use of deception in the process of debriefing, which is a common feature of deception research, they may feel that their trust has been violated. Consequently, deception of patients may have deleterious effects on the willingness of patients to volunteer for future clinical research. More importantly, by undermining patients' faith in the truthfulness of physicians, deception might interfere with the future medical care of those who have experienced deceptive research.

Finally, deception in research raises ethical concern because it can be corrupting for the professionals who practice it, and for those who witness it. According to an ancient perspective in moral philosophy, moral character depends on habits of conduct [33]. The use of deception in research may interfere with the disposition not to lie or deceive persons.

This problem is compounded when the study design requires deception at the initiation of the trial as well as repeated deception of participants while conducting the research. Those who witness deception, especially if performed or sanctioned by professionals in positions of authority, may develop skewed perceptions of the ethics of deception, which may have negative consequences for the development of moral character. In sum, deception in research is prima facie wrongful, and it may be harmful not only to those who are deceived but also to those who practice or witness it.

The American Psychological Association's guidelines [34] are perhaps the most prominent attempt to reconcile the use of deception with the ethical norms of human participant research. According to guideline 8.07 (Deception in Research), "(a) psychologists do not conduct a study involving deception unless they have determined that the use of deceptive techniques is justified by the study's significant prospective scientific, educational, or applied value and that effective nondeceptive alternative procedures are not feasible; (b) psychologists do not deceive prospective participants about research that is reasonably expected to cause physical pain or severe emotional distress; (c) psychologists explain any deception that is an integral feature of the design and conduct of an experiment to participants as early as is feasible, preferably at the conclusion of their participation, but no later than at the conclusion of the data collection, and permit participants to withdraw their data."

We have argued elsewhere that these three conditions are not sufficient to address the ethical concerns raised by deceptive research [25,26]. In particular, these conditions fail to address the fact that concealing the use of deception itself may affect individuals' decision to participate in research and precludes individuals from deciding whether they want to participate in deceptive research. To be sure, the use of debriefing may mitigate the potential harmful consequences of deceitful communication by explaining the rationale for deception. However, just as compensation for damages caused by negligence or restitution for crime does not cancel an infringement of a person's rights, debriefing does not cancel the violation of the principle of respect for persons. To consider how these ethical concerns arise in actual practice, and what steps might be taken to address them, it will be helpful to consider specific examples of the use of deception in placebo research (Table S1 [see "Supporting Information," below—eds.]).

Examples of Deception in Placebo Research

First, in an experiment investigating suggestion and expectation relating to placebo analgesia, 13 women with irritable bowel syndrome were recruited, and were subjected to visceral pain evoked by rectal distention, using a balloon attached to a rectal catheter. The experiment took place under five experimental conditions: (1) natural history (no intervention relating to or disclosure about the pain stimulus), (2) rectal placebo (a sterile surgical lubricant placed on the balloon, described as effective in relieving pain), (3) rectal lidocaine, (4) oral lidocaine, and (5) rectal nocebo (a placebo intervention accompanied by a disclosure that the intervention often causes increased pain) [13]. Notably, the research report stated that "the gastroenterologist who performed the study was the doctor the patients normally consulted in the clinic."

The investigators described their disclosure to the participants as follows: "The patients were told that four drugs that reduced and increased pain in relation to IBS [irritable bowel syndrome], respectively, were being tested, and that they had been proven effective in preliminary studies" [13]. In reality, the participants were administered two different forms of only one drug, along with two placebos. Hence, the participants were deceived by being informed that they would receive drugs that in fact were placebo interventions.

Second, investigators recruited patients with asthma, from an academic medical center, to participate in an experiment examining changes in forced expiratory volume in one second following administration of inhaled saline described deceptively as either a bronchoconstrictor or a bronchodilator [12]. The purpose was to determine the impact of suggestion on a placebo intervention in patients identified as suggestible or suggestion-resistant, based on a validated rating scale. The disclosure to the research participants was described in the article reporting the experimental results as follows: "Patients were contacted via telephone and informed that the investigators were hoping to understand how medications produce beneficial effects in asthma, including whether telling subjects about the potential effects of various medications would alter response to these agents. Patients were not told that they would be exposed to placebo interventions." The study thus used elaborate deception, which involved an inaccurate account of the nature of the research and false descriptions of a placebo intervention. It is therefore puzzling that the authors reported that "all patients gave informed consent to participate in the study," especially since there was no indication that the participants were informed that deception would be employed. Instead, the participants were debriefed about the study at the end of the experiment.

Authorized Deception

Can deceptive research be made compatible with informed consent? Use of deception is not consistent with fully informed consent. If participants are told the true purpose of research and the nature of all procedures, there would be no deception. However, participants can be informed prior to deciding whether to volunteer for a study that the experimental procedures will not be described accurately or that some features of these procedures will or may be misleading or deceptive [25,26]. This approach, which we call "authorized deception," permits research participants to decide whether they wish to participate in research involving deception and, if so, to knowingly authorize its use. Authorized

deception is compatible with the spirit of informed consent. It fosters respect for persons, despite the use of deception, by alerting prospective participants to the fact that some or all participants will be deliberately deceived about the purpose of the research or the nature of research procedures.

For example, investigators using the balanced placebo design to study expectancy and pharmacological effects of dexamfetamine described the informed consent disclosure as follows: "For ethical reasons it was stated in the consent form that '. . . some information and/or instructions given [to the participant] may be inaccurate'" [15]. This statement recognizes the ethical force of authorized deception, but does not seem to go far enough. As illustrated above, the balanced placebo design involves lying to participants in two arms of the study: some participants are told that they are being administered a particular drug when in fact they receive placebo, and others that they are being administered placebo when in fact they receive the drug. Consequently, it is at best an understatement to describe the disclosure in this experiment as possibly involving "inaccurate" information. It would be more accurate to inform the prospective participants that some research participants will be misled or deceived.

Variants of the authorized deception approach have been advocated, and sometimes evaluated experimentally, since the 1970s [23,35–37]; however, it has not become a routine feature of research using deception [38]. In order to solicit informed authorization for the use of deception, the informed consent document could be worded as follows: "You should be aware that the investigators have intentionally misdescribed certain aspects of the study. This use of deception is necessary to obtain valid results. However, an independent ethics committee has determined that this consent form accurately describes the major risks and benefits of the study. The investigator will explain the misdescribed aspects of the study to you at the end of your participation."

When deception of study participants is necessary and justified by the scientific value of the study, the use of authorized deception makes the process of deceptive research transparent. Participants are informed that they will be misled or deceived, though obviously the exact nature of the deception cannot be disclosed. They are assured that the research has been reviewed and approved by an ethics oversight committee that has no vested interest in the research in question, and that no important risks, other than the risks of the deception itself, have been concealed. Finally, they are informed that debriefing will occur.

Methodological Objections and the Need for Future Study

One possible objection to the technique of authorized deception is that it is liable to defeat the purpose of using deception to obviate potentially biased responses of research participants to research interventions. Informing participants that deception will occur (particularly in a study that involves administration of a placebo) is apt to make them suspicious and wary, thus possibly contributing to biased data. This methodological risk is avoided in most deceptive research, which does not employ this technique, provided that prospective participants do not otherwise suspect that deception will be used. However, limited available research indicates that the anticipated biased results from disclosing the possibility of deception do not necessarily occur.

Holmes and Bennett assessed this methodological concern experimentally. Psychology students were exposed to a deceptive experiment in which they were falsely informed that two to eight "painful electric shocks" would be administered at random times after a red signal light appeared [35]. No shocks actually were administered. Measures of self-reported anxiety and physiological arousal (pulse and respiration rates) were obtained. Prior to the deceptive shock intervention, one experimental group was informed that deception is occasionally used in psychology experiments to assure unbiased responses. The other group exposed to the deceptive shock intervention did not receive any information about the possibility of deception. No outcome differences were observed for participants informed of the possibility of deception versus those not informed.

The information about deception in this experiment, however, falls short of the authorized deception approach that we recommend. It disclosed to prospective participants that deception is a possibility in "a few experiments," rather than informing them that deception would actually be employed for all or some participants in the particular experiment in which they were invited to enroll. In contrast, Wiener and Erker directly tested the authorized deception approach, described as "prebriefing," in an experiment evaluating attributions of responsibility for rape based on transcripts from an actual rape trial [37]. Participants (68 undergraduate psychology students) were either correctly informed or misinformed about the jury verdict regarding the defendant's guilt. Half of participants received an informed-consent document stating that "you may be purposefully misinformed." The other half was not alerted to the possibility of deception. No differences on attribution of responsibility were observed depending on whether or not the participants were prebriefed about the use of deception.

A second methodological objection to authorized deception is that it has the potential to reduce the comparability to previous research on placebo mechanisms that did not employ this technique. There is no way to avoid this problem. But to argue that consequently the authorized deception approach should not be adopted would suggest that past ethical lapses justify current ethically deficient practice. Finally, disclosure of the use of deception may lead to reduced participant enrollment, making it more difficult to complete valuable studies and possibly reducing their generalizability. At the extreme, it is possible that too few prospective participants will be willing to volunteer, especially for experiments recruiting patients. One clinical research study using the authorized deception approach (in this case, informing participants that details about the purpose of the research were withheld) found no substantial impact on enrollment [39]. This remains to be studied further. But if this approach reduces participant enrollment, it would indicate that eligible prospective participants do not wish to be deceived, casting doubts on the legitimacy of using deception without disclosing its use.

The results of psychology experiments that alerted participants to the possibility of deception and used prebriefing are encouraging, but may not be generalizable to the situation of patients in clinical research. The null findings obtained by Weiner and Erker and Holmes and Bennett need to be interpreted with caution [35,37]. Given that their study participants were psychology undergraduates, even those who were not prebriefed about the use of deception could have anticipated that they might be deceived [32].

Accordingly, the effects of the authorized deception approach on study outcomes merit investigation with respect to research on the placebo effect in a clinical setting. For example, a methodological experiment comparing the authorized deception approach to the traditional approach that does not reveal the use of deception might be attached to a study using the balanced placebo design to evaluate expectation effects relating to placebo analgesia among patients recovering from surgery. Patients would be randomized to the two methods of disclosure, which would be assessed in terms of their impact on reported pain relief among patients in the various arms of the underlying study. This would allow investigators to examine the extent to which the authorized deception approach biases the study outcomes. It might be desirable to conduct such a methodological experiment in connection with a diversity of underlying studies of the placebo effect and in various patient populations.

We suspect that the use of authorized deception will not bias studies of the placebo effect. Hence, the results of such experiments have the potential to pave the way for important research to proceed that uses the balanced placebo design in the clinical setting along with the authorized deception approach—research that otherwise might be rejected by ethics review committees, owing to concerns about using deception in clinical research. If authorized deception does produce some bias, decisions will have to be made by investigators and ethics review committees about the importance of this bias in compromising the validity of the research compared to the importance of respecting the autonomy of research participants. Conducting studies to estimate the extent of the bias will facilitate and inform these decisions.

If the use of authorized deception proved to produce seriously biased results, then it might be argued that it would be unethical to use the balanced placebo design in clinical research, owing to the extensive deception involved. Nevertheless, some aspects of the role of expectancy in therapeutic responses could still be evaluated in an ethical manner by using nondeceptive research paradigms in clinical settings [20,40,41], such as comparing an open versus closed [10,42] or an open versus double-blind administration of a therapeutic agent [11]. The problem with these experimental paradigms, however, is that because they do not fully manipulate expectancy and pharmacology in a factorial design (as does the balanced placebo design), they do not permit a rigorous evaluation of drug versus expectancy effects and their interaction.

Remaining Qualms about Deceptive Research

Deceptive research involving patients in the clinical setting might be considered unethical even when all pertinent safeguards are in place, including the use of authorized deception. This is because deception, even if authorized in advance, violates the ethical framework of the clinician-patient relationship, which is based on trust. It may be argued that clinician investigators who deceive patients in the course of research are acting fraudulently. Accordingly, professional ethics precludes participation in deceptive research.

This objection, however, confuses the ethics of clinical research with the ethics of medical care [43,44]. Clinical research aims at developing generalizable knowledge in order to improve medical care in the future. Promoting the medical best interests of particular patients is not part of the primary purpose of clinical research. Clinical research also departs from the ethics of medical care in the methods it uses, such as randomization, double-blind procedures, placebo controls, and the justification of risks. Nearly all clinical research, especially research that is not aimed at evaluating the efficacy or safety of treatment interventions, poses risks to participants that are not offset by potential medical benefits. Accordingly, the researcher is not functioning as a therapist in the context of clinical research. It follows that deceptive behavior that would be fraudulent in clinical practice is not necessarily unethical in clinical research. The informed-consent process should clarify that the research in question is different from and outside the purview of medical care. The use of authorized deception in this context makes research involving deception consistent with ethical guidelines appropriate to clinical research.

This objection cannot be so readily dismissed, however, if the investigator or members of the team of investigators include clinicians who have a prior therapeutic relationship with research participants, as in the experiment described earlier involving patients with irritable bowel syndrome [13]. When investigators simultaneously have both therapeutic and research roles, it is difficult, if not impossible, to avoid the violation of medical ethics constituted by deception, even if adequate safeguards are in place to make the deception justifiable in the context of research. In addition, the potential for negative consequences to patients from deception is likely to be greater in this situation. It is not clear why it would be necessary for a clinician having a prior therapeutic relationship with participants to conduct valuable research on the placebo effect. For example, in the case of Vase et al.'s irritable bowel syndrome experiment, an experienced clinician would be needed to safely administer the rectal distention procedure; however, someone other than the treating physician could be recruited to perform this function.

Conclusion

Research aimed at elucidating the placebo effect promises to produce valuable knowledge concerning the psychological and neurobiological dimensions of healing. Insights gleaned from this research may contribute to the development of clinical interventions that can enhance the therapeutic efficacy of existing treatments. Experiments investigating the placebo effect, however, evoke legitimate ethical concerns, owing to the use of deception.

Key safeguards to assure the ethical design and conduct of deceptive placebo research include (1) prior review and approval by an independent research ethics committee to determine that the use of deception is methodologically necessary and that the study protocol offers sufficient value to justify the risks it poses to participants, including the use of deception; (2) disclosure in the informed-consent document that the study involves the use of deception; and (3) debriefing of participants at the conclusion of research participation. To contribute to public accountability, articles reporting the results of research using deception should describe briefly adherence with these participant-protection guidelines [45,46]. As in all clinical research, an acceptable balance must be struck between promoting valuable knowledge and protecting the rights and well-being of participants.

SUPPORTING INFORMATION
Table S1. Clinical Studies on the Placebo Effect Involving Deception.
Found at: www.plosmedicine.org/article/fetchSingleRepresentation.action?uri=info:doi/10.1371/journal.pmed.0020262.st001.

REFERENCES
1. Kleinman A, Guess HA, Wilentz JS (2002) An overview. In: Guess HA, Kleinman A, Kusek JW, Engel LW, editors. The science of the placebo: Towards an interdisciplinary research agenda. London: BMJ. pp. 1–32.
2. Harrington A, editor (1997) The placebo effect: An interdisciplinary exploration. Cambridge (Mass.): Harvard University Press.
3. Kirsch I (1985) Response expectancy as a determinant of experience and behavior. Am Psychol 40: 1189–1202.
4. Pollo A, Amanzio M, Arslanian A, et al. (2001) Response expectancies in placebo analgesia and their clinical relevance. Pain 93: 77–84.
5. Stewart-Williams S, Podd J (2004) The placebo effect: Dissolving the expectancy versus conditioning debate. Psychol Bull 130: 324–340.
6. Wager TD, Rilling JK, Smith EE, et al. (2004) Placebo-induced changes in fMRI in the anticipation and experience of pain. Science 303: 1162–1167.
7. Mayberg HS, Silva JA, Brannan SK, et al. (2002) The functional neuroanatomy of the placebo effect. Am J Psychiatry 159: 728–737.
8. de la Fuente-Fernández R, Schulzer M, Stoessl AJ (2004) Placebo mechanisms and reward circuitry: Clues from Parkinson's disease. Biol Psychiatry 56: 67–71.
9. National Institutes of Health (2001) Elucidation of the underlying mechanisms of placebo effect. Bethesda: National Institute of Health.

Available at: http://grants1.nih.gov/grants/guide/rfa-files/RFA-AT-02-002.html.

10. Benedetti F, Maggi G, Lopiano L, et al. (2003) Open versus hidden medical treatments: The patient's knowledge about a therapy affects the therapy outcome. Prev Treat 6(1): article 1a. Found at: psycnet.apa.org/journals/pre/6/1/1a/.

11. Benedetti F, Pollo A, Lopiano L, et al. (2003) Conscious expectation and unconscious conditioning in analgesic, motor, and hormonal placebo/nocebo responses. J Neurosci 23: 4315–4323.

12. Leigh R, MacQueen G, Tougas G, Hargreave FE, Bienstock J (2003) Change in forced expiratory volume in 1 second after sham broncho-constrictor in suggestible but not suggestion-resistant asthmatic subjects: A pilot study. Psychosom Med 65: 791–795.

13. Vase L, Robinson ME, Verne GN, Price DD (2003) The contributions of suggestion, desire, and expectation to placebo effects in irritable bowel syndrome patients. An empirical investigation. Pain 105: 17–25.

14. Swartzman LC, Burkell J (1998) Expectations and the placebo effect in clinical drug trials: Why we should not turn a blind eye to unblinding, and other cautionary notes. Clin Pharmacol Ther 64: 1–7.

15. Mitchell SH, Laurent CL, de Wit H (1996) Interaction of expectancy and the phenomenological effects of d-amphetamine: Subjective effects and self-administration. Psychopharmacology (Berl) 125: 371–378.

16. McKay D, Schare ML (1999) The effects of alcohol and alcohol expectancies on subjective reports and physiological reactivity: A meta-analysis. Addict Behav 24: 633–647.

17. Kirsch I, Weixel LJ (1988) Double-blind versus deceptive administration of placebo. Behav Neurosci 102: 319–323.

18. Perkins K, Sayette M, Conklin C, Caggiula A (2003) Placebo effects of tobacco smoking and other nicotine intake. Nicotine Tob Res 5: 695–709.

19. Curran HV, Brignell C, Fletcher S, Middleton P, Henry J (2002) Cognitive and subjective dose-response effects of acute oral Delta 9-tetrahydrocannabinol (THC) in infrequent cannabis users. Psychopharmacology (Berl) 164: 61–70.

20. Kirsch I (2003) Hidden administration as ethical alternatives to the balanced placebo design. Prev Treat 6(1): article 5c. Found at: psycnet.apa.org/journals/pre/6/1/5c/.

21. Caspi O (2002) When are placebo medication side effects due to the placebo phenomenon? JAMA 287: 2502.

22. Rohsenow DJ, Marlatt GA (1981) The balanced placebo design: Methodological considerations. Addict Behav 6: 107–122.

23. Milgram S (1977) Subject reaction: The neglected factor in the ethics of experimentation. Hastings Cent Rep 7(5): 19–23.

24. Vedantum S (2004 June 7) Human responses to technology scrutinized: Emotional interactions draw interest of psychologists and marketers. Washington Post; Sect A: 14.

25. Wendler D (1996) Deception in medical and behavioral research: Is it ever acceptable? Milbank Q 74: 87–114.

26. Wendler D, Miller FG (2004) Deception in the pursuit of science. Arch Intern Med 164: 597–600.

27. Fleming M, Bruno M, Barry K, Fost N (1989) Informed consent, deception, and the use of disguised alcohol questionnaires. Am J Drug Alcohol Abuse 15: 309–319.

28. Broder A (1998) Deception can be acceptable. Am Psychol 53: 805–806.

29. Kimmel AJ (1988) In defense of deception. Am Psychol 53: 803–805.

30. Ortman A, Hertwig R (1997) Is deception acceptable? Am Psychol 52: 746–747.

31. Ortman A, Hertwig R (1998) The question remains: Is deception acceptable? Am Psychol 53: 806–807.

32. Gallo PS, Smith S, Mumford S (1973) Effects of deceiving subjects on experimental results. J Soc Psychol 89: 99–107.

33. Aristotle (2004) Nichomachean ethics. Thomson JAK, translator; Tredennick H, Barnes J, editors. London: Penguin Books.

34. American Psychological Association (2002) Ethical principles of psychologists and code of conduct. Am Psychol 57: 1060–1073.

35. Holmes DS, Bennett DH (1974) Experiments to answer questions raised by the use of deception in psychological research. I. Role playing as an alternative to deception. II. Effectiveness of debriefing after a deception. III. Effect of informed consent on deception. J Pers Soc Psychol 29: 358–367.

36. Bok S (1978) Lying: Moral choice in public and private life. New York: Random House.

37. Wiener RL, Erker PV (1986) The effects of prebriefing misinformed research participants on their attributions of responsibility. J Psychol 120: 397–410.

38. Sieber JE, Iannuzzo R, Rodriguez B (1995) Deception methods in psychology: Have they changed in 23 years? Ethics Behav 5: 67–85.

39. Boter H, van Delden JJM, de Haan RJ, Rinkel GJE (2004) Patients' evaluation of informed consent to postponed information: Cohort study. BMJ 329: 86–87.

40. Colloca L, Benedetti F (2004) The placebo in clinical studies and in medical practice. In: Price DD, Bushnell MC, editors. Psychological methods of pain control: Basic science and clinical perspectives. Seattle: IASP Press. pp. 187–205.

41. Price DD (2001) Assessing placebo effects without placebo groups: An untapped possibility? Pain 90: 201–203.

42. Amanzio M, Pollo A, Maggi G, Benedetti F (2001) Response variability to analgesics: A role for non-specific activation of endogenous opioids. Pain 90: 205–215.

43. Miller FG, Rosenstein DL (2003) The therapeutic orientation to clinical trials. N Engl J Med 348: 1383–1386.

44. Miller FG (2004) Research ethics and misguided moral intuition. J Law Med Ethics 32: 111–116.

45. Pittinger DJ (2002) Deception in research: Distinctions and solutions from the perspective of utilitarianism. Ethics Behav 12: 117–142.

46. Miller FG, Rosenstein DL (2002) Reporting of ethical issues in publications of medical research. Lancet 360: 1326–1328.

45

Inclusion of Authorized Deception in the Informed Consent Process Does Not Affect the Magnitude of the Placebo Effect for Experimentally Induced Pain

ANDREA L. MARTIN AND JOEL D. KATZ

Andrea L. Martin and Joel D. Katz, "Inclusion of Authorized Deception in the Informed Consent Process Does Not Affect the Magnitude of the Placebo Effect for Experimentally Induced Pain," Pain 2010;149:208–215.

1. Introduction

Placebos have the potential to enhance the therapeutic outcome of medical interventions and are a source of important variability to be considered in clinical trials designed to evaluate treatment efficacy [14]. However, the methodology by which placebo effects are investigated has raised some ethical concerns [5,10,14,15]. Because placebo analgesia is strongly influenced by the recipient's expectations [16–18], clinical and experimental studies typically rely on the use of deception regarding the purpose of the research and/or the nature of the treatment being administered, thereby leading the participants to believe that they are receiving a physically active treatment when in fact they are receiving a placebo

[14]. This use of deception is often justified on the grounds that full disclosure about the purpose of the research or the experimental procedures may influence the participants' responses and thus jeopardize scientific knowledge [14]. As such, deception is often seen as a necessary means of promoting the internal and external validities of placebo research [13].

However, as Miller and colleagues [13,15] highlight, use of deception conflicts with ethical principles of human experimentation as it: (1) violates the principle of respect for persons by failing to disclose relevant information that might affect an individual's decision to volunteer for a research study; (2) may manipulate individuals to participate in research that they would not have; and (3) may cause distress and lack of trust in research when the deception is revealed. Furthermore, the American Pain Society position statement on the use of placebos in clinical pain management highlights, "deception of patients about clinical treatments violates the right of patients to consent to or refuse treatment" ([22] p. 216).

Miller and colleagues [14,15,26] advocate an alternate approach to the consent process in deceptive research. The participants are informed, prior to deciding whether to participate in a study that some features of the study will or may be misleading or deceptive. They call this form of consent "authorized deception," since the participants are alerted to the presence of deception in the research and thus knowingly permit its use if they decide to participate [15]. Additionally, the participants may be offered the opportunity to withdraw their data after they have been informed about the true nature of the study as a means of restoring participant autonomy [14].

Criticisms of the authorized deception approach are that it may create suspicion, thus resulting in biased data [15], reduce participant enrollment [2,15] and/or cause anxiety [4]. Providing participants the opportunity to withdraw their data also may limit the generalizability of research findings [26] and introduce a participation bias.

The present study was designed to provide an evidence-based evaluation of the authorized deception methodology in experimentally induced placebo analgesia. The participants were randomly assigned to an authorized deception group or a non-authorized deception group. Key outcome variables included assessment of differences in participant enrollment, magnitude of the placebo effect, mood, satisfaction with the research experience, attitudes toward researchers, beliefs regarding respect/infringement of individual rights, and willingness to participate in future research of this kind.

2. Methods
2.1. Participants

Participants comprised 40 adults (28 females and 12 males; mean age = 21.18, SD = 3.34 yrs) recruited from flyers posted around the University campus. Prospective participants un-

derwent an initial telephone screen to rule out any medical conditions or medication use that might interfere with pain sensitivity or increase risk of unnecessary discomfort during thermal sensory testing. Individuals were excluded if they reported an ongoing pain problem, high blood pressure, circulatory problems, diabetes, heart disease, asthma, seizures, frostbite, past trauma to the hands or arms, lupus, other large or small joint disease or injury, or use of analgesics, anti-inflammatory medications, psychoactive drugs and/or antihistamines. The York University Research Ethics Board reviewed and approved the study protocol. The participants received $20 for their involvement in the study.

2.2. Apparatus
2.2.1. EXPERIMENTAL SETTING

The experiment took place on campus in a room set up with medical equipment to resemble a physician's office including an examination table, privacy curtain, medical scale for measuring height and weight, blood pressure cuff, metal equipment tray, containers of cotton balls, tongue depressors, plastic syringes, rubbing alcohol, and wall posters depicting the musculoskeletal system, symptoms of neuropathic pain and the pathophysiology and anatomy of arthritis and knee injury.

2.2.2. MEDOC THERMAL SENSORY ANALYZER

Heat pain was induced by means of a Medoc TSA-II thermal stimulator (Ramat Yishai, Israel). The TSA-II is a computerized device designed to measure sensory thresholds to vibration and temperature (e.g., warm, cold, heat-induced pain and cold-induced pain). The TSA-II is used in a variety of clinical disorders (e.g., diabetes, peripheral neuropathy) to obtain a quantitative evaluation of the integrity of both small (A-delta and C) and large diameter (A-beta) sensory nerve fibers. The TSA-II is capable of delivering thermal stimuli that range from approximately 0 to 50 °C. A thermode is attached to the participant's skin with a Velcro strap and heat stimuli of various temperatures are administered. A participant-initiated button press stops the rise in temperature and the thermode rapidly returns to room temperature at a rate of ~4 °C/s. In the present study, thermal stimuli of 5 s duration were applied to the skin through a thermode with a contact area 3 cm². The temperature of the thermode rose rapidly (4 °C/s) from a baseline temperature of 35 °C to a pre-programmed peak temperature where it remained for 5 s before returning to baseline.

2.2.3. PLACEBO CREAM

The same over-the-counter hypoallergenic moisturizer cream (Glaxal Base), which does not contain an active analgesic agent, was used for both the placebo cream and the control cream. The creams were visible in two plastic syringes on a metal medical tray with the labels 'Alevocaine™' and 'Control Cream.' The experimenter wore latex gloves while handling, applying, and removing the creams. The creams were removed with an alcohol swab.

2.3. Response Measures

2.3.1. NUMERIC RATING SCALE (NRS)—PAIN

The participants were asked to rate the intensity of pain stimuli using an 11-point, self-report, numeric rating scale (NRS) [7] ranging from 0 to 10, with endpoints representing *no pain* (0) and *the most intense pain imaginable* (10). The participants were asked to choose the number that best corresponded to the intensity of each heat pain stimulus they received. The NRS provides a simple, efficient and minimally intrusive measure of pain intensity. This scale is commonly used in clinical settings [1] and is the preferred pain rating scale among patients [27]. The NRS is highly correlated ($r = 0.94$) with the visual analog scale [1] and is sensitive to change following pharmacological interventions [7].

2.3.2. PROFILE OF MOOD STATES (POMS)

The profile of mood states (POMS) [12] is a widely used, 65-item self-report scale designed to measure affective mood states and their fluctuations in medical patients, psychiatric outpatients, normal adults, and college students. Each item is rated on a 5-point scale ranging from *not at all* (0) to *extremely* (4). The *right now* rating period was used for the present study. The POMS yields a total mood disturbance (TMD) score and 6-factor analytic-derived scales, including (1) tension–anxiety, (2) depression–dejection, (3) anger–hostility, (4) vigor–activity, (5) fatigue–inertia, and (6) confusion–bewilderment. The POMS has excellent internal consistency ($\alpha = 0.84$–0.95) and fair test-retest reliability ($r = 0.43$–0.53) over a 6-week period in patients receiving psychiatric treatment [11]. Evidence of the predictive and construct validity of the POMS has been demonstrated in brief psychotherapy research, cancer research, controlled outpatient drug trails, studies on sports and athletes, and studies of response to emotion-inducing conditions in healthy populations [11].

2.3.3. NUMERIC RATING SCALE (NRS)—ATTITUDES

A numeric rating scale (ranging from 0 to 10) was used to assess participants' attitudes across four domains: (1) satisfaction with the research experience, (2) feelings toward researchers who plan and run studies such as the present one, (3) the extent to which they felt that their individual rights were respected while taking part in the study, and (4) their willingness to participate in similar research in the future.

2.4. Procedure

The participants were randomly assigned to one of two groups using the randomization program available at www.randomization.com: authorized deception group or non-authorized deception group. An experimenter wearing a white lab coat greeted the participants upon arrival for the study. The participants were provided with a consent form, and the experimenter verbally described the study following a standard script. The participants in both groups were told that the investigators were examining the effectiveness of a new topical anesthetic cream called Alevocaine™ which had been shown to reduce pain in some individuals; and that the Alevocaine™ cream would be compared against a regular moisturizer cream. The details of the thermal stimulator and the method of assessing the effectiveness of the cream by means of painful heat stimuli were described and the participants were told that they could discontinue participation in the study at any time without negative consequences.

The authorized deception group and the non-authorized deception group received identical information in the consent form with the exception of one paragraph added to the end of the consent form for the authorized deception group. In this paragraph, prospective participants were informed, prior to deciding whether to volunteer for the study, that some aspects of the study were being intentionally misdescribed. Specifically, the following statement, recommended by Miller et al. [15], was included at the end of the consent form for the authorized deception group:

> You should be aware that the investigators have intentionally misdescribed certain aspects of the study. This use of deception is necessary to obtain valid results. However, an independent ethics committee has determined that this consent form accurately describes the major risks and benefits of the study. The investigators will explain the misdescribed aspects of the study to you at the end of your participation (p. 856).

The experimenter also repeated this statement verbally when reviewing the study procedures with the participant to ensure that all participants in the authorized deception group were aware of this information.

Following the consent procedures, the participants in both the authorized deception and non-authorized deception groups completed the POMS and a demographic and pain history questionnaire. The participants were then brought into a laboratory room set-up to resemble a physician's office and underwent four consecutive stages of thermal sensory testing involving a set of familiarization trials, calibration trials, conditioning trials, and test trials [19].

2.4.1. FAMILIARIZATION TRIALS

In order to familiarize participants with the range of temperatures, one trial each of 44, 45, 47, and 49 °C stimuli was delivered in ascending order on the ventral side of the participant's right forearm.

2.4.2. CALIBRATION TRIALS

The participants then underwent a series of calibration trials similar to that of Price and colleagues [19] to control for individual differences in pain perception. A series of 16 thermal stimuli ranging between 44 and 49 °C was administered in a random order and the participants were asked to rate the pain intensity of each stimulus on a 0–10 NRS. At the end of the calibration trials, a regression equation was calculated for each participant in order to predict thermal intensity (temperature in °C) from verbal pain intensity report (NRS pain ratings). This calculation was used to determine the temperature corresponding to each individual's NRS pain rating of 6 and 3, which varied among participants depending on their own personal perception of pain. These two stimulus levels (i.e., temperatures) were used in all subsequent trials and were specific to each individual.

2.4.3. CONDITIONING TRIALS

A plastic template was used to mark two squares on the ventral side of the participant's right forearm. Two square adhesive patches with the center cut out were applied to these two areas to demarcate the two locations on the arm where the creams were applied (Fig. 45.1). In line with previous research [17,23–25], a conditioning procedure was used in which the intensity of heat pain stimuli was surreptitiously lowered during conditioning trials for the placebo cream (i.e., Alevocaine™ cream). That is, in order to create the impression of analgesic efficacy (i.e., pain relief) when testing in the area of skin where the placebo cream was applied, the temperature was surreptitiously lowered to a level corresponding to the participant's NRS pain rating of 3. When testing in the area of skin where the control cream was applied, the temperature was administered at a level corresponding to the participant's NRS pain rating of 6. The participants were asked to verbally rate the intensity of each stimulus using the 0–10 NRS. One block of four thermal stimuli was administered for each cream at each of the two locations according to a randomized counterbalanced design, such that each participant received eight conditioning trials for each cream.

2.4.4. TEST TRIALS

Immediately following the conditioning trials, the participants received one final test trial with each cream. The stimulus intensity for the test trials was the same for both the placebo (Alevocaine™) and the control creams. That is, for the test trial, the stimulus intensity was raised to a temperature corresponding to a pain rating of 6 for the "Alevocaine™" condition. The magnitude of the placebo analgesic effect was determined by comparing the test trial pain ratings for the placebo versus the control cream.

2.5. Post-Test Interview and Debriefing

Following the test trials and before the debriefing process, the participants were asked a series of questions about their feelings concerning the research procedures they had just undergone and their thoughts about the Alevocaine™ cream. The participants in the authorized deception group were asked to describe how they had felt when they read in the

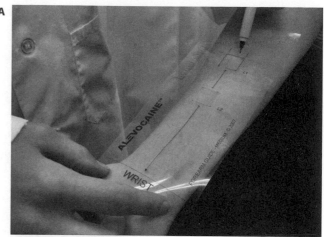

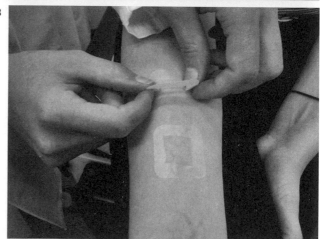

Fig. 45.1. (A) Plastic template used to mark two squares on the ventral side of the participant's right forearm. (B) Adhesive patches used to demarcate the two locations on the arm where the creams were applied.

consent form that certain aspects of the study were being intentionally misdescribed and that the use of deception was necessary to obtain valid results. They were also asked if they wondered what aspect(s) of the study had been misdescribed and if so, what these aspects might have been.

The participants in both the authorized deception and non-authorized deception groups were asked "At any point during the study: did you wonder if Alevocaine™ had side effects that we weren't telling you about; did you wonder if Alevocaine™ was another drug that we didn't tell you about; and, did you wonder if Alevocaine™ might not be a real drug?" If the participants answered yes to any of these questions they were asked "When did you start to wonder this?" "Did this thought make you feel more anxious?" and "Did this thought influence your pain ratings during the study? (And if so, how?)"

Following this set of questions, the participants were given a debriefing form describing the true purpose of the study and the nature of the placebo cream. In the debriefing form the participants were also offered the opportunity to withdraw their data from the study if they felt concerned or uncomfortable about the fact that they had been intentionally deceived. When given the debriefing form, the participants in the authorized deception group were told, "As you are aware, there were certain aspects of this study that I was not able to explain fully to you at the beginning of your participation. I would like to give you a debriefing form now that will explain the purpose of the study and outline the aspects that I was not able to tell you about at the beginning." The participants in the non-authorized deception group were told, "There were aspects of this study that I was not able to explain fully to you at the beginning of your participation. I would like to give you a debriefing form now that will explain the purpose of the study and outline the aspects that I was not able to tell you about at the beginning."

Immediately after the participants finished reading the debriefing forms they were asked to complete the POMS a second time to assess any changes in mood following their participation in the study and the debriefing procedures. A brief set of questions was then administered to both groups to assess their attitudes about the research experience (see Section 2.3.3). Additionally, the participants in the authorized deception group were re-read the same paragraph from the consent form alerting them to the presence of deception in the study and were asked, "Having participated now, would you rather not have been informed of this at the beginning of the study?" The participants in the non-authorized deception group were read this same paragraph and were asked, "Having participated now, would you rather have been informed of this [i.e., alerted to the presence of deception] at the beginning of the study?"

3. Results

3.1. Magnitude of the Placebo Effect

The magnitude of the placebo effect for each group was calculated by subtracting the pain intensity rating for the placebo cream from the pain intensity rating for the control cream during the final trial (i.e., when the temperature was the same for both creams). The resulting placebo response score represents the change in pain intensity rating due to the administration of the placebo [17]. Both the authorized deception and the non-authorized deception groups obtained positive scores averaging 1.05 (SD = 1.43) and 1.40 (SD = 2.35), respectively, indicating a less painful response to the placebo cream than to the control cream (i.e., a placebo effect).

In order to determine whether there was a difference in the magnitude of the placebo effect between the authorized deception group and the non-authorized deception group, a 2 × 2 between-within analysis of variance (ANOVA) was conducted, using group (authorized deception and non-authorized deception) as the between-subjects factor and cream (placebo and control) as the within-subjects repeated measures factor. ANOVA results revealed a non-significant group × cream interaction, $F(1,38) = 0.32$, $p = 0.57$. The main effect of cream (Placebo/Control), $F(1,38) = 15.87$, $p < 0.001$,

indicated significantly lower pain ratings for placebo ($M \pm SD = 5.10 \pm 2.50$) as compared to control cream ($M \pm SD = 6.33 \pm 2.09$) across both groups. The group effect was not significant, $F(1,38) = 0.41$, $p < 0.53$. Taken together, these results indicate that both groups showed a significant placebo effect, the magnitude of which did not differ significantly between the authorized deception and non-authorized deception groups (Fig. 45.2).

3.2. Mood

Means and standard deviations for each of the POMS scales are presented in Table 45.1. A series of between-within ANOVAs were conducted on each of the following POMS scales using time (post-consent vs. post-debrief) as the within-subjects factor and group (authorized deception and non-authorized deception) as the between-subjects factor: (1) tension–anxiety, (2) depression–dejection (3) anger–

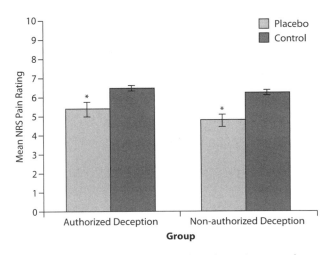

Fig. 45.2. Mean pain ratings for the placebo (Alevocaine™) and control creams in the authorized deception and non-authorized deception groups. Error bars represent standard errors. Data indicate a significant placebo effect for each group. * $p < 0.001$ comparing placebo (Alevocaine™) with control.

Table 45.1.

Means and standard deviations of POMS scores for authorized deception and non-authorized deception groups at time 1 (post-consent) and time 2 (post-debriefing)

POMS scale	Authorized deception group		Non-authorized deception group	
	Time 1 M (SD)	Time 2 M (SD)	Time 1 M (SD)	Time 2 M (SD)
T–A	5.45 (3.68)	4.05 (2.48)	6.60 (3.76)	4.15 (2.08)
D–D	4.80 (7.58)	1.7 (3.88)	5.35 (10.05)	3.20 (6.86)
A–H	2.45 (3.66)	1.35 (2.37)	4.30 (8.29)	2.00 (3.31)
V–A	11.80 (6.99)	12.35 (10.92)	11.70 (5.93)	11.15 (5.63)
F–I	5.15 (4.58)	3.50 (3.49)	6.50 (5.46)	4.45 (4.59)
C–B	5.65 (3.57)	3.75 (2.40)	5.70 (3.63)	3.95 (2.98)
TMD	11.70 (22.18)	2.00 (18.17)	16.75 (30.24)	6.60 (19.66)

Note: T–A = tension–anxiety; D–D = depression–dejection; A–H = anger–hostility; V–A = vigor–activity; F–I = fatigue–inertia; C–B = confusion–bewilderment; TMD = total mood disturbance.

Table 45.2.

POMS between-within ANOVA results with group (authorized deception and non-authorized deception) and time (post-consent and post-debrief)

POMS scale	Time 1 M (SD)	Time 2 M (SD)	Time 1–Time 2 change (within-subjects effect)
Tension–anxiety	6.03 (3.72)	4.10 (2.26)	$F(1,38) = 21.04, p < 0.001$
Depression–dejection	5.08 (8.79)	2.45 (5.56)	$F(1,38) = 15.86, p < 0.001$
Anger–hostility	3.38 (6.40)	1.68 (2.86)	$F(1,38) = 5.71, p = 0.02$
Vigor–activity	11.75 (6.40)	11.75 (8.60)	$F(1,38) = 0.00, p = 1.00$
Fatigue–inertia	5.83 (5.02)	3.98 (4.05)	$F(1,38) = 18.88, p < 0.001$
Confusion–bewilderment	5.68 (3.55)	3.85 (2.68)	$F(1,38) = 31.34, p < 0.001$
Total mood disturbance	14.23 (26.30)	4.30 (0.39)	$F(1,38) = 23.90, p < 0.001$

Note: "Time 1," post-consent; "Time 2," post-debrief; "Time 1" and "Time 2" represent average scores on each scale after collapsing across groups.

Table 45.3.

Means, standard deviations and MANOVA results for attitude variables across the study groups

Variable	Authorized deception M (SD)	Non-authorized deception M (SD)	Between-group differences
Satisfaction with their research experience	8.45 (1.00)	7.85 (1.84)	$F(1,38) = 1.64, p = 0.21$
Feelings toward researchers who plan and run studies like this, involving deception	8.60 (1.43)	8.45 (1.54)	$F(1,38) = 0.10, p = 0.75$
Extent to which they felt that their individual rights were respected throughout their participation in the study	9.65 (0.81)	9.70 (0.57)	$F(1,38) = 0.05, p = 0.82$
Willingness to participate in research of this kind in the future	9.40 (1.31)	8.65 (1.53)	$F(1,38) = 2.76, p = 0.11$

hostility, (4) vigor–activity, (5) fatigue–inertia, (6) confusion–bewilderment, and (7) total mood disturbance. Neither the group main effect nor the group × time interaction effect was significant for any of the mood scales. The time effect revealed significant improvements from post-consent to post-debrief for all the mood scales, with the exception of the vigor–activity scale, which remained unchanged (Table 45.2). These results indicate significant improvements, independent of group, over time for tension–anxiety, depression–dejection, anger–hostility, fatigue–inertia, confusion–bewilderment, and total mood disturbance.

3.3. Attitudes

A multivariate analysis of variance was conducted to examine group differences across the four attitude variables: (1) satisfaction with the research experience, (2) feelings toward researchers who plan and run studies like this, (3) the extent to which the participants felt that their individual rights were respected while taking part in the study, and (4) willingness to participate in research of this kind in the future. Overall, the participant ratings averaged eight (out of 10) or greater for each of the four attitude variables indicating a high degree of satisfaction with their experience in the study, positive feelings toward researchers, feeling that their individual rights had been respected and a high degree of willingness to participate in future research of this kind. Significant group differences were not observed for any of the four attitudes' variables (Table 45.3).

3.4. Enrollment, Withdrawal from the Study, and Feelings about Deception

Study enrollment, retention of the participants, and withdrawal of the data were not affected by the authorized deception procedure (Fig. 45.3). Specifically, none of the prospective participants in the authorized deception group decided against participating in the study after learning in the consent form that they would be deceived if they were to participate in the study. Similarly, all prospective participants in the non-authorized deception groups agreed to participate in the study after reading the informed consent form. No participants from either group withdrew from the study and none of the participants in either group took up our offer to remove their data from the study after the debriefing process.

At the end of the study, just prior to the debriefing process, the participants in the authorized deception group were asked how they felt when they read in the consent form that certain aspects of the study had been intentionally misdescribed and that this use of deception was necessary to obtain valid results. Almost all the participants (90%) reported feeling curious and intrigued upon hearing that certain aspects of the study had been intentionally misdescribed. Few subjects reported experiencing negative reactions such as feelings of anxiety (30%), uncertainty (10%) and anger (5%). Most participants (85%) reported wondering what parts of the study had been misdescribed to them.

Chi-squared analysis did not reveal a significant difference in the proportion of the participants in the authorized decep-

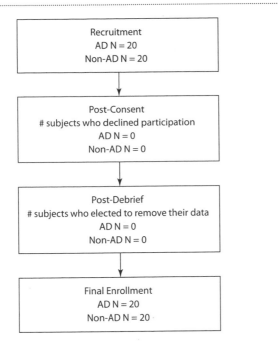

Fig. 45.3. Flowchart depicting participant recruitment and final enrollment for the two groups. AD = authorized deception group; non-AD = non-authorized deception group.

Table 45.4.

Phase of experiment at which participants in each group retrospectively reported wondering if Alevocaine™ was not a real drug

Phase of experiment	AD	Non-AD
Before coming into the study	2	1
While reading the consent form	1	0
While completing the questionnaires at the beginning	1	0
While the creams were being tested	4	5
Now (i.e., when asked)	1	1
Total no. of subjects	9	7

Note: AD = authorized deception group; non-AD = non-authorized deception group.

Table 45.5.

Comments from participants in the authorized deception and non-authorized deception groups expressing a negative reaction to the use of deception

Group	Comments
AD	"I would have been angry if there was deception and you didn't tell me."
AD	"It's good to know [about the deception]. If not I would have been angry. I was in another study with deception and they didn't tell me and I felt angry."
AD	"[I] would be angry."
AD	"I'm very glad you had that clause in there at the beginning so I could ask my questions and feel okay about participating. I would have wondered why you didn't warn me otherwise."
AD	"I would feel cheated if you hadn't told me."
AD	"[I] would prefer to know about the deception. It made me feel more comfortable. If you didn't tell me I would have felt disappointed and more anxious at the end, wondering, what else didn't they tell me?"
AD	"I would have been disappointed if you hadn't told me."
Non-AD	"It's better to know as much as you can. I would be more cautious about future research. I would do it but I'd be looking for deception."

tion (9/20) and non-authorized deception (7/20) groups who wondered if Alevocaine™ might not be a real drug, χ^2 (1) = 0.42, p = 0.52. The stage of the experiment at which these participants wondered about the veracity of the Alevocaine™ is presented in Table 45.4. Six participants in the authorized deception group reported wondering if Alevocaine™ might not be a real drug during the actual experiment; however, these numbers did not differ from those in the non-authorized deception group where five participants also reported wondering about the veracity of the Alevocaine™ while the creams were being tested. These results suggest that any suspicion about the true nature of the creams was likely not due to the fact that the authorized deception group had been alerted to the presence of deception in the study.

At the end of the study, following the debriefing, the paragraph that was included in the consent form for the authorized deception group, alerting them to the presence of deception in the study, was read to all participants. The participants in the non-authorized deception group were asked, "Having participated now, would you *rather* have been informed of this?" while the participants in the authorized deception group were asked, "Having participated now, would you *rather not* have been informed of this?" In the non-authorized deception group, three participants reported that they would rather have been informed of the deception at the outset of the study and one of these participants stated that she would be more cautious about future research as a result of her experience with the deception in this study (Table 45.5). However, 17 participants in the non-authorized deception group reported that they would not rather have been informed of the deception at the outset of the study. Of these 17, 10 felt that knowing about the deception would have made them suspicious, thus biasing their responses and negatively impacting the outcome of the study, and seven stated that they did not have a strong preference for one set of instructions over the other or felt that it was more interesting to find out at the end.

In contrast, 19 out of 20 participants in the authorized deception group reported that they would have preferred to be alerted, as they had been, to the presence of deception in the study. Upon further questioning, of these 19 participants, 13 expressed a clear preference to have been alerted to the deception and seven of these 13 stated they would have experienced a negative reaction to the study, such as anger, disappointment, and feeling as though they had been cheated had they not been warned about the use of deception (Table 45.5). The other six of these 19 participants stated that they did not have a strong preference for one set of instructions over the other. The one participant who reported a preference not to have known about the deception felt that the research findings would be more accurate if the participants were not warned about the use of deception.

4. Discussion

The present study sought to investigate an alternate approach to participant consent in placebo research involving the use of deception. Authorized deception is designed to alert the participants to the presence of deception in the research, without informing them about the exact nature of the deception [13–15,26]. The results of the present study show that the magnitude of the placebo effect did not differ significantly between the participants who were informed about the presence of deception and those who were not. While it is possible that some degree of temporal summation occurred across study trials such that pain increased with subsequent thermal stimuli [6] this would have occurred in both study groups and thus should not account for any differences, or lack thereof, between the authorized deception and the non-authorized deception groups.

Authorized deception has been proposed as a more ethical approach to placebo research since it allows the participants the opportunity to decide whether or not they are willing to volunteer for a study that involves deception [15]. Although authorized deception does not replace full informed consent, it is designed to promote the autonomy of research participants by giving them a fair opportunity to withdraw from a study knowing that deception will be involved [14]. Another measure to promote autonomy in deceptive research is to provide the participants the opportunity to withdraw their data after having learned the true nature of the study during the debriefing process [14].

The results of the present study do not support the concerns that authorized deception has adverse effects on key outcome variables, thus compromising the scientific validity of the data and introducing bias. Important indicators of whether the use of authorized deception is a viable alternative to the traditional approach of informed consent (i.e., non-authorized deception) in placebo research of this nature include potential detrimental effects on recruitment and retention of participants as well as participants' decisions to withdraw their data following debriefing. The present results indicate that use of authorized deception did not have a negative impact on any of these measures; enrollment and retention of the participants were identical between the two groups and none of the participants in the present study chose to withdraw their data when given the option to do so after the debriefing process (Fig. 45.2).

There is little literature regarding participant decisions to withdraw data when offered the opportunity [13]. However, the present results are in line with at least one other study which examined the placebo response in relation to asthma in a clinical population and found none of the 55 patients accepted the offer to withdraw their data [8]. The present findings support the use of authorized deception and granting participants the option to withdraw their data as two methods of enhancing the ethical principles of placebo research without compromising the scientific validity and generalizability of the research findings.

The results of the present study also do not support the suggestion that alerting subjects to the use of deception results in increased anxiety [4]. While a few participants reported experiencing some anxiety upon hearing aspects of the study had been intentionally misdescribed, the vast majority (90%) reported feeling curious and intrigued. Furthermore, there were no differences in mood between the two groups (as measured by the POMS and verbal self-report) following the debriefing when the true nature of the creams and the purpose of the study were revealed.

We hypothesized that the non-authorized deception group would demonstrate a worsening of mood relative to the authorized deception group following the debriefing since the former group had not been warned about the use of deception in the study. We therefore expected these participants to report a negative reaction to the realization that what they thought was an active drug was actually a placebo. However, contrary to this expectation, both groups exhibited improvements in mood across the study. These findings are similar to those of Chung and colleagues [3] who found reductions in anxiety, frustration and fear after revealing to the participants the magnitude of their placebo response in relation to experimentally induced pain.

These improvements in mood may represent an artifact of repeat testing or may reflect participants' relief at having completed the study [3]. Positive interactions with the experimenter throughout the study may have also contributed to improvements in mood. One limitation of the present study is the lack of a true baseline measure of mood prior to the authorized deception intervention. This would have allowed for an assessment of mood changes resulting from the authorized deception intervention; however, given that the intervention involved altering the informed consent process and therefore took place before consent had been obtained, from an ethical standpoint, it was not possible to obtain a prior baseline assessment of mood.

Another potential concern with the use of authorized deception is that it may create suspicion in research participants, thus resulting in biased data [15]. Although a small proportion of the participants in the authorized deception group questioned the true nature of the Alevocaine™ cream, this was no greater than that of the non-authorized deception group, suggesting that any suspicion about the authenticity of the cream was not related to the authorized deception manipulation. Suspicion, expressed by some participants, about the authenticity of the cream could have been related to various factors; including, not experiencing a noticeable reduction in pain when the Alevocaine™ cream was applied, or the fact that the study was advertised as a 'Health Psychology' study and as a primarily undergraduate population, research participants may have been familiar with psychological research involving deception [13].

Interestingly, 13 participants in the authorized deception group expressed a clear preference to be alerted to the presence of deception in the study compared to only three participants in the non-authorized deception group. Several explanations may account for these findings. It is possible that the participants did not have strong feelings about the use of deception in the research. To the extent that this is true, it is important to note that this may be specific to the present population, which consisted predominantly of healthy undergraduate students who we would not expect to have a vested interest in the outcome of the study or the efficacy of the 'drug' under investigation.

Other studies have found that the use of deception in psychological research is not distressing to many subjects [20,21]; however, healthy undergraduate students may have different attitudes toward being deceived than patients participating in a clinical trial [9]. The degree to which an individual is troubled by deception may depend on the extent to which the deceived relies on the deceiver [26]. As such, the present findings may not generalize to clinical populations who are likely more vulnerable to deception, often placing considerable faith and trust in clinical investigators.

It is also possible that the participants in the non-authorized deception group downplayed the negative effects they experienced as a result of the deception and thus our findings may not have accurately captured their true feelings. Participants may, as a means of "saving face" [26], minimize the effects of deception or choose not to report them, particularly when they are asked by the very experimenter who has just deceived them. This explanation may also account for the finding that more than a third of participants in the authorized deception group reported that they would have experienced a negative reaction had they not been warned about the use of deception, while none of the participants in the non-authorized deception group reported actually experiencing such a reaction. It is also possible that the prior warning about the use of deception may have engendered a greater sense of partnership with and trust in the experimenters, thus allowing the authorized deception group to more openly share any negative feelings.

Other data from the authorized deception group also support the use of the authorized deception methodology in placebo research. Over half the participants in this group reported that they preferred to be warned about the use of deception at the outset of the study, prior to agreeing to participate. Numerous participants expressed gratitude for the openness with which they were informed of the deception and some participants reported that they would have likely felt some anger or resentment had they not been warned (Table 45.5).

5. Conclusions

Taken together, the results of the present study suggest that alerting participants to the presence of deception in experimental pain studies on placebo analgesia does not affect the magnitude of the placebo effect, recruitment and retention of participants, nor does it result in any significant psychological harm. Indeed, the majority of participants who received this form of consent preferred it to the traditional approach of not alerting participants to the presence of deception. These findings support the use of authorized deception in laboratory-based studies of placebo analgesia and suggest that it is a viable and ethically preferable method of informed consent compared to the traditional approach. Studies are needed to examine the effect of authorized deception in clinical trials and other placebo research within a clinical setting.

REFERENCES

[1] Bijur PE, Latimer CT, Gallagher EJ. Validation of a verbally administered numerical rating scale of acute pain for use in the emergency department. Acad Emerg Med 2003;10:390–392.

[2] Boter H, van Delden JJM, de Haan RJ, Rinkel GJE. Patients' evaluation of informed consent to postponed information: cohort study. Br Med J 2004;329:86.

[3] Chung SK, Price DD, Verne GN, Robinson ME. Revelation of a personal placebo response: its effects on mood, attitudes and future placebo responding. Pain 2007;132:281–288.

[4] Dawson AJ. Methodological reasons for not gaining prior informed consent are sometimes justified. Br Med J 2004;329:87.

[5] Evans M. Justified deception? The single blind placebo in drug research. J Med Ethics 2000;26:188–193.

[6] Granot M, Granovsky Y, Sprecher E, Nir R, Yarnitsky D. Contact heat-evoked temporal summation: tonic versus repetitive-phasic stimulation. Pain 2006;122:295–305.

[7] Katz J, Melzack R. Measurement of pain. Surg Clin North Am 1999;79:231–252.

[8] Kemeny ME, Rosenwasser LJ, Panettieri RA, et al. Placebo response in asthma: a robust and objective phenomenon. J Allergy Clin Immunol 2007;119:1375–1381.

[9] Korn JH. Judgments of acceptability of deception in psychological research. J Gen Psychol 1987;114:215–216.

[10] Kotzalidis GD, Pacchiarotti I, Manfredi G, et al. Ethical questions in human clinical psychopharmacology: should the focus be on placebo administration? J Psychopharmacol 2008;22:590–597.

[11] McNair DM, Heuchert JWP. Profile of mood states: technical update. North Tonawanda, N.Y.: Multi-Health Systems Inc.; 2003.

[12] McNair DM, Lorr M, Droppleman LF. Manual for the profile of mood states. San Diego, Calif.: Educational and Industrial Testing Service; 1971.

[13] Miller FG, Gluck JP, Wendler D. Debriefing and accountability in deceptive research. Kennedy Inst Ethics J 2008;18:235–251.

[14] Miller FG, Kaptchuk TJ. Deception of subjects in neuroscience: an ethical analysis. J Neurosci 2008;29:4841–4843.

[15] Miller FG, Wendler D, Swartzman LC. Deception in research on the placebo effect. PLoS Med 2005;2(9):e262.

[16] Montgomery G, Kirsch I. Mechanisms of placebo pain reduction: an empirical investigation. Psych Sci 1996;7:174–176.

[17] Montgomery GH, Kirsch I. Classical conditioning and the placebo effect. Pain 1997;72:107–113.

[18] Price DD, Finniss DG, Benedetti F. A comprehensive review of the placebo effect: recent advances and current thought. Annu Rev Psychol 2008;59:565–590.

[19] Price DD, Milling LS, Kirsch I, et al. An analysis of the factors that contribute to the magnitude of placebo analgesia in an experimental paradigm. Pain 1999;83:147–156.

[20] Seber JE, Iannuzzo R, Rodriguez B. Deception methods in psychology: have they changed in 23 years? Ethics Behav 1995;5:67–85.

[21] Soliday E, Stanton AL. Deceived versus nondeceived participants' perceptions of scientific and applied psychology. Ethics Behav 1995:87–104.

[22] Sullivan M, Terman GW, Peck B, et al. APS position statement on the use of placebos in pain management. J Pain 2005;6:215–217.

[23] Voudouris N, Peck C, Coleman G. Conditioned placebo responses. J Pers Soc Psychol 1985;48:47–53.

[24] Voudouris N, Peck C, Coleman G. Conditioned response models of placebo phenomena: further support. Pain 1989;38:109–116.

[25] Voudouris N, Peck C, Coleman G. The role of conditioning and verbal expectancy in the placebo response. Pain 1990;43:121–128.

[26] Wendler D, Miller FG. Deception in the pursuit of science. Arch Intern Med 2004;164:597–600.

[27] Williamson A, Hoggart B. Pain: a review of three commonly used pain rating scales. J Clin Nurs 2005;14:798–804.

46

False Hopes and Best Data

Consent to Research and the

Therapeutic Misconception

PAUL S. APPELBAUM, LOREN H. ROTH, CHARLES W. LIDZ, PAUL R. BENSON, AND WILLIAM J. WINSLADE

Paul S. Appelbaum, Loren H. Roth, Charles W. Lidz, Paul R. Benson, and William J. Winslade, "False Hopes and Best Data: Consent to Research and the Therapeutic Misconception," *Hastings Center Report* 1987;27(2):20–24.

Following a suicide attempt, a young man with a long history of tumultuous relationships and difficulty controlling his impulses is admitted to a psychiatric hospital. After a number of days, a psychiatrist approaches the patient, explaining that he is conducting a research project to determine if medications may help in the treatment of the patient's condition. Is the patient interested, the psychiatrist asks? The answer: "Yes, I'm willing to do anything that might help me."

The psychiatrist returns over the next several days to explain the project further. He tells the patient that two medications are being used, along with a placebo; medications and placebo are assigned randomly. The trial is double blinded; that is, neither physician nor patient will know what the patient is receiving until after the trial has been completed. The patient listens to the explanation and reads and signs the consent form. Since the process of providing information and obtaining consent seems, on the surface, exemplary, there appears to be little reason to question the validity of the consent.

Yet when the patient is asked why he agreed to be in the study, he offers some disquieting information. The medication that he will receive, he believes, will be the one most likely to help him. He ruled out the possibility that he might receive a placebo, because that would not be likely to do him much good. In short, this man, now both a patient and a subject, has interpreted, even distorted, the information he received to maintain the view—obviously based on his wishes—that every aspect of the research project to which he had consented was designed to benefit him directly. This belief, which is far from uncommon, we call the "therapeutic misconception." To maintain a therapeutic misconception is to deny the possibility that there may be major disadvantages to participating in clinical research that stem from the nature of the research process itself.

Research Risks and the Scientific Method

The unique aspects of clinical research include the goal of creating generalizable knowledge; the techniques of randomization; and the use of a study protocol, control groups, and double-blind procedures. Do these elements create a body of risks or disadvantages for research subjects? The answer lies in understanding how the scientific method is often incompatible with one of the first principles of clinical treatment-the value that the legal philosopher Charles Fried calls "personal care."[1]

According to the principle of personal care, a physician's first obligation is solely to the patient's well-being. A corollary is that the physician will take whatever measures are available to maximize the chances of a successful outcome. A failure to adhere to this principle creates at least a potential disadvantage for the clinical research subject: there is always a chance that the subject's interests may become secondary to other demands on the physician-researcher's loyalties.[2] And the methods of science inhibit the application of personal care.

Randomization, an important element of many clinical trials, demonstrates the problem. The argument is often made that comparisons of multiple treatment methods are legitimately undertaken only when the superiority of one over the other is unknown; thus the physician treating a patient in one of these trials does not abandon the patient's personal care, but merely allows chance to determine the assignment of treatments, each of which is likely to meet the patient's needs.[3]

But as Fried and others have noted, it is very unlikely that two treatments in a clinical trial will be identically desirable *for a particular patient*. The physician may have reason to suspect, for example, that a given treatment is more likely to be efficacious for a particular patient, even if overall evidence of greater efficacy is lacking. This suspicion may be based on the physician's previous experience with a subgroup of patients, the patient's own past treatment experience, the family history of responsiveness to treatment, or idiosyncratic elements in the patient's case. Subjects may have had previous unsatisfactory responses to one of the medications in a clinical trial, or may display clinical characteristics that suggest that one class of medications is more likely to benefit them than another.

Ordinarily, these factors would guide the therapeutic approach. But in a randomized study physicians cannot allow these factors to influence the treatment decision, and efforts to control for such factors in the selection of subjects, while theoretically possible, are cumbersome, expensive, and may bias the sample. Thus reliance on randomization represents an inevitable compromise of personal care in the service of attaining valid research results. There are at least two reports in the literature of physicians' reluctance to refer patients to randomized trials because of the possible decrement in the level of personal care.[4]

The use of a study protocol to regulate the course of treatment—essential to careful clinical research—also impedes the delivery of personal care. Protocols often indicate the pattern and dosages of medication to be administered or the blood levels to be attained. Even if they allow some individualization of medication, changes in time or magnitude may be limited. Thus patients who do not respond initially to a low dose of medication may not receive a higher dose, as they would if they were being treated without a protocol; on the other hand, patients experiencing side effects, which could be controlled by lowering their dosage, yet which are not so severe as to require withdrawal from the study, cannot receive the relief they would get in a therapeutic setting.

Analogously, adjunctive medications or forms of therapy, which may interfere with measurement of the primary treatment effect, are often prohibited. The exclusion of adjunctive medications, such as sleeping medications or decongestants, may increase a patient's discomfort. The requirement for a "wash-out" period, during which subjects are kept drug free, may place previously stable patients at risk of relapse even before the experimental part of the project begins. And alternating placebo and active treatment periods may mean that a patient who responds well to a medication must be taken off that drug for the purposes of the study; conversely, patients who improve on placebo must be subject to the risks of active medication. In sum, the necessary rigidities of an experimental protocol often lead investigators to forgo individualized treatment decisions.

The need for control groups or placebos and double-blind procedures can produce similar effects. In the therapeutic setting patients will rarely receive medications that are deliberately designed to be pharmacologically ineffective; the ethics of those occasional situations when placebos are employed clinically are hotly disputed.[5] Yet, placebos are routinely employed in clinical investigations, without the intent of benefiting the individual subject.

Similarly, clinicians in a nonresearch setting will never allow them-selves to remain ignorant of the treatment patients are receiving. Double-blind procedures, however, are necessary to ensure the integrity of a research study, even if they delay recognition of side effects or drug interactions, or have other adverse consequences.

Are these disadvantages so important that they should routinely be called to the attention of research subjects? That issue raises an empirical question: how prevalent is the therapeutic misconception?

Studies on Consent

Our findings suggest that research subjects systematically misinterpret the risk/benefit ratio of participating in research because they fail to understand the underlying scientific methodology.[6]

This conclusion is based on our observations of consent transactions in four research studies on the treatment of psychiatric illness, and our interviews with the subjects immediately after consent was obtained. The studies varied in the extent of the information they provided to subjects. Two of the studies compared the effects of two medications on a psychiatric disorder (one used, in addition, a placebo control group). A third study examined the relative efficacy of two dosage ranges of the same medication. And a fourth examined two different social interventions in chronic psychiatric illness, compared with a control group.

The populations in these studies ranged from actively psychotic schizophrenic patients to nonpsychotic, and in some cases, minimally symptomatic, borderline, and depressed patients. Our questions were based on information included on the consent form with regard to the understanding of randomized or chance assignment; and the use of control groups, formal protocols, and double-blind techniques. Eighty-eight patients comprised the final data pool, but since all of the issues addressed here were not relevant to each project the sample size varied for each question.

We found that fifty-five of eighty subjects (69 percent) had no comprehension of the actual basis for their random assignment to treatment groups, while only twenty-two of eighty (28 percent) had a complete understanding of the randomization process. Thirty-two subjects stated their explicit belief that assignment would be made on the basis of their therapeutic needs. Interestingly, many of these subjects constructed elaborate but entirely fictional means by which an assignment would be made that was in their best interests. This was particularly evident when information about group assignment was limited to the written consent forms and not covered in the oral disclosure; subjects filled vacuums of knowledge with assumptions that decisions would be made in their best interests.

Similar findings were evident concerning other aspects of scientific design. With regard to nontreatment control groups and placebos, fourteen of thirty-three (44 percent) subjects failed to recognize that some patients who desired treatment would not receive it. Concerning use of a double-blind, twenty-six of sixty-seven subjects (39 percent) did not understand that their physician would not know which medication they would receive; an additional sixteen of sixty-seven subjects (24 percent) had only partially understood this. Most striking of all, only six of sixty-eight subjects (9 percent) were able to recognize a single way in which joining a protocol would restrict the treatment they could receive. In the two drug studies in which adjustment of medication dosage was tightly restricted, twenty-two of forty-four subjects (50 percent) said explicitly that they thought their dosage would be adjusted according to their individual needs.

Two cases illustrate how these flaws in understanding affect the patient's ability to assess the benefits of the research. The first demonstrates the effect of a complete failure to recognize that scientific methodology has other than a therapeutic purpose. The second demonstrates a more subtle influence of a therapeutic orientation on a subject who understands the overall methodology but has certain blindspots.

In the first case, a twenty-five-year-old married woman with a high-school education was a subject in a randomized, double-blind study that compared the use of two medications and a placebo in the treatment of a nonpsychotic psychiatric disorder. When interviewed, she was unsure how it would be decided which medication she would receive, but thought that the placebo would be given only to those subjects who "might not need medication." The subject understood that a double-blind procedure would be used, but did not see that the protocol placed any constraints on her treatment. She said that she considered this project not an "experiment," a term that implied using drugs whose effects were unknown. Rather, she considered this to be "research," a process whereby doctors "were trying to find out more about you in depth." She decided to participate because, "I needed help and the doctor said that other people who had been in it had been helped." Her strong conviction that the project would benefit her carried through to the end of the study. Although the investigators rated her a nonresponder, she was convinced that she had improved on the medication. She attributed her improvement in large part to the double-blind procedures, which kept her in the dark as to which medication she was receiving, thereby preventing her from persuading herself that the medication was doing no good. She was quite pleased about having participated in the study.

In the same study, another subject was a twenty-five-year-old woman with three years of college. At the time of the interview, she had minimal psychiatric symptoms and her understanding of the research was generally excellent. She recognized that the purpose of the project was to find out which treatment worked best for her group of patients. She spontaneously described the three groups, including the placebo group, and indicated that assignment would be at random. She understood that dosages would be adjusted according to blood levels and that a double-blind would be used. When asked directly, however, how *her* medication would be selected, she said she had no idea. She then added, "I hope it isn't by chance," and suggested that each subject would probably receive the medication she needed. Given the discrepancy between her earlier use of the word "random" and her current explanation, she was then asked what her understanding was of "random." Her definition was entirely appropriate: "by lottery, by chance, one patient who comes in gets one thing and the next patient gets the next thing." She then began to wonder out loud if this procedure was being used in the current study. Ultimately, she concluded that it was not.

In this case, despite a cognitive understanding of randomization, and a momentary recognition that random assignment would be used, the subject's conviction that the investigators would be acting in her best interests led to a distortion of an important element of the experimental procedure and therefore of the risk/benefit analysis.

The comments of colleagues and reports by other researchers have persuaded us that this phenomenon extends to all clinical research. Bradford Gray, for example, found that a number of subjects in a project comparing two drugs for the induction of labor believed, incorrectly, that their needs would determine which drug they would receive.[7] A survey of patients in research projects at four Veterans Administration hospitals showed that 75 percent decided to participate because they expected the research to benefit their health.[8] Another survey of attitudes toward research in a combined sample of patients and the general public revealed the thinking behind this hope: when asked why people in general should participate in research, 69 percent cited benefit to society at large and only 5 percent cited benefit to the subjects; however, when asked why *they* might participate in a research project, 52 percent said they would do it to get the best medical care, while only 23 percent responded that they would want to contribute to scientific knowledge.[9] Back in the psychiatric setting, Lee Park and Lino Covi found that a substantial percentage of patients who were told they were being given a placebo would not believe that they received inactive medication,[10] and Vincenta Leigh reported that the most common fantasy on a psychiatric research ward was that the research was actually designed to benefit the subjects.[11]

Responding to the Problem

Should we do anything about the therapeutic misconception? It could be argued that as long as the research project has been peer-reviewed for scientific merit and approved for ethical acceptability by an institutional review board (IRB), the problem of the therapeutic misconception is not significant enough to warrant intervention. In this view, some minor distortion of the risk/benefit ratio has to be weighed against the costs of attempting to alter subjects' appreciation of the scientific methods. Such costs include time expended and the delay in completing research that will result when some subjects decide that they would rather not participate.

Whether we accept this view depends on the value that we place on the principle of autonomy that underlies the practice of informed consent. Autonomy can be overvalued when it limits necessary treatment, as it may, for example, in the controversy over the right to refuse psychotropic medications. There, we believe, patients' interests would best be served by giving claims to autonomy lesser weight.[12] But when we enter the research setting, limiting subjects' autonomy becomes a tool not for promoting their own interests, but for promoting the interests of others, including the researcher and society as a whole. We are not willing to accept such limitations for the benefit of others, particularly when, as described below, there may exist an effective mechanism for mitigating the problem.

Assuming that one agrees that distortions of the type we have described in subjects' reasoning are troublesome and worthy of correction, is such an effort likely to be effective? One might point to the data just presented to argue that little can be done to ameliorate the problem. The investigator in one of the projects we studied offered his subjects detailed and extensive information in a process that often extended over several days and included one session in which the entire project was reviewed. Despite this, half the subjects failed to grasp that treatment would be assigned on a random basis, four of twenty misunderstood how placebos would be used, five of twenty were not aware of the use of a double-blind, and eight of twenty believed that medications would be adjusted according to their individual needs. Is it not futile, then, to attempt to disabuse subjects of the belief that they will receive personal care?

Various theoretical explanations of our findings could support this view. Most people have been socialized to believe that physicians (at least ethical ones) always provide personal care.[13] It may therefore be very difficult, perhaps nearly impossible, to persuade subjects that this encounter is different, particularly if the researcher is also the treating physician, who has previously satisfied the subject's expectations of personal care. Further, insofar as much clinical research involves persons who are acutely ill and in some distress, the well-known tendency of patients to regress and entrust their well-being to an authority figure would undercut any effort to dispel the therapeutic misconception.

In response, more of our data must be explored. In each of the studies we observed, one cell of subjects was the target of an augmented informational process, which supplemented the investigator's disclosures to subjects with a "preconsent discussion." This discussion was led by a member of our research team who was trained to teach potential subjects about such things as the key methodologic aspects of the research project, especially methods that might conflict with the principle of personal care.

By introducing a neutral discloser, distinct from the patient's treatment team, we shifted the emphasis of the disclosure to focus on the ways in which research differs from treatment. Of the subjects who received this special education, eight of sixteen (50 percent) recognized that randomization would be used, as opposed to thirteen of the fifty-one (25 percent) remaining subjects; five of five (100 percent) understood how placebos would be employed in the single study that used them, compared with eleven of the fifteen (73 percent) remaining subjects; nine of sixteen (56 percent) comprehended the use of a double blind while only fifteen of fifty-one (31 percent) remaining subjects did so; and five of seventeen (29 percent) initially recognized other limits on their treatment as a result of constraints in the protocol, compared with one of the fifty-one (2 percent) other subjects.

Our data suggest that many subjects can be taught that research is markedly different from ordinary treatment. Other efforts to educate subjects about the use of scientific methodology offer comparably encouraging results.[14] There is no reason to believe that subjects will refuse to hear clear-cut efforts to dispel the therapeutic misconception.

Novel approaches such as we employed may be one thing, of course, while routine procedures are something else. Perhaps our data derive from an unusually gifted group of patient-subjects. Will the complexity of explaining the principle of the scientific method defy understanding by most research subjects?

Undercutting the therapeutic misconception, thereby laying out some of the major disadvantages of any clinical research project, is probably much simpler than it seems. About the goals of research, subjects could be told: "Because this is a research project, we will be doing some things differently than we would if we were simply treating you for your condition. Not all the things we do are designed to tell us the best way to treat *you*, but they should help us to understand how people with your condition in *general* can best be treated." About randomization: "The treatment you receive of the three possibilities will be selected by chance, not because we believe that one or the other will be better for you." About placebos: "Some subjects will be selected at random to receive sugar pills that are not known to help the condition you have; this is so we can tell whether the medications that the other patients get are really effective, or if everyone with your condition would have gotten better anyway."

One can quibble about the wording of specific sections, and complexities can arise with particular projects, but the concepts underlying scientific methodology are in reality quite simple. And as long as subjects understand the key principles of how the study is being conducted, investigators can probably omit some of the detail that currently clogs consent forms and confuses subjects about the minor risks that accompany the experimental procedures, such as blood drawing. Overall, then, we may end up with a much simpler consent process when we focus on the issue of personal care.

Who should have the task of explaining the therapeutic misconception to subjects? Clearly, investigators should be encouraged to discuss such issues with subjects and to include them on consent forms, but several problems arise here. First, it is decidedly not in investigators' self-interest for them to disabuse potential subjects of the therapeutic misconception. Experienced investigators, as we have reported elsewhere,[15] view the recruitment of research subjects as an intricate and extended effort to win the potential subject's trust. One of our subjects in this study described the process in these words: "It was almost as if they were courting me . . . everything was presented in the best possible light." One could argue that it is unrealistic to expect investigators to raise additional doubts about the benefits that subjects can expect; any effort in that regard will result in resistance by investigators, particularly those who have yet to internalize the justifications for informed consent in general.

Second, even investigators who recognize the desirability of subjects making informed decisions may have great trouble conveying this particular information. When a researcher tells subjects that he or she is not selecting the treatment that will be given or that the medications being used may be no more effective than a placebo, the researcher is confessing uncertainty over the best approach to treatment, as well as the likely outcome. Harold Bursztajn and colleagues have argued that the essential uncertainty of all medical practice is precisely what physicians need to convey in both research and treatment settings.[16] Yet, as Jay Katz points out, physicians have been systematically socialized to underplay or ignore uncertainty in their discussions with patients.[17] In a recent report of physicians' reluctance to enter patients in a multicenter breast cancer study, 22 percent of the principal investigators cited as a major obstacle to enrolling subjects difficulty in telling patients that they did not know which treatment was best.[18]

Third, few researchers who are also clinicians feel comfortable acknowledging, even to themselves, that the course of treatment may not be optimally therapeutic for the patient. Thus, there appear such statements as the following, which recently was published in The Lancet: "A doctor who contributes to randomized treatment trials should not be thought of as a research worker, but simply as a clinician with an ethical duty to his patients not to go on giving them treatments without doing everything possible to assess their true worth."[19] The author concludes that since randomized trials are not really research, there is no need to obtain any informed consent from research subjects. Although this conclusion may be extreme, the example emphasizes the difficulties of getting investigators to admit to themselves, much less to their patient-subjects, the limits they have accepted on the delivery of personal care.

If there is concern with particular protocols, IRBs might consider supplementing the investigators' disclosure and the "courtship" process with a session in which the potential subject reviews risks and benefits with someone who is not a member of the research team. (John Robertson has proposed a similar approach, albeit out of other concerns.[20])

The neutral explainer would be responsible to the IRB and would be trained to emphasize those aspects of the research situation about which the IRB has the greatest concern. This approach might be especially appropriate when the investigator is also the subject's treating physician and the methodology used is likely to be interpreted as therapeutic in intent. The model we employed of using a trained educator (nurses are natural candidates for the job) worked well. It is certainly more manageable and less disruptive than the oft-heard suggestions that patient advocates or con-sent monitors sit in on every inter-action between subject and investigator.

There may be advantages to using a trained, neutral educator, apart from aiding subjects' decision-making. Subjects' perceptions of the research team as willing to "level with them," even to the point of explaining why it might not be in subjects' interests to participate in the study, may increase their trust and cooperation. On the other hand, failure to deal with the therapeutic misconception during the consent process could increase distrust of researchers and the health care system in general, if subjects later come to feel they were "deceived," as a few did in the studies we observed. Enough experiences of this sort could further heighten public antipathy to medical research, particularly if they are publicized as some have been.[21] The scientific method is a powerful tool for advancing knowledge, but like most potent clinical procedures it has side effects that must be attended to, lest the benefits sought be overwhelmed by the disadvantages that accrue. With careful planning, the therapeutic misconception can be dispelled, leaving the subjects with a much clearer picture of the relative risks and benefits of participation in research.

REFERENCES

1. Charles Fried, *Medical Experimentation: Personal Integrity and Social Policy* (New York: American Elsevier Publishing Co., 1974).
2. Arthur Schafer, "The Ethics of the Randomized Clinical Trial," *New England Journal of Medicine* 307 (1982), 719–724.
3. "Consent: How Informed?" *The Lancet* 323(1984), 1445–1447.
4. Kathryn M. Taylor, Richard G. Margolese, and Colin L. Soskolne, "Physicians' Reasons for Not Entering Eligible Patients in a Randomized Clinical Trial of Surgery for Breast Cancer," *New England Journal of Medicine* 310 (1984), 1363–1367; Mortimer J. Lacher, "Physicians and Patients as Obstacles to Randomized Trial," *Clinical Research* 26 (1978), 375–379.
5. Sissela Bok, "The Ethics of Giving Placebos," *Scientific American* 231:5 (1974), 17–23.
6. Paul S. Appelbaum, Loren H. Roth, and Charles W Lidz, "The Therapeutic Misconception: Informed Consent in Psychiatric Research," *International Journal of Law and Psychiatry* 5 (1982), 319–329; Paul Benson, Loren H. Roth, and William J. Winslade, "Informed Consent in Psychiatric Research: Preliminary Findings from an Ongoing Investigation," *Social Science and Medicine* 20 (1985), 1331–1341.
7. Bradford H. Gray, *Human Subjects in Medical Experimentation: A Sociological Study of the Conduct and Regulation of Clinical Research* (New York: John Wiley & Sons, 1975).
8. Henry W. Riecken and Ruth Ravich, "Informed Consent to Biomedical Research in Veterans Administration Hospitals," *JAMA* 248 (1982), 344–348.

9. Barrie R. Cassileth, Edward J. Lusk, David S. Miller, and Shelley Hurwitz, "Attitudes toward Clinical Trials among Patients and the Public," *Journal of the American Medical Association* 248 (1982), 968–970.

10. Lee C. Park and Lino Covi, "Nonblind Placebo Trial: An Exploration of Neurotic Patients' Responses to Placebo When Its Inert Content is Disclosed," *Archives of General Psychiatry* 12 (1965), 336–345.

11. Vincenta Leigh, "Attitudes and Fantasy Themes of Patients on a Psychiatric Research Unit," *Archives of General Psychiatry* 32 (1975), 598–601.

12. Paul S. Appelbaum and Thomas G. Gutheil, "The Right to Refuse Treatment: The Real Issue Is Quality of Care," *Bulletin of the American Academy of Psychiatry and the Law* 9 (1982), 199–202.

13. Cassileth et al., "Attitudes toward Clinical Trials."

14. Jan M. Howard, David DeMets, and the BHAT Research Group, "How Informed Is Informed Consent? The BHAT Experience," *Controlled Clinical Trials* 2 (1981), 287–303.

15. Paul S. Appelbaum and Loren H. Roth, "The Structure of Informed Consent in Psychiatric Research," *Behavioral Sciences and the Law* 1:3 (1983), 9–19.

16. Harold Bursztajn, Richard I. Feinbloom, Robert M. Hamm, and Archie Brodsky, *Medical Choices, Medical Chances: How Patients, Families, and Physicians Can Cope with Uncertainty* (New York: Free Press, 1984).

17. Jay Katz, *The Silent World of Doctor and Patient* (New York: Free Press, 1984).

18. Taylor, et al., "Physicians' Reasons for Not Entering."

19. Thurston B. Brewin, "Consent to Randomized Treatment," *The Lancet* 320 (1982), 919–921.

20. John A. Robertson, "Taking Consent Seriously: IRB Intervention in the Consent Process," *IRB: A Review of Human Subjects Research* 4:5 (1982), 1–5.

21. Dava Sobel, "Sleep Study Leaves Subject Feeling Angry and Confused," *New York Times* (July 15, 1980), p. C-1.

SECTION B. CLINICAL PRACTICE

47
The Use of Placebo Interventions in Medical Practice

A National Questionnaire Survey of Danish Clinicians

ASBJØRN HRÓBJARTSSON AND MICHAEL NORUP

Asbjørn Hróbjartsson and Michael Norup, "The Use of Placebo Interventions in Medical Practice—A National Questionnaire Survey of Danish Clinicians," *Evaluation and the Health Professions* 2003;26:153–165.

The use of a placebo intervention outside clinical research is generally regarded as unethical because it often constitutes deceit of a patient (Rawlinson, 1985). The extent to which placebo interventions are actually used in clinical medicine is not clear. As early as 1945, Pepper (1945) noted that "the giving of a placebo—when, how, what—seems to be a function of the physician, which, like certain functions of the body, is not to be mentioned in polite society" (p. 411).

Previously conducted surveys of the actual clinical use of placebos have been few and based on nonrandom, relatively small samples of mostly hospital-based doctors (Berger, 1999; Ernst and Abbot, 1997; Goldberg, Leigh, and Quinlan, 1979; Goodwin, Goodwin, and Vogel, 1979; Gray and Flynn, 1981; Hofling, 1955; Lynøe, Mattsson, and Sandlund, 1993; Shapiro and Struening, 1973; Thomson and Buchanan, 1982). These studies reported an overall low use of placebos but indicated possible greater use in general practice.

Not all doctors find placebo treatments unethical. An article in *Scientific American* by Brown (1998) concluded that "we should respect the benefits of placebos . . . and bring the full advantage of these benefits into our everyday practices" (p. 95). Similarly, a *British Medical Journal* editorial by Oh (1994) concluded that "doctors might consider giving a placebo when active treatment is both costly and likely to confer only marginal or transient benefit" (p. 70).

We suspected that the clinical use of placebos in Denmark could be noticeable, especially outside of hospital settings. The primary aims of this study were to estimate the proportion of doctors who use placebo interventions in their daily clinical practice and to compare this proportion between private practice and hospital settings. Our secondary aims were to investigate which type of placebo interventions were used, and which clinical conditions were involved, as well as the physicians' attitudes toward placebos, and their reasons for using them.

Method

Sample

The study was conducted from May 1999 to August 1999. The department of registration of the Danish Medical Association drew a computer-generated random sample of 286 doctors enlisted as general practitioners, 286 clinicians enlisted as specialists in private practice, and 286 members enlisted as hospital clinicians.

The sample size was based on our predefined aim of detecting a 15% difference among the three types of clinicians with respect to the proportion who had used placebo during the past year. We accepted a risk of a Type I error of 5% and of a Type II error of 10% (Altman, 1991, chap. 10).

Questionnaire

The participants received a letter explaining the purpose of the anonymous study, a questionnaire, and a stamped and numbered return envelope. We emphasized that we were only concerned with the clinical use of placebo interventions, not their role in scientific investigations. Furthermore, we characterized a placebo treatment as an intervention not considered to have any "specific" effect on the condition treated, but with a possible "unspecific" effect. The physicians agreeing with this characterization were asked to fill in the whole questionnaire, whereas those disagreeing were asked to fill in only the section on background information.

We then asked whether placebo interventions in general would have effects on both symptoms and signs, effects only on symptoms, or no effects. We also asked how often during the last year they had used saline injections, B vitamins, antibiotics, sedatives, or physiotherapy (for example, massage, heat, and ultrasound for soft tissue ailments and physical exercises after surgery) in clinical situations in which the expected effect of the pharmacological or "specific" content of the interventions was negligible. We then asked the participants to indicate if they considered any of the examples given not to be placebos and inquired how often they had used other placebo treatments. Additionally, we asked the participants to provide examples of clinical situations in which they had used placebos and to give reasons for use of placebos. Finally, we asked whether they, in general, found placebo interventions ethically acceptable.

On return, the envelope was separated from the questionnaire. Thus, the questionnaire could no longer be connected with any specific person, but the number on the envelope in combination with the original address list enabled us to identify the respondents. A first reminder was sent to the nonrespondents after two weeks. Participants not responding to this were mailed a new copy of the questionnaire a week later, and a final reminder was sent after another three weeks.

Earlier versions of the questionnaire were tested in two pilot studies each involving 30 physicians. Their responses led us to expand the introduction to the questionnaire and to make small adjustments in the phrasing of several questions.

Data Analysis

We recorded how often the respondents reported to have treated patients with saline injections, B vitamins, antibiotics, sedatives, or physiotherapy in situations in which the effect of the pharmacological or specific content of the treatments was expected to be negligible. After summing the number of these interventions, we subtracted any of the above treatments that the respondents did not regard as placebo interventions. We further added the number of times the respondents reported to have used "other placebos." On this basis, we divided the respondents into (a) nonusers of placebo treatments, (b) occasional users (1–10 times within the past year), and (c) frequent users (more than 10 times within the past year). The data in the individual questionnaires were transferred to a statistical software package, SPSS 9.0. We checked for systematic data entry errors by comparing the data from a randomly selected sample of questionnaires with the corresponding electronic data. The frequency of unanswered questions was noted. Respondents who did not answer the questions on the use of placebos were considered nonusers.

We used Fischer's exact test (Altman, 1991, chap. 15) to compare proportions. The p values are two-tailed, and all results are presented with 95% confidence intervals.

Table 47.1.
Use of placebo interventions

Frequency of Clinicians Reporting Use of Placebo Interventions during the Past Year	General Practitioners (n=182)	Hospital-Based Physicians (n=185)	Private Specialists (n=136)
Nonusers	14% (9–19)	46% (39–53)	59% (51–67)
Users	86% (81–91)	54% (47–61)	41% (33–49)
Occasional (1–10 times)	38% (31–45)	44% (37–51)	31% (23–39)
Frequent (>10 times)	48% (41–55)	10% (6–14)	10% (5–15)

Note: Ninety-five percent confidence intervals in parentheses. N_{total}=503.

Results
The Study Population

Early in the study, we discovered that 86 of the 286 doctors classified by the Danish Medical Association as specialists in private practice were in fact primarily working in hospitals. We accepted the slight decrease in statistical power and withdrew the 86 from the study. The final study population, therefore, consisted of 772 physicians.

Return Rate

Of 772 questionnaires, 672 (86%) were returned. Of these, 127 (16%) were blank, whereas 545 (71%) were filled in. A total of 505 respondents agreed with the characterization of a placebo intervention presented in the questionnaire, whereas 40 respondents disagreed. Two of the 505 were excluded, as they worked neither in hospitals nor in practice. The remaining 503 respondents (65%) were classified as general practitioners, hospital-based doctors, or private specialists, according to the information they provided (Table 47.1). There were no significant differences among respondents and nonrespondents with respect to age, sex, or workplace (data not shown).

Use of Placebo

Placebo treatments were reported to have been used at least once within the last year by 86% of general practitioners, 54% of hospital doctors, and 41% of private specialists, p < .001 (Table 47.1). We found that 48% of general practitioners reported use of placebos more than 10 times within the last year, as compared with 10% in the other two groups (p < .001).

Seventy percent of general practitioners reported having used placebos in the form of antibiotics within the last year and roughly 50% in the form of B vitamins, physiotherapy, or sedatives (Table 47.2). Thirty-three percent of the hospital-based doctors reported having used a placebo in the form of antibiotics and roughly 25% in the form of sedatives or physiotherapy. Among the private specialists, the number reporting use was low for all five placebo examples.

A total of 226 of the respondents (45%) provided us with their own examples of clinical situations in which they had used placebos. Ninety respondents reported to have used placebos as analgesics—for example, physiotherapy, block-

Table 47.2.
Types of placebo interventions

Placebo Interventions Reported to Have Been Used at Least Once during the Past Year	General Practitioners (n=182)	Hospital-Based Physicians (n=185)	Private Specialists (n=136)
Antibiotics	70% (63–77)	33% (26–40)	18% (11–25)
Physiotherapy	59% (52–66)	24% (18–30)	13% (7–19)
Sedatives	45% (38–52)	24% (18–30)	10% (5–15)
B vitamins	48% (41–55)	10% (6–14)	9% (4–13)
Saline injections	5% (2–8)	1% (0–2)	0%
Other	26% (20–32)	14% (6–19)	15% (9–21)

Note: Ninety-five percent confidence intervals in parentheses. N_{total}=503.

Table 47.3.
Reason for use of placebo interventions

At Least One Placebo Intervention Had Been Given for the Following Reasons:	General Practitioners (n=182)	Hospital-Based Physicians (n=185)	Private Specialists (n=136)
Follow the wish of the patient and avoid conflict	70% (63–77)	46% (39–53)	42% (34–50)
Take advantage of an effect of placebo	48% (41–55)	22% (16–28)	32% (24–40)
Avoid discontinuing another physician's prescription	40% (33–47)	27% (21–33)	18% (12–24)
Avoid telling that treatment possibilities are exhausted	36% (29–43)	11% (6–16)	17% (11–23)
Test whether a condition is functional or organic	25% (19–31)	13% (8–18)	15% (6–21)
Other	9% (5–14)	6% (3–9)	7% (3–11)

Note: Ninety-five percent confidence intervals in parentheses. N_{total}=503.

ades, ultrasound, analgesics in insufficient dosage, and saline injections. Antibiotics were used against viral infections by 86 respondents. Furthermore, vitamins were used as placebos against fatigue by 32 respondents, whereas 28 doctors treated cough and chronic obstructive lung disease with different placebos, for example, mucolytic drugs, β_2-receptor stimulants, or unspecific cough mixtures. In addition, various other conditions and treatments were reported by no more than 10 respondents. These included treatment of terminal cancer with prednisone or physiotherapy; B vitamins against multiple sclerosis, loss of hair, and neuritis; antidepressives for conditions not considered depressions; quinine against restless legs; and cyclizine for tinnitus and vertigo. The reason reported most often in all groups for giving a placebo treatment was to avoid conflicts with patients by complying with their treatment preferences (Table 47.3).

When excluding placebo physiotherapy, the proportion of users was somewhat smaller in all groups, but the overall conclusion did not change (data not shown). The group of hospital-based doctors consisted of both specialists and nonspecialists. The hospital-based specialist and the private specialist did not differ significantly regarding the frequency of placebo users, whereas the proportion of younger hospital-based nonspecialists using placebo was higher than the proportion among the specialists (p = .001) but lower than the proportion among the general practitioners (p < .001).

Attitudes toward Placebo Interventions

There was no major difference between the three types of clinicians with regard to belief in the effect of placebo (p = .09). Placebo treatments were considered to have an effect only on subjective symptoms by 51% of the respondents; 32% believed in an effect on both subjective symptoms and objective signs, whereas 9% did not believe in any effect. The remaining 8% either did not respond to the questions or responded "don't know." There was also no significant difference between the three types of clinicians with regard to their ethical standpoint on placebo treatments (p = .10). Placebo treatments were considered ethically acceptable by 46%, whereas 40% thought it unethical, and 14% did not know or left the question unanswered. A total of 32% used placebo treatments, found them ethically acceptable, and believed that they have an effect. Forty-six percent of the general practitioners belonged to this group, compared to 24% of hospital doctors and 23% of private specialists (p < .001). Approximately 4% held the opposite combination of views, as they regarded placebo interventions unethical, did not use them, and did not believe in an effect. Seventy-four percent of the respondents who regarded placebo treatments ethically acceptable reported that they had used placebo treatments within the last year. Of the respondents who found placebo treatments unethical, 50% reported they still had prescribed them.

Discussion

Close to 90% of the general practitioners reported that they had used placebo interventions at least once and roughly 50% to have used it more than ten times within the last year. Hospital-based doctors and private specialists reported to have used placebo infrequently. The most frequently reported reason for the use of placebos was to avoid a confrontation with the patient. A typical placebo intervention was antibiotics for viral infections. Approximately 30% of doctors believed in an effect of placebo interventions on objective outcomes, and about 50% found clinical placebo interventions ethically acceptable.

Representativeness of the Survey

The survey was based on a random sample of clinically working members of the Danish Medical Association. The randomization was conducted by a third party. As many as 94% of Danish doctors are members of the association (T. Østerlund, personal communication, 1999). So, there is little risk of an unrepresentative sample.

The response rate was 65%, which is higher than the mean response rate of 54% in questionnaires sent to American doctors (Asch, Jedrziewski, and Christakis, 1997). We found no difference between respondents and nonrespondents with respect to age, sex, and clinical specialties, but we cannot exclude the possibility that the 35% who did not respond differed in their use of placebos from the respondents. In the extreme case, the 104 nonresponding general practitioners never used placebos. However, the overall proportion of general practitioners who had used placebo interventions within the past year would still be approximately 55%, and 30% would have used placebos ten times or more. So even if the proportion of nonusers among the nonrespondents was high, there would still be a considerable number of general practitioners using placebo.

The findings must be confined to a Danish setting. Prescription habits are probably substantially influenced by the cultural or national settings, but it would still surprise us if our main conclusion is primarily a result of national peculiarity. Other (national) surveys could explore to which extent our results are reproducible.

Reporting Bias

Clinical use of placebos has negative connotations with fraud and unscientific conduct, and it is likely that most studies based on self-reported retrospective data of social behaviors with negative connotations underestimate real behavior. Furthermore, it seems likely that we would have found a higher use of placebo intervention if we had included more than the five examples of placebo interventions specifically asked for in the questionnaire. Our aim was, however, to estimate the proportion of placebo users among clinicians, not the total use. This is a dichotomous question, which is probably less influenced by these sorts of bias.

The Concept of Placebo Is Ambiguous

In randomized clinical trials, placebo control interventions are designed to have the appearance of the experimental intervention but without the essential or 'specific' content (for example, a drug) or procedure (for example, a surgical intervention) that is being tested. In clinical practice, there is no experimental intervention that serves as a benchmark, and placebos are problematic to define in a satisfying way. This gives rise to several problems for any attempt to study use of placebo in the clinic.

One problem concerns the distinction found in the medical literature between placebo in a narrow sense, referring to a sham intervention, and placebo in a broader sense, covering various context factors within the doctor-patient relationship, for example, a doctor's positive attitude (Hróbjartsson, 2002; Thomas, 1987).We addressed this problem by designing the questionnaire so that the participants would commit themselves to placebo in the narrow sense. First, we characterized placebo as an intervention and not as a context factor. Second, we avoided using the phrase "placebo effect,"

which is also associated with the doctor-patient relationship in the broader sense. Only 40 respondents disagreed with our characterization of placebo. Furthermore, most respondents who provided examples of placebos they had used mentioned pharmacological interventions, for example, vitamin tablets, thus reflecting the narrow meaning of the term. Only 9 out of 226 doctors provided examples that demonstrated they thought of placebo in its broad sense, for example, a warm doctor-patient interaction or an open consultation atmosphere.

Another problem is connected to the distinction between pure and impure placebos. Pure placebos are interventions with essential components that are inert (for all clinical conditions), for example, lactose tablets. Impure placebos (or "active placebos") are interventions with essential components that are inert for the clinical problem for which the interventions are prescribed but not for other conditions, for example, antibiotics for viral infections. Although this distinction is well established in the literature, some clinicians may be reluctant to accept impure placebos as true placebos. If our results are affected by this reluctance, the proportion of placebo users is underestimated, because most of the examples we presented were of impure placebos. The fact that most of the examples of placebo treatments given by the respondents were of impure placebos suggests, however, that such reluctance is probably not widespread.

A third problem concerns the distinction between "specific" and "nonspecific" effects used in our operational characterization of placebo. Whereas this distinction is relatively clear in connection with pharmacological interventions, it is less obvious in connection with nonpharmacological treatments such as physiotherapy. Variations in the interpretations of the word *specific* could potentially have resulted in inclusion of interventions not generally regarded placebos (Hróbjartsson, 2002). However, the impact of placebo physiotherapy on our overall assessment was small.

Placebo and Decisions under Uncertainty

A fourth problem is connected to the uncertainty of diagnosis and therapeutic effectiveness in real clinical situations. If a doctor chooses to prescribe antibiotics, for example, penicillin, although he or she is fairly convinced that the infection is viral, this can be described either as a safeguard against the worse-case scenario (if the diagnosis is sufficiently uncertain and the potential harm sufficiently dramatic) or as a placebo intervention (if the diagnosis in a practical sense is certain, and the possibility of an effect of penicillin is negligible). Furthermore, depending on the belief of the doctor, the use of a drug without clear documentation of a therapeutic effect may be described either as an attempt to take advantage of a possible but undocumented therapeutic effect of the drug or as a placebo intervention. In some borderline situations, the integration of the diagnostic and therapeutic uncertainties is highly intricate, and the precise beliefs and intentions of the doctor can be impossible to clarify. However, we find it likely that when asked in a questionnaire, a doctor prefers to categorize many of the unclear prescription scenarios in the way she or he finds most acceptable. We also find it likely that a placebo prescription is less acceptable to the majority of clinicians than the use of interventions that are safeguards against worst-case scenarios or interventions that lack documented effect. Thus, it seems likely that this kind of situation does not account for a large proportion of the use of placebo reported in our study.

Other Studies

We found nine previous questionnaire studies that investigated how often placebos are used clinically or the attitudes toward placebo interventions. Six studies surveyed hospital-based physicians or nurses and found that between 10% and 80% had used placebos but mostly quite infrequently (Berger, 1999; Ernst and Abbot, 1997; Goldberg et al., 1979; Goodwin et al., 1979; Gray and Flynn, 1981; Hofling, 1955). One study made no distinction between the use of placebo in randomized trials and in clinical practice (Shapiro and Struening, 1973). Two studies presented hypothetical case stories (Lynøe et al., 1993; Thomson and Buchanan, 1982). Thomson and Buchanan (1982) found that more than 40% of general practitioners would use placebos "at least rarely" in five of eight clinical scenarios. Lynøe et al. (1993) focused on the ethics of prescribing placebos and was the only study in which participants were sampled randomly.

Why Do General Practitioners Prescribe Placebos?

We anticipated that general practitioners and specialists in private practice would have similar patterns of placebo prescriptions, but the hypothesis was not confirmed. In contrary, our findings indicate that the type of patient could be more important than institutional setting. General practitioners encounter nonscreened patients who tend to return several times with chronic problems and with minor ailments that often cannot be clearly diagnosed. In situations in which a firm diagnosis is not found or an efficient treatment does not exist, some general practitioners may be tempted to treat a patient with a placebo, especially if the patient indicates that "something has to be done" and the doctor feels there is not the time for a detailed explanation or lengthy discussion. It is notable that the main reason for use of placebo reported by the respondents was to appease a patient and not primarily to induce an effect of placebo.

The primary argument for the use of placebos considered in the literature is that placebos are reported to induce important clinical effects (Beecher, 1955; Brown, 1998; Lasagna, 1986). The widespread belief in important effects of placebos is, however, not based on good evidence. Detailed examination (Kienle and Kiene, 1997) of some of the most quoted placebo studies revealed severe methodological shortcomings. Furthermore, a systematic review (Hróbjarts-son and Gøtzsche, 2001) of 114 randomized trials comparing placebo with no treatment found no evidence of important effects on binary or objective outcomes and a moderate effect on subjective continuous outcomes; for example, pain could not be clearly distinguished from possible bias.

Conclusion

The proportion of doctors reporting more than occasional use of placebo intervention was fairly high among general practitioners but not among hospital-based doctors or specialists in private practice. The reason reported most often for the use of placebo treatments was to avoid conflict with the patient. Half of the doctors reported that they found placebo interventions ethically acceptable. Thus there seems to exist a tension between the prevailing rejection of placebo interventions in the medical literature and the actual clinical praxis by Danish doctors.

REFERENCES

Altman, D. G. (1991). Practical statistics for medical research. London: Chapman & Hall.

Asch, D. A., Jedrziewski, M. K., and Christakis, N. A. (1997). Response rates to mail surveys published in medical journals. Journal of Clinical Epidemiology, 50, 1129–1136.

Beecher, H. K. (1955). The powerful placebo. Journal of the American Medical Association, 159, 1602–1606.

Berger, J. T. (1999). Placebo medication use in patient care: A survey of medical interns. Western Journal of Medicine, 170, 93–96.

Brown, W. A. (1998). The placebo effect. Scientific American, 278(1), 90–95.

Ernst, E., and Abbot, N. C. (1997). Placebos in clinical practice: Results of a survey of nurses. Perfusion, 10, 128–130.

Goodwin, J. S., Goodwin, J. M., and Vogel, A. V. (1979). Knowledge and use of placebos by house officers and nurses. Annals of Internal Medicine, 9, 106–110.

Goldberg, R. J., Leigh, H., and Quinlan, D. (1979). The current status of placebo in hospital practice. General Hospital Psychiatry, 1, 196–201.

Gray, G., and Flynn, P. (1981). A survey of placebo use in a general hospital. General Hospital Psychiatry, 3, 199–203.

Hofling, C. K. (1955). The place of placebos in medical practice. GP, 11, 103–107.

Hróbjartsson, A. (2002). What are the main methodological problems in the estimation of placebo effects? Journal of Clinical Epidemiology, 55, 430–435.

Hróbjartsson, A., and Gøtzsche, P. C. (2001). Is the placebo powerless? An analysis of clinical trials comparing placebo treatment with no treatment. New England Journal of Medicine, 344, 1594–1602.

Kienle, G. S., and Kiene, H. (1997). The powerful placebo effect: Fact or fiction? Journal of Clinical Epidemiology, 50, 1311–1318.

Lasagna, L. (1986). The placebo effect. Journal of Allergy and Clinical Immunology, 78, 161–164.

Lynøe, N., Mattsson, B., and Sandlund, M. (1993). The attitudes of patients and physicians towards placebo treatment—A comparative study. Social Science and Medicine, 36, 767–774.

Oh, V. M. S. (1994). The placebo effect: Can we use it better? British Medical Journal, 309, 69–70.

Pepper, O. H. P. (1945). A note on the placebo. American Journal of Pharmacy, 17, 409–412.

Rawlinson, M. C. (1985). Truth-telling and paternalism in the clinic: Philosophical reflections on the use of placebos in medical practice. In L. White, B. Tursky, and G. E. Schwartz (Eds.), Placebo: Theory, research, mechanisms (pp. 403–418). New York: Guilford.

Shapiro, A. K., and Struening, E. L. (1973). The use of placebos: A study of ethics and physicians attitudes. *Psychiatry in Medicine*, 4, 17–29.

Thomas, K. B. (1987). General practice consultations: Is there any point in being positive? *British Medical Journal*, 294, 1200–1202.

Thomson, R. J., and Buchanan, W. J. (1982). Placebos and general practice: Attitudes to, and the use of, the placebo effect. *New Zealand Medical Journal*, 95, 492–494.

48

Prescribing "Placebo Treatments"

Results of National Survey of U.S. Internists and Rheumatologists

JON C. TILBURT, EZEKIEL J. EMANUEL, TED J. KAPTCHUK, FARR A. CURLIN, AND FRANKLIN G. MILLER

Jon C. Tilburt, Ezekiel J. Emanuel, Ted J. Kaptchuk, Farr A. Curlin, and Franklin G. Miller, "Prescribing 'Placebo Treatments': Results of National Survey of U.S. Internists and Rheumatologists," BMJ 2008;337:a1938.

Introduction

Before 1960, administration of inert substances to promote placebo effects or to satisfy patients' expectations of receiving a prescribed treatment was commonplace in medical practice.[1-3]

With the development of effective pharmaceutical interventions and the increased emphasis on informed consent, the use of placebo treatments in clinical care has been widely criticised.[4,5] Despite the persistent controversy surrounding the use of placebo treatments, there are few systematic data concerning physicians' attitudes towards and use of placebo treatments in the United States.[6-8] The few contemporary surveys from other countries suggest that more than half of physicians prescribe placebo treatment.[9-11]

To further inform ethical discussions about the appropriateness of recommending placebo treatments, we examined the attitudes and behaviours regarding placebo treatments among a national sample of clinically active internists and rheumatologists in the United States.

Methods

Study Population

Using the 2006 American Medical Association masterfile, we randomly selected 1200 physicians listed with the primary specialties of internal medicine (600) or rheumatology (600): a group of physicians who commonly treat patients with debilitating chronic clinical conditions that are notoriously difficult to manage. In June 2007, an independent survey research firm posted a confidential, self-administered survey, a $20 (£11, €15) incentive, and a letter outlining the voluntary nature of participation. Participants were assured that their identities would not be disclosed to investigators. Those who did not respond to the first survey were sent a second six weeks later. Of the 1200 physicians who were sent questionnaires, 679 responded (overall response rate 57%), of whom 334 specialised in internal medicine (56% response rate) and 345 in rheumatology (58% response rate).

Survey Instrument

The questions on use of placebo treatment were incorporated into a survey that covered other topics related to complementary and alternative medicine. The survey was developed through a formal process and included a review of existing surveys on the use of placebo treatments.[9,12] Because the term "placebo" and behaviours surrounding its use can be contentious, we devised a series of non-judgmental questions beginning with broad questions that avoided the term "placebo" and then gradually gained more specificity, culminating in items whose responses used a clear definition of a "placebo treatment." By constructing a series of items in this manner we allowed respondents to describe their attitudes and experiences as accurately as possible.

The first set of three items began with a hypothetical scenario in which a dextrose tablet was shown in clinical trials to be superior to a no-treatment control group. Respondents were then asked to rate the likelihood of their personally recommending this treatment to non-diabetic patients with fibromyalgia; how often they recommend a therapy "primarily because you believe it will enhance the patient's expectation of getting better"; and whether recommending treatments in this manner was "obligatory," "permissible," "permissible in rare circumstances," or "never permissible." Respondents were then asked to indicate which of several treatments they had used within the past year primarily as a placebo treatment, defined as a treatment whose benefits derive from positive patient expectations and not from the physiological mechanism of the treatment itself; and how they typically described placebo treatments to patients.

Data Management and Analysis

We used descriptive statistics to examine physicians' characteristics as well as frequencies of reported behaviours and attitudes. We used multivariate logistic regression to determine if any characteristics of participants were independently associated with regularly prescribing placebo treatments. For this analysis our dependent variable was recommending treatments "primarily to promote patient expectations" at least two to three times a month based on self-reporting.

Results

The mean age of the 679 respondents was 51 years (range 28–88), 73% (477/652) were men, and 81% (526/648) were white. Overall, respondents most commonly reported a group practice setting (49%, 334/679), followed by solo practice (27%, 186/679), academic (14%, 96/679), and institutional (4%, 28/679). Respondents and non-respondents did not differ significantly according to age, sex, race, practice setting, or specialty.

Table 48.1.

Attitudes and behaviours related to prescribing placebos among 679 US general internists and rheumatologists

Question and Categories of Response	No. (%*)
How likely are you to recommend sugar pill proved to be better than no treatment for fibromyalgia?	
Very likely	160/654 (24)
Moderately likely	221/654 (34)
Unlikely	205/654 (31)
Definitely not	68/654 (10)
How often do you recommend treatment primarily to enhance patient expectation?	
Never	129/646 (20)
≤1/month	219/646 (34)
2–3/month	182/646 (28)
≥1/week	116/646 (18)
Is it appropriate to recommend treatment primarily to promote patients' expectations?	
Obligatory	19/642 (3)
Permissible	380/642 (59)
Permissible only in rare circumstance	197/642 (31)
Never permissible	46/642 (7)

Note: *Based on actual numbers.

Table 48.2.

Treatments used as placebo in past year and how they are described to patients among 679 US general internists and rheumatologists

Question and response items	No. (%*)
Recommended as "placebo treatment" in past year:	
At least one of any type	370/679 (55)
Over-the-counter analgesics	267/648 (41)
Vitamins	243/648 (38)
Sedatives	86/652 (13)
Antibiotics	85/644 (13)
Saline	18/623 (3)
Sugar pills	12/642 (2)
How placebo treatments are typically described to patients:	
Not used	285/637 (45)
Medicine	62/352 (18)
Placebo	18/352 (5)
Medicine with no known effects for your condition	31/352 (9)
Medicine not typically used for your condition but might benefit you	241/352 (68)

Note: *Based on actual numbers of respondents. All 679 respondents answered most questions. Percentages reflect 352 responses of 637 respondents who deemed the question relevant. The 285 respondents who marked "irrelevant—I do not prescribe placebo treatments" were not included in these percentages.

Discussion

Summary of Major Findings

Between 46% and 58% of U.S. internists and rheumatologists engage in recommending placebo treatments as defined. To accurately assess attitudes and behaviours relating to placebo treatments, we asked the physicians about recommending placebo treatments in four distinct ways: response to a hypothetical case, self-reported behaviour without the term "placebo treatment," self-reported behaviour with the term "placebo treatment," and inclusion of "I never use placebo treatments" as a response option in our item related to communication with patients. The first two of these were asked without introducing the term "placebo" to allow the most candid and unbiased responses. The third and fourth were asked after a careful definition of a "placebo treatment." The similar rates across these four different measures indicate that our findings are unlikely to be the result of question framing, wording, or the specific definition of placebo treatment used.

Relation to Other Studies

Our results are consistent with the findings of other studies. Recently, Sherman and Hickner surveyed a convenience sample of 231 academic physicians in the Chicago area and found that 45% had used placebo treatments in clinical practice.[8] Indeed, 8% indicated using placebo treatment more than ten times in the past year. A Danish survey reported that 86% of 545 general practitioners used a placebo treatment at least once within the past year, and 48% reported using placebo

When asked if they would recommend a dextrose tablet for a patient with fibromyalgia if trials had shown such treatment to be superior to no treatment, most respondents (58%, 381/654) said they would be very likely or moderately likely to recommend it. Similarly, 46% (298/646) reported actually recommending a treatment primarily to promote patient expectations at least two to three times a month. The physicians' ethical judgments were also favourable toward the use of placebo treatments, and 62% (399/642) said recommending treatments in this manner was ethically obligatory or permissible (Table 48.1).

Within the previous year, 55% (370/679) of physicians reported having recommended at least one placebo treatment (including "active" and "inactive"). Active placebo treatments were more commonly reported, such as over-the-counter analgesics (41%), vitamins (38%), antibiotics (13%), and sedatives (13%). Only 2% recommended "sugar pills" and 3% saline (Table 48.2).

When asked to describe how they typically introduce placebo treatments to their patients, 45% (285/637) reported never recommending placebo treatments, implying that 55% (352/637) agreed that they had recommended a placebo treatment as defined. Among these 352, about 68% (241) said they usually describe placebo treatments as "a medicine not typically used for your condition but might benefit you," (Table 48.2).

After we controlled for all other characteristics, neither age, sex, race, specialty, practice setting, nor region was independently and significantly associated with having recommended a placebo treatment.

treatments more than ten times in the past year.[12] Smaller surveys from Israel, the UK, Sweden, and New Zealand report similar results.[9–11]

Unresolved Questions

Few of the physicians we surveyed recommend inert placebo treatments. The reasons for this are unclear. It might no longer be possible for physicians to write a prescription for a sugar or bread pill. Without the existence of pharmacies to create such pills, and a lack of actual pills being marketed for such use, physicians could not prescribe them routinely even if they wanted to do so. Or they might have understandable reservations about recommending so called "inactive" or "inert" placebo treatments, fearing these treatments are inherently deceptive and are not amenable to contemporary standards of informed consent.

Yet these data also suggest the desire to promote positive therapeutic expectations among patients is prevalent among the surveyed physicians. The responses suggest a preference for active placebo treatments. Recommending relatively innocuous treatments such as vitamins or over-the-counter analgesics to promote positive expectations might not raise serious concerns about detrimental effects to patients' welfare. Prescribing antibiotics and sedatives when they are not medically indicated, however, could have potentially important adverse consequences for both patients and public health. In the absence of knowing the physicians' indication or motivation for recommending placebo treatments, the interpretation of our findings remains speculative. These issues deserve further investigation.

Limitations

The cross-sectional, self-reported design might not have accurately estimated the actual frequency of recommending placebo treatments. The moderate response rate (57%) also limits our ability to make exact estimates of the behaviour in the entire population of these groups of physicians; and our findings might not be generalisable to attitudes and behaviours in other medical specialties. Furthermore, because these items were included in a survey on complementary and alternative medicine, it is possible that the physicians who chose to respond were more favourably disposed to prescribe placebo treatments than most physicians. However, our findings are consistent with the results of other published studies concerning physicians' use of placebo treatments.

Conclusions

U.S. internists and rheumatologists commonly recommend "placebo treatments." Vitamins and over-the-counter analgesics are the most commonly prescribed. Physicians who use placebo treatments may not be fully transparent with their patients about their use. Whether, or under what circumstances, recommending or prescribing placebo treatments is appropriate remains a topic for ethical and policy debates.

REFERENCES

1 Cabot RC. The use of truth and falsehood in medicine: an experimental study. *Am Med* 1903;5:344–349.
2 Conferences on therapy. The use of placebos in therapy. *N Y State J Med* 1946;17:722–727.
3 Findley F. The placebo and the physician. *Med Clin North Am* 1953;37:1821–1826.
4 Bok S. The ethics of giving placebos. *Sci Am* 1974;231(5):17–23.
5 American Medical Association. *Placebo use in clinical practice*. CEJA Report 2-I-06. Available at: www.ama-assn.org/ama1/pub/upload/mm/369/ceja_recs_2i06.pdf.
6 Goodwin JS, Goodwin JM, Vogel AV. Knowledge and use of placebos by house officers and nurses. *Ann Intern Med* 1979;91:106–110.
7 Berger JT. Placebo medication use in patient care: a survey of medical interns. *West J Med* 1999;170:93–96.
8 Sherman R, Hickner J. Academic physicians use placebos in clinical practice and believe in the mind-body connection. *J Gen Intern Med* 2008;23:7–10.
9 Nitzan U, Lichtenberg P. Questionnaire survey on use of placebo. *BMJ* 2004;329:944–946.
10 Gray G, Flynn P. A survey of placebo use in a general hospital. *Gen Hosp Psychiatry* 1981;3:199–203.
11 Thomson RJ, Buchanan WJ. Placebos and general practice: attitudes to, and the use of, the placebo effect. *N Z Med J* 1982;95:492–494.
12 Hróbjartsson A, Norup M. The use of placebo interventions in medical practice—a national questionnaire survey of Danish clinicians. *Eval Health Prof* 2003;26:153–165.

49
The Ethics of Giving Placebos

SISSELA BOK

Sissela Bok, "The Ethics of Giving Placebos," *Scientific American* 1974;231(5):17–23. (See Sissela Bok's more recent work on the ethics of placebo use: Bok S. *Lying: Moral Choice in Public and Private Life*. New York: Vintage Books, 1999 [1978], pp. 61–68; and, Bok S. Ethical issues in use of placebo in medical practice and clinical trials. In: Guess HA, Kleinman A, Kusek JW, Engel LW (eds.). *The Science of the Placebo: Toward an Interdisciplinary Research Agenda*. London: BMJ Books, 2002, pp. 53–74—eds.)

In 1971 a number of Mexican-American women applied to a family-planning clinic for contraceptives. Some of them were given oral contraceptives and others were given placebos, or dummy pills that looked like the real thing. Without knowing it the women were involved in an investigation of the side effects of various contraceptive pills. Those who were given placebos suffered from a predictable side effect: ten of them became pregnant. Needless to say, the physician in charge did not assume financial responsibility for the babies. Nor did he indicate any concern about having bypassed the "informed consent" that is required in ethical experiments with human beings. He contented himself with the observation that if only the law had permitted it, he could have aborted the pregnant women!

The physician was not unusually thoughtless or hardhearted. The fact is that placebos are so widely prescribed for therapeutic reasons or administered to control groups in experiments, and are considered so harmless, that the fundamental issues they raise are seldom confronted. It appears to me, however, that physicians prescribing placebos cannot consider only the presumed benefit to an individual patient or to an experimental subject at a particular time. They must also take into account the potential risks, both to the patient or the experimental subject and to the medical profession. And the ethical dilemmas that are inherent in the various uses of placebos are central to such an estimate of possible benefits and risks.

The derivation of "placebo," from the Latin for "I shall please," gives the word a benevolent ring, somehow placing placebos beyond moral criticism and conjuring up images of hypochondriacs whose vague ailments are dispelled through adroit prescriptions of beneficent sugar pills. Physicians often give a humorous tinge to instructions for prescribing these substances, which helps to remove them from serious ethical concern. One authority wrote in a pharmacological journal that the placebo should be given a name previously unknown to the patient and preferably Latin and polysyllabic, and "it is wise if it be prescribed with some assurance and emphasis for psychotherapeutic effect. The older physicians each had his favorite placebic prescriptions—one chose tincture of Condurango, another the Fluid-extract of *Cimicifuga nigra*." After all, are not placebos far less dangerous than some genuine drugs? As another physician asked in a letter to *The Lancet*: "Whenever pain can be relieved with two milliliters of saline, why should we inject an opiate? Do anxieties or discomforts that are allayed with starch capsules require administration of a barbiturate, diazepam or propoxyphene?"

Before the 1960s placebos were commonly defined as just such pharmacologically inactive medications as salt water or starch, given primarily to satisfy patients that something is being done for them. It has only gradually become clear that any medical procedure has an implicit placebo effect and, whether it is active or inactive, can serve as a placebo whenever it has no specific effect on the condition for which it is prescribed. Nowadays fewer sugar pills are prescribed, but X rays, vitamin preparations, antibiotics and even surgery can function as placebos. Arthur K. Shapiro defines a placebo as "any therapy (or component of therapy) that is deliberately or knowingly used for its nonspecific, psychologic or psychophysiologic effect, or that . . . , unknown to the patient or therapist, is without specific activity for the condition being treated."

Clearly the prescription of placebos is intentionally deceptive only when the physician himself knows they are without specific effect but keeps the patient in the dark. In considering the ethical issues attending deception with placebos I shall exclude the many procedures in which physicians have had—or still have—misplaced faith; that includes most of the treatments prescribed until this century and a great many still in use but of unproved or even disproved value.

Considering that in the past most therapies had little or no specific effect (yet sometimes succeeded thanks to faith on the part of healers and sufferers) and that we now have more effective remedies, it might be thought that the need to resort to placebos would have decreased. Improved treatment and diagnosis, however, have raised the expectations of patients and health professionals alike and consequently the incidence of reliance on placebos has risen. This is true of placebos given both in experiments and for therapeutic effect.

Modem techniques of experimentation with humans have vastly expanded the role of placebos as controls. New drugs, for example, are compared with placebos in order to distinguish the effects of the drug from chance events or effects associated with the mere administration of the drug. They can be tested in "blind" studies, in which the subjects do not know whether they are receiving the experimental drug or the placebo, and in "double-blind" studies, in which neither the subjects nor the investigators know.

Experiments involving humans are now subjected to increasingly careful safeguards for the people at risk, but it will be a long time before the practice of deceiving experimental subjects with respect to placebos is eradicated. In all the studies of the placebo effect that I surveyed in a study initiated as a fellow of the Interfaculty Program in Medical Ethics at Harvard University, only one indicated that those subjected to the experiment were informed that they would receive placebos; indeed, there was frequent mention of intentional deception. For example, a study titled "An Analysis of the Placebo Effect in Hospitalized Hypertensive Patients" reports that "six patients . . . were asked to accept hospitalization for approximately six weeks . . . to have their hypertension evaluated and to undertake a treatment with a new blood pressure drug . . . . No medication was given for the first five to seven days in the hospital. Placebo was then started."

As for therapeutic administration, there is no doubt that studies conducted in recent decades show placebos can be effective. Henry K. Beecher studied the effects of placebos on patients suffering from conditions including postoperative pain, angina pectoris and the common cold. He estimated that placebos achieved satisfactory relief for about 35 percent of the patients surveyed. Alan Leslie points out, moreover, that "some people are temperamentally impatient and demand results before they normally would be forthcoming. Occasionally, during a period of diagnostic observation or testing, a placebo will provide a gentle sop to their impatience and keep them under control while the important business is being conducted."

A number of other reasons are advanced to explain the continued practice of prescribing placebos. Physicians are acutely aware of the uncertainties of their profession and of how hard it is to give meaningful and correct answers to patients. They also know that disclosing uncertainty or a pessimistic prognosis can diminish benefits that depend on faith and the placebo effect. They dislike being the bearers of uncertain or bad news as much as anyone else. Sitting down to discuss an illness with a patient truthfully and sensitively may take much-needed time away from other patients. Finally, the patient who demands unneeded medication or operations may threaten to go to a more co-operative doctor or to resort to self-medication; such patient pressure is one of the most potent forces perpetuating and increasing the resort to placebos.

There are no conclusive figures for the extent to which placebos are prescribed but clearly their use is widespread: Thorough studies have estimated that as many as 35 to 45 percent of all prescriptions are for substances that are incapable of having an effect on the condition for which they are prescribed. Kenneth L. Melmon and Howard F. Morrelli, in their textbook *Clinical Pharmacology*, cite a study of treatment for the common cold as indicating that 31 percent of the patients received a prescription for a broad-spectrum or medium-spectrum antibiotic, 22 percent received penicillin and 6 percent received sulfonamides—"none of which could possibly have any beneficial specific pharmacological effect on the viral infection per se." They point out further that thousands of doses of vitamin B-12 are administered every year "at considerable expense to patients without pernicious anemia," the only condition for which the vitamin is specifically indicated.

In view of all of this it is remarkable that medical textbooks provide little analysis of placebo treatment. In a sample of nineteen popular recent textbooks in medicine, pediatrics, surgery, anesthesia, obstetrics and gynecology only three even mention placebos, and none of them deal with either the medical or the ethical dilemmas placebos present. Four out of six textbooks on pharmacology consider placebos, but with the exception of the book by Melmon and Morrelli they mention only the experimental role of placebos and are completely silent on ethical issues. Finally, four out of eight standard texts on psychiatry refer to placebos, again without ever mentioning ethical issues.

Yet little thought is required to see the dilemma placebos should pose for physicians. A placebo can provide a potent, although unreliable, weapon against suffering, but the very manner in which it can relieve suffering seems to depend on keeping the patient in the dark. The dilemma is an ethical one, reflecting contrary views about how human beings ought to deal with each other, an apparent conflict between helping patients and informing them about their condition.

This dilemma is pointed up by the concept of informed consent: the idea that the individual has the right to give prior consent to, and even to refuse, what is proposed to him in the way of medical care. The doctrine is recognized in proliferating "bills of rights" for patients. The one recommended by the American Hospital Association states, for example, that the patient has the right to complete, understandable information on his diagnosis, treatment and prognosis; the right to whatever information is needed so that he can give informed consent to any treatment; the right to refuse treatment to the extent permitted by law.

Few physicians appear to consider the implications of informed consent when they prescribe placebos, however. One reason is surely that the usefulness of a placebo may be destroyed if informed consent is sought, since its success is assumed to depend specifically on the patient's ignorance and suggestibility. Then too the substances employed as placebos have been considered so harmless, and at the same time so potentially beneficial, that it is easy to assume that the lack of consent cannot possibly matter. In any case health professionals in general have not considered the possibility that the prescription of a placebo is so intrinsically misleading as to make informed consent impossible.

Some authorities have argued that there need not be any deception at all. Placebos can be described in such a way that no outright verbal lie is required. For example: "I believe these pills may help you." Lawrence J. Henderson went so far as to maintain that "it is meaningless to speak of telling the truth, the whole truth and nothing but the truth to a patient . . . because it is . . . a sheer impossibility . . . . Since telling the truth is impossible, there can be no sharp distinction between what is false and what is true."

Can one really think of prescribing placebos as not being deceptive at all as long as the words are sufficiently vague? In order to answer this question it is necessary to consider the nature of deception. When someone intentionally deceives another person, he causes that person to believe what is false. Such deception may be verbal, in which case it is a lie, or it may be nonverbal, conveyed by gestures, false visual cues or the myriad other means human beings have devised for misleading one another. What is common to all intentional deception is the intent to deceive and the providing of misleading information, whether that information is verbal or nonverbal.

The statement that a placebo may help a patient is not a lie or even, in itself, deceitful. Yet the circumstances in which a placebo is prescribed introduce an element of deception. The setting in a doctor's office or hospital room, the impressive terminology, the mystique of the all-powerful physician prescribing a cure—all of these tend to give the patient faith in the remedy; they convey the impression that the treatment prescribed will have the ingredients necessary to improve the patient's condition. The actions of the physician are therefore deceptive even if the words are so general as not to be lies. Verbal deception may be more direct, but all kinds of deception can be equally misleading.

The view that merely withholding information is not deceptive is particularly inappropriate in the case of placebo prescriptions because information that is material and important is withheld. The crucial fact that the physician may not know what the patient's problems are is not communicated. Information concerning the prognosis is vague and information about the specific way in which the treatment may affect the condition is not provided. Henderson's view fails to make the distinction between such relevant information, which it is usually feasible to provide, and infinite details of decreasing importance, which to be sure can never be provided with any completeness. It also fails to distinguish between two ways in which the information reaching the patient may be altered: it may be withheld or it may be distorted. Often the two are mingled. Consider the intertwining of distortion, mystification and failure to inform in the following statement, made to unsuspecting recipients of placebos in an experiment performed in a psychiatric outpatient clinic: "You are to receive a test that all patients receive as part of their evaluation. The test medication is a nonspecific autonomous nervous system stimulant."

Even those who recognize that placebos are deceptive often dispel any misgivings with the thought that they involve no serious deception. Placebos are regarded as being analogous to the innocent white lies of everyday life, so trivial as to be quite outside the realm of ethical evaluation. Such liberties with language as telling someone that his necktie is beautiful or that a visit has been a pleasure, when neither statement reflects the speaker's. honest opinion, are commonly accepted as being so trivial that to evaluate them morally would seem unduly fastidious and, from a utilitarian point of view, unjustified. Placebos are not trivial, however. Spending for them runs into millions of dollars. Patients incur greater risks of discomfort and harm than is commonly understood. Finally, any placebo uses that are in fact trivial and harmless in themselves may combine to form nontrivial practices, so that repeated reliance on placebos can do serious harm in the long run to the medical profession and the general public.

Consider first the cost to patients. A number of the procedures undertaken for their placebo effect are extremely costly in terms of available resources and of expense, discomfort and risk of harm to patients. Many temporarily successful new surgical procedures owe their success to the placebo effect alone. In such cases there is no intention to deceive the patient; physician and patient alike are deceived. On occasion, however, surgery is deliberately performed as a placebo measure. Children may undergo appendectomies or tonsillectomies that are known to be unnecessary simply to give the impression that powerful measures are being taken or because parents press for the operation. Hysterectomies and other operations may be performed on adults for analogous reasons. A great many diagnostic procedures that are known to be unnecessary are undertaken to give patients a sense that efforts are being made on their behalf. Some of these carry risks; many involve discomfort and the expenditure of time and money. The potential for damage by an active drug given as a placebo is similarly clear-cut. Calvin M. Kunin, Thelma Tupasi and William A. Craig have described the ill effects—including death—suffered by hospital patients as a result of excessive prescription of antibiotics, more than half of which they found had been unneeded, inappropriately selected or given in incorrect dosages.

Even inactive placebos can have toxic effects in a substantial proportion of cases; nausea, dermatitis, hearing loss, headache, diarrhea and other symptoms have been cited. Stewart Wolf reported on a double-blind experiment to test the effects of the drug mephenesin and a placebo on disorders associated with anxiety and tension. Depending on the symptom studied, roughly 20 to 30 percent of the patients were better while taking the pills and 50 to 70 percent were unchanged, but 10 to 20 percent were worse—"whether the patient was taking mephenesin or placebo." A particularly serious possible side effect of even a harmless substance is dependency. In one case a psychotic patient was given placebo pills and told they were a "new major tranquilizer without any side effects." After four years she was taking 12 tablets a day and complaining of insomnia and anxiety. After the self-medication reached 25 pills a day and a crisis had occurred, the physician intervened, talked over the addictive problem (but not the deception) with the patient and succeeded in reducing the dose to two a day, a level that was still being maintained a year later. Other cases have been reported of patients becoming addicted or habituated to these substances to the point of not being able to function without them, at times even requiring that they be stepped up to very high dosages.

Most obvious, of course, is the damage done when placebos are given in place of a well-established therapy that is clearly indicated for the patient's condition. The Mexican-American women I mentioned at the outset, for example, were actually harmed by being given placebo pills in the guise of contraceptive pills. In 1966 Beecher, in an article on the ethics of experiments with human subjects, documented a case in which 109 servicemen with streptococcal respiratory infections were given injections of a placebo instead of injections of penicillin, which was already known to prevent the development of rheumatic fever in such patients and which was being given to a larger group of patients. Two of the placebo subjects developed rheumatic fever and one developed an acute kidney infection, whereas such complications did not occur in the penicillin-treated group.

There have been a number of other experiments in which patients suffering from illnesses with known cures have been given placebos in order to study the course of the illness when it is untreated or to determine the precise effectiveness of the known therapy in another group of patients. Because of the very nature of their aims the investigators have failed to ask subjects for their informed consent. The subjects have tended to be those least able to object or defend themselves: members of minority groups, the poor, the institutionalized and the very young.

A final type of harm to patients given placebos stems not so much from the placebo itself as from the manipulation and deception that accompany its prescription. Inevitably some patients find out that they have been duped. They may then lose confidence in physicians and in bona fide medication, which they may need in the future. They may even resort on their own to more harmful drugs or other supposed cures. That is a danger associated with all deception: its discovery leads to a failure of trust when trust may be most needed. Alternatively, some people who do not discover the deception and are left believing that a placebic remedy works may continue to rely on it under the wrong circumstances. This is particularly true with respect to drugs, such as antibiotics, that are used sometimes for their specific action and sometimes as placebos. Many parents, for example, come to believe they must ask for the prescription of antibiotics every time their child has a fever.

The major costs associated with placebos may not be the costs to patients themselves that I have discussed up to this point. Rather they may be costs to new categories of patients in the future, to physicians who do not abuse placebo treatment and to society in general.

Deceptive practices, by their very nature, tend to escape the normal restraints of accountability and so can spread more easily. There are many instances in which an innocuous-seeming practice has grown to become a large-scale and more dangerous one; warnings against "the entering wedge" are often rhetorical devices but may sometimes be justified when there are great pressures to move along the undesirable path and when the safeguards against undesirable developments are insufficient. In this perspective there is reason for concern about placebos. The safeguards are few or nonexistent against a practice that is secretive by its very nature. And there are ever stronger pressures—from drug companies, patients eager for cures and busy physicians—for more medication, whether it is needed or not. Given such pressures the use of placebos can spread along a number of dimensions.

The clearest danger lies in the gradual shift from pharmacologically inert placebos to more active ones. It is not always easy to distinguish completely inert substances from somewhat active ones and these in turn from more active ones. It may be hard to distinguish between a quantity of an active substance so low that it has little or no effect and quantities that have some effect. It is not always clear to physicians whether patients require an inert placebo or possibly a more active one, and there can be the temptation to resort to an active one just in case it might also have a specific effect. It is also much easier to deceive a patient with a medication that is known to be "real" and to have power. One recent textbook in medicine goes so far as to advocate the use of small doses of effective compounds as placebos rather than inert substances—because it is important for both the doctor and the patient to believe in the treatment! The fact that the dangers and side effects of active agents are not always known or considered important by the physician is yet another factor contributing to the shift from innocuous placebos to active ones.

Meanwhile the number of patients receiving placebos increases as more and more people seek and receive medical care and as their desire for instant, push-button alleviation of symptoms is stimulated by drug advertising and by rising expectations of what "science" can do. Reliance on placebic therapy in turn strengthens the belief that there really is a pill or some other kind of remedy for every ailment. As long ago as 1909 Richard C. Cabot wrote, in a perceptive paper on the subject of truth and deception in medicine: "The majority of placebos are given because we believe the patient . . . has learned to expect medicine for every symptom, and without it he simply won't get well. True, but who taught him to expect a medicine for every symptom? He was not born with that expectation . . . . It is we physicians who are responsible for perpetuating false ideas about disease and its cure . . . . With every placebo that we give we do our part in perpetuating error, and harmful error at that."

A particularly troubling aspect of the spread of placebos is that it now affects so many children. Parents increasingly demand pills, such as powerful stimulants, to modify their children's behavior with a minimum of effort on their part; there are some children who may need such medication but many receive it without proper diagnosis. As I have mentioned, parents demand antibiotics even when told they are unnecessary, and physicians may give in to the demands. In these cases the very meaning of "placebo" has shifted subtly from "I shall please the patient" to "I shall please the patient's parents."

Deception by placebo can also spread from therapy and diagnosis to experimental applications. Although placebos can be given nondeceptively in experimentation, someone who is accustomed to prescribing placebos therapeutically without consent may not take the precaution of obtaining such consent when he undertakes an experiment on human subjects. Yet therapeutic deception is at least thought to be for the patient's own good, whereas experimental deception may not benefit the subject and may actually harm him; even the paternalistic excuse that the investigator is deceiving the patient for his own good then becomes inapplicable.

Finally, acceptance of placebos can encourage other kinds of deception in medicine such as failure to reveal to a patient the risks connected with an operation, or lying to terminally ill patients. Medicine lends itself with particular ease to deception for benevolent reasons because physicians are so clearly more knowledgeable than their patients and the patients are so often in a weakened or even irrational state. As Melvin Levine has put it, "the medical profession has practiced as if the truth is, in fact, a kind of therapeutic instrument [that] . . . can be altered or given in small doses . . . [or] not used at all when deemed detrimental to the patients . . . . Many physicians have utilized truth distortion as a kind of anesthetic to promote comfort and ease treatment." Such practices are presumably for the good of patients. No matter how cogent and benevolent the reasons for resorting to deception may seem, when those reasons are considered in secret, without the consent of the doctored, they tend to be reinforced by less benevolent pressures, self-deception begins to blur nice distinctions and occasions for giving misleading information multiply.

Because of all these ways in which placebo usage can spread it is impossible to look at each incident of manipulation in isolation. There are no water-tight compartments in medicine. When the costs and benefits of any therapeutic, diagnostic or experimental procedure are weighed, not only the individual consequences but also the cumulative ones must be taken into account. Reports of deceptive practices inevitably filter out, and the resulting suspicion is heightened by the anxiety that threats to health always create. And so even the health professionals who do not mislead their patients are injured by those who do and the entire institution of medicine is threatened by practices lacking in candor, however harmless the results may appear to be in some individual cases.

What should be the profession's attitude with regard to placebos? In the case of most experimental applications there are ways of avoiding deception without abandoning placebo controls. Subjects can be informed of the nature of the experiment and of the fact that placebos will be administered; if they then consent to the experiment, the use of placebos cannot be considered surreptitious. Although the subjects in a blind or double-blind experiment will not know exactly when they are receiving placebos or even whether they are receiving them, the initial consent to the experimental design, including placebos, removes the ethical problems having to do with deception. If, on the other hand, there are experiments of such a nature that asking subjects for their informed consent to the use of placebos would invalidate the results or cause too many subjects to decline, then the experiment ought not to be performed and the desired knowledge should be sought by means of a different research design.

As for the diagnostic and therapeutic use of placebos, we must start with the presumption that it is undesirable. By and large, given the principle of informed consent as well as concern for human integrity, no measures that affect someone's health should be undertaken without explanation and permission. Placebos are not so trivial as to be unworthy of ethical evaluation; they carry a definite possibility of harm and discomfort to patients as well as high collective costs; as a result placebo prescriptions present a more serious inroad on patient decision making than has been appreciated up to now. Surreptitious diagnostic and therapeutic administration of placebos should therefore be ruled out whenever possible.

The prohibition should not be absolute, however. In some cases the balance of benefit over cost is so overwhelming that reasonable people would choose to be deceived. There is no clear formula that will quickly reveal in each case whether the benefits will greatly outweigh the possible harm. Much of the problem can be avoided if care is taken to avoid placebos if possible and to observe the following principles in the remaining cases: (1) Placebos should be used only after a careful diagnosis; (2) no active placebos should be employed, merely inert ones; (3) no outright lie should be told and questions should be answered honestly; (4) placebos should never be given to patients who have asked not to receive them;

(5) placebos should never be used when other treatment is clearly called for or all possible alternatives have not been weighed.

If placebo medicine is to be thus limited, the information provided to both medical personnel and patients will have to change radically. Placebos, so often resorted to and yet so rarely mentioned, will have to be discussed from scientific as well as ethical points of view during medical training. Textbooks will have to confront the medical and ethical dilemmas analytically and exhaustively. Similarly, much education must be provided for the public. There must be greater stress on the autonomy of the patient and on his right to consent to treatment or to refuse treatment after being informed of its nature. Understanding of the normal courses of illnesses should be stressed, including the fact that most minor conditions clear up by themselves rather quickly. The great pressure patients exert for more medication must be countered by limitations on drug advertising and by information concerning the side effects and dangers of drugs.

I have tried to show that the benevolent deception exemplified by placebos is widespread, that it carries risks not usually taken into account, that it represents an inroad on informed consent, that it damages the institution of medicine and contributes to the erosion of confidence in medical personnel.

Honesty may not be the highest social value; at exceptional times, when survival is at stake, it may have to be set aside. To permit a widespread practice of deception, however, is to set the stage for abuses and growing mistrust. Augustine, considering the possibility of giving official sanction to white lies, pointed out that "little by little and bit by bit this will grow and by gradual accessions will slowly increase until it becomes such a mass of wicked lies that it will be utterly impossible to find any means of resisting such a plague grown to huge proportions through small additions."

50
The Lie That Heals
The Ethics of Giving Placebos

HOWARD BRODY

Howard Brody, "The Lie That Heals: The Ethics of Giving Placebos," *Annals of Internal Medicine* 1982;97:112–118.

The debate over whether it is ethical for physicians to prescribe placebos for patients has surfaced at intervals in the medical literature since the 19th century. Because traditional oaths and codes of ethics are silent on this issue, physicians taking a stand on placebo use have been unable to appeal to authority and have been prompted to develop original and often highly creative moral arguments. Although these arguments deserve review simply as an often-neglected feature of medical history, they also require critical reexamination in light of two recent developments. The first is the awakening of experimental interest in the placebo effect, and a gradual reconceptualization of placebo phenomena to recognize their pervasiveness as part of medical practice (1). The second is the emphasis in contemporary medical ethics of individual rights and patient autonomy in the doctor-patient relationship (2–4), leading to the rejection of many paternalistic assumptions previously thought to justify medical deception (5).

Placebos and the Placebo Effect

"An empiric oftentimes, and a silly chirurgeon, doth more strange cures than a rational physician . . . because the patient puts his confidence in him," Robert Burton wrote in 1628 (6), showing that at least by Renaissance times physicians appreciated the power of the imagination and expectation to change bodily states and to cure disease. In 1785 Benjamin Franklin led a commission to investigate Mesmer's animal magnetism and, in a series of elegant experiments, showed that the subjects' imagination was the most important factor in explaining the bizarre effects and miraculous cures attributed to that practice (7). Physicians were not reluctant to take advantage of this phenomenon by prescribing medications thought to be pharmacologically inert when no specific remedy was indicated. Thomas Jefferson wrote to Dr. Casper Wistar in 1807, "One of the most successful physicians I have ever known, has assured me, that he used more of bread pills, drops of colored water, and powders of hickory ashes, than of all other medicines put together" (8).

The contemporary era of placebo research began with the adoption of the double-blind controlled trial as the standard experimental method in the 1940s; subsequent findings on the placebo effect have been reviewed extensively (1,9–13). Whenever a supposedly inert treatment is used in an experimental situation, 30% to 40% of subjects can be expected to show some benefit from the placebo treatment (9). The pattern of the response to placebo typically resembles the pharmacologic findings of active drug responses (14). In one study of the effect of both clofibrate and placebo on cholesterol level and cardiovascular mortality, those control subjects who reliably took their placebos showed lower cholesterol and reduced mortality compared with their less compliant counterparts (15). Placebo response is not limited to the patient's subjective experience; placebos alter laboratory values and other measures of objective physiologic change (16). Although placebos are commonly thought of primarily as pain relievers, virtually all potentially reversible symptoms and diseases that have been investigated in double-blind studies show some response to placebo—including diabetes (17), angina pectoris (18), and malignant neoplasms (19). Placebos can also cause many of the same side effects seen with active medication (20,21). For all these reasons it is impossible to use placebo response to distinguish between a real, organic symptom and a symptom that is "all in the patient's head," although the myth to the contrary still persists (22).

From an early focus on attempting to elucidate the "personality type" of persons who react to placebos (which failed in part because the same person may respond or fail to respond to placebo in different circumstances [9]), attempts to understand placebo phenomena have shifted to a broader approach to factors in the doctor-patient relationship, in the overall situational context, and in the cultural background (23–29). It has become more clear that whatever happens when a patient gets better after ingesting a sugar pill also happens to some degree whenever the patient receives a pharmacologically potent treatment within a supportive healing relationship; that at least some of the symptom relief that follows administration of the active treatment arises from emotional and symbolic factors. That is, the placebo effect pervades much of medical practice even when no placebo has been used.

For example, when meprobamate, phenobarbital, and placebo were administered blindly to anxious patients, the two pharmacologically active drugs were clearly superior to placebo when administered by a physician who had confidence in the drugs' efficacy and who was viewed by the subjects as supportive; the drugs and placebo showed no difference when administered by a less supportive and more skeptical physician. Subjects of the first physician also showed more overall symptom relief (30). It is reasonable to suspect, then, that when the family physician prescribes decongestants for a viral upper Respiratory infection, some of the patient's symptom relief is due to the pharmacologic action of the drug, but some is also due to the emotional support of the doctor-patient relationship, the doctor's confirmation and legitimization of the illness, and the reassurance that the symptoms do not represent something more serious than a bad cold.

Definitions

The expanded concept of the placebo effect just described makes it undesirable to have the definition of "placebo effect" totally dependent on the definition of "placebo." The following definitions may serve satisfactorily for our purposes: The placebo effect is the change in the patient's condition that is attributable to the symbolic import of the healing intervention rather than to the intervention's specific pharmacologic or physiologic effects; a placebo is a form of medical therapy, or an intervention designed to simulate medical therapy, that is believed to be without specific activity for the condition being treated, and that is used either for its symbolic effect or to eliminate observer bias in a controlled experiment. It is worth recalling here that although the sugar pill is cited as the paradigm case of placebo use, any medical treatment, including such diverse techniques as surgery (31) and biofeedback (32), can function as a placebo.

Another useful distinction uses the terms "pure" and "impure" placebos. A pure placebo, such as a lactose pill or a saline injection, is totally without pharmacologic potency. An impure placebo has some pharmacologic properties, but these are not relevant to the current circumstances and the treatment is used solely for its psychologic effect. Common examples are thyroid, vitamin B12, and penicillin, when used in patients who do not have hypothyroidism, pernicious anemia, or bacterial infections, respectively.

Placebos and Deception

Jefferson said of the use of bread pills and drops of colored water in 1807, "It was certainly a pious fraud" (8). Subsequent writers, including physicians, philosophers, and scientists, have adopted widely divergent positions on the ethics of giving placebos (33). All authorities, however, are agreed on one point—if there is an ethical problem in therapeutic use of placebos, the problem is that of deception. This agreement in turn arises from a shared assumption about how placebos are typically used in clinical practice, which will be called here the "traditional use" of placebos. In the traditional use, the physician administers a treatment known to him or her to be without pharmacologic potency; but the physician either tells or allows the patient to believe that the treatment has such potency. It is further assumed in the traditional-use model that the patient's false belief in the potency of the treatment is essential for the placebo effect to occur (34–36).

Enough has already been said about the recently expanded concept of the placebo effect to call the traditional-use model into question on several counts. However, the bulk of the medical literature on the ethics of placebos accepts this model as a given. Hence, to do justice to most of the arguments offered by physicians for and against placebo use, the traditional-use model must form the point of departure. In a subsequent section, the ethical position that results from replacing the traditional model with the expanded concept will be considered.

It will be most convenient to survey first the arguments offered against placebo use, as these assume that deception is generally wrong, and that it is just as wrong (if indeed not worse) when encountered in medicine as when encountered elsewhere in life. Next, arguments in favor of placebo use can be investigated to see how successfully they defuse the deception issue.

Arguments against Placebos

It is standard in modern writings on medical ethics to oppose placebo use because it represents a specific instance of the more general issue of patient deception (2,3,5,37,38). The value of avoiding deception is grounded in the more basic values of the autonomy and dignity of the individual patient. The basic idea is that of moral reciprocity. We generally wish that other people treat us in a manner that shows their respect for us as persons; and this entails that they not use manipulation or deception on us, even if they judge the results to be for our own good. If we are to regard our patients as our moral equals and to respect their dignity as persons, we are similarly prohibited from practicing deception or manipulation on them.

This line of reasoning is most at home in the context of a deontologic or duty-based ethical theory. Deception is condemned because it violates an a priori moral rule—a priori because the rule appeals to the very nature of our beings (that is, persons deserving respect) rather than to the good or bad consequences of our actions. Appeal to duty and to moral rule has always been a popular mode of argument. Thus one medical editor (39) wrote in 1885, "physicians . . . cannot always tell the plain truth to a patient without injuring him. It should be the rule of . . . life, however, to be straightforward and candid. Therefore, we say that placebos should be . . . rarely, if ever; prescribed." Describing the characteristics of the trustworthy and virtuous physician, the writer concluded, "We venture to say that such a man would not find it necessary to keep a polychromatic assortment of sugar pills in his closet."

This commentator explicitly rejects an argument from consequences—at times, indeed, being truthful may injure patients. But more basic than negative consequences is the a priori "rule of . . . life," which in the 19th century was closely tied to concepts of virtue and gentlemanly conduct, and hence truthfulness.

Other physicians, however, have been uncomfortable with a priori appeals and have preferred a utilitarian mode of argument, demanding to be shown that placebo use, generally applied, would lead to a net increase in unhappiness over happiness for all concerned. Among many adopting a utilitarian stand, the most articulate and forceful was Richard C. Cabot, best known today as originator of the clinicopathologic conferences of the Massachusetts General Hospital, but in his day an innovative writer on medical ethics as well as on medicine, and holder of the Chair of Social Ethics at Harvard University in addition to his medical appointment (40). Cabot (41) rejected an a priori approach to issues of truth and falsehood—"you will notice I am not now arguing that a lie is, in itself and apart from its consequences, a bad thing"—but felt that the negative consequences of placebo use condemned the practice. The obvious short-range consequence occurred when the patient discovered the deception and lost trust in the physician. True, it was probable in any single case that the physician would not be found out; but Cabot (41) rejoined, "Is it good for us as professional men to have our reputations rest on the expectation of not being found out?"

But Cabot (41) was much more concerned about the long-range consequences of creating unhealthy public attitudes toward medicine and medications:

> The majority of placebos are given because we believe that the patient will not be satisfied without them. He has learned to expect medicine for every symptom and without it he simply won't get well. True, but who taught him to expect a medicine for every symptom? He was not born with that expectation. He learned it from an ignorant doctor who really believed it. . . . It is we physicians who are responsible for perpetuating false

ideas about disease and its cure . . . and with every placebo that we give we do our part in perpetuating error, and harmful error at that.

Cabot elsewhere (42) stated even more bluntly, "Placebo giving is quackery." He concluded (41) that in general the negative consequences of placebo use outweighed the positive; but that placebos could be justified in some rare cases:

> No patient whose language you can speak, whose mind you can approach, needs a placebo. I give placebos now and then . . . to Armenians and others with whom I cannot communicate, because to refuse to give them would create more misunderstandings, a falser impression, than to give them. The patient will think that I am refusing to treat him at all; but if I can get hold of an interpreter and explain the matter, I tell him no lies in the shape of placebos.

Another more recent commentator reflected on both the occasional justification for giving placebos, and the rarity with which such a case ought to arise: "Some patients are so unintelligent, neurotic, and inadequate as to be incurable, and life is made easier for them by a placebo." Then, paraphrasing an earlier commentator (43), he concluded: "It has been said that the use of placebos is in inverse ratio to the combined intelligences of patient and doctor" (44).

In assessing the consequences of placebo use as a general policy, one should note the tendency of deception to multiply itself, and the need to cover up for the original lie. Prescribing placebos now involves ensuring the complicity of the nurse, the pharmacist, and all other parties to the prescription. There is also the problem of setting a fee for the placebo prescription—if too high, then someone will appear to be making an unjustified profit from deception; if too low, the deception may inadvertently be discovered. It may be more for such mundane reasons and not out of any increased ethical insight that the use of totally inert medicines like lactose pills has declined once physicians stopped dispensing their own drugs. In more recent times, fear of lawsuits may also have played a role.

Arguments for Placebos

Deceptive or not, placebos have in fact been widely administered by practicing physicians, and to many the fascinating power of the body to respond to purely symbolic interventions seemed too potent a therapeutic tool to pass up. A number of commentators have tried to give a formal justification for placebo use. Once again, two general moral approaches have been used. For the deontologist, the force of the moral rule against deception cannot be denied; so it must be argued either that the deception rule does not properly apply to the placebo case, or that other moral rules may mitigate it. The utilitarian may calculate all the good consequences attributable to placebos, and argue (or assume) that these outweigh the evils of deception. For each of these attempts at justification, however, the placebo opponents have had a ready and generally persuasive reply.

First, one may forthrightly deny that placebo use need involve deception by the physician. This position, while occasionally alluded to (45), is seldom stated explicitly in the medical literature; but it is frequently encountered in debate and discussion among physicians. It is usually argued that if the physician tells the patient that a sugar pill is morphine or penicillin, he is guilty of an outright and unethical lie. But if he administers the pill with a noncommittal statement, such as, "This pill will make you feel much better," he has not deceived the patient; any false beliefs result from the patient's deceiving himself and are not the moral responsibility of the physician: "should a patient become suspicious . . . , the therapist need only give an honest evasion, rather than a lie" (36).

Richard Cabot (41) attacked this and other arguments defending medical practices that mislead the patient by stating, "a true impression, not certain words literally true, is what we must try to convey." By way of fleshing out Cabot's objection, it may be acknowledged that what counts as deception may be dependent on the norms and expectations associated with particular social settings. For instance, when we go to the theater and see Mark Twain reading from Huckleberry Finn, we do not consider ourselves to have been deceived when we discover he is a cleverly made-up actor. We may then ask whether the clinical setting is one of those special social situations where creating a false impression by deliberate misdirection does not count as deception. Cabot appears to have assumed that a patient may reasonably expect in that setting that, if a drug or other treatment is given, it is selected for its pharmacologic potency for the patient's condition. It also seems reasonable to assume that the patient will not expect that the physician will specifically name the treatment—the patient is accustomed to receiving pills alluded to by the physician merely as "an antibiotic" or "a decongestant," but these remedies are still assumed by the patient to be pharmacologically potent. One may then conclude that if the physician prescribes an inert pill and conceals this from the patient by verbal misdirection, he has violated these legitimate patient expectations and is guilty of deception; the special nature of the clinical setting gives no license for creating a false impression in this manner.

Legal backing (46) for Cabot's argument comes with the characterization of the physician-patient relationship as a fiduciary one, in which one party assumes a special responsibility to look out for the best interests of the other. "Where a person sustains toward others a relation of trust and confidence, his silence when he should speak, or his failure to disclose what he ought to disclose, is as much a fraud in law as an actual affirmative false representation" (47).

Still, the physician is not responsible for false beliefs the patient may bring into the encounter, if the physician has taken no action to cause those beliefs (48,49); how far the physician's duty extends to dispel those false beliefs, if they do not lead directly to health-threatening behavior, is an interesting ethical question in itself. What is the physician's duty toward the patient who arrives with a firmly entrenched belief in the therapeutic and preventive powers of vitamins, and asks the physician to recommend a good daily vitamin supplement? This patient harbors a false belief, and energetic and prolonged discussion from the physician might mitigate or dispel it. But this reeducation seems hardly worth the effort, given the low probability of harm and the (presumed) low readiness of the patient to assimilate the new information. Thus the postulated duty not to create false beliefs in the patient by one's words or actions need not imply a more onerous duty to seek out and dispel all the false beliefs the patient may have acquired elsewhere.

Second, the placebo advocate may admit that placebos as traditionally used involve deception, but still insist that this use is ethically justified. Social practice recognizes a class of deceptions called white lies, which are felt to be essentially harmless because of their innocuous content and benign motivation (50). Even if the special circumstances of medical practice do not automatically permit out-and-out deception, it still seems to be the case that many partial truths or euphemisms are appropriate. For example, proper supportive care of the cancer patient seeking some hope to mitigate the frightening diagnosis calls for a somewhat slanted presentation emphasizing the potential gains from therapy, not merely for a listing of the 5-year survival statistics.

But a problem in including placebos in the category of white lies is that what counts as a white lie is fairly well demarcated by social convention; otherwise anyone uttering a falsehood, however blatant, could excuse his act by claiming it was "only a white lie." Members of society are thus in effect forewarned about this practice and, if they choose to ask their friends how their new hats or ties look on them, they can be said to have given at least implied consent to any white lie that results. By contrast, the traditional-use model assumes that knowledge of the lie will be restricted to the medical profession, lest placebos lose their effectiveness with wider publicity. Recipients of the so-called white lie are therefore systematically excluded from any knowledge of the existence of this practice, and they have no opportunity to challenge questionable uses of placebo deception by reference to generally accepted social norms and limits. This would make placebo use morally suspect in a way that the usual white lies are not.

Leslie (51) attempted to justify placebo deception in a similar fashion: "There is a fine line of distinction between the words, *deception* and *deceit* . . . deceit implies blameworthiness whereas deception does not necessarily do so . . ." Leslie emphasized the benign intent of the physician and offered as an analogy a magician practicing sleight of hand to entertain an audience. But Bok (50) has emphasized that the supposedly benign intent of the person doing the lying, and the expected value of the resulting benefits, often look very different from the perspective of the person being lied to. The audience choosing voluntarily to witness the magician's performance can weigh for themselves the degree of deception, the intent, and the value of the benefits; the patient in

the traditional-use model of placebos is denied this opportunity. (It may in fact be argued that the magic show is not "deception" at all, as any reasonably well informed person knows what goes on at such events and is not fooled in any substantive way.) Thus, Leslie is either merely asserting that some deceptions are justified and others are not, without giving any arguments to prove that placebos belong in the justified category; or else his "fine line" between deception and deceit is so fine as to escape attention altogether.

All this discussion of justified and unjustified deception, however, may seem pointless to the pragmatic physician who adopts the traditional use of placebos merely because it can benefit the patient. By this pragmatic view, either the physician's duty not to deceive is of no moral concern at all, or else it is far outweighed by the much stronger duty to benefit the patient—a duty which, Veatch (38) has argued, has dominated the so-called Hippocratic ethical tradition in medicine to the unwarranted exclusion of other, equally rational moral considerations. This view has gained added impetus since the recent wave of research described above, showing the extent and frequency of placebo responses. The pragmatic approach has been further bolstered by research linking the placebo response to endorphins (52). Because endorphins function primarily in analgesia, and because, as was noted above, the placebo response is not limited to pain, this endorphin research really provides a very limited account of the physiologic means by which placebos may exert their effects. But to the uncritical medical mind, the identified biochemical basis for some placebo responses has somehow made the whole placebo issue suddenly respectable. (Shapiro [53] discovered in an informal survey that negativism toward placebo use among physicians correlated with greater age, private rather than academic practice, and nonparticipation in clinical research.)

In this setting, the placebo advocate may attribute, rightly or wrongly, several false beliefs to the person who argues against placebo use. The opponent of placebos may be thought to believe: that placebos really do not work, or work only for a limited number of medical conditions; that some pharmacologically active remedy exists for all conditions, so that the doctor who prescribes a placebo is automatically withholding the "correct" drug; or that any treatment that works by psychologic mechanisms is thereby inferior to a treatment that works by biochemical means. As we saw, ethical concern over placebos does not depend on any of these false assumptions, yet placebo opponents are still sometimes labeled as if their arguments ran contrary to modern scientific medicine. It may have been a mistaken attribution of these false beliefs that led a distinguished investigator of the placebo response (54) to characterize as "oft-quoted but fatuous" one of the better recent papers (55) offering arguments of the sort first used by Cabot.

One could, of course, offer a utilitarian counter-attack to Cabot (41) and contend that he had miscalculated the likelihood and the Severity of the various consequences of placebo use. But any balanced view of the pros and cons makes this a remote possibility. First, if past studies are reliable, only 30% to 40% of patients will respond to placebo positively. Second, even though lactose can be expected to have fewer toxic effects than active drugs, placebo side effects and even addiction do periodically occur. Finally, even if one rejects these considerations, one is still left with the long-range consequences Cabot predicted—a public conditioned to look for the cure for all ills in a bottle of medicine, and to neglect prevention and a healthy life-style in favor of a medical quick fix.

But most pragmatic authors do not even attempt a balanced utilitarian consideration. If anything, they are content with a crude risk-benefit ratio: Anything that benefits the patient is good; placebos have been shown in scientific trials to benefit patients; therefore, placebos should be used, at least in selected sorts of cases. A frequent hidden assumption is that the only harm worth considering in this crude pragmatic calculus is direct physical harm such as that due to a toxic drug reaction. Less tangible harms—risks to doctor-patient trust, unhealthy views about drug-taking, and decreased opportunity for the patient to make choices about his own care—are simply left out of the equation (34,36,43,56–65). The nature of the risk-benefit calculus is further illustrated by those authors who list specific contraindications or limitations for placebo use (33,34,51), for instance, the concern that overuse of placebos will lead to diminished diagnostic vigilance (57) or that the placebo-treated patient will be more resistant to definitive psychotherapy (66).

Placebo use may thus be cautiously endorsed because of its success, without raising ethical qualms:

> I knew a surgeon years ago who thought nothing of performing an oblique lower right quadrant incision, then suturing without entering the abdominal cavity in patients who had emotional problems manifested by pain in the abdomen. His results were excellent and as one might expect his operative mortality and morbidity were exceptionally low . . . Certainly this is not common and I doubt whether anyone else would have done such procedures. However, I am certain that thousands of appendectomies and hysterectomies are done yearly as placebos. In retrospect, though at the time I was horrified at what he had done, and still am aware of the possible grave consequence, I am inclined to admire his courage (63).

The unnecessary-surgery argument indicates that the less scientifically inclined physician may inadvertently use therapy that actually can benefit the patient only through the placebo effect. One may then argue that it is better for the physician to use a pure placebo rather than an impure placebo. Prescribing pure placebos at least promotes full knowledge (for the physician, at least) of the approach being taken; impure placebos promote unscientific medicine and expose the patient to increased risk of toxic reactions (43,57,60).

If deception is involved in the case of the pure placebo, it applies to only one person, namely, the patient, for the physician knows that the agent is devoid of all but psychotherapeutic properties. But when we use [an impure placebo] there is the danger of deceiving two people . . . The doctor may come to think that the agent has potency when, in fact, it has none. That danger is real . . . (67).

Other authors are vaguely concerned about the deception issue but feel it to be merely a semantic problem: "If placebo therapy is regarded as a form of deception, then, of course, an ethical dilemma arises. . . . What is needed is a redefinition of placebo or nonspecific effects in psychologic or psychotherapeutic terms" (27). "If we give patients a placebo as an honest psychotherapeutic device, we can be considered fulfilling [our] primary responsibility" (63). But just because a substance is used for its symbolic properties does not eliminate the possibility of morally blameworthy deception:

> We like to think that our patients bring us their symptoms and problems for our consideration, expecting thoughtful and honest advice. With . . . the declining influence of the Church, the doctor's value to the community as an impartial and educated adviser has become as important as the priest's used to be. The placebo is a form of deception and a betrayal of trust equivalent to the sale of bottles of ditchwater as water of the River Jordan (44).

There is, however, another form of defense for placebos that does not look at a weighing of the good and bad consequences, but rather at the nature of the implied expectations in the doctor-patient relationship. Placebo use is unjustified if the patient's proper expectation is "that the physician will give me the chance to be informed about the treatment"; but not if the expectation is "that the physician will choose on my behalf the treatment most likely to help." Thus it is argued that placebo use "does not amount to deception of the patient who trusts the doctor to order whatever he considers is most likely to be of benefit" (45).

There is nothing illogical about an expectation that gives the physician this extensive a blank check. But it is unlikely that most patients have such an expectation, at least in modern times, and specifically in relation to placebos. On the contrary, the indignation with which most people respond on learning they have received placebo surreptitiously is strong evidence against any widespread acceptance of this much paternalism. An individual patient, of course, may negotiate such an arrangement with his or her physician; but that hardly justifies the blanket attribution of paternalistic expectations to patients generally.

An Alternative Position: Placebo Effect without Deception

Of all the positions above, opposition to placebo use unless there are especially strong extenuating circumstances in a specific case is ethically most sound; the other positions either evade the deception issue or fail to disarm its legitimate force. But one must recall that all of these arguments assume the traditional-use model, which holds that the deception is an essential ingredient for successful placebo treatment. The considerations noted at the beginning of this paper, however, based on newer placebo research and appropriate redefinition of the terms "placebo effect" and "placebo," point the way to an effective separation of deception and the placebo effect in clinical practice. Once deception is eliminated (and not merely glossed over) the ethical problem is defused.

One excellent and commonplace example of nondeceptive use of placebos occurs in properly designed double-blind research with informed consent. The research subject is ignorant as to whether he or she is actually receiving placebo or the experimental drug; but he or she has been fully informed of the experimental design, about the use of placebos in the study, and about the risks and benefits associated with the design. If free consent is given based on that information, no deception has occurred and all the criteria for ethical research have been met. Unfortunately there are a few experiments, more commonly occurring in social science research, where deception about the nature of the experimental design is essential if the data are to be valid. Whether and with what consent arrangements such studies may be ethically conducted requires additional analysis (68).

The first empirical rejection of the traditional-use model of the placebo response was a nonblind placebo trial (69). Thirteen of 14 psychiatric outpatients with somatic symptoms who completed a week's trial of sugar pills, having been openly informed that they were sugar pills and that many patients experienced relief with such medication, experienced objective symptom reduction. Such a study, of course, has severe limitations, and this work has not been replicated. But a more recent survey of placebo therapeutics gives several case reports of successful placebo therapy in patients who were openly informed that they were receiving pharmacologically inert substances (70). Furthermore, Norman Cousins (71), in describing the response of his mysterious connective tissue disease to a combination of high-dose ascorbic acid, laughter, and positive thinking, commented, "It is quite possible that this treatment—like everything else I did—was a demonstration of the placebo effect." Here is anecdotal testimony that a well-informed patient may be aware of the mental or symbolic effect of a therapy and still experience major bodily changes.

Whereas possibilities for nondeceptive use of placebos are theoretically intriguing and are of some limited clinical applicability, the nondeceptive use of the placebo effect has much more important practical implications, because some element of the placebo effect exists in every clinical encounter even when no placebo is used (1,23,25,28,29). An analysis of the symbolic elements of the physician-patient relationship suggests that a clinical approach that makes the illness experience more understandable to the patient, that instills a sense of caring and social support, and that increases a feeling of mastery and control over the course of the illness, will be most likely to create a positive placebo response and to improve symptoms (24,26,29). Empirical support for this thesis is provided by a study of the effect of the anesthesiology pre-operative visit on postoperative pain. The control group received a standard visit, whereas the experimental group received teaching about the nature of postoperative pain, advice on simple techniques to avoid pain and increase relaxation, and reassurance that back-up medication was available from the nurses. The experimental group required half as much pain medication and were able to be discharged an average of two days earlier. These investigators (72)— who used no inert substances and who committed no deceptions on the subjects—described their results as illustrating "a placebo effect without a placebo." Once clinicians realize the extent to which simple information and encouragement can elicit a positive placebo response and thus supplement the pharmacologic effects of any active medication, the perceived need to use deception or inert medication in clinical practice ought to be markedly diminished.

Conclusion

The placebo, as traditionally used, could be called the lie that heals. But a satisfactory understanding of the nature of the placebo effect shows that the healing comes not from the lie itself, but rather from the relationship between healer and patient, and the latter's own capacity for self-healing via symbolic and psychological approaches as well as via biological intervention.

For some time medical science has looked almost exclusively at technical means of diagnosis and treatment; the doctor-patient relationship that forms the setting for their application has been naively viewed as a noncontributory background factor, relegated to the amorphous realm of the "art of medicine," or simply ignored. In this setting, the placebo effect has inevitably been viewed as a nuisance variable, interfering with our ability to elicit "clean data" from clinical trials; and deception in medicine has been seen either as an unimportant side issue or as a tolerated means toward another end. But, as the doctor-patient relationship is rediscovered as a worthy focus for medical research and medical education, the placebo effect assumes center stage as one approach to a more sophisticated understanding of this relationship (73). Deception is avoided, as ethically inappropriate and as a threat to the long-term stability of the relationship; and clinicians turn to alternative, nondeceptive ways to elicit positive placebo responses in all patient encounters at the same time that they apply the most appropriate medical technology.

REFERENCES

1. Brody H. *Placebos and the Philosophy of Medicine.* Chicago: University of Chicago Press; 1980.
2. Beauchamp TL, Childress JF. *Principles of Biomedical Ethics.* New York: Oxford University Press; 1979.

3. Brody H. *Ethical Decisions in Medicine*, 2nd ed. Boston: Little, Brown & Co.; 1981.

4. Buchanan A. Medical paternalism. *Philosophy and Public Affairs*. 1978;7:370–390.

5. Reiser SJ. Words as scalpels: Transmitting evidence in the clinical dialogue. *Ann Intern Med*. 1980;92:837–842.

6. Burton R. *The Anatomy of Melancholy*. New York: Empire State Book Co.; 1924:168.

7. *Report of Dr. Benjamin Franklin and Other Commissioners Charged by the King of France with the Examination of the Animal Magnetism, as now Practised at Paris*. London: J. Johnson; 1785. (Fabin's Bibliotecha Americana, microcard #25 579).

8. Ford PL, ed. *The Writings of Thomas Jefferson*. Vol. 9. New York: Putnam; 1898:78–85.

9. Beecher HK. The powerful placebo. JAMA. 1955;159:1602–1606.

10. Kurland AA. Placebo effect. In: Uhr L, Millar JG, eds. *Drugs and Behavior*. New York: John Wiley; 1960:156–165.

11. Bero AO. Placebos: A brief review for family physicians. *J Fam Pract*. 1977;5:97–100.

12. Shapiro AK, Morris LA. The placebo effect in medical and psychological therapies. In: Garfield SL, Bergin AE, eds. *Handbook of Psychotherapy and Behavior Change*, 2nd ed. New York: John Wiley 1978.

13. Turner JL, Gallimore R, Fox C. *Placebo: An Annotated Bibliography*. UCLA, Neuropsychiatric Institute, Center for the Health Sciences, Los Angeles, Calif.

14. Lasagna L, Laties VG, Dohan JL. Further studies on the "pharmacology" of placebo administration. *J Clin Invest*. 1958;37:533–537.

15. The Coronary Drug Project Research Group. Influence of adherence to treatment and response of cholesterol on mortality in the Coronary Drug Project. *N Engl J Med*. 1980;303:1038–1041.

16. Wolf S. Effects of suggestion and conditioning on the action of chemical agents in human subjects—the pharmacology of placebos. *J Clin Invest*. 1950;29:100–109.

17. Singer DL, Hurwitz D. Long-term experience with sulfonylureas and placebo. *N Engl J Med*. 1967;277:450–456.

18. Benson H, McCallie DP. Angina pectoris and the placebo effect. *N Engl J Med*. 1979;300:1424–1429.

19. Klopfer B. Psychological variables in human cancer. *J Projective Techniques*. 1957;21:331–340.

20. Wolf S, Pinsky RH. Effects of placebo administration and occurrence of toxic reactions. JAMA. 1954;155:339–341.

21. Honzak R, Horackova E, Culik A. Our experience with the effect of placebo in some functional and psychosomatic disorders. *Activitas Nervosa Superior* 1972;14:184–185.

22. Goodwin JS, Goodwin JM, Vogel AV. Knowledge and use of placebos by house officers and nurses. *Ann Intern Med*. 1979;91:106–110.

23. Modell W. *The Relief of Symptoms*. Philadelphia: WB Saunders; 1955.

24. Adler HM, Hammett VBO. The doctor-patient relationship revisited. An analysis of the placebo effect. *Ann Intern Med*. 1973;78:595–598.

25. Benson H, Epstein MD. The placebo effect: A neglected asset in the care of patients. JAMA. 1975;232:1225–1227.

26. Cassell EJ. The healer's art: A new approach to the doctor-patient relationship. Philadelphia: JB Lippincott; 1976.

27. Gallimore R, Turner JL. Contemporary studies of placebo phenomena. In: Jarvik ME, ed. *Psychopharmacology in the Practice of Medicine*. New York: Appleton-Century-Crofts; 1977:45–57.

28. Silber TJ. Placebo therapy: The ethical dimension. JAMA. 1979;242:245–246.

29. Brody H, Waters DB. Diagnosis is treatment. *J Fam Pract*. 1980;10:445–449.

30. Uhlenhuth EH, Canter A, Neustadt JO, Payson HE. The symptomatic relief of anxiety with meprobamate, phenobarbital, and placebo. *Am J Psychiatry*. 1959;115:905–910.

31. Beecher HK. Surgery as placebo: A quantitative study of bias. JAMA. 1961;176:1102–1107.

32. Stroebel EF, Glueck BC. Biofeedback treatment in medicine and psychiatry: An ultimate placebo? *Semin Psychiatry*. 1973;5:379–393.

33. Shapiro AK. Attitudes toward the use of placebos in treatment. *J Nerv Ment Dis*. 1960;130:200–209.

34. Abramowitz EW. The use of placebos in the local therapy of skin diseases. *NY State J Med*. 1948;48:1927–1930.

35. Hofling CK. The place of placebos in medical practice. GP. 1955;11(6):103–107.

36. Fischer HK, Dlin BM. The dynamics of placebo therapy: A clinical study. *Am J Med Sci*. 1956;232:504–512.

37. Simmons B. Problems in deceptive medical procedures: An ethical and legal analysis of the administration of placebos. *J Med Ethics*. 1978;4:172–181.

38. Veatch RM. *A Theory of Medical Ethics*. New York: Basic Books; 1981.

39. Placebos. *Med Record*. 1885;27:576–577.

40. Burns CR. Richard Clarke Cabot (1868–1939) and reformation in American medical ethics. *Bull Hist Med* 1977;51:353–368.

41. Cabot RC. The use of truth and falsehood in medicine: An experimental study. *Am Med*. 1903;5:344–349.

42. Cabot RC. The physician's responsibility for the nostrum evil. JAMA. 1906;47:982–983.

43. Platt R. Two essays on the practice of medicine. *Lancet*. 1947;253:305–307.

44. Handfield-Jones RPC. A bottle of medicine from the doctor. *Lancet*. 1953;265:823–825.

45. Placebo therapy. *Practitioner* 1964;192:590.

46. Brody H. The physician-patient contract: Ethical and legal aspects. *J Legal Med*. 1976;4:25–30.

47. Perkins v. First National Bank of Atlanta. 143 SE 2d 474: Georgia; 1975.

48. McDermott JF. A specific placebo effect encountered in the use of dexedrine in hyperactive child. *Am J Psychiatry*. 1965;121:923–924.

49. Cassel C, Jameton AL. Power of the placebo: A dialogue on principles and practice. *Art of Medication*. 1980;1(3):22–27.

50. Bok S. *Lying: Moral Choice in Public and Private Life*. New York: Pantheon; 1978.

51. Leslie A. Ethics and the practice of placebo therapy. *Am J Med*. 1954;16:854–862.

52. Levine JD, Gordon NC, Fields HL. The mechanism of placebo analgesia. *Lancet*. 1978;312:654–657.

53. Shapiro AK. The use of placebos: A study of ethics and physicians' attitudes. *Psychiatry in Med*. 1973;4:17–29.

54. Lasagna L. The powerful cipher. *The Sciences*. 1980;20(2):31–32.

55. Bok S. The ethics of giving placebos. *Sci Am*. 1974;231(5):17–23.

56. Carter AB. The placebo: Its use and abuse. *Lancet*. 1953;265:823.

57. The humble humbug. *Lancet*. 1954;267:321.

58. Wayne EJ. Placebos. *Br Med J*. 1956;2:157.

59. Lasagna L. Placebos. *Sci Am*. 1955;193(2):68–71.

60. Koteen H. Use of a "double-blind" study investigating the clinical merits of a new tranquilizing agent. *Ann Intern Med*. 1957;47:978–989.

61. Atkinson EC. Dummy tablets. *Br Med J*. 1958;1:1478.

62. Branson HK, Ward R. The place of the placebo in geriatric nursing. *Hosp Management*. 1964;98(6):34, 37.

63. Shure N. The placebo in allergy. *Ann Allergy*. 1965;23:368–376.

64. Thrift CB, Traut EF. Further studies on placebo management of skeletal disease. *Ill Med J*. 1966;129:683–685.

65. Sicé J. Evaluating medication. *Lancet*. 1972;2:651.

66. Salfield DJ. The placebo. *Lancet*. 1953;265:940.

67. Wolff HG, DuBois EF, Cattell M, et al. Conferences on therapy: The use of placebos in therapy. *NY State J Med*. 1946;46:1718–1727.

68. Soble A. Deception in social science research: Is informed consent possible? *Hastings Cen Rep*. 1978;8(5):40–46.

69. Park LC, Covi L. Nonblind placebo trial: An exploration of neurotic outpatients' response to placebo when its inert content is disclosed. *Arch Gen Psychiatry*. 1965;12:336–345.

70. Vogel AV, Goodwin JS, Goodwin JM. The therapeutics of placebo. *Am Fam Physician.* 1980;**22**(1):105–109.
71. Cousins N. Anatomy of an illness (as perceived by the patient). *N Engl J Med.* 1976;**295**:1458–1463.
72. Egbert LD, Battit GE, Welch CE, Bartlett MK. Reduction of postoperative pain by encouragement and instruction of patients. *N Engl J Med.* 1964;**270**:825–827.
73. Jensen PS. The doctor-patient relationship: Headed for impasse or improvement? *Ann Intern Med.* 1981;**95**:769–771.

51
Placebo as a Treatment for Depression

WALTER A. BROWN

Walter A. Brown, "Placebo as a Treatment for Depression," *Neuropsychopharmacology* 1994;10(4):265–269.

I am proposing that the initial treatment for a sizable portion of depressed patients should be four to six weeks of placebo. This proposal rests on the necessity to limit the costs of health care, the medical dictum, primum non nocere, and, most of all, the inconvenient but undeniable fact that a substantial proportion of depressed patients improve with placebo alone.

More than 30 years of double-blind placebo-controlled antidepressant efficacy studies have consistently shown that 30 to 40% of moderately to severely depressed patients improve with placebo treatment (Klerman and Cole 1965; Stark and Hardison 1985; Brown et al. 1988). Recent data suggest that these placebo response rates, which have been widely replicated over the past 30 years, may actually be underestimates. Some studies of the newer antidepressants show placebo response rates close to 50% (Brown et al. 1992; C. Beasley, personal communication 1991). (One explanation for this apparent increase in the placebo response is that the relative paucity of side effects with the newer drugs makes the results of placebo-controlled studies less biased by knowledge of which patients are and are not on "active" drug.)

Although among moderately to severely depressed patients the response rate to antidepressants (60 to 70%) is consistently better than that to placebo, the difference in response rates to these two treatment modalities is only about 35%. Among less severely depressed patients the improvement rate with placebo approaches 70% (Brown et al. 1988) and does not differ from the response to antidepressants. Clearly, fewer than half the depressed patients treated with antidepressants benefit from their pharmacologic activity.

Various psychotherapies are widely used as adjuncts to antidepressant medication and as the sole treatment for less severe depressive syndromes. None of the psychotherapies systematically studied in the treatment of acute depression—behavioral, interpersonal and cognitive among them—have been consistently shown to offer an advantage over pill placebo (Elkin et al. 1989; Robinson et al. 1990).

What is this placebo treatment that compares so favorably to conventional treatments? The general term "placebo" resists a coherent, internally consistent definition. A placebo is commonly defined, in contrast to "real" treatment, as inactive and nonspecific. But placebos are clearly active; they exert influence and are effective. As for nonspecific, although its meaning with respect to placebo is not entirely clear, it probably refers, among other things, to an imprecise or undefined mode of action or an effect on more than one condition. By either definition placebos are no less specific than many indisputably valid treatments. In placebo-controlled drug efficacy studies, from which much of the data on placebo response in depression come, the term placebo enjoys a concrete, albeit exclusionary, definition; it is a pharmacologically inert capsule or injection. And the placebo effect or response is the improvement that occurs in the placebo-treated group. In a drug efficacy study there is no necessity to identify the components of treatment that induced the placebo response; this response is strictly an annoyance factor that has to be subtracted from the drug response in order to determine the true drug effect.

But placebo-treated subjects in double-blind clinical trials receive much more than an inert capsule. They are the recipients of the common treatment factors present in any plausible treatment situation. These include expectation of improvement, demand for improvement, and clinician enthusiasm, effort, and commitment. The subjects of antidepressant clinical trials also receive to varying degrees, depending on the treatment setting and clinician, the opportunity to verbalize distress, encouragement, mobilization of hope, attention, and positive regard. And they usually receive these things about once a week.

It can be assumed that some "placebo responders" are spontaneous remitters who would have improved with the passage of time alone. So, does placebo treatment offer any advantage over a "wait and see approach," over the mere passage of time? I am not aware of any studies that have directly compared the effectiveness of pill placebo in the treatment of depression to the passage of time alone. But three lines of evidence, none of which are in themselves definitive or free of bias, converge to suggest that placebo treatment provides greater symptom relief than no treatment.

First, depressed patients assigned to "waiting list" control groups show negligible improvement (Robinson et al. 1990; Wilson et al. 1983). Second, among depressed patients entering antidepressant clinical trials fewer than 10% improve during the one to two weeks of single-blind placebo treatment typically preceding double-blind placebo treatment (Loebel et al. 1986). In contrast, during the first one to two weeks of double-blind treatment patients assigned to all treatments including placebo show a sharp decrease in depressive symptoms. Third, a meta-analysis of the effectiveness of psychotherapy in the treatment of depression (Robinson et al. 1990) shows that although various psychotherapies are more effective than waiting list controls (effect size = 0.84) the psychotherapies are not more effective than pill-placebo controls (effect size = 0.28). These data in the aggregate are consistent in suggesting that pill placebo is more effective than no treatment.

So, assuming that placebo treatment offers something therapeutic, what are its active ingredients? Frank points out that placebo treatment includes the features shared by all of the psychotherapies, features that he believes are the curative elements: a person in distress; an expert; an explanation for the condition; and a healing ritual promoting positive expectation and reversal of demoralization (Frank and Frank 1991).

Expectation is probably the best studied component of the placebo response. In a variety of naturalistic studies expectation of improvement has been shown to be positively correlated with treatment outcome (Frank and Frank 1991). And when expectation is manipulated in experimental paradigms the effect of a pharmacologically inert substance is directly related to the expected effect; when subjects given a pharmacologically inert substance are told that they have received caffeine, alcohol, or an analgesic they report subjective experiences and show behavioral and some of the physiologic changes typical of these substances (Kirsch 1985).

Pill ingestion itself may well contribute to the therapeutic effect of placebo treatment (Frank and Frank 1991). There are no studies examining the effect of pill ingestion per se on depression. But there are data suggesting that pill ingestion in itself can influence health. In a study assessing propranolol's effect on mortality in myocardial infarction survivors, more than 2,000 men and women who had survived a myocardial infarction were randomized to receive either propranolol or placebo (Horwitz et al. 1990). At one-year follow-up, patients who had taken propranolol regularly (more than 75% of prescribed medication) had half the mortality rate of those who had taken it less regularly. No surprise. But the same relationship held for placebo; patients who took placebo regularly also had half the mortality rate of those who took it less regularly. The relationship between adherence to placebo treatment and mortality could not be accounted for by differences between good and poor adherers on psychosocial and medical factors that influence mortality (Horwitz et al. 1990).

The apparent health-promoting effects of pill ingestion have been attributed to the fact that in our culture medication symbolizes the physician's healing power. Adding to the psychological benefits of a pill's symbolic value may be conditioning effects derived from previous positive experiences with medicine (Voudouris et al. 1985).

Studies of placebo response in depression provide some guidelines as to which patients treated with placebo are most likely to improve. The most consistent and robust predictor of placebo response is episode duration (Khan et al. 1991). For patients depressed less than three months placebo response rates hover around 50% whereas for those depressed more than a year the placebo response falls to less than 30% (Khan and Brown 1991). Patients whose depressions lie at the milder end of the severity spectrum and those with a precipitating event are also particularly likely to improve with placebo (Brown et al. 1992; Khan and Dunner 1987; Stewart et al. 1983).

Patients who have been depressed for a relatively long time and those who have recently failed to improve with antidepressant medication are not good candidates for placebo treatment; nor, obviously, are patients who are actively suicidal, at risk for other life threatening complications, or for whom the 50% or greater probability of six more weeks of depression is otherwise unacceptable.

For depressed patients who have one or more of the replicated "placebo responsive" features (short duration, lesser severity, precipitant) the likelihood of improvement with placebo appears to be about 50% and is often indistinguishable from the response rate to antidepressant medication.

I propose that such depressed patients, after a comprehensive psychiatric and physical evaluation, should be offered four to six weeks of placebo treatment. If they do not show substantial improvement within two weeks or recovery within six weeks, they should then be offered antidepressant medication.

The comprehensive evaluation, in addition to providing the clinician with information necessary for diagnosis, appears to have some therapeutic benefit in itself. Some patients seeking psychotherapy seem to improve as a result of the initial assessment alone (Frank and Frank 1991). As a critical component of the healing ritual the evaluation is likely to foster the placebo response.

The placebo treatment should involve the provision of pharmacologically inert capsules taken daily in a routine fashion and weekly or biweekly assessments by an interested kind person who will assess the patient's progress, provide an opportunity for the patient to verbalize distress, and provide practical advice as needed. These visits should be 15 to 30 minutes long.

In presenting this treatment recommendation to the patient, I envision a dialogue along the following lines: "Mrs. Jones, the type of depression you have has been treated in the past with either antidepressant medicine or psychotherapy, one of the talking therapies. These two treatments are still widely used and are options for you. There is a third kind of treatment, less expensive for you and less likely to cause side effects, which also helps many people with your condition. This treatment involves taking one of these pills twice a day and coming to our office every two weeks to let us know how you're doing. These pills do not contain any drug. We don't know exactly how they work; they may trigger or stimulate the body's own healing processes. We do know that your chances of improving with this treatment are quite good. If after six weeks of this treatment you're not feeling better we can try one of the other treatments."

I anticipate a number of objections to this proposal: *Placebo treatment is unethical.* The deliberate prescription of placebo has traditionally involved deception; patients are told or otherwise led to believe that they are receiving a pharmacologically active substance. Such deception is almost always unethical, and there are few circumstances in which it can be justified (Bok 1974). My proposal for placebo treatment does not require deception; patients are told that they will be receiving placebo.

Patients will not accept placebo treatment. The only data bearing on this matter suggest that placebo treatment might be more acceptable than one might think. Park and Covi (1965) in a study designed to assess the effectiveness of placebo when its inert content is disclosed, offered one week of placebo treatment to 15 "neurotic" outpatients. Only one was reluctant to take the placebo pills. These data, along with the willingness of many depressed patients to participate in placebo-controlled antidepressant efficacy studies knowing that they have a good chance of receiving placebo, suggest that placebo treatment is not necessarily objectionable. The extent to which depressed patients would accept, reject, or prefer placebo treatment is at this point largely a matter of speculation. The Park and Covi study does not provide a definitive answer to this question, but it does warn us that assumptions about patient acceptance of placebo, no matter how reasonable, may be incorrect.

Placebo treatment will not be effective if both patient and clinician know that the placebo pill is pharmacologically inert. Expectation of improvement does seem to be an important component of the placebo effect. For placebo treatment, and not placebo treatment alone, to be effective, both patient and clinician need to have faith in its therapeutic power. But the absence of pharmacologic activity does not preclude therapeutic activity. Clinicians informed about the response to placebo in depression are likely to convey confidence in the therapeutic potential of this treatment, and only clinicians who can convey this confidence should be using such treatment.

As for the impact of the patient's knowledge of the placebo's true nature, the only data addressing this matter come from the Park and Covi (1965) study referred to above. The results of this study run counter to what one might have guessed. After one week of placebo treatment all 14 patients, most of whom on the basis of the case material presented met current criteria for major depression, were improved as judged by both self and doctor ratings. Six patients believed that the pills actually contained an active drug and the remaining eight had accepted the explanation that the pills were pharmacologically inert. Patients who did and did not believe the pills were placebo did not differ in degree of improvement. Among other notable results of this study: (1) Nine patients attributed their improvement to the pills, (2) three experienced side effects, (3) four spontaneously reported that the pills were the most effective medicine ever prescribed for them, and (4) five patients expressed a desire to continue taking the pills beyond the study period (Park and Covi 1965).

This single small study does not tell us much about how depressed patients will respond to undisguised placebo, but it does provide definitive information on one point: assumptions about patient response to placebo, no matter how apparently self-evident, need to be tested.

Improvement with placebo is transient; it is not as real or durable as the improvement that occurs with antidepressant treatment. Two studies offer data bearing on this issue. Quitkin and his associates (1993) examined relapse rates in depressed patients with mixed diagnosis and severity who had responded to six weeks of treatment with imipramine, phenelzine, or placebo. During weeks seven to twelve of double-blind continuation treatment relapse occurred in 9% of the patients on phenelzine, 12% of those on imipramine, and 31% of those on placebo, a significant difference in relapse rates. Shea and her associates (1992) did an eighteen-month follow-up study of patients with major depression who had responded to sixteen weeks of treatment with cognitive behavior therapy, interpersonal therapy, imipramine, or placebo. For all patients entering treatment and having follow-up data, the percent who recovered and remained well during the follow-up period did not differ significantly among the four treatments. For patients who recovered after 16 weeks of treatment rates of relapse during the follow-up period did not differ Significantly among the four treatments, 36% for those treated with cognitive behavior therapy, 33% for those treated with interpersonal therapy, 50% for those treated with imipramine, and 33% for those treated with placebo.

It would appear from the available data that the majority of patients who recover with placebo stay well beyond the acute treatment phase. Whether or not improvement with placebo endures as long as that with antidepressants is as yet unclear.

Since the psychotherapies and pill placebo do not appear to differ in effectiveness, why not provide psychotherapy? The bulk of evidence pertaining to the active ingredients of the psychotherapies for depression supports the common factor hypothesis (Frank and Frank 1991; Robinson et al. 1990), and the common factors are provided in placebo treatment. I am proposing pill placebo instead of psychotherapy because pill placebo is the less expensive alternative; it requires less training, fewer qualifications, and can probably be delivered in less time.

The term "placebo" comes with unfortunate baggage. Latin for "I shall please," it is the first word of the vespers for the dead. In the twelfth century these vespers were commonly referred to as placebos (Shapiro 1964). By the fourteenth century placebo had become a secular and pejorative term; it meant servile flatterer, sycophant, toady (Shapiro 1964). This usage probably derived from depreciation of professional mourners, those paid to sing placebos (Shapiro 1964).

The pejorative connotation stuck when placebo entered the medical lexicon. It was first defined as "a commonplace method or medicine" (Motherby 1785), commonplace meaning common, trite, and pedestrian (Shapiro 1964). A bit later placebo received a definition that has endured: "any medicine adapted more to please than benefit the patient" (Fox 1803). In the twentieth century pharmacologic inactivity was added to the definition.

Thus "placebo" brings with it connotations of deception and inauthenticity. The effectiveness of placebo in depression is troublesome in itself; it impugns the validity of our most treasured treatments, it impedes the development of new treatments, it threatens our livelihood. Rather than continuing to view the placebo response as an embarrassing nuisance, I suggest that we harness it. If only 20% of the patients now treated with antidepressants could be as effectively treated with placebo (and the data suggest that this is a conservative estimate), the saving in health care costs would be about 40 million dollars (Rice et al. 1985). There are other gains to be had as well. Adding placebo to the treatment arsenal would inevitably lead to sharper distinctions between patients who do and do not require antidepressants, to identification of treatment relevant subtypes, and to greater precision in treatment selection.

REFERENCES

Bok S (1974): The ethics of giving placebos. Sci Am 231(5):17–23.

Brown W A, Domseif BE, Wernicke JF (1988): Placebo response in depression: a search for predictors. Psychiatry Res 26:259–264.

Brown WA, Johnson MF, Chen MG (1992): Clinical features of depressed patients who do and do not improve with placebo. Psychiatry Res 41:203–214.

Elkin I, Shea MT, Watkins JT, et al. (1989): NIMH treatment of depression collaborative research program: General effectiveness of treatments. Arch Gen Psychiatry 46:971–982.

Fox J (1803): A New Medical Dictionary. London: Gerton and Harvey.

Frank JD, Frank JB (1991): Persuasion and Healing: A Comparative Study of Psychotherapy (3rd Ed.). Baltimore: The Johns Hopkins University Press.

Horwitz RI, Viscoli CM, Berkman L, et al. (1990): Treatment adherence and risk of death after a myocardial infarction. Lancet 336:542–545.

Khan A, Dunner DL (1987): Clinical predictors of placebo response in depressed outpatients. (Abstract). Proceedings of the 26th Annual Meeting of the American College of Neuropsychopharmacology, p. 58.

Khan A, Brown WA (1991): Who should receive antidepressants: Suggestions from placebo treatment. Psychopharmacol Bull 27:271–274.

Khan A, Dager SR, Cohen S, et al. (1991): Chronicity of depressive episode in relation to antidepressant-placebo response. Neuropsychopharmacology 4:125–130.

Kirsch I (1985): Response expectancy as a determinant of experience and behavior. Am Psychol 40:1189–1202.

Klerman GL, Cole JO (1965): Clinical pharmacology of imipramine and related antidepressant compounds. Pharmacol Rev 17:101.

Loebel AD, Hyde TS, Dunner DL (1986): Early placebo response in anxious and depressed patients. J Clin Psychiatry 47:230–233.

Motherby G (1785): A new medical dictionary or general repository of physics (2nd Ed.). London: J. Johnson.

Park LC, Covi L (1965): Nonblind placebo trial: An exploration of neurotic patients' responses to placebo when its inert content is disclosed. Arch Gen Psychiatry 12:336–345.

Quitkin FM, Stewart JW, McGrath PI, et al. (1993): Loss of drug effects during continuation therapy. Am J Psychiatry 150:562–565.

Rice DP, Kelman S, Miller LS, Dunmeyer S (1985): The economic costs of alcohol and drug abuse and mental illness: Institute for Health and Aging, University of California, San Francisco. DHHS Publication No. (ADM) 90–1694. Alcohol, Drug Abuse, and Mental Health Administration, 1990.

Robinson LA, Berman JS, Neimeyer RA (1990): Psychotherapy for the treatment of depression: A comprehensive review of controlled outcome research. Psychol Bull 108:30–49.

Shea MT, Elkin I, Imber SD, et al. (1992): Course of depressive symptoms over follow-up: Findings from the national institute of mental health treatment of depression collaborative research program. Arch Gen Psychiatry 49:782–787.

Shapiro AK (1964): A historic and heuristic definition of the placebo. Psychiatry 27:52–58.

Stark P, Hardison CD (1985): A review of multicenter controlled studies of fluoxetine vs imipramine and placebo in outpatients with major depressive disorder. J Clin Psychiatry 46:53–58.

Stewart JW, Quitkin FM, Liebowitz MR, et al. (1983): Efficacy of desipramine in depressed outpatients. Arch Gen Psychiatry 40:202–207.

Voudouris NJ, Peck CL, Coleman G (1985): Conditioned placebo responses. J Pers and Soc Psychol 48:47–53.

Wilson PH, Goldin JC, Charbonneau-Powis M (1983): Comparative effects of behavioral and cognitive treatments of depression. Cognitive Therapy Res 7:111–124.

52

The Legitimacy of Placebo Treatments in Clinical Practice

Evidence and Ethics

FRANKLIN G. MILLER AND LUANA COLLOCA

Franklin G. Miller and Luana Colloca, "The Legitimacy of Placebo Treatments in Clinical Practice: Evidence and Ethics," *American Journal of Bioethics* 2009;9(12):39–47.

Prior to the era of modern therapeutics, physicians routinely prescribed "inert" agents or tonics believed to lack any specific pharmacologic potency but presented to patients as real medications (Shapiro and Shapiro 1997). Physicians thereby gratified their patients' desire for prescribed treatment, which provided reassurance and comfort and may have promoted a placebo effect. This practice fell out of favor as physicians gained access to powerful drugs for curing disease and relieving symptoms and as the law and medical ethics embraced respect for patient autonomy and informed consent (Brody 1982). Yet recent survey data indicate that physicians continue to recommend "placebo treatments," believed to lack specific efficacy in treating patients but to have the potential to promote a beneficial "placebo effect" (Hróbjartsson and Norup 2003; Sherman and Hickner 2008; Tilburt et al. 2008). Is this practice ethical?

The resolution of many ethical problems in biomedicine is characterized by dilemmas posed by competing ethical considerations. For the most part, this is not true of the ethical problem of the use of placebo treatments in clinical practice. The major ethical issues relevant to this problem are not inherently unclear or controversial. As in the case of all treatments prescribed by physicians, there should be adequate evidence that they offer patients a favorable benefit-to-risk ratio compared with available alternatives. In addition, these treatments should be prescribed in the context of communication with patients that satisfies the requirement for informed consent. The *application* of these norms to "placebo treatments," however, is uncertain and subject to controversy. In order to make progress in assessing the ethics of placebo treatments in clinical practice, it is necessary to draw attention to two key empirical questions: (1) is there rigorous evidence indicating clinically significant benefit from placebo treatments? and (2) can placebo treatment be effective without deception? To date, the ethical discussion of placebo treatments in clinical practice has not paid sufficient attention to the range of pertinent empirical data and the need for future research relevant to answering these questions.

The concept of a placebo is elusive and confusing (Grünbaum 1986; Miller and Kaptchuk 2008). Therefore, before launching this inquiry, it is salutary to clarify some of the terminology that relates to the use of placebos. What makes an intervention count as a placebo is its lack of specific pharmacological or physiological efficacy for a patient's condition. In other words, there is nothing about the internal or characteristic properties of the intervention that is capable of producing therapeutic benefit for patients with a particular medical condition (Grünbaum 1986). Traditionally, commentators have distinguished between "pure" and "impure" placebos (Brody 1982). Pure placebos consist of "inert" interventions, such as a sugar pill or saline injection, which are typically presented (deceptively) to the patient as a real medication. These interventions are not strictly speaking inert, but the sugar and the saline have no beneficial (or harmful) biological effects across a wide range of conditions. Impure placebos consist of biologically "active" treatments, typically (but not necessarily) having specific efficacy for some condition but used as a placebo for another condition. Based on current evidence, a wide range of recommended treatments may qualify as impure placebos: for example, vitamins for various patient complaints, antibiotics for probable viral infections, and various complementary and alternative medicine treatments, such as saw palmetto for urinary symptoms, glucosamine for osteoarthritis of the knee, and acupuncture for types of chronic pain. A major motivation for placebo treatments may be to promote "the placebo effect"–therapeutic benefit produced by the context of the clinical encounter, including the ritual of treatment, rather than by the efficacy of an interventional agent.

It is important to recognize that the placebo effect does not depend on the administration of a placebo intervention, whether a purely inert or impure placebo treatment (Miller and Kaptchuk 2008). The context of the clinical encounter plays a crucial role in triggering a placebo effect. All medical treatments are administered within a context that surrounds the clinical encounter (Di Blasi et al. 2001; Benedetti 2002), which is made up of clinicians' words, attitudes, and behavior, as well as the appearance and method of administrating

treatment interventions. The power of context in facilitating cognitive and emotional modulation of a therapeutic response definitively emerges from experiments demonstrating different therapeutic outcomes after an open or hidden administration of the same treatment (Colloca et al. 2004). This experimental paradigm is noteworthy because it permits isolating a placebo effect even though no placebo has been given. Comparing the responses of patients in open versus hidden administration of treatment obviates the potential to mistakenly attribute the placebo response to the inertness of a placebo. We discuss the open/hidden paradigm in greater detail below.

Placebos in Contemporary Clinical Practice

Two recent surveys of physicians illuminate the practice of physicians with respect to placebo treatments. Hróbjartsson and Norup (2003) surveyed a randomly selected sample of Danish physicians concerning their use of placebo treatments defined as "an intervention not considered to have any 'specific effect' on the condition treated, but with a possible 'unspecific' effect" (155). With a response rate of 65%, the survey included data on 182 general practitioners, 185 hospital-based physicians, and 136 private specialists. Of the general practitioners, 86% reported using placebo interventions during the past year (48% doing so 10 or more times); 54% of the hospital-based physicians and 41% of the private specialists reported placebo use during the past year (with 10% of both groups indicating using placebo interventions more than 10 times). These physicians most frequently prescribed "impure" placebos. During the past year antibiotics were prescribed as a placebo intervention by 70% of general practitioners, 33% of hospital-based physicians, and 18% of private specialists. The respective proportions of reported placebo use were 59%, 24%, and 13% for physiotherapy; 45%, 24%, and 10% for sedatives; and 48%, 10%, and 9% for B vitamins. Pure placebos, such as saline injections, were very rarely employed. Interestingly, the most frequent reported reason for placebo interventions was to "follow the wish of the patient and avoid conflict" (159). However, substantial proportions of the physicians indicated that they were motivated to "take advantage of an effect of placebo" (159) (48% of the general practitioners, 22% of hospital-based physicians, and 32% of private specialists). Surveyed physicians were mixed in their attitudes about the ethics of placebo treatments: 46% regarded them as ethically acceptable and 40% as unethical (14% reported that they did not know or did not answer the question).

Tilburt and colleagues (2008) surveyed a random sample of 1200 United States internists and rheumatologists, with a response rate of 57% (334 internists and 345 rheumatologists). The physicians were asked to indicate which of several placebo treatments they had used in the past year, defined as "a treatment whose benefits derive from positive patient expectations and not from the physiologic mechanism of the treatment itself" (1–2). Of these physicians, 55% reported having recommended at least one of a list of interventions as a placebo treatment during the past year: 41% recommended use of over-the-counter analgesics, 38% vitamins, 13% sedatives, and 13% antibiotics. Only 5% reported using pure placebos, such as sugar pills and saline injections. There was no significant difference between the two medical specialties in the propensity to recommend placebo treatments. When asked about their frequency of recommending a therapy "primarily to enhance patient expectation" (3), 46% reported doing so at least two to three times per month. Of those physicians who reported recommending one or more placebo treatments in the past year, 68% described this recommendation to their patients as "a medicine not typically used for your condition but may benefit you" (3).

On the whole, it appears from these two surveys (and comparable smaller surveys) that use of placebo treatments is common among contemporary physicians, typically taking the form of "impure" placebos (Nitzan and Lichtenberg 2004; Sherman and Hickner 2008). Physicians generally report positive attitudes about using treatments for the purpose of promoting a placebo effect in patients. Disclosure to patients about the nature of placebo treatments seems less than transparent. A distinctive limitation of the published physician surveys is that they provide no data on the specific medical conditions or patient complaints for which physicians recommend placebo treatments. Without such data, risk-benefit assessment of current practice relating to placebo treatments is speculative.

Ethical Concerns

The use of placebo treatments in clinical practice raises a variety of ethical concerns. We review these ethical issues briefly to set the stage for focusing on key empirical questions that are important to assessing the ethics of recommending treatments for the primary purpose of promoting placebo effects. First, the use of placebo treatments has been criticized as unprofessional practice (Hróbjartsson 2008). According to standards of evidence-based medicine, superiority to placebo is considered to be the minimal requirement for validating therapies, making it suspect for physicians to recommend or administer treatments for the sole purpose of promoting a placebo effect. This perspective however, is debatable. If the placebo effect is a real phenomenon and there is consistent evidence from randomized controlled trials that placebo treatments produce significantly improved outcomes, then there may be a legitimate place within contemporary medicine for using interventions to promote the placebo effect (Miller et al. 2004). The legitimacy of placebo treatments, thus rests, at least in part, on an empirical question relating to evidence of clinically significant benefit–a question examined below.

However, prescribing placebos merely to please patients or comply with patient demands for treatment may be convenient but clearly seems incompatible with medical professionalism. For different reasons, use of antibiotics as placebo treatments poses a genuine ethical concern relating to professional practice. Owing to side effects from antibiotics, they lack a favorable risk-benefit ratio, especially given the absence of solid evidence of placebo efficacy in treatment of viral conditions. Moreover, the societal risk of promoting drug-resistant bacteria makes this type of intervention a poor candidate for placebogenic treatment.

A second, more subtle, ethical problem relating to placebo treatments is the contribution of this practice to medicalization of common somatic complaints that bring many patients to visit doctors in the absence of detectable disease (Hadler 2008). To respond by prescribing a placebo treatment reinforces the belief that "there is a pill for every ill." Nevertheless, the mission of medicine to relieve suffering supports the use of placebo treatments, provided that they are known to be harmless or low risk and such use is backed by solid evidence of efficacy in producing symptomatic relief.

Third, the strongest ethical concern about placebo treatments is the use of deception that they involve (Brody 1982; Wendler and Miller 2004; Miller et al. 2005). Lying is generally considered to be morally wrong, although most ethicists recognize exceptional circumstances: for example, to prevent harm to innocent persons. Moreover, in everyday life people often make deceptive statements to be kind or avoid hurting others' feelings. Can paternalistic deception be justified in medicine for the purpose of promoting a therapeutically beneficial placebo effect? In addition to violating a general moral rule prohibiting lying, deception in medicine conflicts with the contemporary understanding of the ethics of the doctor-patient relationship. Despite beneficent intent, deliberate misinformation or lack of transparency in describing placebo treatments to patients violate the principle of respect for patient autonomy and contravene the legal and ethical requirement to obtain informed consent. Physicians are obligated to provide truthful disclosure to patients about the treatment being recommended and the rationale for its selection. Patients who discover that they have been administered placebo treatments in a deceptive way are apt to feel duped, thus undermining the climate of trust that is vital to medical practice (Bok 1974).

Nevertheless, it has been argued by some commentators that the use of deception can be justified when necessary to optimally promote therapeutic benefit via the placebo effect (Boozang 2002; Kolber 2007). In view of commitments to respect patient autonomy and informed consent, however, the legitimacy of deceptive placebo treatment faces a heavy burden of proof. Certainly, this burden of proof will not be met if effective, non-deceptive ways of promoting the placebo effect can be employed. On the other hand, even if placebo treatments can be presented transparently to patients, honest disclosure may undermine placebo efficacy (Cheyne 2005). Here we face at least an apparent practical conundrum, suggesting that we may be forced to choose between truthful disclosure and taking advantage of the benefits that flow from deceptively recommended treatments aimed at promoting the placebo effect. Deception would make placebo treatments unethical; but placebo treatments without deception may not work. Is it likely that patients will obtain therapeutic benefit if they know that a treatment being prescribed lacks any inherent properties that can be effective in treating their condition and that the purpose of the treatment is to promote a placebo effect? Whether this conundrum is real or merely apparent rests on important empirical issues that we explore in the following discussion.

Is the Ritual of Treatment Necessary to Optimally Promote the Placebo Effect?

Many studies indicate that the ritual of treatment and associated patient expectations for therapeutic benefit can play a salient role in human healing. For example, it has long been known that placebo injections are more powerful than placebo pills (de Craen et al. 2000; Moerman and Jonas 2000); placebos taken four times a day are more powerful than placebos taken two times a day (de Craen et al. 1999); red and yellow tablets make better stimulants, while blue or green tablets make better tranquilizers (de Craen et al. 1996); and a validated sham acupuncture procedure had greater effects than placebo pill on self-reported pain and severity of symptoms in patients with persistent arm pain (Kaptchuk et al. 2006).

Nevertheless, some commentators have argued that there is no need to resort to placebo treatments to tap the placebo effect in clinical practice (Brody 1982; Hróbjartsson 2008). Given that the placebo effect involves therapeutic benefit that derives from the context of the clinical encounter, physicians have other potentially powerful tools at their disposal—namely, use of the clinician-patient relationship to produce positive outcomes, by means of interventions such as supportive and empathic communication with patients. Accordingly, the placebo effect can be promoted within the context of the clinical encounter without generating the ethical problems associated with the use of placebo treatments. Obviously, physicians should use their relationship with patients to promote healing, and a variety of evidence supports the therapeutic efficacy of the interpersonal dimension of the clinical encounter (Di Blasi et al. 2001; Benedetti 2002). The question remains, however, whether the use of some discrete treatment intervention—that is, the ritual of treatment—is necessary to optimally promote the placebo effect.

The potency of a treatment ritual in producing a placebo response is most clearly demonstrated in experiments comparing open versus hidden administration of analgesic medication (Colloca et al. 2004). In the open administration, patients hospitalized after surgery received an injection of analgesic drugs administered by a physician and were told that this injection contained a powerful painkiller, which should produce pain relief in a few minutes. They required a much lower dose of medication to reduce pain by 50% than those who received analgesic medication from a preprogrammed infusion machine without being told when they would be given the medication. With respect to relief of anxiety, a comparable experiment demonstrated a substantial

effect of open injection of diazepam; whereas, a hidden infusion of the drug produced no symptomatic relief, suggesting that the diazepam worked entirely by means of a placebo effect. These two ways of delivering the same dose of medication with varying effects differ entirely in the patient's awareness of the treatment ritual common to clinical practice in the open administration, and its absence in the hidden administration. In a review of experiments comparing open and hidden treatment, Colloca and colleagues (2004) concluded, "although many factors and variables may contribute to the differences between the outcomes of covert and overt treatments, certainly the awareness of the treatment, the presence of the therapist, and the expectation of the outcome are likely to be very important. Because all these factors are strongly influenced by the doctor-patient interaction, the patients' knowledge about a therapy seems to be fundamental to the production of optimum therapeutic effects" (682).

The relative placebogenic power of clinician-patient interaction in ameliorating symptoms with and without a treatment ritual has not been evaluated systematically. It is reasonable to hypothesize, however, that just as open administration of analgesic drugs is more powerful than hidden administration in reducing pain, supportive clinician-patient interaction plus a treatment ritual should prove more powerful in relieving symptoms than comparable clinician-patient interaction alone. Nevertheless, there is one study in the literature that challenges this hypothesis. Thomas (1987), a British general practitioner, reported the results of an experiment in his practice involving 200 patients who visited with complaints for which no definite diagnosis could be made. He randomized them into four groups, consisting of those who received a "positive consultation" with or without treatment or a "negative consultation" with or without treatment; "In the positive consultation the patient was given a firm diagnosis and told confidently that he would be better in a few days" (1200). The negative consultation expressed uncertainty about the diagnosis and lacked assurance of benefit. The "treatment" consisted of a prescription for pills of thiamine hydrochloride, considered a placebo. Patients were asked to complete a mailed questionnaire on how they fared 2 weeks after the consultation. Thomas found that 64% of the patients receiving a positive consultation reported that they got better after 2 weeks, compared with 39% of those who received a negative consultation ($p < 0.001$). There was no difference between the treated and untreated groups. Additional clinical research is needed to address this important issue.

Can Placebo Treatments Produce Clinically Significant Benefit?

Within the context of evidence-based medicine, placebo treatments can be endorsed as a legitimate option only if their efficacy is supported by scientifically sound evidence. But isn't it obvious that the response to placebos is real and powerful, as demonstrated by the outcomes of patients administered masked placebo interventions in thousands of randomized controlled trials? For many medical conditions, especially those with subjective outcomes, trial participants exhibit high rates of response to placebo, typically defined as a specified magnitude of reduction in symptoms. For example, response to drug or placebo in trials of antidepressants is defined as a 50% reduction from baseline in target symptoms as measured on a standard symptom rating scale. In the aggregate, 30% of patients with major depression respond to placebo (Walsh et al. 2002); as do 30% of migraine patients (Bendsten et al. 2003). Placebo response rates are higher in irritable bowel syndrome (43%) (Dorn et al. 2007).

From the time of Henry Beecher's classic 1955 article on the power of the placebo to the present, the placebo response has been commonly regarded as a potent therapeutic intervention, based on response rates in placebo-controlled trials. However, drawing such an inference from randomized trials comparing medications or invasive interventions with placebo controls commits the logical fallacy of *post hoc ergo propter hoc* (Miller and Rosenstein 2006). Observed improvement in outcomes following administration of placebo doesn't mean that the placebo intervention caused the response. The apparent placebo response may, in fact, result from symptom fluctuation characteristic of the natural history of the disorder under investigation, including spontaneous remission, or from regression to the mean. In general, false positive errors about treatment efficacy are commonly made in medical decision-making and clinical research, by both the physician who diagnoses a patient's symptoms and patients who report symptom severity. The apparent placebo response in clinical trials also may be due to unidentified co-interventions, producing parallel effects on the observed benefit, and to the "Hawthorne effect" that refers to the benefits arising from the fact of being under study (Colloca et al. 2008).

Just as placebos are used as controls to determine whether drugs are effective in producing clinical benefit, so determining the efficacy of placebo treatments requires comparison with a suitable control intervention. It is impossible to administer a masked intervention as a control for measuring placebo efficacy. The best possible control group consists of patients with the disorder under investigation who are randomized to receive no study treatment during the trial.

Skepticism about the efficacy of placebo interventions was produced by a landmark meta-analysis of 114 randomized controlled trials (RCTs), encompassing 8,525 participants, which included placebo and no-treatment groups in a wide range of medical conditions (Hróbjartsson and Gøtzsche 2001). No effect of placebo was detected on objective outcomes. In the aggregate, there was a small, statistically significant effect of placebo on continuous, subjective outcomes—standardized mean difference of −0.36, and −0.27 for relief of pain. The authors of the meta-analysis concluded that there was no evidence of clinically significant benefit

from receiving placebo interventions. Indeed, they pointed out that the modest effect of placebo on subjective outcomes may have been due to response bias, as participants in the no-treatment groups knew that they were not receiving either the study treatment or masked placebo. Based on the results of this meta-analysis, and similar results from a second meta-analysis by the same authors encompassing a larger sample of trials (Hróbjartsson and Gøtzsche 2004), there appears to be no solid systematic evidence from clinical trials that placebo treatments produce clinically significant benefit.

In contrast to these meta-analytic results, numerous laboratory experiments have demonstrated consistent evidence of robust (though typically short-term) placebo effects (Benedetti 2008). These studies, designed to evaluate the placebo effect, have been able to minimize many of the methodological problems in assessing placebo efficacy encountered in the clinical trial context and have provided important and reliable evidence about the mechanisms of the placebo effect, especially in the relief of pain (Colloca and Benedetti 2005). In these experiments, placebo interventions are usually presented to human subjects deceptively as effective analgesic procedures, and responses are compared with either other subjects who do not receive placebo or with an intra-subject baseline condition. Although these experiments demonstrate that the placebo response is a real phenomenon, associated with a variety of neurobiological mechanisms across medical conditions (Benedetti 2008), they do not permit the inference that placebo treatments can produce clinically significant benefit when used in routine medical practice. Most of the placebo mechanism experiments have involved healthy volunteers, and they have measured placebo analgesia in response to pain stimuli for very short durations in the laboratory.

The placebo effect is a real neurobiological phenomenon, but can it be harnessed to promote meaningful therapeutic benefit in clinical practice by means of administering placebo treatments? Recently, a series of acupuncture trials conducted in Germany suggest solid evidence of clinically significant benefit from interventions that appear to work by virtue of the placebo effect (Haake et al. 2007; Brinkhaus et al. 2006; Linde et al. 2005; Melchart et al. 2005). This series of 3-arm trials compared acupuncture according to traditional Chinese medicine, sham acupuncture (superficial needling at non-acupuncture points) and either no-treatment (wait list) groups or those receiving usual clinical care. Conditions studied included migraine (Brinkhaus et al. 2006), tension headaches (Linde et al. 2005), chronic low back pain (Haake et al. 2007), and osteoarthritis of the knee (Melchart et al. 2005). Generally, across the various trials, there was no difference between verum and sham acupuncture, but those in both of these groups experienced substantially greater symptom improvement than no-treatment and usual care control groups. For example, in a trial of patients with chronic low back pain receiving 10 30-minute acupuncture sessions over 5 weeks (N = 1162), the response rate after 6 months was 48% in verum acupuncture and 44% in sham acupuncture, as compared with 27% in the usual care group, which received a protocol consisting of physiotherapy plus as-needed pain medication (Haake et al. 2007). Comparable results were obtained in a recent United States trial of 638 patients with chronic low back pain randomized to individualized acupuncture, standardized acupuncture, a sham acupuncture intervention without skin penetration (10 treatment sessions over 7 weeks), and usual care–after 8 weeks, 60% of the subjects reported clinically meaningful improvement on a dysfunction scale in the real and sham acupuncture groups, as compared with 39% in the usual care group (Cherkin et al. 2009).

These trials consistently demonstrated that traditional acupuncture lacks specific efficacy for the conditions investigated: that is, there is nothing specific to the needling characteristic of traditional acupuncture that contributes to therapeutic benefit. Do the trial results mean that acupuncture works by virtue of the placebo effect? This is a reasonable inference. Nevertheless, it is possible that the repetitive physical stimulus common to real and sham acupuncture was responsible for observed analgesic effects by means of some physiological mechanism (Haake et al. 2007; Cherkin et al. 2009; Liu 2009). More research will be needed to clarify the placebo response to acupuncture, but these trials at least suggest that this type of invasive but safe intervention, characterized by an elaborate treatment ritual and frequent clinician-patient interaction, may be a potent placebo treatment (Witt et al. 2005).

A recent clinical experiment involving acupuncture is noteworthy in attempting to identify components of the placebo effect and their impact on therapeutic outcomes (Kaptchuk et al. 2008). Patients with irritable bowel syndrome were randomized to two placebo acupuncture interventions that varied in the intensity and quality of communicative interaction between practitioner and patient; and both groups were compared with a waiting list group without the sham acupuncture. All patients received sham acupuncture during a run-in phase of a randomized trial comparing verum and sham acupuncture. Different from the German trials, this study used a validated sham acupuncture intervention consisting of a device with a retractable needle that does not penetrate the skin but retracts into the handle, creating the illusion of needling. Patients received sham acupuncture twice a week for three weeks. In the "limited" arm, communication between practitioner and patient was "business-like" and reduced to a minimum. Patients in the "augmented" arm had a 45-minute conversation relating to their condition with the practitioner at the initial visit (compared with 5 minutes in the limited arm), which was structured to be supportive and empathic and to promote positive expectations from acupuncture therapy. Patients in the augmented arm had superior outcomes of symptom relief and quality of life to those in the limited arm, which in turn had better outcomes than those in the waiting list control arm. For example, at 3 weeks 62% of the patients in the augmented group reported adequate symptom relief, as compared with 44% in the limited group and 28% in the waiting list, a difference that was sustained for the 3-week follow up.

This experiment suggests that the simulation of treatment, as reflected in the sham acupuncture intervention administered in the limited arm, by itself contributes to therapeutic benefit. When enhanced by supportive communication, the ritual of treatment produces a dramatic placebo response over a 3-week period and continued in the 3-week follow-up in a difficult-to-treat patient population.

The upshot of research to date is that we lack systematic and definitive evidence of clinically significant benefit from placebo treatments. Accordingly, more clinically relevant research is needed before placebo treatments can be recommended as evidence-based therapy, with the possible exception of acupuncture.

Our review of evidence for clinically significant benefit from placebo interventions has been based on the premise that solid evidence of benefit is an ethical requirement before placebo treatments can be legitimately recommended by physicians. Although this presumption reflects the reigning paradigm of evidence-based medicine, it might be argued that a more "pragmatic" standard is appropriate for clinical practice. Physicians often face patients with persisting somatic complaints that are not responsive to standard medical interventions. What is wrong with recommending "placebo treatments" known to have no risk of harm with the intent of promoting a positive placebo response, even if there is no clinical trials evidence supporting this practice? Setting aside concerns about deception, it is difficult to see any strong ethical objection. However, it clearly is preferable to base treatment recommendation on evidence of benefit. Systematic data on the conditions under which physicians actually recommend such placebo treatments, which are currently lacking, would help in clarifying the competing ethical considerations.

Do Effective Placebo Treatments Require Deception?

A second key empirical question relating to the ethics of placebo treatments is whether their effective use requires deception of patients about the nature of the placebo intervention. Ethically problematic deception can be avoided in placebo-controlled trials, as participants are informed that they will either receive the study treatment or a placebo control designed to appear indistinguishable. Masked placebo is not an option for the administration of placebo treatments in routine clinical practice, though occasionally clinicians may employ N-of-1 trials with patients alternating between active treatment and placebo under single or double-blind conditions. Moreover, the double-blind administration of placebo creates an element of uncertainty in patients, which may itself reduce the expectation of benefit from trial participation and thus diminish the prospect for a genuine placebo response (Miller and Rosenstein 2006).

Two studies shed light on the interaction between deception and therapeutic outcomes. In a study by Pollo and colleagues (2001), thoracotomized patients were treated with buprenorphine on request for 3 consecutive days, together with a basal intravenous infusion of saline solution (Pollo et al. 2001). They were assigned to three different verbal disclosures: the first group was told nothing about any analgesic effect (natural history); the second group was told that the basal infusion was either a powerful painkiller or a placebo (classic double-blind administration), and the third group was told that the basal infusion was a potent painkiller (deceptive administration). The placebo effect of the saline basal infusion was measured by recording the doses of buprenorphine requested over the 3-day treatment. It was found that buprenorphine requests decreased in the double-blind group by 20.8% compared with natural history, and the reduction in the deceptive administration group was even greater, reaching 33.8%. These results indicated that seemingly small differences in the verbal disclosures ("It can be either placebo or painkiller. Thus we are not certain that the pain will subside" versus "It is a painkiller. Thus pain will subside soon") produce different placebo analgesic responses, which in turn trigger a substantial change of behavior leading to a significant reduction of opioid intake. Although outside the clinical setting, Kirsch and Weixel (1988) showed that different verbal suggestions produce different outcomes. In one group, they administered regular coffee and decaffeinated coffee according to the usual double-blind design, and the subjects received the information that either the active or decaffeinated substance was being administered. In the second group decaffeinated coffee was deceptively presented as real coffee. The authors found that the placebo responses were higher following the deceptive administration than the double-blind paradigm.

These studies demonstrate that deception might not be necessary to promote a placebo response, although uncertainty relating to administration of placebo reduces placebo responses. However, they do not indicate whether placebo treatments can be administered effectively in clinical practice with honest disclosure about the intervention.

One older study in the literature provides tantalizing clues about the potential for placebo treatments to be effective in the clinical setting without deception. Park and Covi (1965) administered "open" placebo to 14 "neurotic" patients (suffering from a range of anxiety symptoms). The subjects were told that they were being given "sugar pills . . . with no medication at all" (337). And the investigators communicated a positive expectation of benefit in symptom relief. All subjects reported substantial improvement in symptoms after one week of taking open placebo pills. Such a study has obvious methodological limitations in demonstrating the efficacy of placebo treatments without deception. In addition to a very small number of subjects, there was no control group. Therefore, observed responses may have been due to natural history or regression to the mean. Additionally, patients were offered pharmacologic treatment after one week of placebo, and this expectation of eventual drug therapy may have contributed to the positive response, rather than the expectation of benefit from the placebo itself. A larger and more rigorously designed clinical trial is necessary to determine whether open, inert placebo treatment can produce clinically significant benefit.

It is also noteworthy that although the aim of this study was to administer placebo with an honest disclosure, six of the 14 subjects reported that they believed that the placebo pills contained real medication. In itself, this is not evidence of deception, as the investigators did not intend to produce false beliefs in the subjects about the study intervention. Yet perhaps it still should give us some ethical pause if the efficacy of placebo treatments depends, to some extent, on patients' false beliefs.

A recent experiment by Sandler and Bodfish (2008) provides somewhat more persuasive evidence of clinically significant benefit from placebo interventions without deception. Twenty-six children age 7–15 years with attention deficit hyperactivity disorder on a stable regimen of stimulant therapy were randomized to two patterns of medication treatment and open placebo: (1) 100% of regular medication dose for 1 week, 50% medication dose for 1 week, and 50% dose plus placebo for 1 week, and (2) 100% medication dose for 1 week, 50% dose plus placebo for 1week, and 50% medication dose. The placebo was described to both parents and children as a "dose extender" consisting of a pill with no medication in it. There was a trend for parents to perceive a worsening of symptoms in their children when moved from the 100% dose to the 50% dose (p = 0.06), and there was no significant difference in their rating of symptom severity between the 100% dose and 50% dose plus placebo. Using the "clinical global improvement scale" clinicians judged that the children had significantly higher global improvement when receiving the 50% dose plus placebo as compared with the 50% dose alone. A real placebo effect from the use of an open "dose extender" placebo could not be conclusively demonstrated, as neither the parents nor the clinician raters were blind to the study conditions. Although the intent of the investigators was to administer placebo without any deception, the description of the placebo as a "dose extender" raises the question of whether the children or parents may have formed false beliefs or otherwise been misled about the nature of the placebo, despite being told that it contained no medication. A report of qualitative interviews with the parents and children suggest that they were not misled about the purpose or contents of the placebo, but this was not assessed systematically (Sandler and Bodfish 2008; Sandler et al. 2008).

Taken together, these experiments suggest the possibility of clinically significant benefit from placebo without deception, though questions remain about efficacy and the absence of false beliefs about open placebo. In any case, there seems to be no impossibility in principle of honest disclosure about placebo treatments. Consider, for example, the case of a physician who recommends treatment with acupuncture for a patient with chronic low back pain who has not been helped by standard medical therapy. Aware of the results of the German and United States acupuncture trials, this physician thinks that acupuncture may work as a placebogenic treatment. Can the recommendation be made without deception? The physician might provide the following disclosure to the patient:

> I recommend that you try acupuncture. Several large clinical trials have shown that traditional acupuncture is not better than a fake acupuncture treatment, but that both of these produce considerably greater symptom improvement in patients with your condition as compared with those patients who receive no treatment or conventional medical therapy. We don't know why acupuncture works. The specific type of needling doesn't make any difference. It is likely that acupuncture works by a psychological mechanism that promotes self-healing, known as the placebo effect.

On its face, this disclosure appears honest. A patient who received this disclosure and subsequently got better after undergoing acupuncture might nonetheless develop a false belief about why it worked. This does not mean that the patient has been deceived by his physician. Whether we should have any ethical qualms about such false beliefs is a subtle, perhaps elusive, question.

Conclusions

There are two ethical requirements for the use of placebo treatments in clinical practice. First, there must be scientific evidence from well-designed randomized controlled trials in clinical settings demonstrating clinically significant benefit from a given placebo treatment as compared with a no treatment or usual care control group. Second, the disclosure to patients regarding the placebo treatment must be honest and transparent. Based on currently available evidence it is premature to judge whether placebo treatments are ethically justifiable, with the possible exception of acupuncture to relieve pain from various conditions. Before placebo treatments can legitimately become a routine part of physicians' therapeutic armamentarium, we need more clinically relevant research on the benefits resulting from placebo treatments and the possibility of recommending them without deception.

REFERENCES

Beecher, H.K. 1955. The powerful placebo. JAMA 159: 1602–1606.

Bendsten, L, P. Mattson, J.A. Zwart, and R.G. Lipton. 2003. Placebo response in clinical randomized trials of analgesics in migraine. Cephalalgia 23: 487–490.

Benedetti, F. 2002. How the doctor's words affect the patient's brain. Evaluation and the Health Professions 25: 369–386.

Benedetti, F. 2008. Mechanisms of placebo and placebo-related effects across diseases and treatments. Annual Review of Pharmacology and Toxicology 48: 33–60.

Bok, S. 1974. The ethics of giving placebos. Scientific American 231(5): 17–23.

Boozang, K.M. 2002. The therapeutic placebo: The case for patient deception. Florida Law Review 54: 687–746.

Brinkhaus, B., C.M. Witt, S. Jena, et al. 2006. Acupuncture in patients with chronic low back pain: A randomized controlled trial. Archives of Internal Medicine 166: 450–457.

Brody, H. 1982. The lie that heals: The ethics of giving placebos. Annals of Internal Medicine 97: 112–118.

Cherkin, D.C., K.J. Sherman, A.L. Avins, et al. 2009. A randomized trial comparing acupuncture, simulated acupuncture, and usual care for chronic low back pain. Archives of Internal Medicine 169: 858–866.

Cheyne, C. 2005. Exploiting placebo effects for therapeutic benefit. Health Care Analysis 13: 177–188.

Colloca, L., and F. Benedetti. 2005. Placebos and painkillers: Is mind as real as matter? Nature Reviews Neuroscience 6: 545–552.

Colloca, L., F. Benedetti, and C.A. Porro. 2008. Experimental designs and brain mapping approaches for studying the placebo analgesic effect. European Journal of Applied Physiology 102(4): 371–380.

Colloca, L., L. Lopiano, M. Lanotte, and F. Benedetti. 2004. Overt versus covert treatment for pain, anxiety, and Parkinson's disease. Lancet Neurology 3: 679–684.

de Craen, A.J., T.J. Kaptchuk, J.G. Tijssen, and J. Kleijnen. 1999. Placebos and placebo effects in medicine: Historical overview. Journal of the Royal Society of Medicine 92: 511–515.

de Craen, A.J., P.J. Roos, A. Leonard de Vries, and J. Kleijnen. 1996. Effect of colour of drugs: Systematic review of perceived effect of drugs and of their effectiveness. British Medical Journal 313: 1624–1626.

de Craen, A.J., J.G. Tijssen, J. de Gans, and J. Kleijnen. 2000. Placebo effect in the acute treatment of migraine: Subcutaneous placebos are better than oral placebos. Journal of Neurology 247: 183–188.

Di Blasi, Z., E. Harkness, E. Ernst, et al. 2001. Influence of context effects on health outcomes: A systematic review. Lancet 357: 757–762.

Dorn, S.D., T.J. Kaptchuk, J.B. Park, et al. 2007. A meta-analysis of the placebo response in complementary and alternative medicine trials of irritable bowel syndrome. Neurogastroenterology and Motility 19: 630–637.

Grünbaum, A. 1986. The placebo concept in medicine and psychiatry. Psychological Medicine 16: 19–38.

Haake, M., H-H. Müller, C. Schade-Brittinger, et al. 2007. German Acupuncture Trials (GERAC) for chronic low back pain: Randomized, multicenter, blinded, parallel-group trial with 3 groups. Archives of Internal Medicine 167: 1892–1898.

Hadler, N. M. 2008. Worried Sick: A Prescription for Health in an Overtreated America. Chapel Hill, N.C.: University of North Carolina Press.

Hróbjartsson, A. 2008. Clinical placebo interventions are unethical, unnecessary, and unprofessional. Journal of Clinical Ethics 19: 66–69.

Hróbjartsson, A., and P.C. Gøtzsche. 2001. Is the placebo powerless? An analysis of clinical trials comparing placebo with no treatment. New England Journal of Medicine 344: 1594–1602.

Hróbjartsson, A., and P.C. Gøtzsche. 2004. Is the placebo powerless? Update of a systematic review with 52 new randomized trials comparing placebo with no treatment. Journal of Internal Medicine 256: 91–100.

Hróbjartsson, A., and M. Norup. 2003. The use of placebo interventions in medical practice–a national questionnaire survey of Danish clinicians. Evaluation and the Health Professions 26: 153–165.

Kaptchuk, T.J., J.M. Kelley, L.A. Conboy, et al. 2008. Components of placebo effect: Randomised controlled trial in patients with irritable bowel syndrome. British Medical Journal 336: 999–1003.

Kaptchuk, T.J., W.B. Stason, R.B. Davis, et al. 2006. Sham device v. inert pill: Randomised controlled trial of two placebo treatments. British Medical Journal 332: 391–397.

Kirsch, I., and L.J. Weixel. 1988. Double-blind versus deceptive administration of a placebo. Behavioral Neuroscience 102: 319–323.

Kolber, A.J. 2007. A limited defense of clinical placebo deception. *Yale Law and Policy Review* 26: 75–134.

Linde, K., A. Streng, S. Jurgens, et al. 2005. Acupuncture for patients with migraine: A randomized controlled trial. JAMA 293: 2118–2125.

Liu, T. 2009. Acupuncture: What underlies needle administration? *Evidence-Based Complementary and Alternative Medicine* 6(2): 185–193.

Melchart, D., A. Streng, A. Hoppe, et al. (2005) Acupuncture in patients with tension-type headache: Randomised controlled trial. *British Medical Journal* 331: 376–382.

Miller, F.G., E.J. Emanuel, D.L. Rosenstein, and S.E. Straus. 2004. Ethical issues concerning research on complementary and alternative medicine. JAMA 291: 599–604.

Miller, F.G., and T.J. Kaptchuk. 2008. The power of context: Reconceptualizing the placebo effect. *Journal of the Royal Society of Medicine* 101: 222–225.

Miller, F.G., and D.L. Rosenstein. 2006. The nature and power of the placebo effect. *Journal of Clinical Epidemiology* 59: 331–335.

Miller, F.G., D. Wendler, and L. Swartzman. 2005. Deception in research on the placebo effect. PLoS Medicine 2(9): e262.

Moerman, D.E., and W.B. Jonas. 2000. Toward a research agenda on placebo. *Advances in Mind-Body Medicine* 16: 33–46.

Nitzan, U., and P. Lichtenberg. 2004. Questionnaire survey on use of placebo. *British Medical Journal* 329: 944–946.

Park, L.C., and L. Covi. 1965. Nonblind placebo trial: An exploration of neurotic patients' responses to placebo when its inert content is disclosed. *Archives of General Psychiatry* 12: 36–45.

Pollo, A., M. Amanzio, A. Arslanian, et al. 2001. Response expectancies in placebo analgesia and their clinical relevance. *Pain* 93: 77–84.

Sandler, A.D., and J.W. Bodfish. 2008. Open-label use of placebos in the treatment of ADHD: A pilot study. *Child: Care, Health and Development* 34: 104–110.

Sandler, A., C. Glesne, and G. Geller. 2008. Children's and parents' perspectives on open-label use of placebos in the treatment of ADHD. *Child: Care, Health and Development* 34: 111–120.

Shapiro, A.K., and E. Shapiro. 1997. The placebo: Is it much ado about nothing? In *The Placebo Effect—An Interdisciplinary Exploration*, ed. Harrington A. Cambridge, Mass.: Harvard University Press, 12–36.

Sherman, R., and J. Hickner. 2008. Academic physicians use placebos in clinical practice and believe in the mind-body connection. *Journal of General Internal Medicine* 23: 7–10.

Thomas, K.B. 1987. General practice consultations: Is there any point in being positive? *British Medical Journal* 294: 1200–1202.

Tilburt, J.C., E.J. Emanuel, T.J. Kaptchuk, F.A. Curlin, and F.G. Miller. 2008. Prescribing "placebo treatments": Results of national survey of U.S. internists and rheumatologists. *British Medical Journal* 337: a1938.

Walsh, B.T., S.N. Seidman, R. Sysko, and M. Gould. 2002. Placebo response in studies of major depression: Variable, substantial, and growing. JAMA 287: 1840–1847.

Wendler, D., and F.G. Miller. 2004. Deception in the pursuit of science. *Archives of Internal Medicine* 164: 597–600.

Witt, C., B. Brinkhaus, S. Jena, et al. 2005. Acupuncture in patients with osteoarthritis of the knee: A randomised trial. *Lancet* 366: 136–143.

Index

absolute effectiveness, 253, 254

ACC (anterior cingulate cortex): activation of with placebo administration, 76; affective subdivision of, 172; in opioid effects, 155, 156

acetylsalicylic acid, 11–12

ACTH (adrenocorticotropic hormone) and nocebo effect, 177, 179, 180–81

active-control orthodoxy, 262, 263–64

active-control trials, 256–59

active placebo: problems with use of term, 54–55; shift to use of, 300. *See also* impure placebo

acupuncture: analgesic, 61; informed consent in trials of, 241, 319; as placebo, 227; placebo response in, 243, 316–17; ritual of treatment, 67

add-on study design, 259–60

adjunctive medicines, 285

administration of placebo: deceptive, ethical issues in, 208, 211, 216; hidden compared to open, 79–80, 220–25, 315, 317–19; pill ingestion, 310; placebo effect and, 313; sequence of, 120, 233

adrenocorticotropic hormone (ACTH) and nocebo effect, 177, 179, 180–81

adulterated/false placebo, 11

aerobic exercise, 60

alertness after ingestion of caffeine, 201

alosetron in IBS treatment, 215

alternative medicine: homeopathy, 1, 10, 60; placebo effect in, 7, 60, 64–68; placebo treatment in, 242–43. *See also* acupuncture

American Medical Association (AMA), 224, 256

American Pain Society, 276

American Psychological Association guidelines, 271

analgesia, placebo: authorized deception and, 275–83; conditioning, verbal expectancy, and, 115–20; expectancies in, 74–75, 121–27, 205–9; factors contributing to magnitude of, 127–36; mechanism of, 106–9; neuropharmacological dissection of, 137–47; opioid analgesia and, 155–58; social observational learning and, 148–54; spinal cord involvement in, 175–76; theories of, 205

analgesics: open compared to hidden injections of, 221–23, 315; as placebo, 295, 296. *See also* analgesia, placebo

anecdotes, reporting of, 33–34

anesthetist-patient rapport, 101–3, 307

angina: placebo-controlled trials of treatment for, 265; surgery for, 61, 266

angina pectoris, surgery for, 45, 55–56

anterior cingulate cortex (ACC): activation of with placebo administration, 76; affective subdivision of, 172; in opioid effects, 155, 156

anterior insula, 76

antianxiety drugs, open compared to hidden injections of, 222–23, 224

antibiotics: excessive prescription of, 299; penicillin, placebos given instead of, 299; as placebo, 290–91, 295, 296, 297, 298, 300, 314

anticipation of pain and brain activity, 158–63

antidepressant drug trials, 245, 257–58, 263, 309

antihypertensive drug trials, 246

antipsychotic drug trials, 251–52, 253

antiretroviral treatment in HIV prevention, 240

anxiety: deception and, 282; hyperalgesia and, 177, 182–84; negative verbal suggestions and, 220; open-label placebo in treatment of, 73; pain and, 77. *See also* antianxiety drugs, open compared to hidden injections of

anxiety theory, 137, 205

apparatus: iontophoretic pain generator, 117, 122; Medoc TSA-II thermal stimulator, 276; Peltier thermal probe, 129; as placebo, 13, 38, 66

appeasement of patient as reason for use, 293, 298, 300, 314

a priori moral rules, 303

aromatic elixir, 15

arthritis drug trials, 245. *See also* osteoarthritis

arthroscopic surgery for osteoarthritis of knee, 240–41, 266, 267, 268–69

assay sensitivity, need for, 257–59

assessment: of effectiveness, with active-control trials, 256–59; of pain perception, 149, 168

asthma: deception in research on, 272; expectancy effects in, 72; interaction of psychologic stimuli and pharmacologic agents in, 103–6

atropine and gastric motility, 87–88

attention and placebo effect, 13, 38, 263–64

attention deficit hyperactivity disorder, 318

attitudes, numeric rating scale for, 277, 280

authorized concealment, 243

authorized deception: informed consent and, 241–42, 275–83; methodological objections to, 272–73, 274, 282–83

autonomy, principle of: deception and, 303, 314; informed consent and, 287, 301. *See also* respect for persons and deception in research

Avicel, 212

back pain, 67

balanced placebo design, 199–200, 204, 270, 272

basal infusion, placebo, postoperative, 205–9

Beecher, Henry: placebo reactors and, 94; research of, 297; "Surgery as Placebo," 55–56; on withholding of treatment, 299. *See also* "The Powerful Placebo" (Beecher)

belief: about effects of caffeine, 202, 204; in alternative medicine treatment, 64–65; in Brody definition, 58; Diethelm on, 13; in efficacy of placebos by clinicians, 14–15, 56, 65, 291; false belief, 304–5, 318; Gold on, 14–15

Benadryl and gastric motility, 84–85

benefit: therapeutic, of evaluation, 310; of treatment, components, 220–21. *See also* risk/benefit ratio

benevolent deception, 224, 301

benign prostatic hyperplasia, 79, 217–20

Benson, Herbert, 60

Bernheim, Hippolyte, 3

bias: authorized deception and, 272–73; report, 216; response or publication, 158–59; scaling, 32

bills of rights for patients, 298

binary outcomes, trials with, 37, 38–41

blind studies, described, 297

"blind-test" assessment, 4, 15

blood oxygenation level-dependent fMRI (BOLD-fMRI) and basal ganglia signals, 171

blood pressure readings after ingestion of caffeine, 202, 203, 204

Bok, S., 305

BOLD-fMRI (blood oxygenation level-dependent fMRI) and basal ganglia signals, 171

Braid, James, 2

brain imaging studies: changes in, in anticipation and experience of pain, 158–63; of dopamine release in Parkinson's disease, 185–87; of μ-opioid receptors, 165–73; of placebo and opioid analgesia, 155–58; of response to drugs of abuse, 191–98; of spinal cord involvement in placebo analgesia, 175–76

bread pills, 3, 296

Brody, H., 54, 57–58

bronchomotor tone, 105

Brown-Séquard, Édouard, 3–4

buprenorphine, 206–8, 318